MW01526814

LIBRARY

College of Physicians and Surgeons
of British Columbia

Soft Tissue Tumors

Soft Tissue Tumors

A Multidisciplinary, Decisional Diagnostic Approach

Edited by

Jerzy Klijanienko
Institut Curie

Réal Lagacé
Centre Hospitalier Universitaire de Québec
Québec, Canada

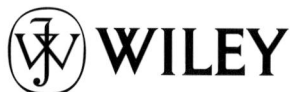

WILEY

A JOHN WILEY & SONS, INC., PUBLICATION

Copyright © 2011 by John Wiley & Sons, Inc. All rights reserved.

Published by John Wiley & Sons, Inc., Hoboken, New Jersey
Published simultaneously in Canada

No part of this publication may be reproduced, stored in a retrieval system, or transmitted in any form
or by any means, electronic, mechanical, photocopying, recording, scanning, or otherwise, except as
permitted under Section 107 or 108 of the 1976 United States Copyright Act, without either the prior
written permission of the Publisher, or authorization through payment of the appropriate per-copy fee to
the Copyright Clearance Center, Inc., 222 Rosewood Drive, Danvers, MA 01923, (978) 750-8400, fax (978)
750-4470, or on the web at www.copyright.com. Requests to the Publisher for permission should be
addressed to the Permissions Department, John Wiley & Sons, Inc., 111 River Street, Hoboken, NJ 07030,
(201) 748-6011, fax (201) 748-6008, or online at http://www.wiley.com/go/permission.

Limit of Liability/Disclaimer of Warranty: While the publisher and author have used their best efforts
in preparing this book, they make no representations or warranties with respect to the accuracy or
completeness of the contents of this book and specifically disclaim any implied warranties of merchant-
ability or fitness for a particular purpose. No warranty may be created or extended by sales representatives
or written sales materials. The advice and strategies contained herein may not be suitable for your
situation. You should consult with a professional where appropriate. Neither the publisher nor author
shall be liable for any loss of profit or any other commercial damages, including but not limited to special,
incidental, consequential, or other damages.

For general information on our other products and services or for technical support, please contact
our Customer Care Department within the United States at (800) 762-2974, outside the United States
at (317) 572-3993 or fax (317) 572-4002.

Wiley also publishes its books in a variety of electronic formats. Some content that appears in print
may not be available in electronic formats. For more information about Wiley products, visit our web site
at www.wiley.com.

Library of Congress Cataloging-in-Publication Data:

  Soft tissue tumors : a multidisciplinary, decisional, diagnostic approach / edited by Jerzy Klijanienko,
Real Lagace.
       p.   ; cm.
Includes bibliographical references.
ISBN 978-0-470-50571-7 (cloth)
1. Soft tissue neoplasms. I. Klijanienko, Jerzy.   II. Lagace, Real.
     [DNLM: 1. Soft Tissue Neoplasms. WD 375]
RC280.S66S72 2010
616.99′4075—dc22   2010036846

Printed in Singapore

10 9 8 7 6 5 4 3 2 1

Contents

Foreword

Cytology began with vaginal sampling, and cervical cancer screening programs gradually made the method adopted worldwide.

Diagnostic cytology gained recognition much later, and fine needle aspiration (FNA) cytology initially raised many controversies, hallmarking the disadvantages compared with the open or core biopsy, which was the considered "gold standard."

Sweden, and the Karolinska Institute in particular, can be considered the cradle of FNA clinical cytology.

Many cytologists, including myself, were trained there and initiated into the management of the sampling in the one-day clinic, examining the patient, reading the clinical chart, and dialoguing with the radiologist.

Nowadays the diagnostic needs of the clinician, and moreover the oncologist, have dramatically increased. There is no more room for just prototypic diagnoses.

Benign versus malignant is no longer enough. Suspicion is banned.

We moved from a contemplative era of morphology to an interpretive era of diagnosis incorporating clinical, epidemiological, and radiological aspects for and against the cytologic criteria.

Medical oncologists ask more information than just morphology for cancer-targeted therapy planning. We enter now into the new era of molecular diagnosis with the detection of recurrent chromosome translocations, imbalances, losses, gain, or amplifications specific to histologic types or clues of individual response to adjuvant therapy and outcome, which are even "stronger" than histological typing.

Molecular methods applied on cytological sampling or microbiopsy are becoming increasingly important for initial diagnosis prior to neoadjuvant, nonsurgical therapy, and the combination of molecular biology with metaphase or interphase cytogenetics is imperative in the integrated diagnosis. Therefore, cytology can contribute to individualizing diagnosis through these molecular analyses.

Fine needle aspiration cytology of mesenchymal lesions is not yet as widely accepted for epithelial lesions, and debate persists on its predictive value and accuracy in subtyping and grading sarcomas. One major drawback is the inexperience of most cytopathologists in the field of soft tissue tumors.

This monograph is addressed to a wide readership of medical specialists (radiologists, medical oncologists, surgeons, biologists, young doctors in training, and of course cytopathologists). Because of the rarity and the apparent complexity of the topic, many surgical pathologists are reluctant to be concerned by this issue. Most of their adverse judgments may be avoided while reading this monograph, which makes FNA patterns in soft tissue seem not that difficult.

This monograph does not compete with well-known and largely recognized classic textbooks dealing with soft tissue tumors (Enzinger and Weiss, WHO fascicule, and others); this book rather must be perceived as a useful original supply in this pathology providing information otherwise unavailable or difficult to locate in a user-friendly format.

The authors with North American or European background (France, Greece, Sweden, USA, and Canada) reflect widely accepted international viewpoints; they founded their expertise on their published research data on new entities and emerging methodologies. They based their long-lasting practice on material collected for half a century in dedicated reference centers such as the Institut Curie in Paris and l'Hôtel-Dieu in Québec City.

The authors aim to cover the diagnostic areas where FNA is feasible today in soft tissue lesions. This includes palpable lesions and lesions sampled using various radiological methods. Correlations with mandatory ancillary techniques are detailed.

This book proposes a new horizon in the diagnosis of soft tissue tumors, putting forward how to obtain an optimal approach for diagnosis in the multidisciplinary team.

The contents are logically organized with the first chapters addressing the utility of clinical history, patient's age, site, and size of the tumor, which are essential in the differential diagnoses; the advantages of an organized multidisciplinary team are emphasized by integrating the clinical data, the radiological features, and the morphological pattern.

Precious advice for obtaining optimal material is developed in the technical chapters. The authors offer to teach a diagnostic method of approach that optimizes health care. Complete decisional trees concerning radiology, FNA, core needle, and immunocyto/histochemistry are proposed; weak points are stressed, errors are analyzed, and troubleshooting is proposed.

The basics of morphologic patterns are then reviewed focusing on the results of optimal nonsurgical sampling in offering opportunities for conventional cytology and histology as well for immunostaining and molecular techniques.

Sampling by FNA or core biopsy is less invasive than open biopsy (violation of anatomical compartments, tissue displacements, and vascular emboli). First line mutilating surgery or open biopsy imperatively submits the patient to delayed healing and histological diagnosis.

Risk of tumor seeding within the needle track is a scarecrow.

FNA cell-rich material (usually 10−20 millions cells through one needle pass) is in many cases much better than microbiopsy for molecular techniques: "cell by cell" analysis for fluorescent in situ hybridization (FISH) and "sorted" tumor cells by fluorescence immunophenotyping (FICTION).

The future is definitely in "small sampling" through both FNA and core for microbiology and molecular genetics.

Obtaining FNA one-day diagnosis allows initial fast treatment while waiting for definitive pathological and genomic results, which is extremely important in pediatric round cell sarcomas/blastematous tumors.

Even if some entities may have a surprisingly characteristic morphology allowing an accurate cytologic typing (like myxoid liposarcoma and synovial sarcoma), identification of translocations and oncogene mutations are requested in several tumor types. Specific molecular findings are detected by reverse transcriptase PCR or ISH. In situ hybridization (ISH) is based on morphology by direct microscopic visualization of probe-specific intranuclear signals. The method allows a targeted detection of genetic aberrations in the nondividing nucleus. The FISH can be applied to isolated cells from aspirated fluids, intraoperative smears, cell cultures, or paraffin-embedded and frozen tissue blocks. PCR and ISH are complementary methods, and optimal diagnostic accuracy can be reached when both are available.

In the two last chapters, all differential diagnoses and pitfalls of a wrong or unlikely diagnosis are reviewed entity by entity.

For a practical point on the benchmark, the chapters of entities were grouped following a predominant cell pattern and not an academic classification, which is based on the putative tissue origin; all these facilitate the diagnosis on small tissue volume. For these reasons, some entities, like MPNST or leiomyosarcoma, may be shown in both low-grade and high-grade chapters. All groups of tumors are supported by a complete bibliography hallmarking, for example, that low-grade tumors (like schwannoma, fibromyxosarcoma, and leiomyosarcoma) being benign or malignant may have identical surgical management—the diagnosis of low-grade tumor allows for "prepared" surgery in good conditions.

This monograph supplemented by numerous high-quality morphology illustrations of both FNA and core needle, will become a precious guide to the cytopathologist in eliminating all the incompatible, improbable, possible diagnoses and in retaining only the likely one.

Alain Verhest, MD, PhD, FIAC

Past President of the International Academy of Cytology
Former Head of the Department of Pathology, Cytology & Cytogenetics
Institut Jules Bordet, Cancer Center of the Untversité Libre de Bruxelles, Belgium

Preface

The purpose of this monograph is to highlight a multidisciplinary approach to soft tissue tumors, based on the combined experience of European and North American clinicians, radiologists, biologists, surgical pathologists, and cytopathologists. It does not have the pretention to cover the wide field of mesenchymal neoplasms and pseudotumors, which is very adequately provided in the well-known classic textbooks. Clinical presentation as well as epidemiology and the importance of a precise diagnosis are presented from the clinician point of view. A chapter is devoted to the radiologic evaluation, which has evolved during the past half-century, particularly the techniques of computed tomography and magnetic resonance imaging that are essential in the diagnosis/decisional trees for pathological sampling and the staging of malignant neoplasms. Special emphasis is given to cytological study of specimens of both fine needle aspiration (FNA) biopsy and core needle biopsy (CNB) because the material that forms the basis of the present book has been collected from the cytopathology files of Curie Institute, Paris. In the last decades, FNA and CNB have been recognized as useful tools in the primary diagnosis of soft tissue tumors. Accordingly, a chapter deals with the optimal methodologies to obtain representative diagnostic material, as well as the advantages and disadvantages of FNA versus CNB.

Ancillary studies such as immunohistochemistry, cytogenetics, and molecular biology are discussed in general chapters, because they are essential to diagnosis in several malignant entities. Given the limitations and the pitfalls of grading malignant soft tissue tumors, the rules for obtaining the highest performance and the reproducibility of the systems are discussed as are the controversies in the literature regarding the grading with aspirates and core needle biopsy specimens. The second part of the monograph deals with different tumors entities that have been grouped according to their principal morphological pattern of presentation, namely low-grade spindle cell, tumors with fibrillary stroma, malignant spindle cell, myxoid, lipomatous, epithelioid, pleomorphic, and round cell.

Nowadays, highly specialized centers with targeted clinical consultations and performant radiological technical plateau adapted to small biopsy consultation, performed either by the radiologist or the pathologist, are habilitated to diagnose and consequently treat most of these tumors. It also allows access to suitable material for cytogenetic and molecular biology investigations, using procedures as less invasive as possible, which preserve an eventual noncontaminated surgical field or the tumor integrity, and that permit radiological monitoring in the follow-up of a given tumor treated by neoadjuvant, nonsurgical procedure.

Since 1920, at Institut Curie, Paris, France, the clinical experience in the diagnosis and management of soft tissue tumors has been recognized. For decades, performant radiological evaluation for both pediatric and adult neoplasias has assessed FNA and CNB performed on-site diagnosis by pathologists in day-to-day practice, which allowed for constituting a large archival collection of mesenchymal neoplasms, both for cytology and for correlation with corresponding histology. Facilities in cytogenetics and molecular biology are of valuable help for reaching a precise diagnosis. The data from different investigations along with discussions in multidisciplinary meetings have resulted in optimal patient management. Different diagnostic approaches based on standardized decisional trees have been developed in cooperation with major Parisian hospitals.

We hope that this book will be a good complement to other publications on the same topic and that it is addressed to all those members of multidisciplinary teams concerned with the diagnosis and management of soft tissue tumors.

Jerzy Klijanienko
Réal Lagacé

Acknowledgments

To my mother – Teresa Pienkowska, MD, PhD and to Marie, Julie and Alice.

I wish to express my appreciation to my colleagues of the Pathology, Radiology, Clinical Oncology, and Pediatrics departments at the Institut Curie; to Dr. Philippe Vielh, former head of the Cytopathology Unit; to Dr. Xavier Sastre-Garau, head of the Department of Pathology who encouraged me in the achievement of this work; to Drs. Paul Fréneaux, Daniel Orbach, Marick Laé, and Vincent Servois, my colleagues of "every day oncology practice" who are strongly involved in the diagnosis of pediatric and adult soft tissue tumors; and to Pr. Jean-Michel Zucker, retired head of Department of Pediatric Oncology. For many years, he was the leader in the introduction of the fine needle technique in the diagnosis of solid pediatric tumors.

Many thanks also to Dr. Antoine Zajdela, former head of Cytopathology Unit at the Institut Curie and a pioneer of Clinical Cytology in France, for collecting a large series of aspirates in connective tissue tumors since 1954. Special acknowledgments go to Drs. Jean-Michel Caillaud, Paris, Svante R Orell, Southern Australia, and Olivier Mir, Paris, for discussions and help in the redaction of this monograph. The contributions of Mrs. Véronique Marck and Eliane Padoy, cytotechnicians, as well as of Patricia Le Mouel for her help in typing and of Mr. Pierre Laborde, Institut Curie, are also greatly acknowledged.

Jerzy Klijanienko

To my wife Jacqueline, children and grandchildren

I express my deep gratitude to Dr. Philippe Vielh, Institut Gustave Roussy, Paris, and former head of The CytopathologyUnit at Institut Curie, who kindly invited me to spend a sabbatical year at Institut Curie, Paris, and guided my candidature to obtain a Mayant-Rotschild award as a visiting professor in 1999–2000. I had the privilege to be initiated by Dr. Alain Aurias and Josette Derré, INSERM U830, into the fascinating novel insights of molecular cytogenetics. I also wish to express my appreciation to Dr. Xavier Sastre-Garau and his staff surgical pathologists who welcomed me in their service to share the interpretation of interesting and problematic cases. Over the years of my professional activity at l'Hôtel-Dieu de Québec, Québec city, Canada, colleagues and residents have forwarded me many bone and soft tissue cases, which enhanced my interest and experience for these lesions. Special thanks also to Dr. Sébastien Labonté and Mrs. Louise Tremblay, Department of Anatomical Patholoy, University Hospital-Hôtel-Dieu de Québec, for their contribution to the final sprint of this monograph.

I thank all of you!

Réal Lagacé

Contributors

CARLOS BEDROSSIAN, MD, PhD (Hon)
Professor of Pathology
Rush University Medical College
Medical Director
Biomedical Concepts
Medical Arts Building
715 Lake St., Ste 302
Oak Park, IL 60301, USA

HERVÉ BRISSE, MD, PhD
Senior Radiologist, in charge of Pediatric Radiodiagnosis at the Institut Curie
Institute Curie, Radiodiagnostic
26 rue d'Ulm
75248 Paris cedex 05, France

JÉRÔME COUTURIER, MD
Head of Cytogenetics Unit, Institut Curie
Institut Curie
26 rue d'Ulm
75248 Paris cedex 05, France

HENRYK A. DOMAŃSKI, MD, PhD
Coordinator of the Cytology Service
University and Regional Laboratories Region Skåne
Department of Pathology
Lund University Hospital
Pathologie
S-221 85 Lund, Sweden

FRANÇOIS GOLDWASSER, MD, PhD
Assistant Professor, Medical Oncologist
Paris Descartes University
Hôpital Cochin, Paris
Hôpital Cochin
27 rue du Faubourg Saint Jacques
75679 Paris cedex 14, France

JERZY KLIJANIENKO, MD, PhD, MIAC
Senior Surgical Pathologist and Medical Oncologist, in charge of Clinical
Cytopathology at the Institut Curie
Institut Curie, Pathologie
26 rue d'Ulm
75248 Paris cedex 05, France

RÉAL LAGACÉ, MD, FRCPC
Emeritus professor of Pathology, Laval University
Centre Hospitalier Universitaire de Québec, Québec, Canada
11 Côte du Palais
Québec G1R 2J6, Canada

STAMATIOS THEOCHARIS, MD, PhD
Assistant Professor
Department of Forensic Medicine and Toxicology
University of Athens, Medical School
75, Mikras Asias Street, Goudi
Athens, Greece, GR 11527

Chapter *1*

Clinical Approach in Soft Tissue Tumors

François Goldwasser

1.1 EPIDEMIOLOGY

Sarcomas are rare malignant tumors that originate from mesenchymal tissue at any body site. Soft tissue sarcomas comprise approximately 1% of malignant tumors [1,2]. There are more than 50 subtypes, pleomorphic sarcoma, liposarcoma, leiomyosarcoma, synovial sarcoma, and malignant peripheral nerve sheath tumor accounting for 75% of the cases. Roughly speaking, 80% of sarcomas originate from soft tissues, whereas the remainder are from bones. More than 10,000 new cases are diagnosed each year in the United States [1,2]. They account for 0.72% of all cancers diagnosed annually, whereas they represent 7% of all cancers in children. In Europe, similar data are reported with almost 8% of neoplasms in children, and almost half of them being less than 5 years of age at diagnosis [3]. Between 1988 and 1997, the age-standardized incidence of soft tissue sarcomas in Europe was 9.1 per million children, with a lower range of affected patients in the western and eastern parts of the continent and a higher one in the northern. The annual incidence is 30 per million [3].

Most soft tissue sarcomas occur in adults older than 55 years. Approximately 50% of bone sarcomas and 20% of soft tissue sarcomas are diagnosed in people younger than 35 years. The gastrointestinal stromal tumor (GIST), the frequency of which has been underestimated, is the most common form of soft tissue neoplasm. Its incidence, prevalence, and clinical aggressiveness also have been underestimated [4]. More recent experience from epidemiologic studies and active GIST therapeutic trials suggest that the annual incidence of GIST in the United States is at least 4000 to 6000 new cases (roughly 7 to 20 cases per million population per year) [4]. Some sarcomas,

Soft Tissue Tumors: A Multidisciplinary, Decisional Diagnostic Approach
Edited by Jerzy Klijanienko and Réal Lagacé
Copyright © 2011 John Wiley & Sons, Inc.

such as leiomyosarcoma, chondrosarcoma, and GIST are more common in adults than in children. Only approximately 500 thigh liposarcomas are diagnosed per year in the United States compared with more than 212,900 adenocarcinomas of the female breast. Thus, the number of adenocarcinomas originating in one anatomic site in women exceeds by almost 500-fold the number of thigh liposarcomas and is 22-fold higher than the total number of soft tissue sarcomas of all pathological varieties, at all anatomical sites, in all age groups, and in both genders.

Most high-grade bone sarcomas, including Ewing sarcoma/peripheral neuroectodermal tumor and osteosarcoma, are much more common in children and young adults. Among children, soft tissue sarcomas are two times more common in Caucasians than in African Americans. Rhabdomyosarcoma is the most frequent childhood soft tissue sarcoma (50%). Population-based data from Connecticut covering the years 1935–1989 have shown an increased incidence of soft tissue sarcomas in both genders, with men being more affected than women. The recent increase of acquired immune deficiency syndrome−related Kaposi sarcoma does not explain the upward trend in soft tissue sarcoma, dating back decades. A similar trend was found in a population-based study including 5802 cases of soft tissue sarcomas in children aged 0–14 years, which was extracted from the database of the Automated Childhood Cancer Information System (ACCIS) and registered in population-based cancer registries in Europe for the period 1978–1997. The incidence of soft tissue sarcomas in children increased by almost 2% per year during the period 1978–1997 as a result of the higher incidence of genitourinary rhabdomyosarcoma [3]. In most cases of soft tissue sarcomas, precise etiology is unknown, although several associated or predisposing factors have been identified, including environmental, physical, biological, and chemical factors.

1.1.1   Previous Local Injury

Soft tissue sarcomas can develop in areas of scar tissue after surgery, burns, fractures, radiation therapy [5–10], chronic irritation, and lymphedema out. The number of cancer patients who live longer after a curative treatment of a primary neoplasm is increasing. Therefore, childhood cancer survivors have an increased risk for developing secondary sarcomas. Postirradiation sarcoma, although uncommon, is more frequent because the number of long-term survivors increases [5]. The risk of subsequent bone cancer among 9170 patients who had survived 2 or more years after the diagnosis of a cancer in childhood has been estimated [6]. As compared with the general population, the patients had a relative risk of 133 (95% confidence interval [CI], 98–176) and a mean ± (standard error [SE]) 20-year cumulative risk of 2.8 ± 0.7% [6]. A large cohort of childhood cancer survivors was followed to determine the true incidence of secondary sarcomas. The history of secondary sarcomas in 14,372 participants in the Childhood Cancer Survivor Study was determined from self-reports in three questionnaires [7]. A total of 108 patients developed sarcomas in a median of 11 years after the initial diagnosis of childhood cancer. The risk of sarcoma was more than nine-fold higher among childhood cancer survivors than among the general population (standardized incidence ratio [SIR] = 9.02, 95% CI = 7.44–10.93). The excess absolute risk of secondary sarcoma was 32.5 per 100,000 person-years (95% CI = 26.1–40.3 per 100,000 person-years). Higher standardized incidence ratios and excess absolute risks were associated with a young age at primary diagnosis, a primary sarcoma diagnosis, and a family history of cancer. In a multivariable model, an increased risk of secondary sarcoma was associated with radiation therapy (relative risk [RR] = 3.1, 95% CI = 1.5–6.2), a primary diagnosis of sarcoma (RR = 10.1, 95% CI = 4.7–21.8), a history of other secondary neoplasms (RR = 2.2, 95% CI = 1.1–4.5), and treatment with higher doses of anthracyclines (RR = 2.3, 95% CI = 1.2–4.3) or alkylating agents (RR = 2.2, 95% CI = 1.1–4.6) [6]. A study attempted to evaluate the risk of soft tissue sarcoma in areas close to previously irradiated anatomic regions in women with breast carcinoma. This population-based, retrospective cohort study allowed identifying 194,798 women who were diagnosed with invasive breast carcinoma between 1973 and 1995. According to data from the Surveillance, Epidemiology and End Results Program (SEER), 54 women in the radiation therapy cohort and 81 women in the nonradiation therapy cohort subsequently developed soft tissue sarcomas. In the radiation therapy cohort, the age-standardized incidence ratios were 26.2 (95% CI=16.5–41.4) for angiosarcoma and 2.5 (95% CI=1.8–3.5) for other sarcomas. In the nonradiation therapy cohort, the age-standardized incidence ratios were 2.1 (95% CI=1.0–4.4) and 1.3 (95% CI=1.0–1.7), respectively. The radiation therapy cohort demonstrated a greater risk for developing both angiosarcoma (RR=15.9, 95% CI=6.6–38.1) (Fig 1.1) and other sarcomas (RR=2.2, 95% CI=1.4–3.3) compared with the nonradiation therapy cohort, and the largest increase was observed in the chest wall/breast. The elevated RR was significant even within 5 years of radiation therapy but reached a maximum between 5 and 10 years. That study also showed that the risk of developing soft tissue sarcoma, especially angiosarcoma, was elevated after radiation therapy in women with breast carcinoma [8]. Eighty patients had a confirmed histologic diagnosis of sarcoma that occurred after radiation therapy during 1975 and 1995. The patients were treated for breast cancer (n = 33, 42%), non-Hodgkin lymphoma (n = 9, 11%), cervical cancer (n = 9, 11%), benign lesions (n = 4, 5%), or other tumors (n = 25, 31%). Sarcoma occurred after a mean latency of 12 years (range, 3–64 years), with most (70%) developing in the soft tissues [9]. In another study, the median dose of radiation delivered to the primary tumor site was 45 Gy, and the median interval between radiotherapy and a diagnosis of sarcoma was 14 years. Seven tumors were located in the anatomical region of the sternum, three were located on the lateral chest wall, and five were located in the thoracic outlet [10].

1.1.2 Exposure to Chemicals

The risk of developing a soft tissue sarcoma increases in patients who have been exposed to carcinogenic agents, particularly polycyclic hydrocarbons, asbestos, dioxin, and vinyl chloride [11–16]. The strongest documented association is related to vinyl chloride. In a case-control study of childhood rhabdomyosarcoma, families of 33 cases and 99 controls were interviewed. An RR of 3.9 was associated with fathers' (but not mothers') cigarette smoking (p =.003). For other cases, children had fewer immunizations than controls, particularly smallpox vaccinations (RR = 0.2; p =.001), and conversely had more preventive infections. An RR of 3.2 (p = .03) was found with exposure to chemicals, as well as with diets including giblets meats (RR of 3.7; p = .004). Mothers of affected children older than 30 years of age at the subject's birth, those to be overaged at childbirth, and the role of antibiotics treatment preceding or during pregnancy also have been assessed. Other findings suggest that low socio-economic status could be associated with an increased risk of rhabdomyosarcoma. All these findings suggest that environmental factors could play an important role in the etiology of childhood rhabdomyosarcoma [11]. Marijuana and cocaine addiction of parents during the year preceding their child's birth has been reported to increase by two-fold to five-fold the risk of rhabdomyosarcoma in their children [12]. Exposure to phenoxyacetic acids has been associated with a roughly three-fold increased risk for soft tissue sarcoma, therefore confirming previous findings, whereas exposure to chlorophenols was not associated with a risk of developing soft tissue sarcomas in this study [13]. The potential role of phenoxy herbicides and chlorophenols in the development of soft tissue sarcomas also has been evaluated. In studies based on population referents, increased risks for soft tissue sarcoma were documented in gardeners (odds ratio [OR] = 4.1), railroad workers (OR = 3.1), as well as construction workers exposed to impregnating agents (OR = 2.3) [14]. Moreover, it also has been demonstrated [15] that soft tissue sarcoma risk, modeled using conditional logistic regression, was associated significantly with high-intensity chlorophenol exposure (OR = 1.79, 95% CI 1.10–2.88). A duration-response trend was evident among more highly exposed subjects (p < .0001). For subjects with 10 or more years of substantial exposure, the odds ratio was 7.78 (95% CI 2.46–24.65). These results suggest that chlorophenol exposure, independent of phenoxyherbicides, may increase the risk of soft tissue sarcoma [16].

1.1.3 Diseases or Conditions

Patients with weakened immune defenses such as human immunodeficiency virus (HIV) infection, congenital (inborn) immune deficiency, or immunosuppressive therapy are at risk for developing soft tissue sarcomas. Kaposi sarcoma is linked to HIV infection. HIV and human herpesvirus 8 has been implicated in the pathogenesis of Kaposi sarcoma. Rare familial syndromes with soft tissue sarcomas sarcoma have been identified. A report from the Cancer Family Registry of the National Cancer Institute allowed retrieving 24 kindreds of a syndrome that includes sarcoma, breast carcinoma, and other neoplasms in young patients. Cancer developed in an autosomal dominant pattern in 151 blood relatives, 119 (79%) of whom were affected before 45 years of age. These young patients had 50 bone and soft tissue sarcomas of diverse histological subtypes and 28 breast cancers. Additional features of the syndrome included an increased incidence of brain tumor (14 cases), leukemia (9 cases), and adrenocortical carcinoma (4 cases) before 45 years of age. These neoplasms also accounted for 73% of the multiple primary cancers occurring in 15 family members. This description led to the discovery of the Li-Fraumeni syndrome, which is related to p53 germline mutations [17,18]. New germline mutations of the p53 gene are rare among patients with "sporadic" sarcoma, whereas they are more frequent in patients whose background includes either multiple primary cancers or a family history of cancer [17]. As many as 7% of children with soft tissue sarcomas have Li-Fraumeni syndrome. The p53 gene seems altered in at least one third of sarcoma patients. In another third of patients, the *MDM2* gene is amplified, resulting in an inhibition of the p53. Soft tissue sarcomas are more frequent among patients with certain inherited conditions including retinoblastoma [19], Li-Fraumeni syndrome, Gardners's syndrome, Werner's syndrome, nevoid basal cell carcinoma syndrome, neurofibromatosis type 1, and some immunodeficiency syndromes. Indeed, these risk factors account for a minority of soft tissue sarcomas, hence, the need for more genetic and environmental investigations.

1.2 CLINICS AND CLINICAL PROFILES

In day-to-day practice, the suspicion/diagnosis of a soft tissue sarcoma is unusual because of the rarity of these neoplasms; most patients seeking medical advice for a soft tissue lump do have a benign neoplastic or non-neoplastic condition. Some clinical presentations should suggest a reference to a specialist (those with a mass larger than 5 cm, as well as pain, increased size, deep to fascia, or a recurrent mass after previous excision). The definitive tests for diagnosing sarcoma are imaging (ultrasound, X-rays, computed tomography [CT] scan, or magnetic resonance imaging [MRI] scan) and a biopsy. It is important that both imaging and biopsy samples should be performed by experienced radiologists and pathologists in the management of soft tissue lesions. Many benign lumps simulate sarcomas, and they are obviously much more frequent. The contribution of pathologists to the multidisciplinary team of sarcomas, management and in the quality control of sarcoma diagnosis is mandatory. The planning of the surgical procedure follows the histological diagnosis. However, some sarcomas will come to be revealed or diagnosed in unexpected situations (e.g., uterine sarcoma in specimens of hysterectomy or GIST in resected abdominal and gastrointestinal masses). Otherwise, surgery should be undertaken under the supervision of a sarcoma specialist multidisciplinary team, even when the surgeon is not a regular member of that team.

1.2.1 Natural History of Soft Tissue Sarcomas

Soft tissue sarcomas can affect any part of the body. The most frequent location is the lower limb, accounting for about half of the cases, although the abdominal space and the retroperitoneum also are affected. Ideally, a definitive diagnosis should be stated in terms of benignancy or malignancy before any other procedure takes place. An initial surgical removal/biopsy is not recommended to avoid the contamination of the tumor bed, particularly for those lumps suspicious of malignancy. It has been demonstrated that the adequacy of an initial surgical resection was an important factor of prognosis, either in terms of recurrence and/or metastasis. Histologic evaluation of the surgical margins is mandatory [20] for both high- and low-grade neoplasms, whether superficial or deep. Approximately 50% of sarcoma patients will suffer a local recurrence and/or metastasis. For most histologic subtypes of soft tissue sarcomas, the most predictive factor of distant metastatic disease is tumor grade [21, 22]. The metastatic potential of low-grade sarcomas is 5–10%, of intermediate-grade sarcomas is 25–30%, and of high-grade sarcomas is approximately 50–60%. Additional histologic features have been used to evaluate tumor grade such as necrosis, pleomorphism, and the number of mitoses per microscopic high power field (HPF). However, some soft tissue sarcomas do not respond to the usual grading criteria; for example, tumors of the Ewing sarcoma/peripheral neuroectodermal tumor family are all high-grade sarcomas, whereas alveolar soft part sarcoma and some well-differentiated synovial sarcomas, although depicting a very low mitotic index and a well-recognized tumor type, are unpredictable in their biologic behavior.

Soft tissue sarcomas of the extremities usually metastasize to the lungs (70% of patients), with liver metastases being rare (<5%). Retroperitoneal and organ-based soft tissue sarcomas have a greater incidence of liver metastases with a similar rate of frequency to lung metastases. Myxoid liposarcoma is an exception, with a tendency to metastasize to other sites rather than to the lungs. Lymph node metastases are rare in soft tissue sarcomas and occur in less than 2–3% of cases, with the exception of synovial sarcoma, epithelioid sarcoma, and clear cell sarcoma of tendon sheath whose incidence of lymph node metastases reaches 20% [23].

Several low-grade soft tissue sarcomas are prone to gain a second clone of neoplastic cells during the course of their progression. These so-called "dedifferentiated sarcomas" depict a different phenotype of variable malignancy and can pursue a more aggressive clinical course [24–28]. In terms of oncogenesis, dedifferentiation is a phenomenon of tumor progression that seems to be time dependent. Dedifferentiation occurs in roughly 10% of well-differentiated liposarcomas of any subtype [25–28]. The risk of dedifferentiation is greater for deep-seated (particularly retroperitoneum) tumors and is significantly less for the limbs. Approximately 90% develop de novo, whereas 10% occur in recurrences. Dedifferentiation to leiomyosarcoma or rhabdomyosarcoma or less-differentiated liposarcoma is predictive of a worse prognosis in terms of recurrences, metastases, and survival. The use of microarray technology to evaluate gene expression profiles in biopsy or surgical specimens will provide newer insights into the pathogenesis of these tumors and therefore allow more precise subclassification and optimize the selection of therapeutic targets [8].

1.2.2   Age at Diagnosis

The age of the patient at the first presentation of a soft tissue tumor could be suggestive of a given type of neoplasm. Rhabdomyosarcoma is the most common soft tissue tumor of childhood and accounts for approximately one half of all soft tissue sarcomas in this age group. Approximately 65% of cases occur in children less than 6 years of age. It is less frequent during the early-to-mid teenage years and is rare in adulthood. The two most common subtypes, embryonal and alveolar, account for at least 80% of all rhabdomyosarcomas. Synovial sarcoma is at the crossroads between the pediatric and the adult age groups. Although children and adults with synovial sarcoma share a similar clinical presentation, their outcome differs, which suggests that factors other than unfavorable clinical features could influence their biological behavior. Whether this difference is related to biological variables or to historically different treatment approaches for pediatric versus adult patients is a matter of debate [29]. In adults, 40% of sarcomas are malignant fibrous histiocytomas and 25% are liposarcomas. Fibrosarcoma incidence peaks at ages 30–39 years (24%), whereas leiomyosarcoma peaks later at ages 50–59 years (25%). Malignant fibrous histiocytoma peaks at ages 60–69 years (21%) with a regular increase in incidence between 30 and 70. Liposarcoma also peaks at ages 60–69 years (22.5%), but a high prevalence of liposarcoma is observed from ages 40 to 80 years. Well-differentiated liposarcoma represents the largest subgroup of malignant adipocytic neoplasms and accounts for about 40–45% of all liposarcomas. It occurs in middle-aged adults with a peak incidence in the sixth decade. Myxoid liposarcoma is a disease of young adults, with a peak incidence in the fourth and fifth decades of life. Although rare, it is the most common form of liposarcoma in patients younger than 20 years old. There is no sex predilection. Most pleomorphic liposarcoma develops in elderly patients (>50 years) with an equal sex distribution.

1.2.3 Tumor Location and Clinical Presentation

Approximately 60% of soft tissue sarcomas develop in the arms and legs, 30% develop in the trunk of the body, and 10% develop in the head and neck.

Rhabdomyosarcomas typically originate in the head and neck region, urinary tract and reproductive organs, as well as the arms and legs. Embryonal rhabdomyosarcoma is generally a localized tumor, with a favorable response to treatment, and it usually gives distant metastases years after the initial diagnosis. When not occurring in the limbs, rhabdomyosarcomas are revealed under different clinical presentation, with a painless lump in the head or neck and symptoms related to the tumor location (e.g., a bulging or a swollen eyelid and even paralysis of the eye muscles, a stuffy or blocked nose, sometimes together with a nasal discharge that contains pus or blood if the sinus is involved with the tumor, and erosion of the skull bones triggering headache and nausea as the tumor gradually grows toward the brain's surface). In the urogenital tract, symptoms and clinical signs such as dysuria, hematuria, the presence of a lump or mass in the vagina, vaginal discharge of blood and mucus, and painless enlargement of the scrotum when the testicle is affected are common.

Synovial sarcomas mostly occur in the vicinity of large joints such as the knees or ankles, although they can originate in other sites, (Fig 1.1). Rare cases of synovial sarcomas of the gastrointestinal tract have been reported, with most of them in the

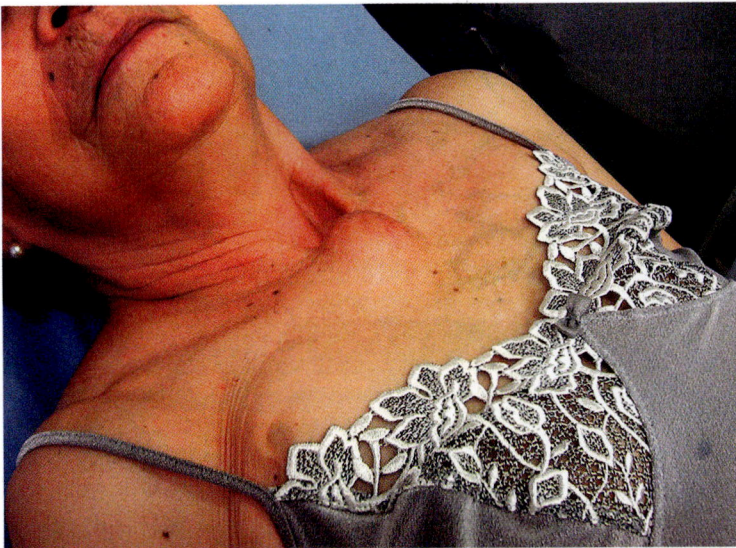

FIG. 1.1 Presternal synovial sarcoma.

esophagus [30]. Synovial sarcomas account for 8–10% of all soft tissue sarcomas. They are characterized by a significant risk for local recurrence, even after a complete surgical excision of a paradoxically well-limited and slowly growing neoplasm. They develop in the vicinity or close to anatomical sites of joints, mostly in the lower limbs (2/3). In a series of 41 patients with synovial sarcoma, a multivariate analysis showed that metastasis at presentation and monophasic tumor subtype affected overall survival. For progression-free survival, monophasic subtype was only one prognostic factor. The study confirmed that histologic subtype is the most important independent prognostic factor of synovial sarcoma regardless of tumor stage [31]. Three histologic subtypes of synovial sarcoma are recognized—biphasic, monophasic, and poorly differentiated tumors. The detection of the characteristic chimeric transcript often contributes to the precision of the histopathological diagnosis, especially when the tumors originate in unusual locations and for the monophasic and poorly differentiated varieties. Previous studies have shown that SYT-SSX1 is the most common SYT-SSX fusion transcript in biphasic synovial sarcomas of the limbs. The detection of a SYT-SSX2 chimeric transcript was confirmed by reverse transcript polymerase chain reaction (RT-PCR) and direct sequencing analysis in both cases. Additional genetic analysis is needed to understand fully the biological and clinical features of synovial sarcoma originating in the thorax [32].

Liposarcomas are mostly neoplasms of the retroperitoneum and the thigh. Well-differentiated liposarcoma occurs most frequently in deep soft tissue of the limbs, especially the thigh (Fig 1.2), followed by the retroperitoneum, the paratesticular area, and the mediastinum. They also can originate in subcutaneous tissues and, very rarely, in the skin (Fig 1.3). The retroperitoneum is the most common anatomic location, outnumbering the soft tissue of extremities by at least 3:1. Other locations include the spermatic cord and, more rarely, the head and neck as well as the

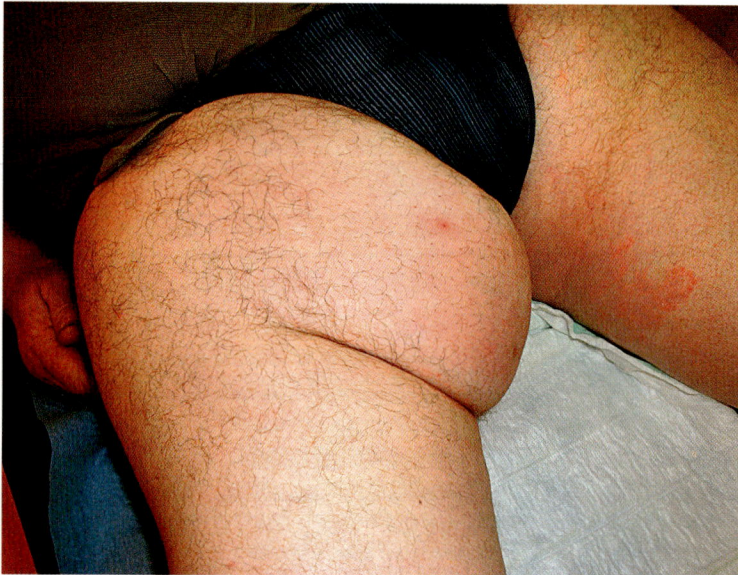

FIG. 1.2 Well-differentiated liposarcoma of the thigh.

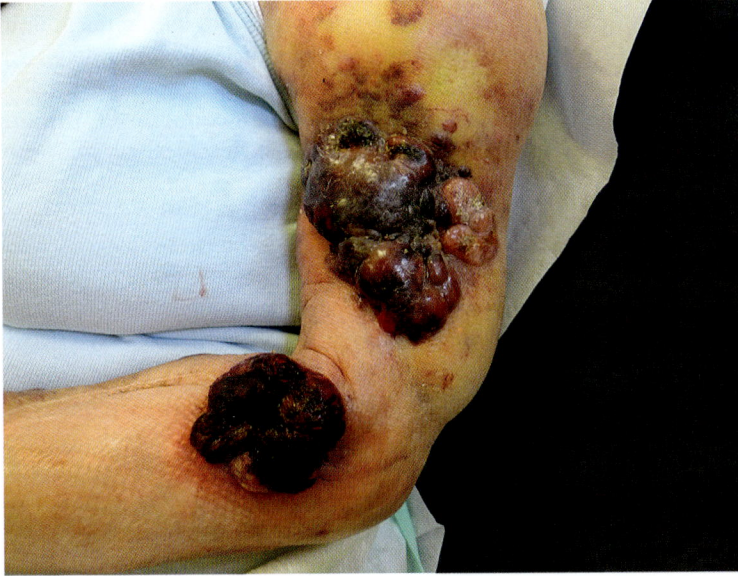

FIG. 1.3 Superficial dedifferentiated liposarcoma in an advanced stage.

trunk. Occurrence in subcutaneous tissue is extremely rare. Atypical lipoma/ well-differentiated liposarcoma usually presents as a deep-seated, painless, and slow-growing enlarging mass of very large size, particularly when developing in the retroperitoneum. Retroperitoneal lesions often are asymptomatic until the tumor has exceeded 20 cm in diameter and may be found incidentally, hence, the poor outcome even for low-grade neoplasms. Initial symptoms are delayed and associated with large tumors and include vague and nonspecific abdominal pain, weight loss, nausea, a sometimes palpable abdominal mass, and compression of the kidney and ureter. Therapeutic management of retroperitoneal sarcomas is challenging because of their location and frequent intimate association with anatomical structures in the retroperitoneum. This proximity of large vessels, visceral organs, axial skeleton, and neural structures may impair significantly the ability to perform a margin-negative resection, which is the optimal potentially curative treatment approach in patients with localized disease. Even in the setting of a complete resection, local recurrence is common.

Dedifferentiated liposarcomas usually present as large painless masses, which may be found incidentally (particularly in the retroperitoneum). In the limbs, the history of a long-standing mass with a recent increase in size is suggestive of dedifferentiation. Radiologic imaging shows a coexistence of both fatty and nonfatty solid components, which in the retroperitoneum may be discontinuous.

Myxoid liposarcoma is the second most common subtype of liposarcoma, accounting for more than one third of liposarcomas and approximately 10% of all adult soft tissue sarcomas. Grossly, it is well circumscribed. It was considered a tumor of intermediate grade with a definite metastatic potential, particularly the round cell variant, but it pursues a relatively indolent behavior [33]. Its therapeutic approach has changed since the demonstration of its sensitivity to trabectidin. Myxoid liposarcoma occurs with a predilection in the deep soft tissues of the extremities and in more than two thirds of cases originates within the musculature of the thigh. It rarely develops primarily in the retroperitoneum or in the subcutaneous tissue. It is prone to recur locally, and one third of patients develop distant metastases particularly with the round cell subtype. In comparison with other types of liposarcoma or other myxoid sarcomas of the extremities, myxoid liposarcoma tends to metastasize to unusual sites, like soft tissue (such as retroperitoneum, opposite extremity, axilla, etc.) or bone (with predilection to spine) locations, even before spreading to lungs. In a significant number of cases, myxoid liposarcoma patients present clinically with synchronous or metachronous multifocal disease. This unusual phenomenon most likely represents a pattern of hematogenous metastases to other sites by tumor cells seemingly incompetent to seed the lungs. The tendency for myxoid liposarcoma to metastasize to other soft tissues in preference to lung parenchyma has been well described [34]. A series of the Royal Marsden Hospital covering a 10-year period and including 50 patients with myxoid liposarcoma, with a median follow-up of 43 months, has shown that the actuarial 5-year soft tissue metastasis rate was 31%, and that the most common sites of myxoid liposarcoma were the retroperitoneum, abdominal wall, and abdominal cavity. In 12 patients with soft tissue metastases, there was a median interval of 23 months after the original diagnosis before the occurrence of the first metastases (range, 0–142 months). The median survival after the first metastasis was 35 months; 6 of the 12 patients died between 6 and 50 months. In this series, any round cell component of the myxoid liposarcoma was associated with a significantly greater risk of metastatic disease (p = .02), which has not been confirmed by other studies. The overall 5-year and 7-year survival rates were 85% and 68%, respectively. Patients with soft tissue metastases had an 11-fold greater risk of dying than those who did not. Therefore, the subset of patients who develop soft tissue metastases have a significantly worse prognosis [34].

Pleomorphic liposarcoma represents the rarest subtype of liposarcoma, accounting for approximately 5% of all liposarcomas and 20% of pleomorphic sarcomas. Pleomorphic liposarcoma tends to occur on the extremities (lower > upper limbs), whereas the trunk and the retroperitoneum are affected less frequently. Rare sites of involvement include the mediastinum, the paratesticular region, the scalp, the abdominal/pelvic cavities, and the orbit. Although most cases originate in deep soft tissues, examples in subcutis are rare. As for other deep-seated sarcomas, most patients complain of a firm, enlarging mass, with many cases presenting a notably short preoperative history. In general, pleomorphic liposarcoma is an aggressive mesenchymal neoplasm showing a 30–50% metastatic rate and an overall tumor associated mortality of 40–50%. Many patients die within a short period of time, and the lung represents the preferred site of metastases. In contrast, dedifferentiated liposarcomas and high-grade myxofibrosarcomas have a prolonged clinical course, whereas pleomorphic myogenic sarcomas of deep soft tissues show an even more aggressive clinical course emphasizing the need for subclassification of pleomorphic sarcomas.

Angiosarcomas occur in the following different clinical settings: tumors of the skin affecting mostly older patients (Figure 1.4), deep soft tissue tumors or organ-based neoplasms, and postradiation tumors. The mean age of patients with angiosarcoma of the scalp is approximately 70 years. The tumor manifested clinically as a bruise-like lesion in early phase and as indurated, erythematous plaque accompanied by nodules, ulcerations, and bleeding in advanced phase. Besides cutaneous

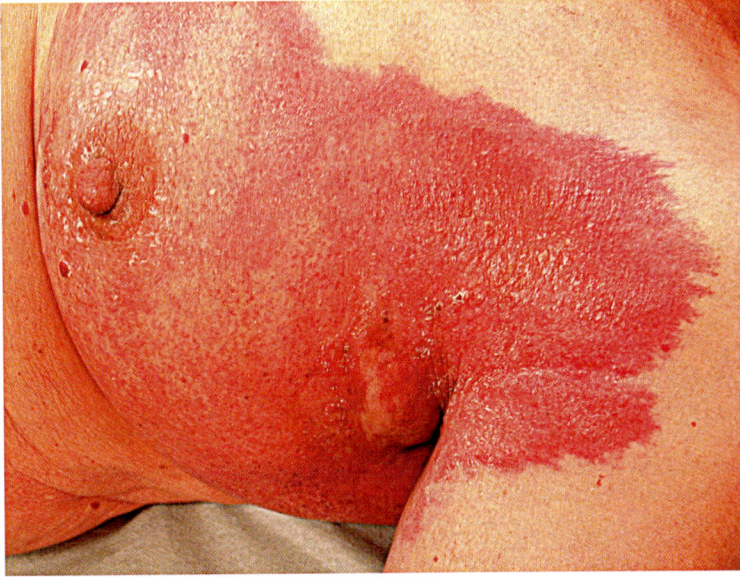

FIG. 1.4 Skin angiosarcoma in a patient with breast carcinoma history.

angiosarcomas, the angiosarcoma of the liver has been described in vinyl chloride workers worldwide [35]. Angiosarcomas are frequently sensitive to Paclitaxel treatments [36].

Hemangiopericytoma is a rare vascular tumor, and its histological distinction from synovial sarcoma and solitary fibrous tumor is a significant problem because they share similar histologic features. As will de discussed later, over the years, it has become a morphologic diagnosis of exclusion. Between July 1982 and February 1998, 62 patients with a diagnosis of primary, recurrent, or metastatic hemangiopericytoma were identified from a prospectively maintained database [37]. Using well-defined and recognized pathologic criteria, including immunohistochemistry and electron microscopy, tumors from 25 of 57 patients had a diagnosis of conventional hemangiopericytoma. At the time of initial presentation, 19 patients had primary tumors, 3 had locally recurrent diseases, and 3 had metastases. The most frequent anatomic sites of occurrence were the extremities, the pelvis, and the head and neck, accounting for 80% of the total cases. Two and 5-year overall survival rates (n = 25) were 93% and 86%, respectively. Patients undergoing complete resection (n = 16) showed a 100% median survival at 60 months. So far, complete tumor resection for patients with conventional hemangiopericytoma is recommended. However, considering their favorable biological behavior, surgical procedures that can generate altered anatomical functions or limb threatening are not recommended [37].

GIST is the most common sarcoma of the intestinal tract. It originates in the stomach, the small gut, and occasionally the large intestine. Rare cases also are reported in other locations, namely the esophagus, the abdominal cavity, and the retroperitoneum. Numerous GISTs are clinically symptomatic (69%), others are incidental findings at surgery (21%) or are found at autopsy (10%). Forty-four percent of symptomatic, clinically detected GISTs were categorized as high risk (29%) or overtly malignant (15%), with tumor-related deaths occurring in 63% of patients and 83% of patients, respectively (estimated median survival of 40 months and 16 months, respectively). Tumor-related deaths occurred in only two of 170 of patients (1.2%) with very-low-risk, low-risk, or intermediate-risk tumors [3].

1.2.4 Paraneoplastic Syndromes

A large variety of sarcomas can reveal or be associated with paraneoplastic syndromes. Neurologic, endocrinologic, dermatologic, and urinary symptoms as well as clinical signs are common [38–40].

The neurologic system is the target of many immunologic paraneoplastic syndromes in sarcoma patients, such as opsoclonus-myoclonus syndromes [38], which are reported in neurofibrosarcoma patients as are antineural antibodies in an anti-Hu syndrome with neurologic deficits [39], and sensorimotor polyneuropathy. Central neurologic symptoms such as dysphasia may reveal a central nervous system vasculitis. Central nervous system vasculitis usually is diagnosed by MRI/ magnetic resonance angiography (MRA) and cerebral angiography. Complete neurologic recovery may be achieved with Prednisone [38–40]. Endocrin manifestations also are very diverse [41–43]. Ectopic hormone productions may induce Cushingoid symptoms [41]. Arterial hypertension may be secondary to renin-producing leiomyosarcomas [42]. Hypoglycemia may be a consequence of a secretion of insulin-like growth factor, which also has been reported in leiomyosarcoma patients [43]. Clinical symptoms of inflammation also are possible. Dermatologic and rheumatologic syndromes also have been reported [44–50], including hand and foot ulceration, fixed cyanosis, and pallor complicating a central nervous system rhabdomyosarcoma and oncogenic osteomalacia. Acrokeratosis paraneoplastica (Bazexs syndrome) is a rare obligate paraneoplastic dermatosis characterized by erythematosquamous lesions localized symmetrically at the acral sites [50]. The condition almost exclusively affects Caucasian men older than 40 years. The surgical removal of a liposarcoma associated with acrokeratosis paraneoplastica shows a parallel regression or the development of the tumor in case of a recurrence of the liposarcoma [50]. Paraneoplastic pemphigus is a rare, life-threatening autoimmune bullous skin disease, which is an obligate paraneoplasm. The patient may present with recalcitrant stomatitis and a generalized lichenoid rash. In renal syndromes, for example, a membranous nephropathy [51–53], proteinuria, may disappear with the remission of the tumor. Nephrotic syndrome and acute renal failure have been associated with embryonal rhabdomyosarcoma. Effective treatment of the sarcoma was associated with sustained remission of the nephrotic proteinuria. A differential diagnosis for proteinuria is the obstruction of the renal veins, frequently caused by thrombosis or tumor processes. Although the obstructive mass initially may be misdiagnosed as thrombosis, positron emission tomography helps to reveal the tumor character of the lesion and a fine needle aspiration (FNA) allows for rapid diagnosis of a leiomyosarcoma originating from the caval or renal veins [54]. Stauffer syndrome [55], a very rare paraneoplastic syndrome, refers to reversible intrahepatic cholestasis in the setting of an abdominal malignancy and also was described in sarcoma patients. Prolonged fever or biological manifestations of inflammation also may be part of a paraneoplastic syndrome [56–58]. A white blood cell count of more than $50 \times 10(9)/l$, not related to bone marrow involvement, is referred to as leukemoid reaction. Pyrexia, leukocytosis, and other inflammatory findings may be associated with a sarcoma showing positive immunostaining for human granulocyte-colony simulating factor (G-CSF). Northern and polymerase chain reaction (PCR) analyses also may detect CSF and its mRNA in the tumor. Therefore, it should be kept in mind, in case of adjuvant chemotherapy, that G-CSF (frequently prescribed to prevent doxorubi-cin-ifosfamide–induced profound neutropenia) shoud be avoided, if the patients had, at initial diagnosis, clinical symptoms or biological manifestations compatible with the presence of G-CSF receptors at the tumor surface.

1.3 CLINICAL DIFFERENTIAL DIAGNOSIS

In most cases, patients with soft tissue sarcoma will complain of a new and persistent lump, usually on an arm, leg, or trunk. This lump may or may not be painful. In patients with physical activity, the lump sometimes is mistaken for an injury related to athletic, professional, or recreational activities. We emphasize the following frequent situations: superficial sarcoma misinterpreted as hematoma or another benign condition and a deep retroperitoneal mass. First-line clinical subdifferentia-tion is important because the different subtypes vary in prognosis and therapeutic strategies [59] and allow for optimal patient management. Soft tissue sarcomas often present as a painless and slowly enlarging mass. Several sarcomas, like synovial sarcoma may be misdiagnosed clinically with other benign conditions, such as the Baker cyst or villonodular pigmented synovitis, considering their deceiving macro-scopic and chronological features. Patients with sarcoma reporting trauma may be considered to have muscular posttraumatic hematomas [60–62]. Thus, posttraumatic intramuscular hematomas should be approached with a high degree of clinical suspicion and be evaluated radiologically (see Chapter 2). Briefly, the ultrasono-graphic investigation in an emergency is useful and may suggest the nature of the lesion [63]. Secondary MRI analysis also can be used as an important diagnostic tool, but both radiological investigations must be interpreted in the context of the clinical history. The MRI may reveal a small tumor mass with enhancement and characterize the hematoma in the lesion in a more precise fashion than does CT. Therefore, MRI imaging is a suitable method for differentiating these soft tissue sarcomas from chronic traumatic hematoma [62]. However, MRI is not sensitive or specific enough to rule out malignancy. As an initial approach, the search for malignant cells using percutaneous fine needle aspiration is indicated. If the cytological diagnosis of a sarcoma is suggested, then a histological biopsy will be considered [61]. Besides intramuscular hematomas, patients may present with hematoma at the site of a visceral sarcoma. For instance, intrathoracic sarcoma may be revealed by a chronic expanding thoracic hematoma [64]. Similarly, chronic subdural hematoma may lead to the diagnosis of subdural rhabdomyosarcoma, granulocytic sarcoma, or other subtypes of sarcoma [65–67].

Retroperitoneal sarcomas account for approximately one third of all retroper-itoneal masses [68–72]. Although most extravisceral large masses in the retroper-itoneum represent a retroperitoneal sarcoma, a differential diagnosis, including lymphoma, testicular neoplasm, germ cell tumor, desmoids, functioning and non-functioning adrenal masses, renal tumor, pancreatic tumor, and gastrointestinal stromal tumor, should be considered [68–72]. Among adrenal masses, exceptionally an adrenal sarcoma is identified as most often either a synovial sarcoma [73] or an angiosarcoma [74]. If visceral invasion is present, then a differential diagnosis should be made that includes tumors of these organs and site-directed endoscopy with or without biopsy, if feasible, to evaluate for intraluminal evidence of involvement (e.g., stomach, duodenum, pancreas, colon). Symptoms suggestive of lymphoma include the classic B symptoms of unexplained fever, drenching night sweats, and weight loss in addition to the symptoms of unexplained pruritus and alcohol-induced pain at the sites of disease. For patients with testicular neoplasms, the physical examination should include a testicular examination for masses and consideration of testicular ultrasound. In addition, if a testicular neoplasm or germ cell tumor is considered then initial laboratory studies should include serum tumor markers, such as alpha fetoprotein (AFP), beta-human chorionic growth hormone (beta-HCG), and lactate dehydrogenase (LDH). The initial diagnostic evaluation of patients who are suspected of having retroperitoneal sarcoma should include a contrast-enhanced CT of the abdomen and pelvis to evaluate the size and extent of the lesion [68]. The use of oral and intravenous contrast is necessary to allow adequate visualization of the surrounding vascular structures, visceral organs, and skeletal structures for the assessment of respectability [68–72]. The CT appearance of liposarcomas typically includes fat-density components, but other retroperitoneal sarcoma histologic findings can be difficult to distinguish from other retroperitoneal tumors. MRI of the abdomen has been evaluated as a method of staging; however, MRI often does not add additional information to that obtained with contrast-enhanced CT of the abdomen. When enhanced-contrast CT is not available, MRI may provide an alternative modality to assess the local disease extent [68]. A biopsy for these lesions in the preoperative setting is controversial if there is a low index of suspicion for other tumors based on the initial evaluation; however, if neoadjuvant therapy is used, then histologic verification is usually necessary. In this event, a CT-guided cytology and biopsy is the preferred diagnostic approach. Surgical resection is considered the only potentially curative treatment modality, and complete surgical resection with negative margins remains the goal of therapy for most patients [69–71]. The likelihood of a negative margin surgical resection depends on several factors, including invasion of adjacent visceral organs, vascular structures, and skeletal structures.

1.4   THE IMPORTANCE OF MOLECULAR DIAGNOSIS AND ITS PERSPECTIVES

Molecular assays are described in Chapter 4. Briefly, the specific gene fusions provide a genetic approach to the differential diagnosis of soft tissue sarcomas. The genetic categories may correspond closely to the standard histopathologic categories. The polymerase chain reaction assays for chimeric transcripts are useful tools for the rapid and objective assessment of pediatric soft tissue sarcomas [75]. However, for many tumors, the histogenesis is controversial [76, 77].

1.5   TREATMENT STRATEGIES

The American Joint Commission on Cancer determines the stage of tumors by assessing the tumor's grade, size, and extension to nearby lymph nodes or to distant organs [78]. The French Federation of Cancer Centers system is a different method that relies on microscopic grading to predict the apparition of metastastatic disease, even when other tests cannot detect that the sarcoma has spread. A high likelihood of metastastatic disease can influence the treatment that is recommended. The Musculoskeletal Tumor Society Staging System assigns tumor stage based on tumor grade, presence of metastases, and whether the tumor has extended beyond the anatomical region. Because muscle groups in the skeleton are divided into separate compartments by "sleeves" of connecting tissue, any growth or spread beyond the compartment of origin can be evidence that a tumor is spreading aggressively. For most soft tissue sarcomas, surgery is the basic treatment. The entire tumor is removed along with a wide excision. Improvements in curative surgery results are dependent on the delay for diagnosis on the conditions of biopsy or first excision [79]. Radiotherapy has a role inside a multimodal strategy [80]. After surgery, continued treatment usually depends on the type of sarcoma, the tumor stage and grade, tumor location, and the patient's age and general health. Tumor grade is the key to the tumor's current spread and future behavior. High-grade soft tissue sarcomas tend to spread early to distant sites. Metastatic disease is common, and conventional chemotherapy provides for only a narrow therapeutic window outside of a few responsive pathological subtypes.

REFERENCES

1. Zahm SH, Fraumeni JF Jr. The epidemiology of soft tissue sarcoma. Semin Oncol 1997, 245: 504–514.

2. Jemal A, Siegel R, Ward E, et al. Cancer statistics, 2007. CA Cancer J Clin 2007, 57: 43–66.

3. Pastore G, Peris-Bonet R, Carli M, Martinez-Garcia C, Sanchez J de Toledo, Steliarova-Foucher E. Childhood soft tissue sarcomas incidence and survival in European children (1978–1997): report from the Automated Childhood Cancer Information System project. Eur J Cancer 2006, 42: 2136–2149.

4. Nilsson B, Bumming P, Meis-Kindblom JM, et al. Gastrointestinal stromal tumors: the incidence, prevalence, clinical course, and prognostication in the preimatinib mesylate era—a population-based study in western Sweden. Cancer 2005, 103: 821–829.

5. Robinson E, Neugut AI, Wylie P. Clinical aspects of postirradiation sarcomas. J Natl Cancer Inst 1988, 80: 233–240.

6. Tucker MA, D'Angio GJ, Boice JD Jr, et al. Bone sarcomas linked to radiotherapy and chemotherapy in children. N Engl J Med 1987, 317: 588–593.

7. Henderson TO, Whitton J, Stovall M, et al. Secondary sarcomas in childhood cancer survivors: a report from the Childhood Cancer Survivor Study. J Natl Cancer Inst 2007, 99: 300–308.

8. Huang J, Mackillop WJ. Increased risk of soft tissue sarcoma after radiotherapy in women with breast carcinoma. Cancer 2001, 92: 172–180.

9. Lagrange JL, Ramaioli A, Chateau MC, et al. Sarcoma after radiation therapy: retrospective multiinstitutional study of 80 histologically confirmed cases. Radiation Therapist and Pathologist Groups of the Federation Nationale des Centres de Lutte Contre le Cancer. Radiology 2000, 216: 197–205.

10. Chapelier AR, Bacha EA, de Montpreville VT, et al. Radical resection of radiation-induced sarcoma of the chest wall: report of 15 cases. Ann Thorac Surg 1997, 63: 214–219.

11. Grufferman S, Wang HH, DeLong ER, Kimm SY, Delzell ES, Falletta JM. Environmental factors in the etiology of rhabdomyosarcoma in childhood. J Natl Cancer Inst 1982, 68: 107−113.

12. Grufferman S, Schwartz AG, Ruymann FB, Maurer HM. Parents' use of cocaine and marijuana and increased risk of rhabdomyosarcoma in their children. Cancer Causes Control 1993, 4: 217−224.

13. Hardell L, Eriksson M. The association between soft tissue sarcomas and exposure to phenoxyacetic acids. A new case-referent study. Cancer 1988, 62: 652−656.

14. Wingren G, Fredrikson M, Brage HN, Nordenskjold B, Axelson O. Soft tissue sarcoma and occupational exposures. Cancer 1990, 66: 806−811.

15. Hoppin JA, Tolbert PE, Herrick RF, Freedman DS, Ragsdale BD, Horvat KR, Brann EA. Occupational chlorophenol exposure and soft tissue sarcoma risk among men aged 30−60 years. Am J Epidemiol 1998, 148: 693−703.

16. Vineis P, Faggiano F, Tedeschi M, Ciccone G. Incidence rates of lymphomas and soft tissue sarcomas and environmental measurements of phenoxy herbicides. J Natl Cancer Inst 1991, 83: 362−363.

17. Li FP, Fraumeni JF Jr, Mulvihill JJ, Blattner WA, Dreyfus MG, Tucker MA, Miller RW. A cancer family syndrome in twenty-four kindreds. Cancer Res 1988, 48: 5358−5362.

18. Toguchida J, Yamaguchi T, Dayton SH, et al. Prevalence and spectrum of germline mutations of the p53 gene among patients with sarcoma. N Engl J Med 1992, 326: 1301−1308.

19. Eng C, Li FP, Abramson DH, et al. Mortality from second tumors among long-term survivors of retinoblastoma. J Natl Cancer Inst 1993, 85: 1121−1128.

20. Singer S, Antonescu CR, Riedel E, et al. Histologic subtype and margin of resection predict pattern of recurrence and survival for retroperitoneal liposarcoma. Ann Surg 2003, 238: 358−370.

21. Costa J, Wesley R, Glatstein E, et al. The grading of soft tissue sarcomas: results of a clinicohistopathologic correlation in a series of 163 cases. Cancer 1984, 53: 530−541.

22. Presant C, Russell W, Alexander R, et al. Soft tissue and bone sarcoma histology peer review: the frequency of disagreement in diagnosis and the need for second pathology opinions. The South Eastern Cancer Study Group Experience. J Clin Oncol 1986, 4: 1658−1661.

23. Fong Y, Coit D, Woodruff J, et al. Lymph node metastasis from soft tissue sarcoma in adults. Ann Surg 1993, 217: 72−77.

24. Lewis JJ, Leung D, Woodruff JM, et al. Retroperitoneal soft-tissue sarcoma: analysis of 500 patients treated and followed at a single institution. Ann Surg 1998, 228: 355−365.

25. Heslin MJ, Lewis JJ, Nadler E, et al. Prognostic factors associated with long-term survival for retroperitoneal sarcoma: implications for management. J Clin Oncol 1997, 15: 2832−2839.

26. Binh MB, Guillou L, Hostein I, et al. Dedifferentiated liposarcomas with divergent myosarcomatous differentiation developed in the internal trunk: a study of 27 cases and comparison to conventional dedifferentiated liposarcomas and leiomyosarcomas. Am J Surg Pathol 2007, 31: 1557−1566.

27. Fabre-Guillevin E, Coindre JM, Somerhausen Nde S, et al. Retroperitoneal liposarcomas: follow-up analysis of dedifferentiation after clinicopathologic reexamination of 86 liposarcomas and malignant fibrous histiocytomas. Cancer 2006, 106: 2725−2733.

28. Gronchi A, Casali PG, Fiore M, et al. Retroperitoneal soft tissue sarcomas: patterns of recurrence in 167 patients treated at a single institution. Cancer 2004, 100: 2448−2455.

29. Sultan I, Rodriguez-Galindo C, Saab R, Yasir S, Casanova M, Ferrari A. Comparing children and adults with synovial sarcoma in the surveillance, epidemiology, and end results program, 1983 to 2005: an analysis of 1268 patients. Cancer 2009, 115: 3537–3547.

30. Makhlouf HR, Ahrens W, Agarwal B, et al. Synovial sarcoma of the stomach: a clinicopathologic, immunohistochemical, and molecular genetic study of 10 cases. Am J Surg Pathol 2008, 32: 275–281.

31. Koh KH, Cho EY, Kim DW, Seo SW. Multivariate analysis of prognostic factors in synovial sarcoma. Orthopedics. 2009, 32: 824.

32. Yano M, Toyooka S, Tsukuda K, et al. SYT-SSX fusion genes in synovial sarcoma of the thorax. Lung Cancer. 2004, 44: 391–397.

33. Patel SR, Burgess MA, Plager C, Papadopoulos NE, Linke KA, Benjamin RS. Myxoid liposarcoma. Experience with chemotherapy. Cancer 1994, 74: 1265–1269.

34. Spillane AJ, Fisher C, Thomas JM. Myxoid liposarcoma—the frequency and the natural history of nonpulmonary soft tissue metastases. Ann Surg Oncol 1999, 6: 389–394.

35. Lee FI, Smith PM, Bennett B, Williams DM. Occupationally related angiosarcoma of the liver in the United Kingdom 1972–1994. Gut 1996, 39: 312–318.

36. Penel N, Bui BN, Bay JO, et al. Phase II trial of weekly paclitaxel for unresectable angiosarcoma: the ANGIOTAX Study. J Clin Oncol 2008, 26: 5269–5274.

37. Espat NJ, Lewis JJ, Leung D, Woodruff JM, Antonescu CR, Shia J, Brennan MF. Conventional hemangiopericytoma: modern analysis of outcome. Cancer 2002, 95: 1746–1751.

38. Stepensky P, Waldman E, Simanovsky N, Fried I, Revel-Vilk S, Resnick IB, Weintraub M. Isolated CNS vasculitis: unusual presentation of relapsed Ewing sarcoma. Pediatr Blood Cancer 2010, 54: 326–328.

39. Mitoma H, Orimo S, Sodeyama N, Tamaki M. Paraneoplastic opsoclonus-myoclonus syndrome and neurofibrosarcoma. Eur Neurol 1996, 36: 322.

40. Deik A, Azizi E, Shapira I, Boniece IR. Supraclavicular extraskeletal myxoid chondro-sarcoma presenting with a sensorimotor polyneuropathy associated with anti-Hu anti-bodies. Oncology (Williston Park) 2009, 23: 718–721.

41. Guran T, Turan S, Ozkan B, Berrak SG, Canpolat C, Dagli T, Eren FS, Bereket A. Cushing's syndrome due to a non-adrenal ectopic adrenocorticotropin-secreting Ewing's sarcoma in a child. J Pediatr Endocrinol Metab 2009, 22: 363–368.

42. Fromme M, Streicher E, Kraus B, Kruse-Jarres J. Arterial hypertension in renin-producing retroperitoneal leiomyosarcoma. Klin Wochenschr 1985, 63: 158–163.

43. Daughaday WH, Emanuele MA, Brooks MH, Barbato AL, Kapadia M, Rotwein P. Synthesis and secretion of insulin-like growth factor II by a leiomyosarcoma with associated hypoglycemia. N Engl J Med 1988, 319: 1434–1440.

44. Pelajo CF, de Oliveira SK, Rodrigues MC, Torres JM. Cutaneous vasculitis as a paraneoplastic syndrome in childhood. Acta Reumatol Port. 2007, 32: 181–183.

45. Lamont EB, Cavaghan MK, Brockstein BE. Oncogenic osteomalacia as a harbinger of recurrent osteosarcoma. Sarcoma 1999, 3: 95–99.

46. Soltani A, Hasani-Ranjbar S, Moayyeri A. Hypocalcemia as a presentation for multifocal osteosarcoma. Pediatr Blood Cancer 2008, 50: 687–689.

47. Tuy BE, Obafemi AA, Beebe KS, Patterson FR. Case report: elevated serum beta human chorionic gonadotropin in a woman with osteosarcoma. Clin Orthop Relat Res 2008, 466: 997–1001.

48. Bosco M, Allia E, Coindre JM, Odasso C, Pagani A, Pacchioni D. Alpha-fetoprotein expression in a dedifferentiated liposarcoma. Virchows Arch 2006, 448: 517–520.

49. Tartaglia F, Blasi S, Sgueglia M, Polichetti P, Tromba L, Berni A. Retroperitoneal liposarcoma associated with small plaque parapsoriasis. World J Surg Oncol 2007, 5: 76.

50. Sator PG, Breier F, Gschnait F. Acrokeratosis paraneoplastica (Bazex's syndrome): association with liposarcoma. J Am Acad Dermatol 2006, 55: 1103–1105.

51. Tourneur F, Bouvier R, Langue J, Saïd MH, Bergeron C, Hermier M, Cochat P. Membranous nephropathy and orbital malignant tumor. Pediatr Nephrol 2000, 14: 53–55.

52. Olowu WA, Salako AA, Adelusola KA, Sowande OA, Adetiloye VA, Adefehinti O, Osasan SA. Focal segmental glomerulosclerosis and nephrotic syndrome in a child with embryonal rhabdomyosarcoma. Clin Exp Nephrol 2008, 12: 144–148.

53. Agha I, Mahoney R, Beardslee M, Liapis H, Cowart RG, Juknevicius I. Systemic amyloidosis associated with pleomorphic sarcoma of the spleen and remission of nephrotic syndrome after removal of the tumor. Am J Kidney Dis 2002, 40: 411–415.

54. Hegner B, Krakamp B, Hedde JP, Brockmann M, Weber M, Schulze-Lohoff E. Positron emission tomography reveals a leiomyosarcoma causing proteinuria. Clin Nephrol 2003, 60: 139–142.

55. Bardia A, Thompson CA, Podratz KC, Okuno SH. Bizarre big belly ball: intraabdominal abscess mimicking stauffer syndrome secondary to uterine leiomyosarcoma. Eur J Gynaecol Oncol 2007, 28: 134–136.

56. Ando J, Sugimoto K, Tamayose K, Ando M, Kojima Y, Oshimi K. Cytokine-producing sarcoma mimics eosinophilic leukaemia. Eur J Haematol 2007, 78: 169–170.

57. Jardin F, Vasse M, Debled M, et al. Intense paraneoplastic neutrophilic leukemoid reaction related to a G-CSF-secreting lung sarcoma. Am J Hematol 2005, 80: 243–245.

58. des Guetz G, Mariani P, Freneaux P, Pouillart P. Paraneoplastic syndromes in cancer: case 2. Leucocytosis associated with liposarcoma recurrence: original presentation of liposarcoma recurrence. J Clin Oncol 2004, 22: 2242–2243.

59. van Vliet M, Kliffen M, Krestin GP, van Dijke CF. Soft tissue sarcomas at a glance: clinical, histological, and MR imaging features of malignant extremity soft tissue tumors. Eur Radiol 2009, 19: 1499–1511.

60. Niimi R, Matsumine A, Kusuzaki K, Okamura A, Matsubara T, Uchida A, Fukutome K. Soft-tissue sarcoma mimicking large haematoma: a report of two cases and review of the literature. J Orthop Surg (Hong Kong) 2006, 14: 90–95.

61. Gomez P, Morcuende J. High-grade sarcomas mimicking traumatic intramuscular hematomas: a report of three cases. Iowa Orthop J 2004, 24: 106–110.

62. Imaizumi S, Morita T, Ogose A, Hotta T, Kobayashi H, Ito T, Hirata Y. Soft tissue sarcoma mimicking chronic hematoma: value of magnetic resonance imaging in differential diagnosis. J Orthop Sci 2002, 7: 33–37.

63. Russo A, Zaottini A. Diagnosis of synovial sarcoma of the knee accidentally revealed by trauma. Role of ultrasound. Differential diagnosis by scar-hematoma. Ann Ital Chir 2009, 80: 151–157.

64. Kwon YS, Koh WJ, Kim TS, Lee KS, Kim BT, Shim YM. Chronic expanding hematoma of the thorax. Yonsei Med J 2007, 48: 337–340.

65. Nejat F, Keshavarzi S, Monajemzadeh M, Mehdizadeh M, Kalaghchi B. Chronic subdural hematoma associated with subdural rhabdomyosarcoma: case report. Neurosurgery 2007, 60: E774–E775.

66. Oertel MF, Korinth MC, Gilsbach JM. Recurrent intracranial sarcoma mimicking chronic subdural haematoma. Br J Neurosurg 2003, 17: 257–260.

67. Smidt MH, de Bruin HG, van't Veer MB, van den Bent MJ. Intracranial granulocytic sarcoma (chloroma) may mimic a subdural hematoma. J Neurol 2005, 252: 498–499.

68. Cohan RH, Baker ME, Cooper C, et al. Computed tomography of primary retroperitoneal malignancies. J Comput Assist Tomogr 1988, 12: 804–810.

69. Windham TC, Pisters PW. Retroperitoneal sarcomas. Cancer Control 2005, 12: 36–43.

70. Thomas JM. Retroperitoneal sarcoma. Br J Surg 2007, 94: 1057–1058.

71. Porter GA, Baxter NN, Pisters PW. Retroperitoneal sarcoma: a population-based analysis of epidemiology, surgery, and radiotherapy. Cancer 2006, 106: 1610–1616.

72. Schwarzbach MH, Hormann Y, Hinz U, et al. Clinical results of surgery for retroperitoneal sarcoma with major blood vessel involvement. J Vasc Surg 2006, 44: 46–55.

73. Just PA, Tissier F, Silvera S, et al. Unexpected diagnosis for an adrenal tumor: synovial sarcoma. Ann Diagn Pathol 2010, 14: 56–59.

74. Invitti C, Pecori Giraldi F, Cavagnini F, Sonzogni A. Unusual association of adrenal angiosarcoma and Cushing's disease. Horm Res 2001, 56: 124–129.

75. Barr FG, Chatten J, D'Cruz CM, et al. Molecular assays for chromosomal translocations in the diagnosis of pediatric soft tissue sarcomas. JAMA 1995, 273: 553–557.

76. Nielsen TO, West RB, Linn SC, et al. Molecular characterisation of soft tissue tumours: a gene expression study. Lancet 2002, 359: 1301–1307.

77. Singer S, Socci ND, Ambrosini G, et al. Gene expression profiling of liposarcoma identifies distinct biological types/subtypes and potential therapeutic targets in well-differentiated and dedifferentiated liposarcoma. Cancer Res 2007, 67: 6626–6636.

78. Greene F, Page D, Norrow M. AJCC cancer staging manual. 6th edition. New York: Springer; 2002.

79. Gutierrez JC, Perez EA, Moffat FL, et al. Should soft tissue sarcomas be treated at high volume centers? An analysis of 4205 patients. Ann Surg 2007, 245: 952–958.

80. O'Sullivan B, Davis AM, Turcotte R, et al. Preoperative versus postoperative radiotherapy in soft-tissue sarcoma of the limbs: a randomised trial. Lancet 2002, 359: 2235–2241.

Chapter *2*

Radiological Diagnostic Approach in Soft Tissue Tumors

Hervé Brisse

2.1 INTRODUCTION

The occurrence of a soft tissue mass is a common clinical situation. Fortunately, benign soft tissue lesions outnumber their malignant counterparts by approximately 100 to 1. Although much more frequent, the benign nature of the lesion should not be presumed systematically, and primary surgical resection therefore is not recommended, even for superficial masses [1]. The rarity of malignant tumors explains the frequently delayed diagnosis and often inadequate initial management by primary excision. The management of primarily resected malignant tumors without preoperative imaging and biopsy raises serious concerns; postoperative changes make it very difficult to identify any residual tumor, and reoperation is usually necessary [2,3]. In the absence of a measurable macroscopic residual disease, the chemosensitivity of the tumor, an essential prognostic factor, no longer can be evaluated, leading to a risk of overtreatment. Finally, when radiotherapy is indicated, the absence of precise local staging can lead to wider safety margins and consequently to local late effects. Apart from certain benign lesions with a typical appearance in clinical examination and/or imaging, upfront diagnostic surgical excision therefore should be avoided.

The radiological patterns of the various tumor types already have been described largely in review articles [4–9] or reference books [10,11]. This section is devoted to presenting a rational diagnostic approach based on clinical and radiological criteria.

Soft Tissue Tumors: A Multidisciplinary, Decisional Diagnostic Approach
Edited by Jerzy Klijanienko and Réal Lagacé
Copyright © 2011 John Wiley & Sons, Inc.

The accuracy of imaging—notably magnetic resonance imaging (MRI)—in the characterization of soft tissue tumors relies on the radiologists' experience. Gielen et al. [12] reviewed, with a centralized approach, the material of 548 untreated and proven soft tissue tumors or tumor-like lesions. Concerning the differentiation between malignant and benign lesions, a sensitivity of 93%, specificity of 82%, negative predictive value (NPV) of 98%, and positive predictive value (PPV) of 60% with an accuracy of 85% were obtained. Concerning phenotype characterization, a sensitivity of 67%, specificity of 98%, NPV of 98%, PPV of 70%, and accuracy of 96% were obtained. For benign lesions, a sensitivity of 75%, specificity of 98%, NPV of 98%, PPV of 76%, and accuracy of 97% were obtained. The phenotype's definition of a malignant tumor had a sensitivity of 37%, a specificity of 96%, an NPV of 96%, a PPV of 40%, and an accuracy of 92%. Finally, a correct diagnosis compared with a histological assessment was proposed in 227 (50%) of the 455 histologically confirmed cases.

2.2 PATIENT MANAGEMENT

A patient presenting a soft tissue mass ideally should be managed in a multi-disciplinary reference center. The role of imaging is essential in these cases, either to confirm its benign nature or, on the contrary, to indicate the necessity of a biopsy if the lesion is potentially aggressive or of a nonspecific appearance.

Clinical examination is still the first step of diagnosis. Age, sex, and the site of the lesion are useful information that lead to diagnosis [8,9]. Tumors can occur anywhere, but some sites can help to guide the diagnosis. Predisposing diseases such as type-1 neurofibromatosis [13,14] must be investigated clinically (Table 2.1).

A size larger than 5 cm, pain, increase in size, and depth beneath the deep fascia are signs associated more frequently with malignancy rather than a benign lesion [15], although they also could be observed in some inflammatory lesions. Systematized dysesthesia should suggest a neurogenic tumor. It is essential to evaluate the clinical growth rate, bearing in mind that rapid growth can be observed in malignant tumors as well as in benign inflammatory lesions. Depending on clinical presentation, the presence of multiple lesions could be suggestive of neurogenic tumors, multiple lipomas, multiple desmoid tumors, myxoma, Kaposi's sarcoma, venous malformations, or metastases.

Clinical examination must assess the consistency, mobility, color, variations of volume with Valsalva manoeuvre (venous malformations), presence of a thrill (arteriovenous malformation), presence of systematized muscle atrophy (neurogenic tumors), and draining lymph nodes (metastatic lymph nodes).

Imaging is not necessary for some superficial lesions whose clinical presentation is sufficient to establish a diagnosis. However, in most cases, imaging is mandatory for diagnostic precision and to assess the local extension of the lesion.

2.3 IMAGING TECHNIQUES

Conventional radiography is of diagnostic value as a first-line investigation, particularly for limb lesions. Analysis of bones could reveal a primary bone lesion

TABLE 2.1 Soft tissue tumors and associated diseases (adapted from [7])

Predisposing disease	Tumors
Neurofibromatosis type 1 (NF1 gene mutation)	Neurofibroma Plexiform neurofibroma Malignant peripheral nerve sheath tumor Rhabdomyosarcoma
Hereditary retinoblastoma (RB1 gene mutation)	Bone and soft tissue sarcomas Melanoma
Antineoplastic treatment (radiotherapy, or alkylating agents)	Sarcomas
Li-Fraumeni syndroma (TP53 gene mutation)	Rhabdomyosarcoma
Beckwith-Wiedemann syndrome	Rhabdomyosarcoma
Gardner's syndrome	Mesenteric fibromatoses
Gorham, Maffucci, and Blue rubber bleb nervus syndromes	Venous malformation
Turner, Noonan, Klippel-Trenaunay-Weber syndromes	Cystic lymphangioma
PHACE syndrome	Haemangioma
Fibrous dysplasia (Mazabraud syndrome)	Myxoma
Carney syndrome	
Familial hypercholesterolemia	Xanthoma

either with a soft tissue extension, contiguous extension to bone, or bone deformity. More rarely, demonstration of bone hypertrophy may indicate an arteriovenous malformation. Analysis of soft tissues is valuable to demonstrate calcifications and fat density areas.

Added to plain films, ultrasound is part of the simple first-line examination for cases clinically and radiologically suggestive; the radiography-US couple allows establishing the diagnosis of some pseudotumors (adenitis, abscess, popliteal cyst, synovial cyst, foreign body, or hematoma), benign tumors (lipomas, infantile hemangioma, or fibromatosis colli), or malformations (vascular). Doppler analysis confirms the avascular nature of cystic lesions or, conversely, assesses the type of blood supply of solid lesions.

MRI is currently the gold standard for evaluation of soft tissue tumors because of its excellent tissue contrast [4,6,16]. It is mandatory before biopsy if the clinico-radiological presentation is nonspecific, if the limits of the lesion are difficult to evaluate, or if the lesion is situated close to the central nervous system (facial or paraspinal mass).

Technically, the choice of coils, imaging planes (at least two orthogonal), and acquisition parameters depends on the size and site of the lesions. The sequences used are T1- and T2-weighted spin echo sequences, a short tau inversion recovery (STIR) leading to fat suppression and combining T1 and T2 effects, T2-weighted gradient echo (very sensitive to magnetic field heterogeneities and useful to detect hemosiderin deposits or vessels with high flow rates), and three-dimensional (3D) T1-weighted GE sequences for dynamic acquisitions. Spectral fat-saturation or selective water-excitation techniques are used to increase the contrast on enhanced T1- and T2-weighted sequences.

Gadolinium chelates are used routinely because some highly necrotic malignant or myxoid lesions can have a pseudocystic appearance. Dynamic MRI, which studies the enhancement kinetics of the lesions, helps to define the nature of the mass and viable tumor areas, which guides the biopsy procedure [17]. The impact of diffusion-weighted sequences is still under evaluation [18–21].

Magnetic resonance (MR) spectroscopy of soft tissue tumors has been restricted to the study of ^{31}P and to the evaluation of the response to chemotherapy [22]. The diagnostic use of proton spectroscopy has been evaluated in preliminary studies [23] but is not used routinely. MR spectroscopy could be helpful in differentiating malignant from benign musculoskeletal tumors by revealing the presence or absence of water-soluble choline metabolites [24].

In view of the performances of MRI, a computed tomography (CT) scan now has an extremely limited role. According to the American College of Radiology guidelines [25], CT still has two indications:

1. Demonstration of calcifications is of major diagnostic value if conventional radiography does not provide this information; for example, when myositis ossificans is suspected, the entity could present a misleading appearance in MRI [26].
2. Lesions of the chest wall and anterior abdominal wall frequently are associated with artifacts on MRI.

Apart from the recognized indication of flurodeoxygluclose positron emission tomography (FDG-PET) for the staging of malignant melanoma, the use of this technique for the investigation of soft tissue masses is very recent, and large-scale prospective series are still necessary to assess its real contribution [27]. A study of musculoskeletal tumors based on standard uptake value measurements has shown that FDG-PET can distinguish benign lesions from aggressive and/or malignant lesions with a sensitivity of 92% and a specificity of 100% [28]. However, there is still some overlap between aggressive and malignant lesions. Positron emission tomography computed tomography (PET-CT) also can contribute to staging [29] and to the diagnosis of local recurrence during subsequent follow-up [30], but further studies still are needed to define the rational use of this technique.

2.4 RADIOLOGIC CHARACTERIZATION

Purely cystic lesions may correspond to pseudotumors (cysts, hematomas, or abscesses) or vascular tumors (macrocystic lymphangiomas). However, some malignant tumors are sometimes very necrotic and can be suspected by the presence of a contrast-enhanced, thick, nodular wall. Some malignant lesions are sometimes homogeneous and well delineated with a low signal intensity on T1-weighted sequences and a very high signal intensity on T2-weighted sequences, and they may be mistaken for cystic lesions, especially synovial sarcomas [31,32] and tumors with a large myxoid component, such as myxoid liposarcomas [33], which emphasizes the importance of systematic contrast-enhanced MR sequences.

Calcifications in a suggestive site are strong arguments in favor of dermoid cysts or subcutaneous pilomatrixomas. Phleboliths (Fig 2.1) indicate a diagnosis of venous malformation. The irregular peripheral calcifications of myositis ossificans also are characteristic (Fig 2.2). However, the presence of calcifications is not always

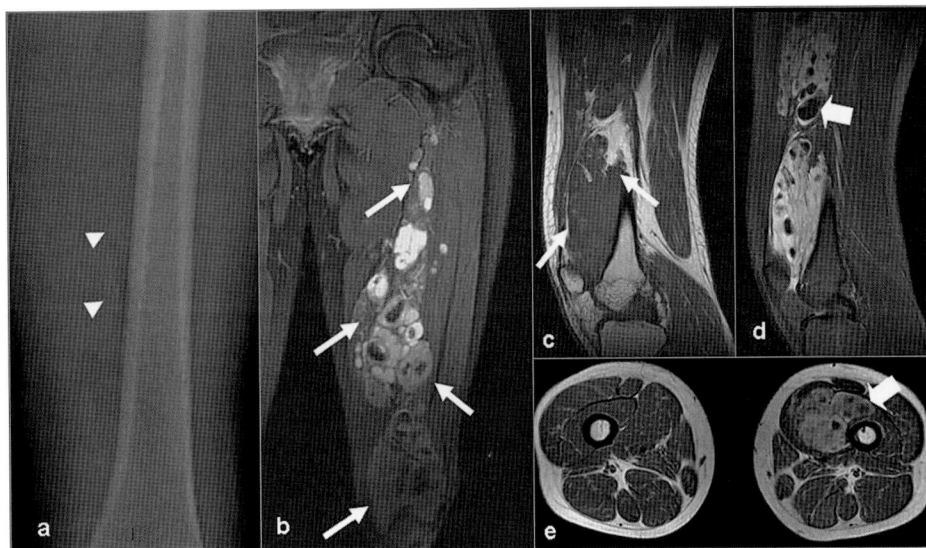

FIG. 2.1 Deep venous malformation of the left thigh. Plain film (a) demonstrates typical phleboliths (arrowheads). MR images of a (b) coronal FS T2-WI, (c) sagittal T1-WI, (d) sagittal FS T2-WI and (e) axial enhanced T1-WI demonstrate a diffuse venous malformation (long arrows) infiltrating the quadriceps femoris. Multiple contiguous cysts are observed, with some including focal spots (short arrows) of low signal intensity on T2-WI that correspond to focal thrombosis or phleboliths. In patients with such typical imaging features, neither FNA nor core needle biopsy (CNB) is required for diagnosis.

indicative of a benign lesion; approximately one half of synovial sarcomas contain amorphous calcifications. The rare osteocartilaginous soft tissue lesions also can contain calcifications (surface-type or periosteal osteosarcomas, extraskeletal osteosarcomas, or chondrosarcomas).

A fatty component in children is suggestive of a benign lesion such as lipoblastoma [34], fibrolipomatous hamartoma, lipoma (Fig 2.3), or dermoid cyst. Liposarcomas usually are not observed before the age of 10 years [11,35]. A lobular internal structure classically is observed in vascular tumors (venous malformations) [36] and lipoblastomas.

Low-signal-intensity areas on T2, although nonspecific, are suggestive of a benign lesion such as benign fibrous tumor, fibromatosis (Fig 2.4) [37,38], benign neurogenic tumor ("target sign" of neurofibromas [39]), venous malformation (phleboliths) (Fig 2.3) [36], or tenosynovial giant cell tumors (hemosiderin deposits) [32].

In MRI, the presence of tortuous vessels with signal voids constitutes an important diagnostic argument in favor of an arteriovenous malformation or hemangioma (Fig 2.5) in children [40].

By ultrasound, the echogenicity and homogeneity of the lesions are nonspecific [41]. Some Doppler criteria can be suggestive of malignancy. Among the various quantitative criteria, the resistance index seems to have a poor predictive value, whereas systolic velocity (>0.5 m/s in favor of malignancy) seems to be more discriminant, but there is an overlap between benign and malignant lesions [42]. The morphological criteria of tumor neovascularization on power Doppler using a

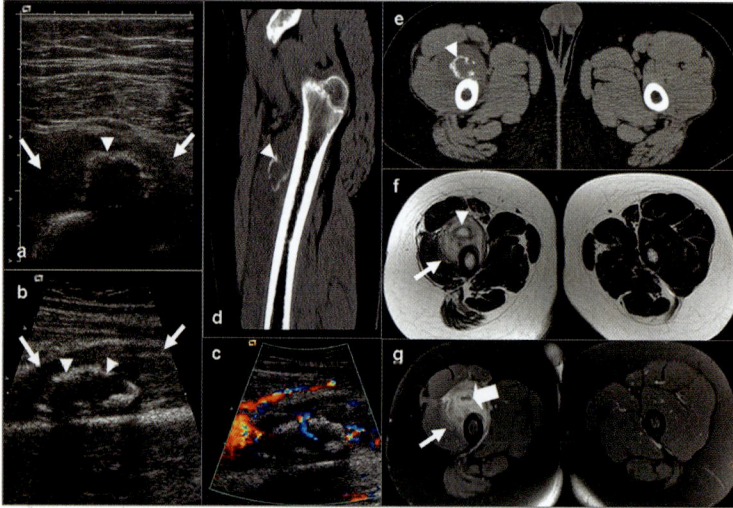

FIG. 2.2 Myositis ossificans of the right quadriceps femoris. Ultrasound examination (a,b) displays a hypoechogenic mass (arrows) containing dense calcifications (arrowheads). Color-Doppler (c) demonstrates peripheral vascularization. Unenhanced CT scans of a (d) sagittal reconstruction and (e) an axial view demonstrate typical peripheral irregular calcifcations located within the vastus intermedius. MRI of a (f) axial T2-WI and an (g) axial enhanced FS T1-WI show diffuse swelling of the vastus intermedius muscle centered by a necrotic area (short arrow) surrounded by calcifcations (arrowhead). In patients with such typical imaging features, neither FNA nor CNB is required for diagnosis.

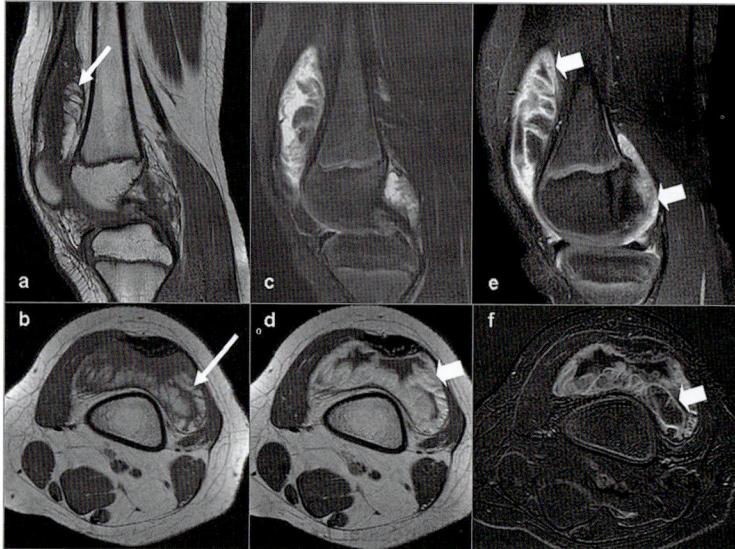

FIG. 2.3 Lipoma arborescens of the left knee. MR images of a (a) sagittal T1-WI, (b) axial T1-WI, (c) sagittal FS T2-WI, (d) enhanced axial T1 WI, (e) sagittal enhanced FS T1-WI, and (f) a enhanced axial T1 WI with subtraction demonstrate hypertrophic synovial villi distended by a tissue of a similar signal to that of subcutaneous fat (long arrows) surrounded by peripheral enhancement (short arrows). The imaging pattern is specific, and CNB is not required for diagnosis.

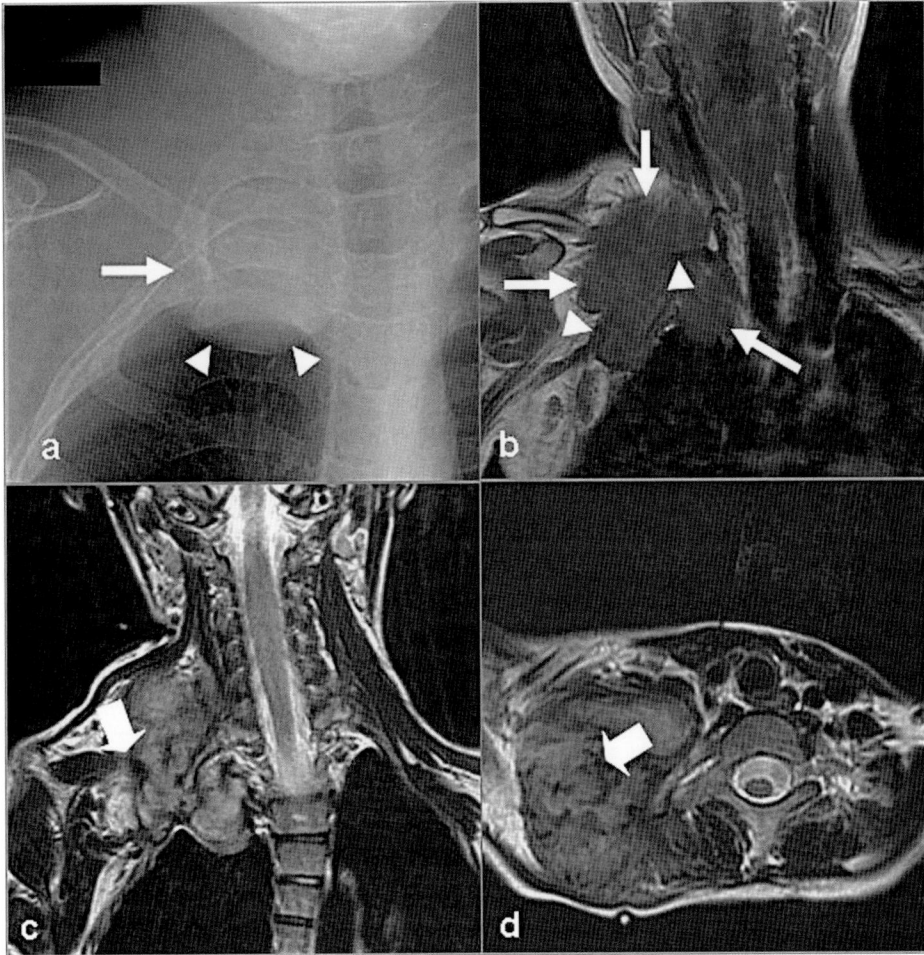

FIG. 2.4 Desmoid tumor of the right cervicothoracic junction. Plain film (a) demonstrates a focal hyperdensity with a mass effect (arrowheads) on the superior lobe of the right lung and focal destruction of the anterior segment of the first rib (arrow). MR images of a (b) coronal T1-WI, (c) coronal T2-WI, and (d) axial T2-WI demonstrate a lobular-shaped mass (long arrows) containing multiple low-signal areas on T2-WI (short arrows) corresponding to dense collagen fibrosis. The right subclavian artery (arrowheads) is encased by the tumor. The MR signal pattern and local agressivness are highly suggestive of a desmoid tumor; however, histologic confirmation (by surgical or CNB) is mandatory.

high-frequency probe have been studied more recently; the disorganized architecture of vessels and images of trifurcations, stenoses, and occlusions are arguments in favor of malignancy. However, these criteria cannot be used for small (1.5 cm) and necrotic lesions [41,42]. The complete absence of any detectable flow within a solid mass is a good criterion in favor of a benign lesion [42].

Although the morphology and the signal are not totally specific [43, 44], MR is considered an accurate method to differentiate between malignant and benign lesions [12]. Criteria in favor of malignancy are size (5 cm) [45,46], absence of low signal intensity on T2-weighted sequences [46], signal heterogeneity on T1-weighted

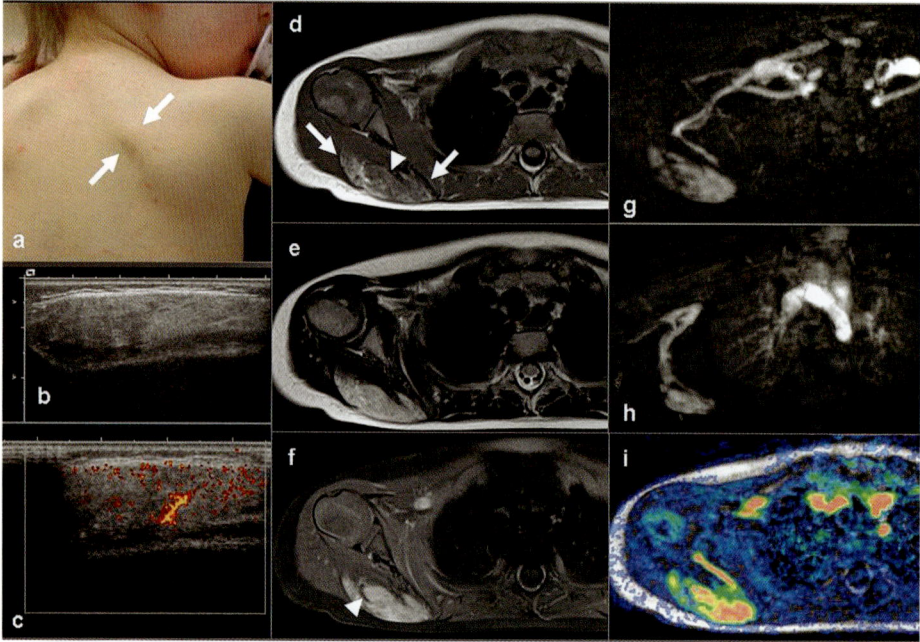

FIG. 2.5 Infantile hemangioma of the posterior chest wall in an infant. Physical examination (a) shows a firm subcutaneaous mass without skin abnormality. Ultrasound examination demonstrates a fusiform hyperechogenic mass (b) containing arterial vessels on Doppler examination (c). Conventional axial MR images of a (d) T1-WI, (e) T2-WI, and (f) enhanced FS T1 WI demonstrate a well-defined mass (long arrows) located between the infraspinatus and the deltoideus containing linear low-signal areas on T2-WI (arrowheads) corresponding to arterial vessels ("flow-voids"). Dynamic MRI with maximum intensity projection (MIP) angiography (g,h) and a parametric image (i) of an enhancement slope demonstrate both the arterial supply (g) and the venous drainage (h) of the mass, and intense, homogeneous, and rapid enhancement after gadolinium injection, comparable with that of arterial vessels. When both clinical and imaging patterns are typical, FNA and CNB are not required for diagnosis. Atypical forms will benefit from FNA because this technique is less aggressive than CNB and is associated with a very low risk of local bleeding.

sequences [46], peripheral and centripetal contrast enhancement (Fig 2.6) [47], and contiguous invasion of bone and/or neurovascular bundles [46]. The circumscribed or noncircumscribed appearance of the lesion and the presence of edema around the tumor are not predictive criteria [6]. However, all MR criteria can be misleading [6]. A predominantly peripheral enhancement also can be observed in benign lesions, and some benign tumors can present radiological signs of marked aggressiveness, especially desmoid fibromatosis, which frequently invades adjacent tissues and bone (Fig 2.4).

The intensity of contrast enhancement and enhancement slopes after dynamic injection (Fig 2.5) are correlated with histological grade but are incompletely predictive because of the overlap between benign and malignant lesions [6,48]. Nevertheless, combined unenhanced static and dynamic contrast-enhanced MR imaging parameters are considered significantly superior to unenhanced MR imaging alone and to unenhanced MR imaging combined with static contrast-enhanced MR

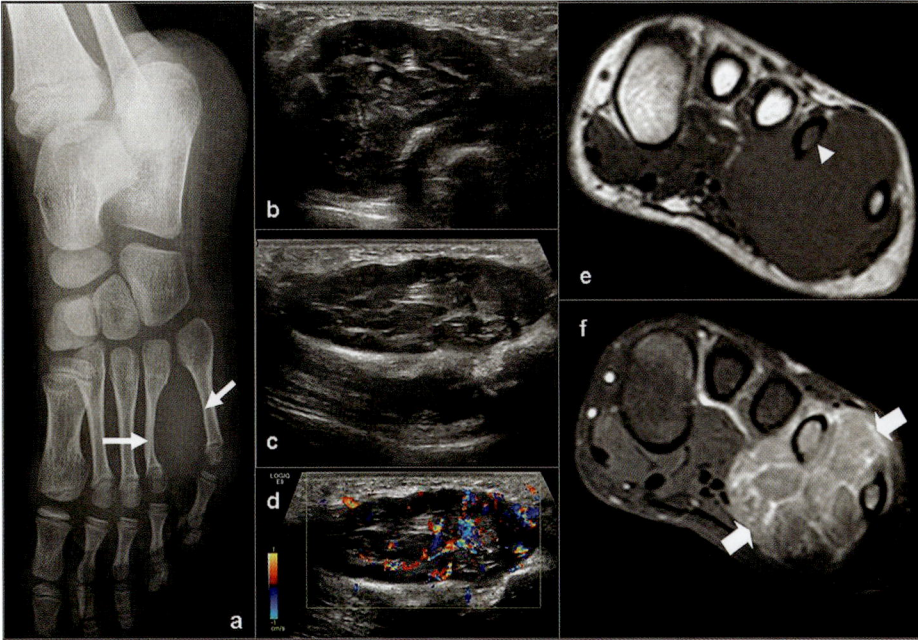

FIG. 2.6 Alveolar rhabdomyosarcoma of the left foot in a 6-year-old boy. Plain film (a) demonstrates a focal hyperdensity of soft tissues with a mass effect on the adjacent metatarsal bones (arrows). Ultrasound (b,c) displays a heterogeneous mass with heterogeneous vascularization on color-Doppler (d). MR images of an (e) axial T1-WI and (f) axial enhanced FS T1-WI demonstrate a well-defined mass with heterogeneous enhancement (arrow), invading the fourth metatarsal bone (arrowhead). Imaging suggests a locally aggressive tumor, but histology is mandatory for characterization. FNA performed before CNB will provide additional material for cytogenetics and molecular biology analyses.

imaging in the prediction of malignancy [49]. The most discriminating criteria on dynamic MRI suggestive of malignancy are an early enhancement (within 6 seconds after arterial enhancement) peripheral or inhomogeneous enhancement, and the shape of the dynamic enhancement curve (rapid initial enhancement followed by a plateau or a washout phase) [49]. Visualization of territories with early, intense contrast enhancement (Fig 2.7) also can be useful to guide the biopsy procedure [17,48].

2.5 TUMOR BIOPSY

2.5.1 Surgical and Core Needle Biopsies.

In the absence of definite signs of benign lesion, a biopsy always should be performed. Consultation with the radiologist, the surgeon, and the pathologist allows for defining the biopsy tract using compartmental anatomy definitions [50,51], the biopsy site- (most suspicious portion) (Fig 2.8) [17] and the appropriate processing of biopsy specimens (tissue preservation for genetic studies). A surgical excisional biopsy or a percutaneous procedure (core needle biopsy) is decided

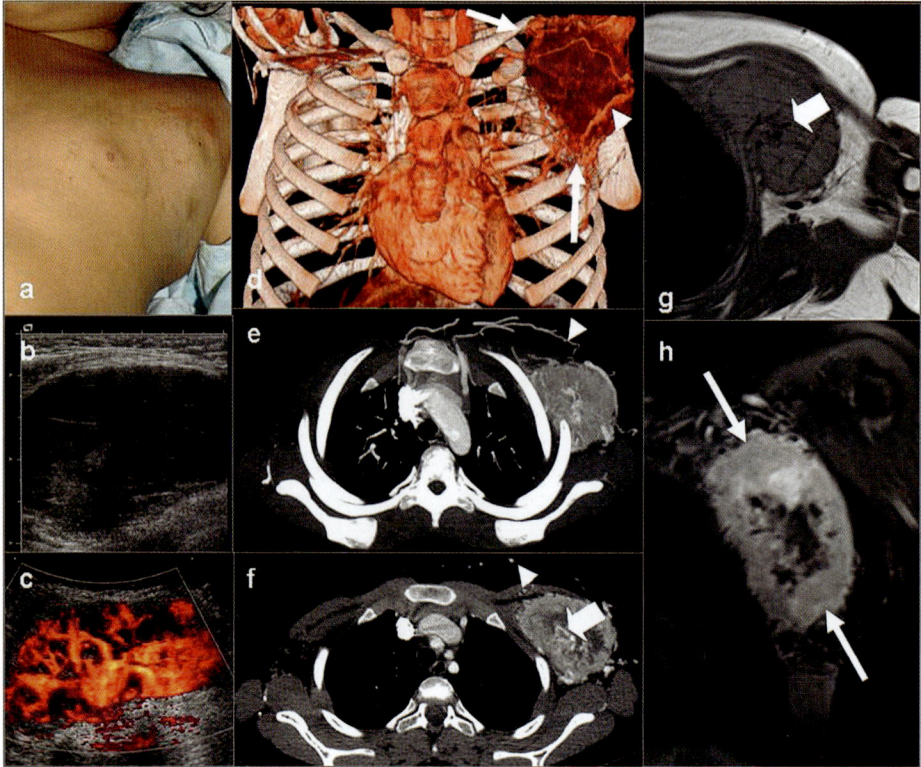

FIG. 2.7 Alveolar soft part sarcoma of the chest wall. Physical examination (a) demonstrates a subcutaneous mass and multiple superficial dilated veins. Ultrasound (b) demonstrates a well-delineated tissular heterogeneous mass containing numerous high-flow vessels on color-Doppler (c). enhanced CT scans of a (d) 3D-volume rendering, (e) axial MIP reconstruction, and (f) axial view demonstrate a highly vascularized tumor (long arrows) with central arteries (short arrows) and multiple peripheral drainage veins (arrowheads) located behind the pectoralis muscles and infiltrating the axillary region. MR images of an (g) axial T1-WI, and a (h) coronal enhanced FS T1-WI demonstrate a well-defined mass with central arteries (short arrow) and a predominantly peripheral enhancement (long arrows). The imaging pattern is suggestive but nonspecific. CNB and FNA are required for definite diagnosis.

according to the size and location of the mass. Although large lesions of the limbs can undergo biopsy easily without image guidance, deep-seated musculoskeletal lesions are difficult to target and benefit from CT or ultrasound (US) guidance. Imaging-guided percutaneous core needle biopsies are performed by trained radiologists, under local or general anesthesia, using CT or US guidance [52–55] (Table 2.2). The procedure ideally should be performed by both the radiologist and the pathologist, the latter being the most qualified to evaluate the specimen quality and to separate the tissue for morphological and biological studies. If the specimen cannot be frozen immediately, then it must not be fixed directly, but should be placed temporarily in a culture medium such as RPMI.

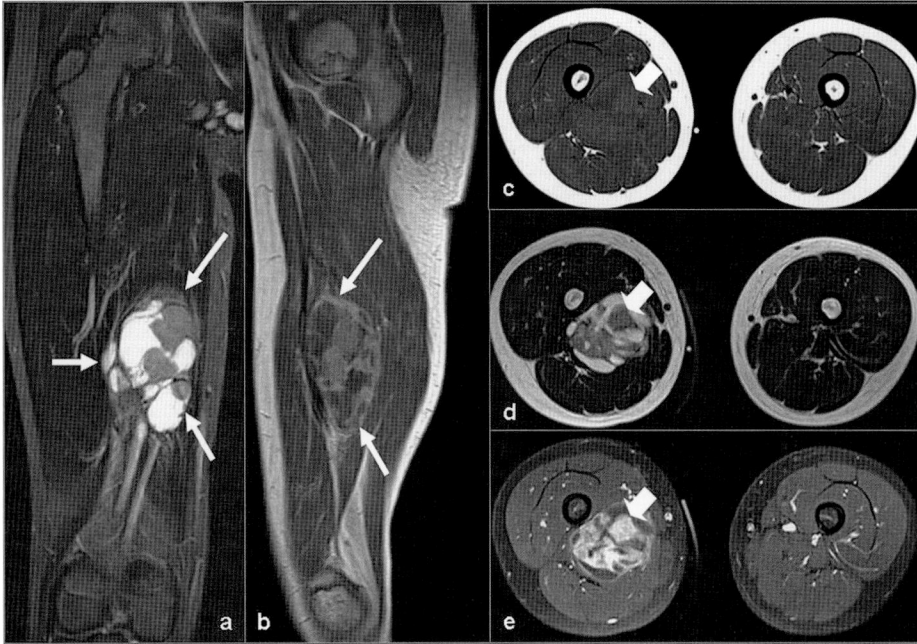

FIG. 2.8 Synovial sarcoma of the right thigh. MR images of a (a) coronal FS T2-WI, (b) sagittal enhanced T1-WI, (c) axial T1-WI, (d) axial T2-WI, and (e) axial enhanced FS T1-WI demonstrate a lobulated mass located in the adductor longus (long arrows). The tumor is of mixed signal intensity with fluid-filled areas and tissular areas of intermediate signal intensities and heterogeneous enhancement (short arrows). CNB must be targeted on tissular areas.

2.5.2 Fine Needle Aspiration

Fine needle aspiration (FNA) usually does not replace biopsy but constitutes an excellent first-line and reliable diagnostic procedure in our experience, provided that it is performed and examined by trained pathologists. It is an inexpensive technique, without almost morbidity [56], and it can be performed under local anesthesia. Using fine needles (23 gauge, 0.6 mm of outer diameter), with ultrasound guidance if necessary, it provides highly contributive cell aspirates [57,58]. In the diagnostic strategy, FNA may be used directly after initial imaging when the decision regarding performing or not a biopsy is debatable (e.g., for clinically and radiologically presumed benign [Figs 2.9 and 2.10] or pseudotumoral lesions, for a highly vascularized lesion at risk for a biopsy, or for suspected relapses). FNA material is excellent for ancillary techniques (this material is tumor-cell rich and stroma-cell poor) and allows for karyotyping and molecular analyses. Cells should be stored in ethylene diaminetetra acetic acid (EDTA).

TABLE 2.2   Diagnostic strategy of soft tissue tumors (adapted from [7])

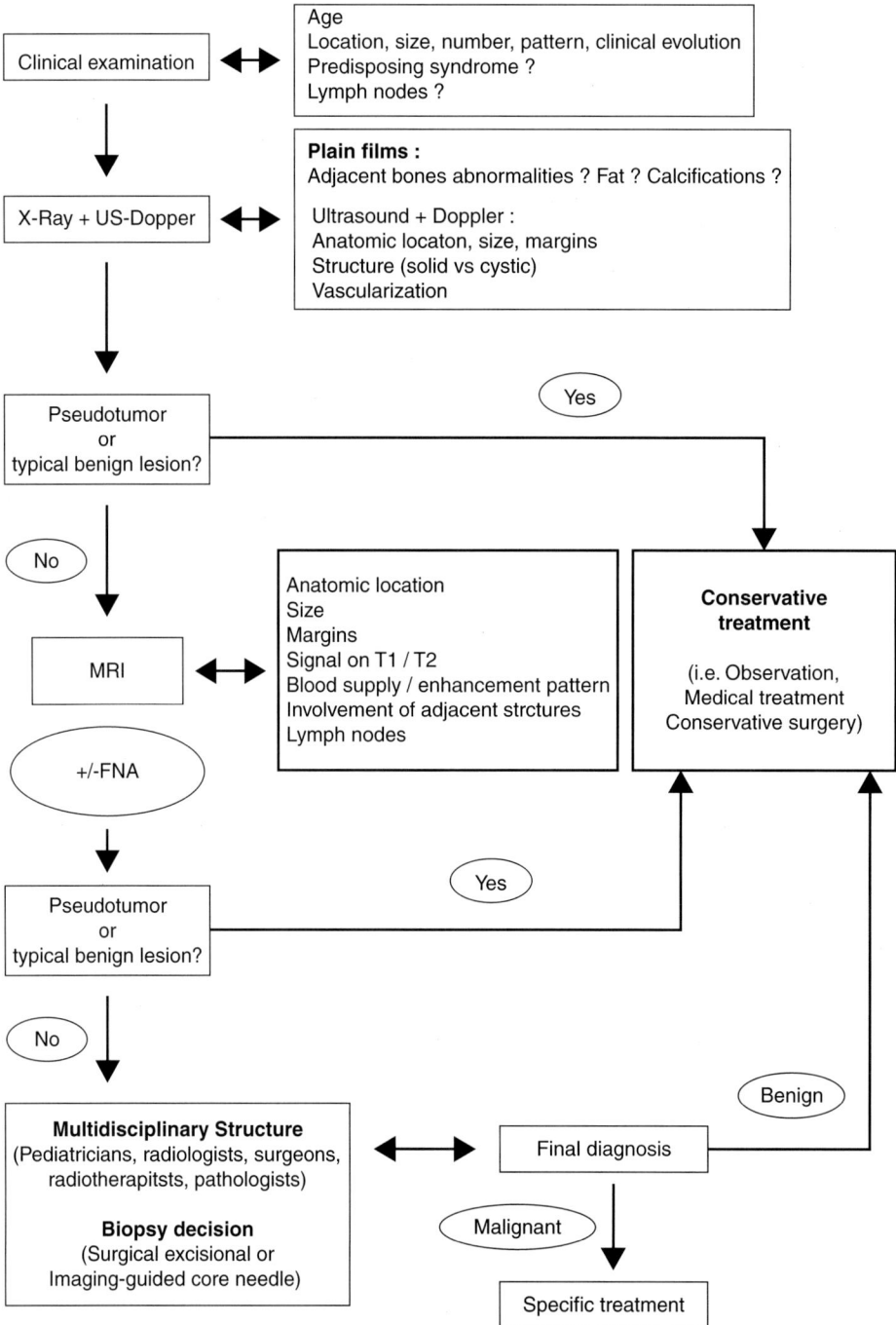

```
┌──────────────────────┐        ┌──────────────────────────────────────────────┐
│ Clinical examination │ ◀──▶   │ Age                                            │
└──────────────────────┘        │ Location, size, number, pattern, clinical evolution │
           │                    │ Predisposing syndrome ?                        │
           ▼                    │ Lymph nodes ?                                  │
                                └──────────────────────────────────────────────┘

                                ┌──────────────────────────────────────────────┐
                                │ **Plain films :**                              │
┌──────────────────────┐        │ Adjacent bones abnormalities ? Fat ? Calcifications ? │
│ X-Ray + US-Dopper    │ ◀──▶   │                                                │
└──────────────────────┘        │ Ultrasound + Doppler :                         │
           │                    │ Anatomic locaton, size, margins                │
           ▼                    │ Structure (solid vs cystic)                    │
                                │ Vascularization                                │
                                └──────────────────────────────────────────────┘
```

Pseudotumor or typical benign lesion?

(Yes)

No

```
┌──────────┐        ┌────────────────────────────────────┐    ┌──────────────────────┐
│   MRI    │ ◀──▶   │ Anatomic location                  │    │ **Conservative**     │
└──────────┘        │ Size                               │    │ **treatment**        │
                    │ Margins                            │    │                      │
( +/-FNA )          │ Signal on T1 / T2                  │    │ (i.e. Observation,   │
                    │ Blood supply / enhancement pattern │    │ Medical treatment    │
                    │ Involvement of adjacent strctures  │    │ Conservative surgery)│
                    │ Lymph nodes                        │    └──────────────────────┘
                    └────────────────────────────────────┘
```

Pseudotumor or typical benign lesion?

(Yes)

No

(Benign)

```
┌────────────────────────────────────┐        ┌──────────────────┐
│ **Multidisciplinary Structure**    │ ◀──▶   │ Final diagnosis  │
│ (Pediatricians, radiologists, surgeons, │    └──────────────────┘
│ radiotherapitsts, pathologists)    │
│                                    │        ( Malignant )
│ **Biopsy decision**                │
│ (Surgical excisional or            │        ┌──────────────────┐
│ Imaging-guided core needle)        │        │ Specific treatment │
└────────────────────────────────────┘        └──────────────────┘
```

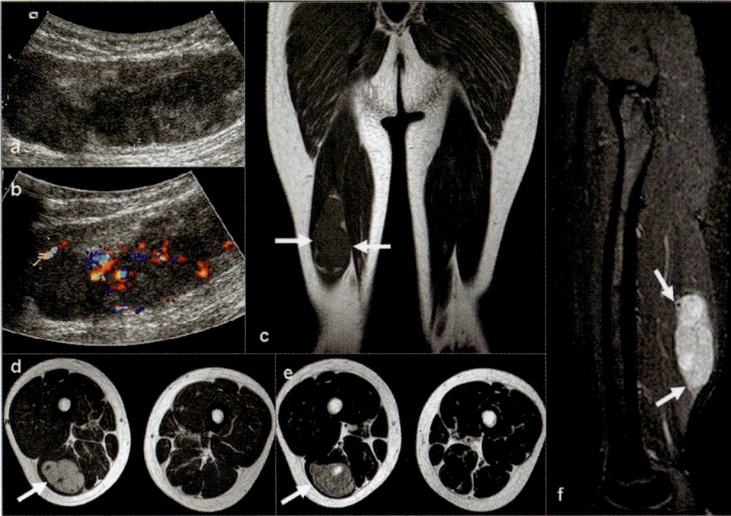

FIG. 2.9 Shwannoma of the right thigh (biceps femoris nerve). Ultrasound (a) shows a fusiform lobular-shaped tissular mass with vascularization on color-Doppler (b). MR images of a (c) coronal T1-WI, (d) axial enhanced T1-WI, (e) axial T2-WI, and (f) sagittal proton density-WI demonstrate a well-delineated fusiform mass located within the biceps femoris (long arrows). Signal intensities and enhancement pattern are nonspecific. The anatomic location and shape suggest a peripheral nerve origin. Histological analysis is mandatory.

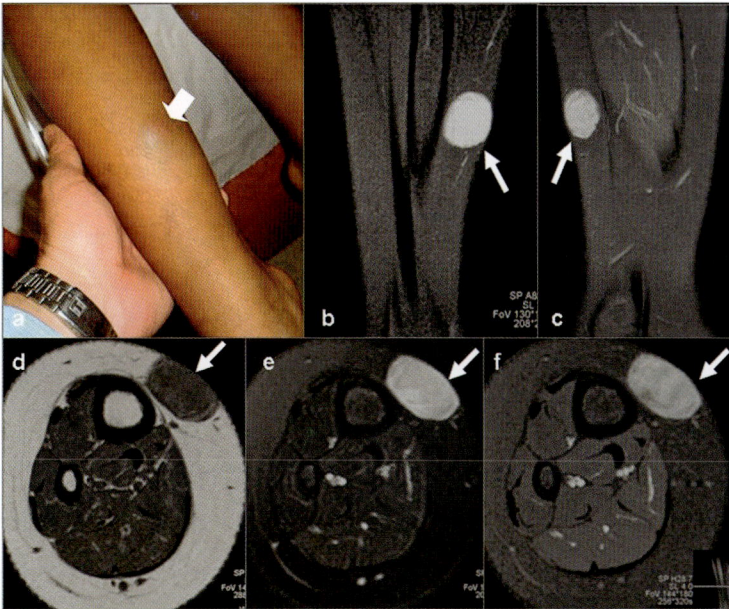

FIG. 2.10 Dermatofibrosarcoma of the right leg. Physical examination (a) demonstrates a subcutaneous firm mass with cutaneous involvement. MR images of a (b) coronal FS T2-WI, (c) sagittal FS PD-WI, (d) axial T1-WI, (e) axial FS T2-WI, and (f) axial enhanced FS T1-WI demonstrate a well-defined mass located within the subcutaneous fat (arrows). The lesion does not show any aggressive pattern; however, the signal intensities and enhancement pattern are nonspecific. Histological analysis is mandatory.

REFERENCES

1. Beaman FD, Kransdorf MJ, Andrews TR, Murphey MD, Arcara LK, Keeling JH. Superficial soft-tissue masses: analysis, diagnosis, and differential considerations. Radiographics 2000, 27: 509−523.

2. Kaste SC, Hill A, Conley L, Shidler TJ, Rao BN, Neel MM. Magnetic resonance imaging after incomplete resection of soft tissue sarcoma. Clin Orthop 2002, 204−211.

3. Davies AM, Mehr A, Parsonage S, Evans N, Grimer RJ, Pynsent PB. MR imaging in the assessment of residual tumour following inadequate primary excision of soft tissue sarcomas. Eur Radiol 2004, 14: 506−513.

4. Kransdorf MJ, Murphey MD. Radiologic evaluation of soft-tissue masses: a current perspective. AJR Am J Roentgenol 2000, 175: 575−587.

5. Laor T. MR imaging of soft tissue tumors and tumor-like lesions. Pediatr Radiol 2004, 34: 24−37.

6. De Schepper AM, De Beuckeleer L, Vandevenne J, Somville J. Magnetic resonance imaging of soft tissue tumors. Eur Radiol 2000, 10: 213−223.

7. Brisse H, Orbach D, Klijanienko J, Freneaux P, Neuenschwander S. Imaging and diagnostic strategy of soft tissue tumors in children. Eur Radiol 2006, 16: 1147−1164.

8. Kransdorf MJ. Benign soft-tissue tumors in a large referral population: distribution of specific diagnoses by age, sex, and location. AJR Am J Roentgenol 1995, 164: 395−402.

9. Kransdorf MJ. Malignant soft-tissue tumors in a large referral population: distribution of diagnoses by age, sex, and location. AJR Am J Roentgenol 1995, 164: 129−134.

10. De Schepper A, De Beuckeleer L, Vandevenne J. Soft tissue tumors in pediatric patients. In: De Schepper A, editior. Imaging of soft tissue tumors. Heidelberg, Springer-Verlag; Germany: 2001, pp. 433−452.

11. Weiss SW, Goldblum JR. Enzinger and Weiss's soft tissue tumors. 5th edition. St. Louis, MO: Mosby; 2008.

12. Gielen JL, De Schepper AM, Vanhoenacker F, Parizel PM, Wang XL, Sciot R, Weyler J. Accuracy of MRI in characterization of soft tissue tumors and tumor-like lesions. A prospective study in 548 patients. Eur Radiol 2004, 14: 2320−2330.

13. Levy AD, Patel N, Dow N, Abbott RM, Miettinen M, Sobin LH. From the archives of the AFIP: abdominal neoplasms in patients with neurofibromatosis type 1: radiologic-pathologic correlation. Radiographics 2005, 25: 455−480.

14. Ferrari A, Bisogno G, Macaluso A, et al. Soft-tissue sarcomas in children and adolescents with neurofibromatosis type 1. Cancer 2007, 109: 1406−1412.

15. Johnson CJ, Pynsent PB, Grimer RJ. Clinical features of soft tissue sarcomas. Ann R Coll Surg Engl 2001, 83: 203−205.

16. Siegel MJ. Magnetic resonance imaging of musculoskeletal soft tissue masses. Radiol Clin North Am 2001, 39: 701−720.

17. Shapeero LG, Vanel D, Verstraete KL, Bloem JL. Fast magnetic resonance imaging with contrast for soft tissue sarcoma viability. Clin Orthop 2002, 212−227.

18. van Rijswijk CS, Kunz P, Hogendoorn PC, Taminiau AH, Doornbos J, Bloem JL. Diffusion-weighted MRI in the characterization of soft-tissue tumors. J Magn Reson Imaging 2002, 15: 302−307.

19. Baur A, Huber A, Arbogast S, Durr HR, Zysk S, Wendtner C, Deimling M, Reiser M. Diffusion-weighted imaging of tumor recurrencies and posttherapeutical soft-tissue changes in humans. Eur Radiol 2001, 11: 828−833.

20. Einarsdottir H, Karlsson M, Wejde J, Bauer HC. Diffusion-weighted MRI of soft tissue tumours. Eur Radiol 2004, 14: 959−963.

21. MacKenzie JD, Gonzalez L, Hernandez A, Ruppert K, Jaramillo D. Diffusion-weighted and diffusion tensor imaging for pediatric musculoskeletal disorders. Pediatr Radiol 2007, 37: 781–788.

22. Kettelhack C, Wickede M, Vogl T, Schneider U, Hohenberger P. 31 Phosphorus-magnetic resonance spectroscopy to assess histologic tumor response noninvasively after isolated limb perfusion for soft tissue tumors. Cancer 2002, 94: 1557–1564.

23. Oya N, Aoki J, Shinozaki T, Watanabe H, Takagishi K, Endo K. Preliminary study of proton magnetic resonance spectroscopy in bone and soft tissue tumors: an unassigned signal at 2.0-2.1 ppm may be a possible indicator of malignant neuroectodermal tumor. Radiat Med 2000, 18: 193–198.

24. Wang CK, Li CW, Hsieh TJ, Chien SH, Liu GC, Tsai KB. Characterization of bone and soft-tissue tumors with in vivo 1H MR spectroscopy: initial results. Radiology 2004, 232: 599–605.

25. Berquist TH, Dalinka MK, Alazraki N, et al. Soft tissue masses. American College of Radiology. ACR Appropriateness Criteria. Radiology 2000, 215 (Suppl): 255–259.

26. Kransdorf MJ, Meis JM, Jelinek JS. Myositis ossificans: MR appearance with radiologic-pathologic correlation. AJR Am J Roentgenol 1991, 157: 1243–1248.

27. Franzius C, Schulte M, Hillmann A, Winkelmann W, Jurgens H, Bockisch A, Schober O. Clinical value of positron emission tomography (PET) in the diagnosis of bone and soft tissue tumors. 3rd Interdisciplinary Consensus Conference "PET in Oncology": results of the Bone and Soft Tissue Study Group. Chirurg 2001, 72: 1071–1077.

28. Feldman F, van Heertum R, Manos C. 18FDG PET scanning of benign and malignant musculoskeletal lesions. Skeletal Radiol 2003, 32: 201–208.

29. Tateishi U, Yamaguchi U, Seki K, Terauchi T, Arai Y, Kim EE. Bone and soft-tissue sarcoma: preoperative staging with fluorine 18 Fluorodeoxyglucose PET/CT and conventional imaging. Radiology 2007, 245: 839–847.

30. Lucas JD, O'Doherty MJ, Wong JC, Bingham JB, McKee PH, Fletcher CD, Smith MA. Evaluation of fluorodeoxyglucose positron emission tomography in the management of soft-tissue sarcomas. J Bone Joint Surg Br 1998, 80: 441–447.

31. Berquist T, Ehman R, King B, Hodgman C, Ilstrup D. Value of MR imaging in differentiating benign from malignant soft-tissue masses: study of 95 lesions. Am J Roentgenol 1990, 155: 1251–1255.

32. Narvaez JA, Narvaez J, Aguilera C, De Lama E, Portabella F. MR imaging of synovial tumors and tumor-like lesions. Eur Radiol 2001, 11: 2549–2560.

33. Sung MS, Kang HS, Suh JS, Lee JH, Park JM, Kim JY, Lee HG. Myxoid liposarcoma: appearance at MR imaging with histologic correlation. Radiographics 2000, 20: 1007–1019.

34. Reiseter T, Nordshus T, Borthne A, Roald B, Naess P, Schistad O. Lipoblastoma: MRI appearances of a rare paediatric soft tissue tumour. Pediatr Radiol 1999, 29: 542–545.

35. Ha TV, Kleinman PK, Fraire A, Spevak MR, Nimkin K, Cohen IT, Hirsh M, Walton R. MR imaging of benign fatty tumors in children: report of four cases and review of the literature. Skeletal Radiol 1994, 23: 361–367.

36. Teo EL, Strouse PJ, Hernandez RJ. MR imaging differentiation of soft-tissue hemangiomas from malignant soft-tissue masses. AJR Am J Roentgenol 2000, 174: 1623–1628.

37. Kingston CA, Owens CM, Jeanes A, Malone M. Imaging of desmoid fibromatosis in pediatric patients. AJR Am J Roentgenol 2002, 178: 191–199.

38. Robbin MR, Murphey MD, Temple HT, Kransdorf MJ, Choi JJ. Imaging of musculoskeletal fibromatosis. Radiographics 2001, 21: 585–600.

39. Bhargava R, Parham DM, Lasater OE, Chari RS, Chen G, Fletcher BD. MR imaging differentiation of benign and malignant peripheral nerve sheath tumors: use of the target sign. Pediatr Radiol 1997, 27: 124–129.

40. Dubois J, Garel L. Imaging and therapeutic approach of hemangiomas and vascular malformations in the pediatric age group. Pediatr Radiol 1999, 29: 879–893.

41. Bodner G, Schocke MF, Rachbauer F, Seppi K, Peer S, Fierlinger A, Sununu T, Jaschke WR. Differentiation of malignant and benign musculoskeletal tumors: combined color and power Doppler US and spectral wave analysis. Radiology 2002, 223: 410–416.

42. Belli P, Costantini M, Mirk P, Maresca G, Priolo F, Marano P. Role of color Doppler sonography in the assessment of musculoskeletal soft tissue masses. J Ultrasound Med 2000, 19: 823–830.

43. Crim JR, Seeger LL, Yao L, Chandnani V, Eckardt JJ. Diagnosis of soft-tissue masses with MR imaging: can benign masses be differentiated from malignant ones? Radiology 1992, 185: 581–586.

44. Moulton JS, Blebea JS, Dunco DM, Braley SE, Bisset GS, 3rd, Emery KH. MR imaging of soft-tissue masses: diagnostic efficacy and value of distinguishing between benign and malignant lesions. AJR Am J Roentgenol 1995, 164: 1191–1199.

45. Tung GA, Davis LM. The role of magnetic resonance imaging in the evaluation of the soft tissue mass. Crit Rev Diagn Imaging 1993, 34: 239–308.

46. De Schepper AM, Ramon FA, Degryse HR. Statistical analysis of MRI parameters predicting malignancy in 141 soft tissue masses. Rofo 1992, 156: 587–591.

47. Ma LD, Frassica FJ, McCarthy EF, Bluemke DA, Zerhouni EA. Benign and malignant musculoskeletal masses: MR imaging differentiation with rim-to-center differential enhancement ratios. Radiology 1997, 202: 739–744.

48. Verstraete KL, Lang P. Bone and soft tissue tumors: the role of contrast agents for MR imaging. Eur J Radiol 2000, 34: 229–246.

49. van Rijswijk CSP, Geirnaerdt MJA, Hogendoorn PCW, et al. Soft-tissue tumors: value of static and dynamic gadopentetate dimeglumine-enhanced MR Imaging in prediction of malignancy. Radiology 2004, 233: 493–502.

50. Anderson MW, Temple HT, Dussault RG, Kaplan PA. Compartmental anatomy: relevance to staging and biopsy of musculoskeletal tumors. AJR Am J Roentgenol 1999, 173: 1663–1671.

51. Toomayan GA, Robertson F, Major NM. Lower extremity compartmental anatomy: clinical relevance to radiologists. Skeletal Radiol 2005, 34: 307–313.

52. Puri A, Shingade VU, Agarwal MG, et al. CT-guided percutaneous core needle biopsy in deep seated musculoskeletal lesions: a prospective study of 128 cases. Skeletal Radiol 2006, 35: 138–143.

53. Liu JC, Chiou HJ, Chen WM, et al. Sonographically guided core needle biopsy of soft tissue neoplasms. J Clin Ultrasound 2004, 32: 294–298.

54. Konermann W, Wuisman P, Ellermann A, Gruber G. Ultrasonographically guided needle biopsy of benign and malignant soft tissue and bone tumors. J Ultrasound Med 2000, 19: 465–471.

55. Shin HJ, Amaral JG, Armstrong D, et al. Image-guided percutaneous biopsy of musculoskeletal lesions in children. Pediatr Radiol 2007, 37: 362–369.

56. Wakely PE Jr, Kardos TF, Frable Wj. Application of fine needle aspiration biopsy to pediatrics. Hum Pathol 1988, 19: 1383–1386.

57. Costa MJ, Campman SC, Davis RL, Howell LP. Fine-needle aspiration cytology of sarcoma: retrospective review of diagnostic utility and specificity. Diagn Cytopathol 1996, 15: 23–32.

58. Willen H, Akerman M, Carlen B. Fine needle aspiration (FNA) in the diagnosis of soft tissue tumours: a review of 22 years experience. Cytopathology 1995, 6: 236–247.

Chapter *3*

Sampling Procedure, Fine Needle Aspiration (FNA), and Core Needle Biopsy (CNB)

Henryk A. Domanski

3.1 ADVANTAGES AND LIMITATIONS OF FNA AND CNB IN SOFT TISSUE LESIONS

Although clinical and radiographic data provide important information in the evaluation of soft tissue lesions/neoplasms, morphologic tissue examination is considered to be a necessary part of the diagnostic evaluation. The standard procedure for obtaining tumor tissue for morphologic evaluation has been an incisional (open) biopsy. An open biopsy most often provides sufficient tissue for a routine histopathological evaluation as well as for ancillary studies such as immunohistochemistry, electron microscopy, cytogenetics, molecular genetics, and DNA-ploidy analysis. There are, however, some disadvantages with open biopsy. There are risks of intraoperative and postoperative complications of which most important are the threat of tumor cells spreading into adjacent compartments and wound infection. An occasional delay in the initiation of therapy during the time that the surgical wound heals is another disadvantage of incisional biopsy, especially in deep-seated soft tissue tumors. In addition, an incisional biopsy can break natural barriers for tumor growth such as muscle fascia, myosepta, periostium, epineurium, and tissue around blood vessels. This adversely can affect subsequent surgical procedures and increase the risk of sequelae.

Soft Tissue Tumors: A Multidisciplinary, Decisional Diagnostic Approach
Edited by Jerzy Klijanienko and Réal Lagacé
Copyright © 2011 John Wiley & Sons, Inc.

Increasing the use of minimally invasive diagnostic procedures in many centers has resulted in better acceptance of fine needle aspiration (FNA) with needles having an outer diameter of 0.4–0.8 mm (27–22 gauge) and core needle biopsy (CNB) with needles having an outer diameter of 1.2–1.4 mm (18–14 gauge). In guidelines published by the Association of Directors of Anatomic and Surgical Pathology, FNA was not recommended as the first-line examination technique in the evaluation of soft tissue tumors [1]. This technique generally has been accepted in the work-up of metastatic and recurrent neoplasms. However, in the past, this question has been revisited, and FNA currently is accepted in many centers as a valuable tool in the initial diagnostic investigation, frequently providing significant diagnostic information that allows treatment initiation or guides the continued diagnostic workup [2–9]. CNB is a more widely accepted biopsy technique in the investigation of soft tissue lesions, including nonneopastic and neoplastic, primary, recurrent, and metastatic and has emerged as a substitute for open biopsy in many centers [10–13].

Compared with open biopsy, both FNA and CNB have some advantages, but they also have some limitations. Both techniques are outpatient procedures, well tolerated by patients and with negligible risk of serious complications. In addition, taking FNA and CNB specimens is done easily, and the technique is simple to learn. The morphological details of cells obtained by FNA, in technically satisfactory smears, is often superior to that observed in core needle and incisional biopsy specimens. When thin needles are used for aspiration, it is relatively easy to obtain multiple samples and samples from different parts of large tumors (by altering the direction of the needle), thereby demonstrating possible tumor heterogeneity and focal necrosis. In comparison, CNB occasionally can sample only a limited area of a large soft tissue tumor and may not provide this information and may result in incorrect tumor grading. Though rapid staining and preliminary reporting is applied more conveniently to aspiration smears, imprint preparations from CNB also can be evaluated quickly (Fig 3.1). It is thus possible to assess FNA and CNB specimen adequacy while the patient waits. If necessary, additional aspirations or biopsies can be performed to obtain material for ancillary studies. One major disadvantage of the FNA technique is a lack of recognizable tissue pattern, making it very difficult or impossible to make a specific histotype diagnosis in some tumors. Although tumor tissue architecture generally is evaluated easily in CNB samples (Figs 3.2 and 3.3), it also can be evaluated in cell blocks prepared from specimens obtained by FNA. In many cases, material from an FNA is sufficient to prepare a cell block in which sections can show microbiopsies with a preserved tissue architecture (Figs 3.4–3.7). This well-established technique can be an important diagnostic tool, but in cases in which a tumor has a collagenous matrix, aspiration often does not yield adequate material for the preparation of cell blocks. In these cases, CNB seems to be a more appropriate method to evaluate tissue architecture.

Thus, the accuracy of FNA in distinguishing benign from malignant soft tissue lesions and sarcoma from other malignancies has been shown to be comparable with that of surgical biopsies, whereas its accuracy in the grading of soft tissue sarcoma and in establishing a specific histological diagnosis has been inferior to surgical biopsies [9,14–18]. The experience at the Sarcoma Center in Lund University Hospital, Lund, Sweden, has shown that for most patients who are referred with a clinical suspicion of sarcoma but in whom it is later proved by FNA examination to be a benign lesion, only one visit to the center was necessary for a therapeutic

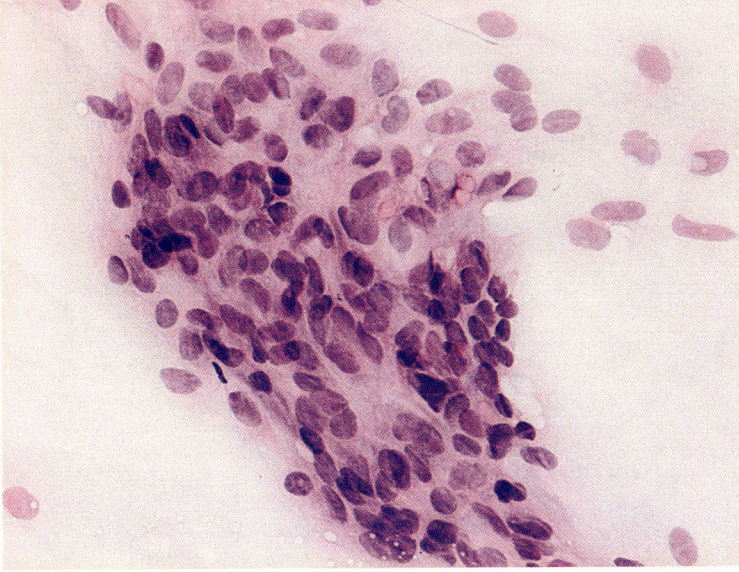

FIG 3.1 Medium power of imprint preparations from CNB of a synovial sarcoma.

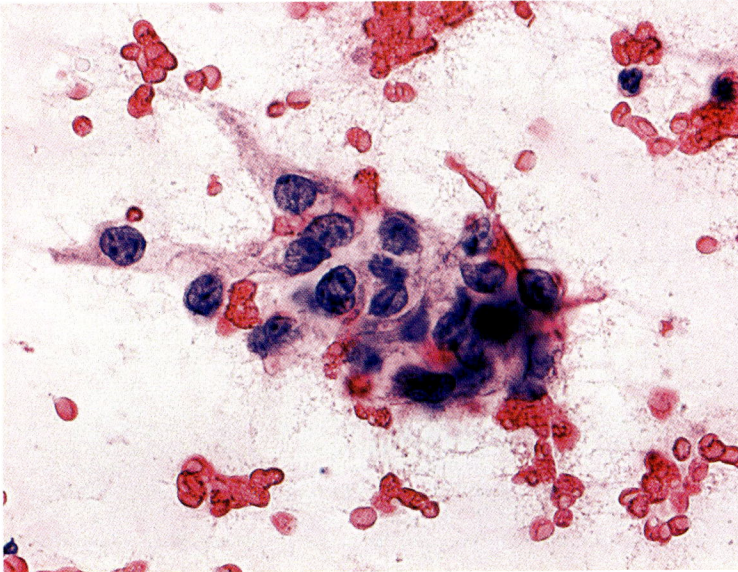

FIG 3.2 FNA smears in angiosarcoma.

decision to be made. In addition, the combined evaluation of clinical and radiological data and FNA has been sufficient for making a treatment decision in most patients with soft tissue sarcomas. Only in a minority of patients was open surgical biopsy necessary before definitive treatment [3,4].

Studies comparing FNA and CNB indicated that the diagnostic accuracy of these techniques is approximately the same or slightly higher for CNB alone. CNB is better

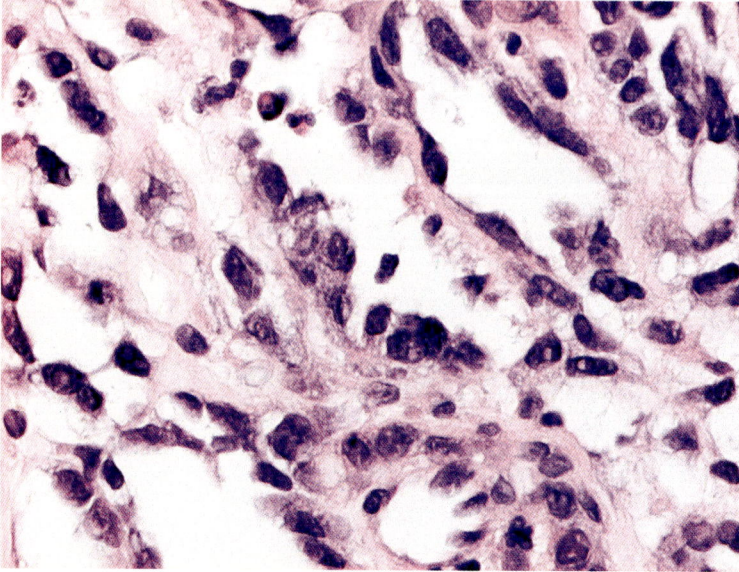

FIG 3.3 CNB in angiosarcoma corresponding to Fig 3.2. Well-preserved tumor tissue architecture.

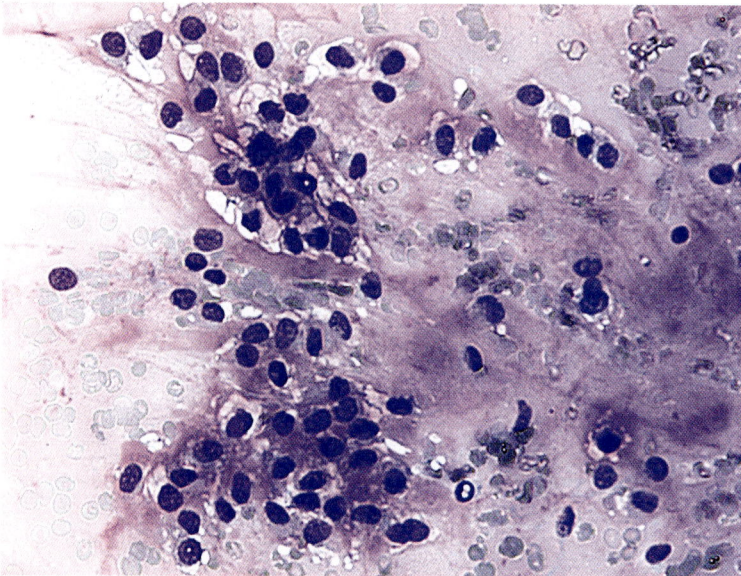

FIG 3.4 FNA smears in extraskeletal myxoid chondrosarcoma.

at ascertaining the histological subtype and grade of soft tissue neoplasms [19–21]. A brief comparison of the major advantages and disadvantages of different biopsy techniques is presented in Table 3.1.

In summary, the main advantages of both FNA and CNB in the primary work-up of soft tissue lesions are that these techniques are simple, quick, and cost effective. Both

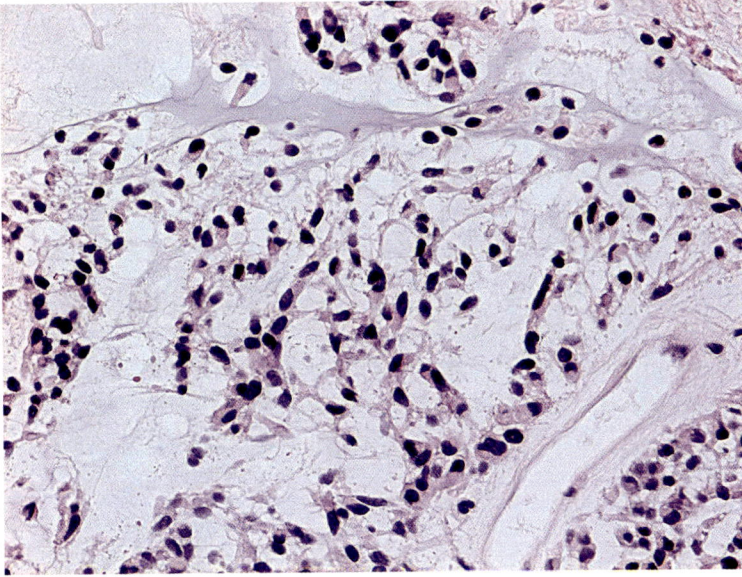

FIG 3.5 Cell block in extraskeletal myxoid chondrosarcoma corresponding to Fig 3.4. Note the preserved tumor tissue architecture in the cell block section.

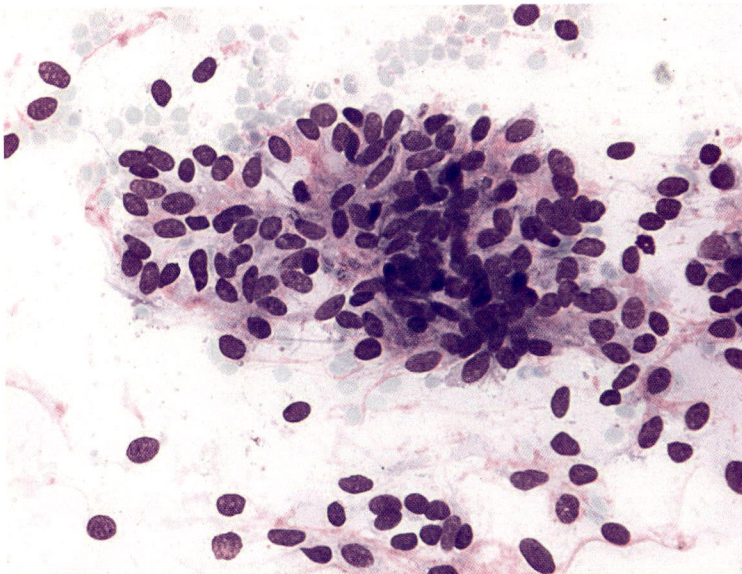

FIG 3.6 FNA smears in dermatofibrosarcoma protuberans.

entail minimal trauma to the tissue (in contrast to open biopsy), and both usually are performed in an outpatient setting. In our experience, the combined FNA and CNB diagnosis in conjunction with clinical and radiological data has a high diagnostic accuracy in the evaluation of soft tissue lesions and has been sufficient for making a treatment decision in most patients with suspicion of soft tissue sarcomas admitted to

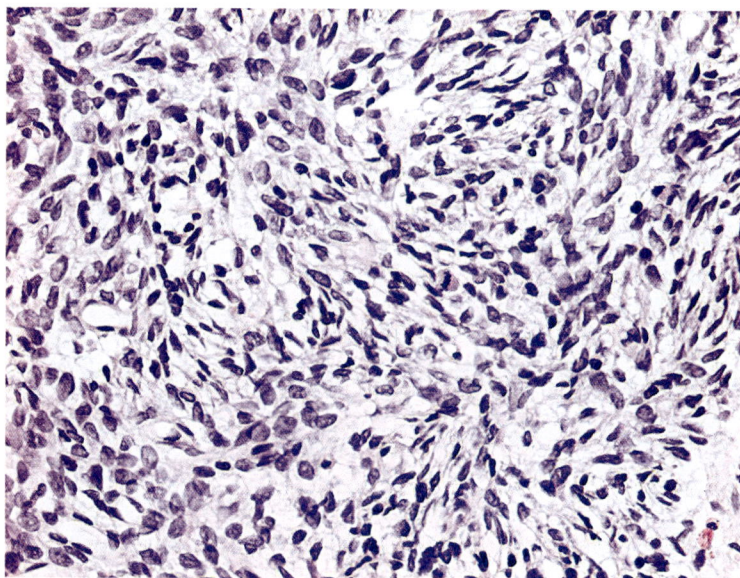

FIG 3.7 Cell block in dermatofibrosarcoma protuberans corresponding to Fig 3.6. Note the preserved tumor tissue storiform pattern in the section from cell block.

TABLE 3.1   Comparison of FNA with other biopsy methods

Characteristics	FNA	CNB	Open biopsy
Technical considerations	Easy procedure (to perform and to learn)	Easy procedure (to perform and to learn)	Complex procedure, most often requires general anaesthesia and operating room/operating staff
Interference with subsequent treatment; Surgical fields disturbed	No	No	Yes
Availability of examination of tissue architecture	Yes (cell block)	Yes	Yes
Speed of interpretation	Fast	Slow	Slow
Availability of ancillary techniques	Yes	Yes	Yes
Accuracy in differentiating benign versus malignant	High	High	High
Accuracy of histologic subtyping [9]	30–75%	75–90%	>95%
Risk of complications	Very low	Low	Higher than FNA and CNB
Cost	Low	Low	High

our center. As FNA and CNB complement each other in the examination of soft tissue lesions [19] the double (FNA/CNB) diagnostic approach permits a combination of cytomorphology and tumor tissue architecture and also yields tumor tissue adequate for various ancillary procedures more often than FNA or CNB alone.

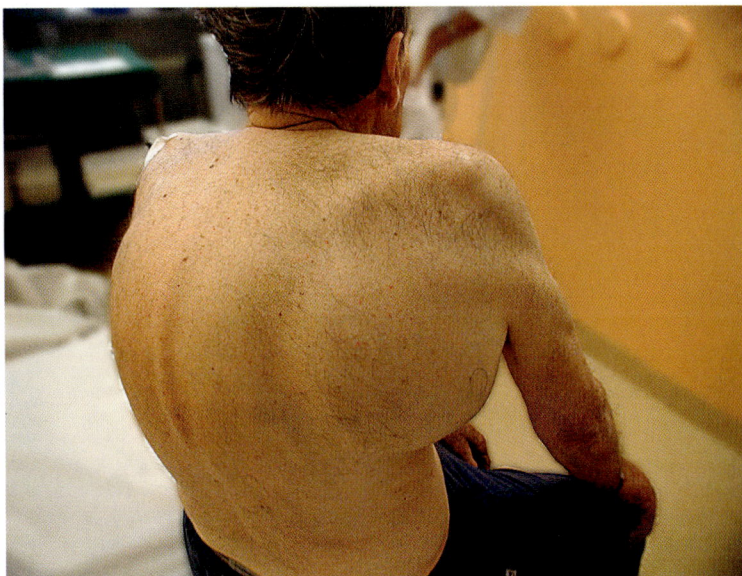

FIG 3.8 Liposarcoma. This tumor is easily accessible to FNA and CNB. The optimal point of biopsy was defined by the circle on the skin.

3.2 TECHNIQUES OF FNA AND CNB AS APPLIED TO SOFT TISSUE LESIONS

The techniques for performing FNA and CNB of soft tissue lesions are similar to those used for other types of lesions. Thorough palpation and estimation of size, site, and consistency of the tumor is essential. If the clinician does not indicate the insertion point/points specifically, then aspiration through the vertex, using the same point of insertion if several punctures are performed, is recommended when examining a suspected sarcoma.

FNA of soft tissue tumors is performed in the same way as for epithelial tumors (Figs 3.8 and 3.9). It usually is not necessary to use a local anaesthetic. A 10-ml syringe and needles of varying lengths may be recommended. The technique of aspirating without suction applied through the syringe, only using the capillary suction of the needle, is seldom successful in soft tissue lesions; this method is more suitable for the aspiration of lesions in such organs as the thyroid, lymph nodes, and skin and subcutis where the connective tissue component does not dominate the lesion. The syringe holder that allows aspiration with one hand may be necessary to obtain sufficient samples from soft tissue tumors. The length of the needle depends on the location of the lesion. For deep-seated intramuscular or intermuscular tumors, a needle with a stylet can be used to avoid unnecessary sampling of subcutaneous fat or other tissue surrounding the tumor. Needles used for the FNA of soft tissues are the same size as those used for aspiration in other organs. Needles larger than 23 or 22 gauge seldom are needed.

As mentioned previously, all passes with the needle preferably would go through the same site in the skin, but the direction of the needle should be changed with each pass to cover different parts of the tumor. The doctor performing the aspiration has to move the needle back and forth at least four or five (but sometimes many) times to

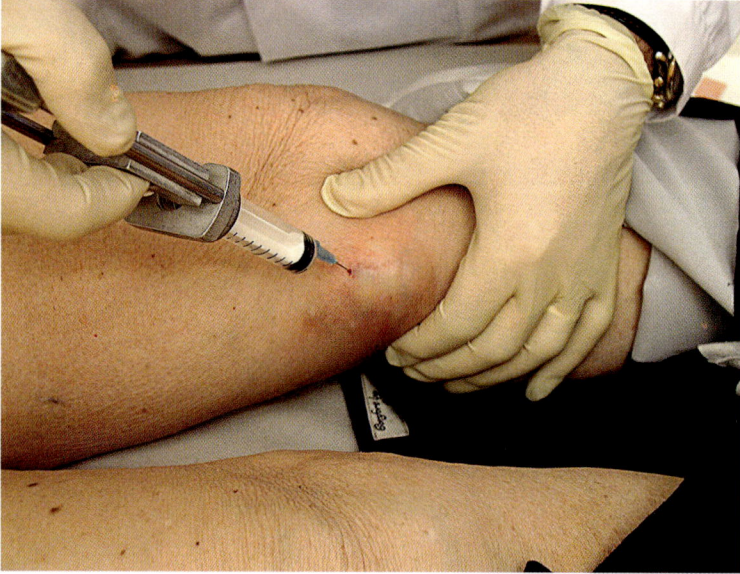

FIG 3.9 FNA aspiration of the knee tumor using the syringe holder.

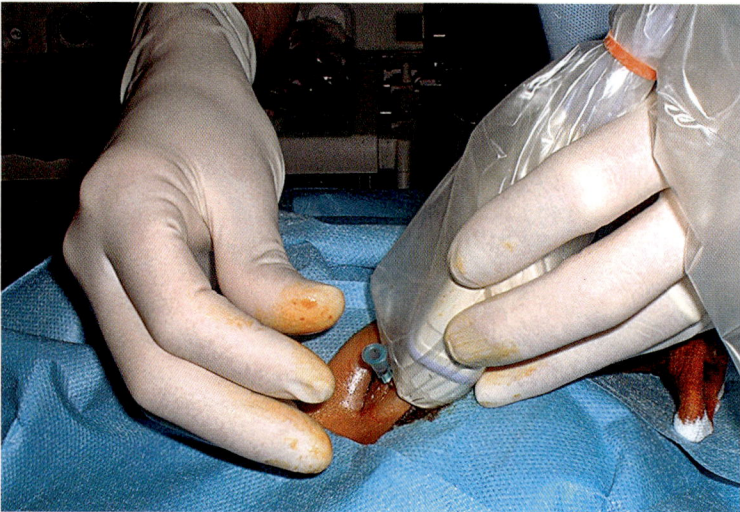

FIG 3.10 Ultrasound-guided FNA of the orbital tumor. In such cases, CNB may be contrindicated.

ensure that sufficient material is obtained for examination. In most cases, it is not necessary to puncture more than five times in this manner to obtain specimens adequate for both routine smears and ancillary studies.

If the mass is cystic, necrotic, or hemorrhagic, then representative diagnostic areas may be difficult to aspirate adequately. Small, deep-seated, inter- or intramuscular lesions may be occasionally difficult to reach with usual needles. Ultrasound guidance and computerized tomography (CT) may be of help in the aspiration (Fig 3.10) and in a CNB of small, deep-seated, as well as cystic and necrotic lesions

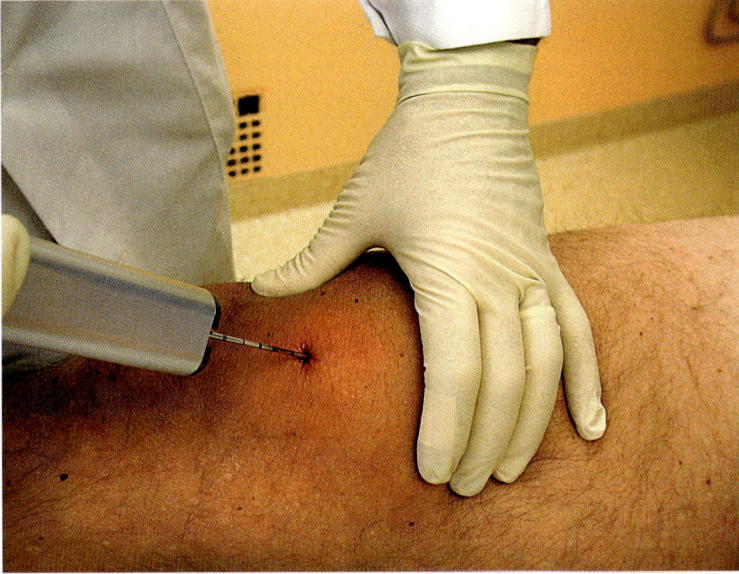

FIG 3.11 CNB of knee tumor. The same case as Figure 3.9.

[22–24]. The person performing the aspiration or CNB sampling, however, should be experienced enough to be able to evaluate whether the material obtained is likely to be representative for the lesions in question.

Both FNA and CNB require skin disinfection using 70% ethanol or iodine swabs. Local anesthesia is necessary in CNB (Fig 3.11) and can be achieved by injecting 1% lidocaine into the skin and subcutaneous/deeper tissue.

3.3 PROCESSING THE FNA AND CNB SAMPLES AND PREPARATION OF THE FNA SPECIMEN FOR ANCILLARY TECHNIQUES

There are many techniques for processing aspiration smears. The most basic point in the preparation of aspiration smears is to spread the specimen, consisting most often of a droplet of bloody fluid admixed with the cellular material, evenly over a glass slide using gentle pressure, usually with a cover slip or another glass slide. The smears may be air-dried and stained with Diff-Quick or May–Grünwald–Giemsa, or wet-fixed (usually in ethanol) and stained with Papanicolau or hematoxylin and eosin stains. The microscopic evaluation of soft tissue lesions should be based on the evaluation of both wet-fixed and air-dried smears. The wet-fixed material is superior for evaluation of nuclear details, whereas air-dried smears give better information about cytoplasmic details and the background matrix.

New techniques for the wet preparation of cytologic specimens such as liquid- and filtration-based preparations (Millipore, SurePath, and ThinPrep) are, in this author's experience, particularly suitable for the preparation of aspirates from soft tissue lesions for ancillary techniques such as immunocytochemistry, and fluorescence in-situ hybridization (FISH) (Fig 3.12). It must be noted that, occasionally,

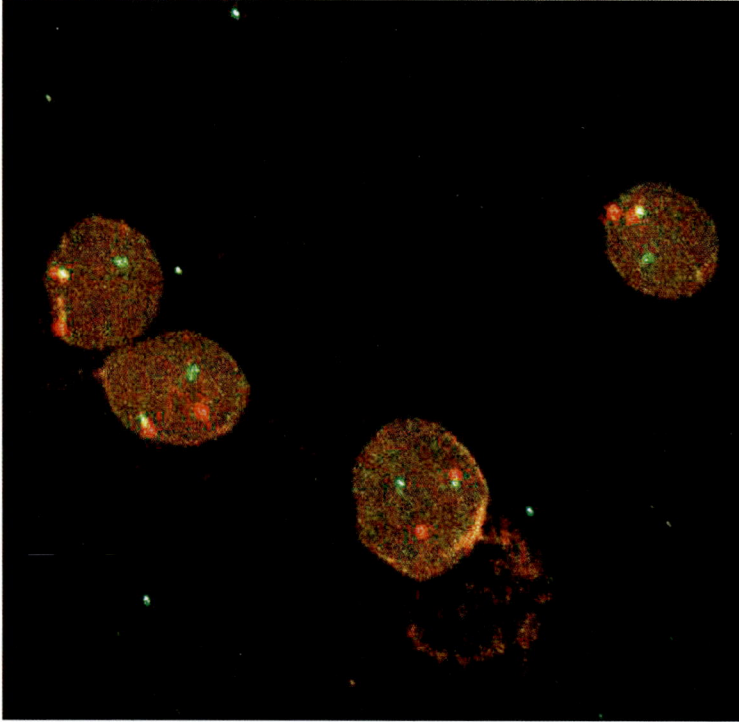

FIG 3.12 FISH performed on FNA smears for synovial sarcoma, Separate red and green signals are indicative of a rearrangement of one copy of the SYT gene region (breakapart probe).

important morphological details of specimens from soft tissue and other tumors, especially myxoid and collagen-rich tumors, may be obscured in liquid-based preparation [25] (Fig 3.13).

The tissue core obtained by CNB usually is fixed in 10% buffered formalin. Cores also may be used for cytogenetic/molecular genetics analysis, electron microscopy, and flow cytometry.

Today, immunocytochemistry is the most common procedure used to complement routine microscopic examination of aspirates. Immunolabeling of cytological material can be difficult to standardize and can vary depending on the method used to prepare cells [26–32]. In general, immunocytochemistry may be performed on any of several types of preparations such as direct smears, cytospin-preparations, cell blocks or liquid-based cytology. Each laboratory should control its technique carefully in this regard. In our experience, the results of immunocytochemical examinations of aspirates are very dependent on the quality of the material, most importantly the number of cells, the presence of necrosis, and the amount of background material. Immunolabeled direct smears can be difficult to evaluate because of the trauma inherent to the technique. Nuclei can be stripped of their cytoplasm, and the background material can contain the fragments and remnants of many different cells (Fig 3.14). Cytocentrifugation is probably the most commonly used technique to prepare cytological material for immunocytochemistry, and in experienced hands, it often has given sufficient results.

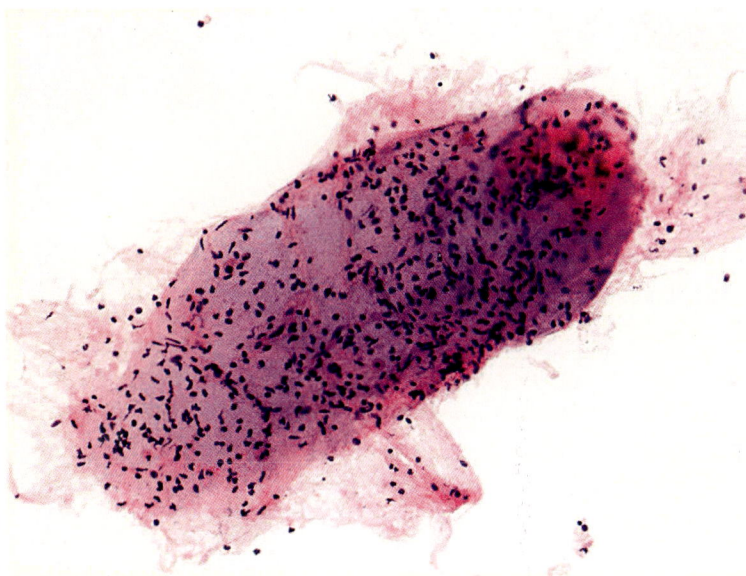

FIG 3.13 Liquid-based preparation of the FNA aspirate from a myxoid liposarcoma. Lipoblasts and characteristic branching capillaries are not evident.

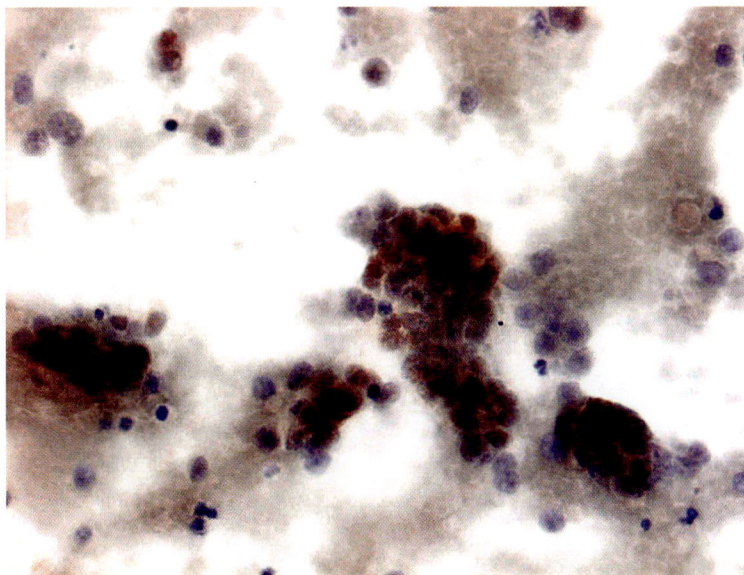

FIG 3.14 Results of the immunostaining of an FNA specimen from rhabdomyosarcoma with an antibody against MyoD1 performed on direct smears.

Our experience and that of many others indicate that cell block preparations from formalin-fixed and paraffin-embedded cells (Fig 3.15), allowing the preparation of histological sections with a quality similar to surgical biopsies (Fig 3.16), is probably the best method of preparation of an FNA specimen from soft tissue lesions for immunocytochemistry (Figs 3.15–3.17) [33]. Cell blocks, prepared from aspirated

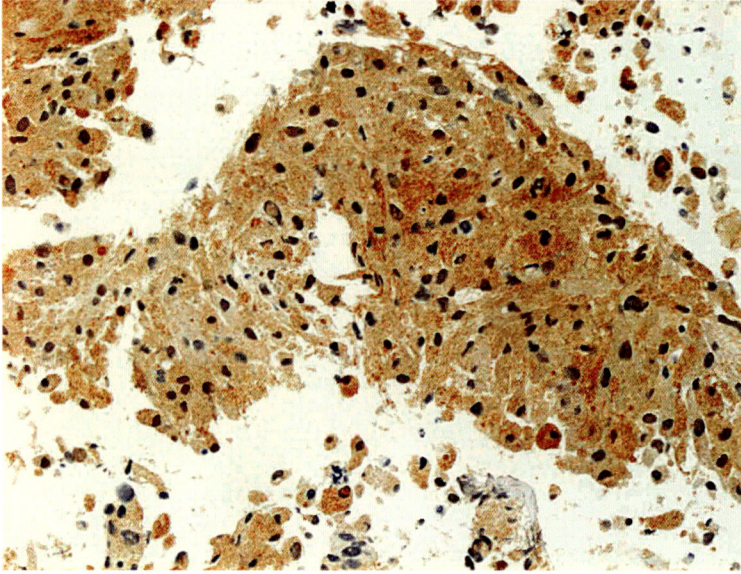

FIG 3.15 Immunocytochemistry on a cell block prepared from aspiration smears. Positive results of immunostains with an antibody against the S-100 protein in FNA from a granular cell tumor.

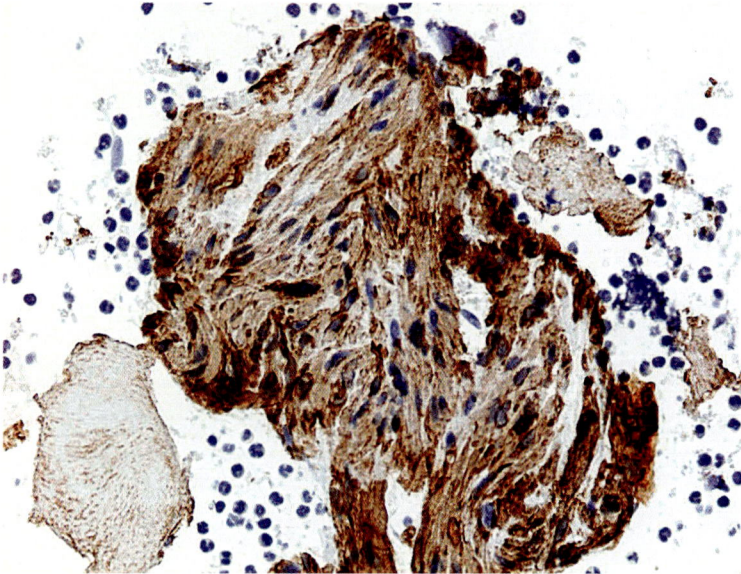

FIG 3.16 Immunocytochemistry on a cell block prepared from aspiration smears. Desmin positivity in leiomyosarcoma.

material, contain a material that looks like minibiopsies (Figs 3.5, 3.7, 3.18, 3.19). The processing of these slides for immunostaining follows the same procedures as for a surgical biopsy. Cell block preparations easily can be compared with subsequent operative specimens (Figs 3.20−3.23).

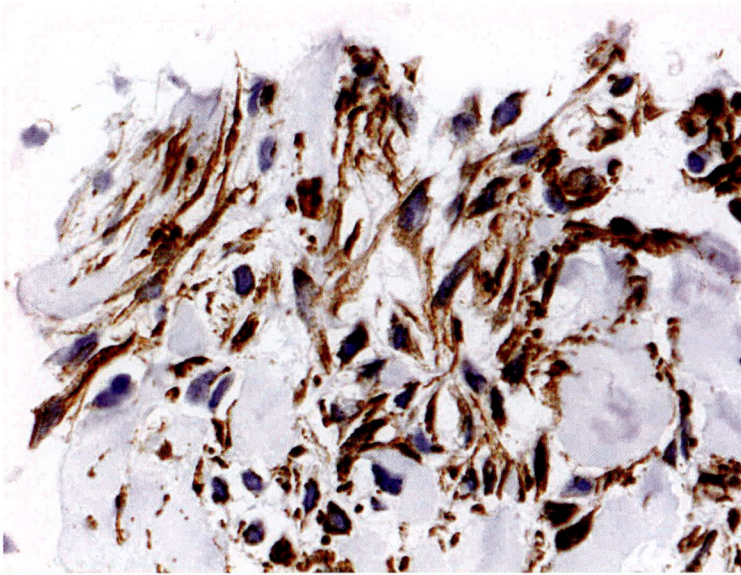

FIG 3.17 Immunocytochemistry on a cell block prepared from aspiration smears. Smooth muscle actin (SMA) is often more sensitive than desmin but is not so specific. Immunostaining for SMA performed on cell block from desmoid tumor.

Recently, some techniques based on liquid-based cytology have become common procedures for preparing cytological material for immunocytochemistry [34−36]. The author has experienced liquid-based preparation for about 8 years and finds the results very promising (Fig 3.24). Compared with cell blocks, however, immunocytochemistry controls in liquid-based cytology systems are more difficult to prepare, control, and maintain. The advantages and disadvantages of various FNA preparations for immunocytochemistry are presented in Table 3.2.

It is important to note that immunocytochemistry in FNA of soft tissue lesions should be used as a complement to the routine cytological examination of the aspirate. Traditional light microscopic examination of air-dried or alcohol-fixed and routinely stained smears should be the basis for cytological diagnosis.

Despite the fact that electron microscopy cannot identify all types of cells in soft tissue tumors, it can reveal certain differentiated structural features and clarify the origin of cells that lack definite signs of differentiation by light microscopy. In certain areas of histopathological and cytological examinations, electron microscopy has been replaced by other techniques, such as immunohistochemistry, cytogenetics, and molecular biology. Electron microscopy still may play a certain role in the classification of the small round cell and spindle cell tumors. It is useful for differentiating spindle cell sarcomas from spindle cell carcinomas and also for determining a specific histotype in myogenic, neurogenic, or fibroblastic/myofibroblastic tumors. Compared with the preparation of cytologic material for immunocytochemistry, the processing of aspirates for electron microscopy is more time consuming. The results of electron microscopy in aspirated cells and cell fragments can be compared favorably with the results observed in biopsy material (Fig 3.25) [37−39].

Flow cytometric as well as static DNA-ploidy analyses can be performed on both cores and aspirated material. DNA analysis has limited diagnostic value in the

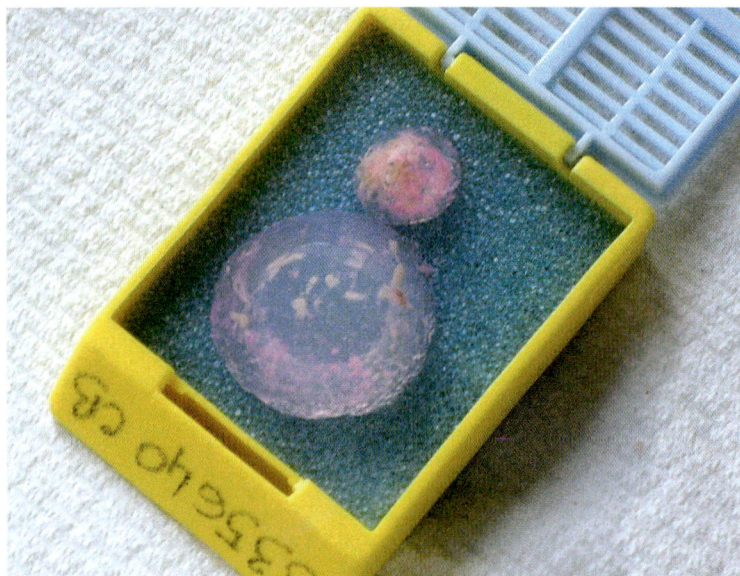

FIG 3.18 Small tissue fragments in a cell block before paraffin inclusion obtained from the aspirate.

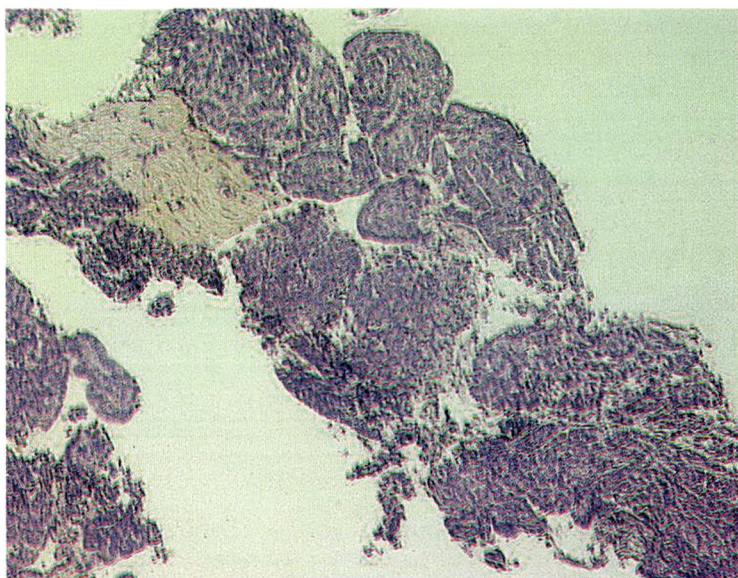

FIG 3.19 Tumor architecture is reproduced on a cell block from an aspirate. A double component, spindle cell, and epithelial is observed clearly in synovial sarcoma. Same case as Fig 3.18.

evaluation of soft tissue tumors. False flow cytometric diploid histograms of soft tissue sarcomas have been reported [40]. In addition, it has been shown that numerous high-grade malignant soft tissue sarcomas may present with a diploid histogram [41].

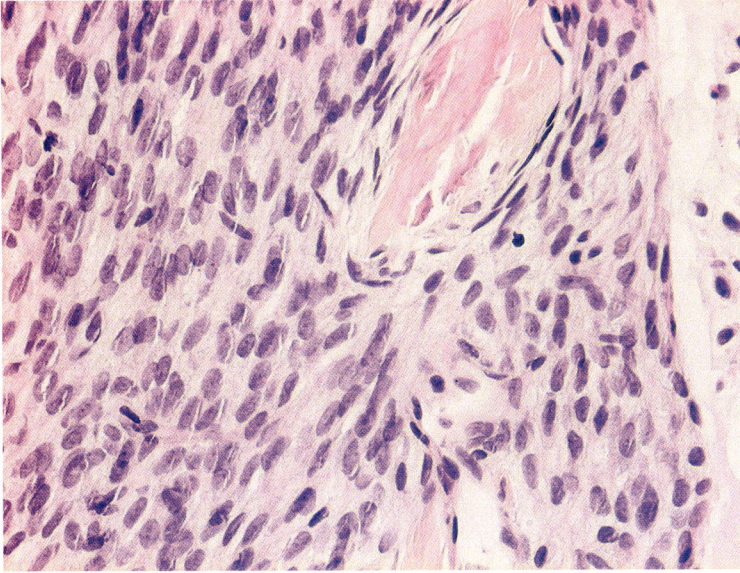

FIG 3.20 Cell block section from synovial sarcoma.

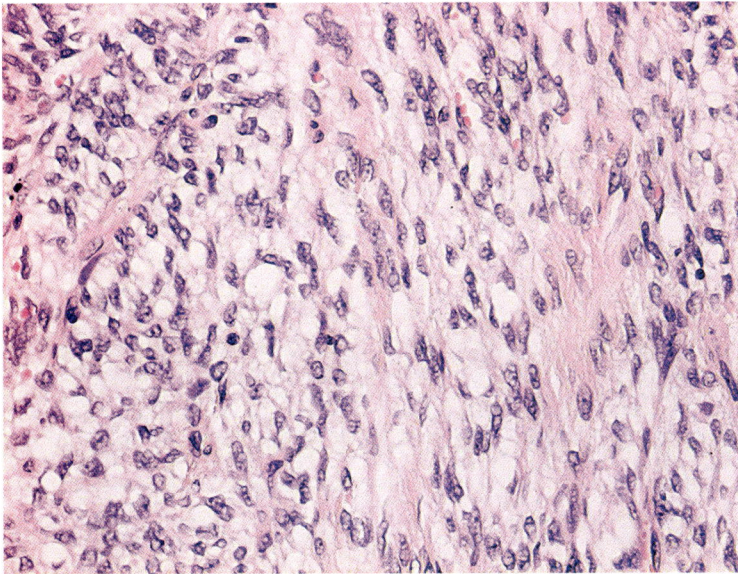

FIG 3.21 Histological section from an operative specimen of synovial sarcoma. Same case as Fig 3.20.

3.4 CHALLENGES IN THE FNA AND CNB OF SOFT TISSUE

Challenges in FNA and CNB diagnoses can be divided into those stemming from the technical aspects of sampling and those caused by difficult differential diagnoses [42].

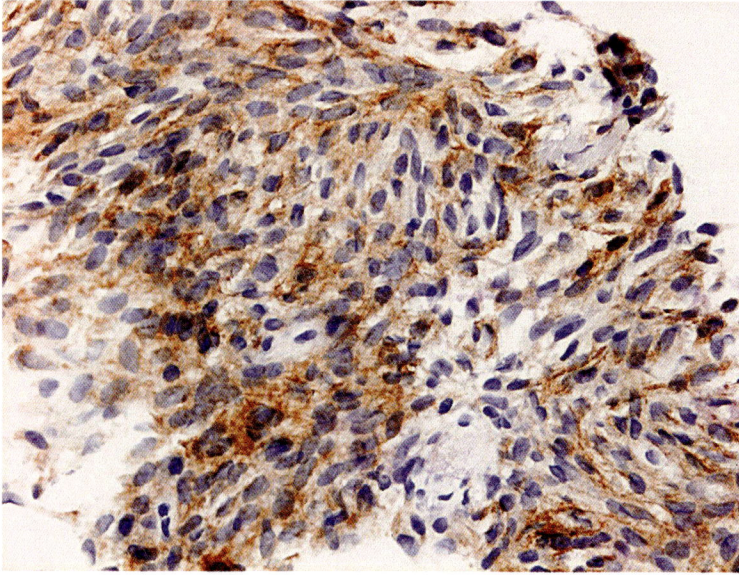

FIG 3.22 Immunostaining for epithelial membrane antigen (EMA) performed on a cell block in synovial sarcoma. Same case as Fig 3.20.

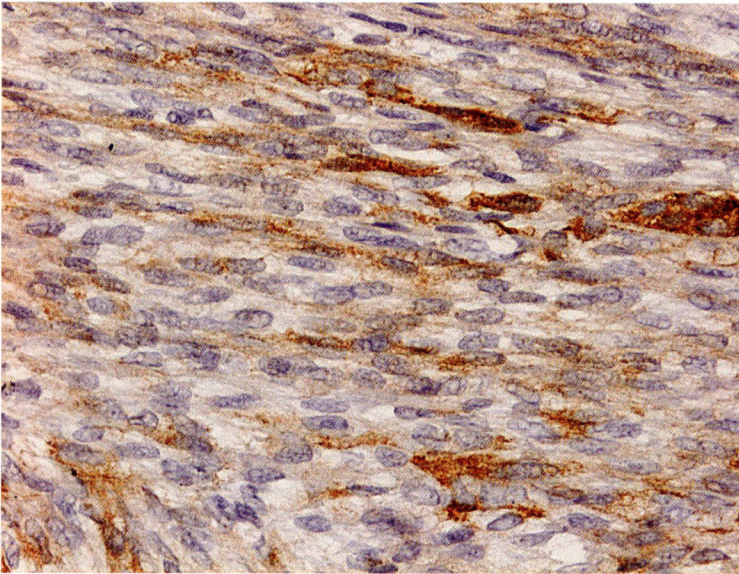

FIG 3.23 Immunostaining for EMA performed on an operative specimen from synovial sarcoma. The results of immunostaining are identical comparison with Fig 3.22.

The amount and quality of aspirated material first may depend on the type, size, and localization of the aspirated lesion/tumor as well as on the technical skill of the aspirator. Poorly preserved and scanty aspiration smears and cores as well as samples obtained from cystic, necrotic, highly collagenous, or hemorrhagic areas of soft tissue sarcomas cause difficulties in the interpretation of microscopical features in the

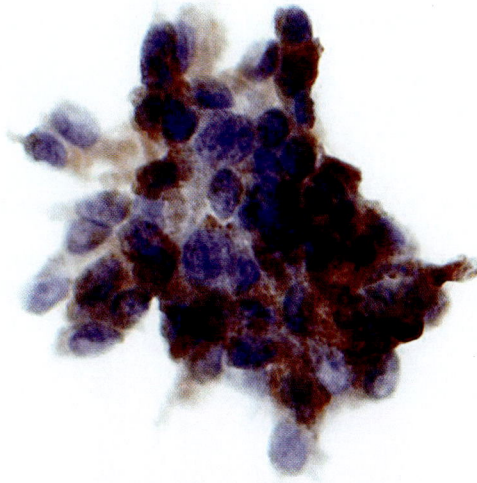

FIG 3.24 EMA positivity in a liquid-based of an preparation of FNA aspirate from a synovial sarcoma.

TABLE 3.2 Advantages and disadvantages of different preparation methods of fine needle aspirates for immunocytochemistry

Preparation method	Advantages	Disadvantages
Direct smear	No specific preparation	Occasionally difficult to evaluate because of cytoplasmic background and stripped nuclei. Only nuclear antibodies suitable.
Cytospin preparation	Universally accepted method for cytochemistry and immunocytochemistry	Risk for false negative result because of focal expression of antibodies
Cell block preparation	Similar to a very small histologic biopsy. Easy to perform controls and to compare with subsequent immunocytochemistry on histological samples	Sometimes difficult to aspirate sufficient material for preparation
Liquid-based cytology	"Clean" background. Monolayer of cells. Material can be saved for further evaluation	Not yet sufficiently evaluated with regard to all antibodies.

routinely stained smears and core sections and limit the usefulness of ancillary techniques. There are different causes of inadequate FNA and CNB specimens, with the most common being that the lesion is missed altogether by the aspirator; cells can be aspirated or cores can be sampled from the tissue surrounding the lesion. Reactive changes in the tissues adjacent to the tumor tissue may mimic neoplasm (i.e., reactive changed adipose tissue may mimic liposarcoma, and reactive fibroblasts/myofibroblasts may be confused with a pleomorphic sarcoma). These problems occur most often when small, deep-seated, inter- or intramuscular lesions are examined. Ultrasound guidance may be of help in the aspiration of small and deep-seated as well as cystic and

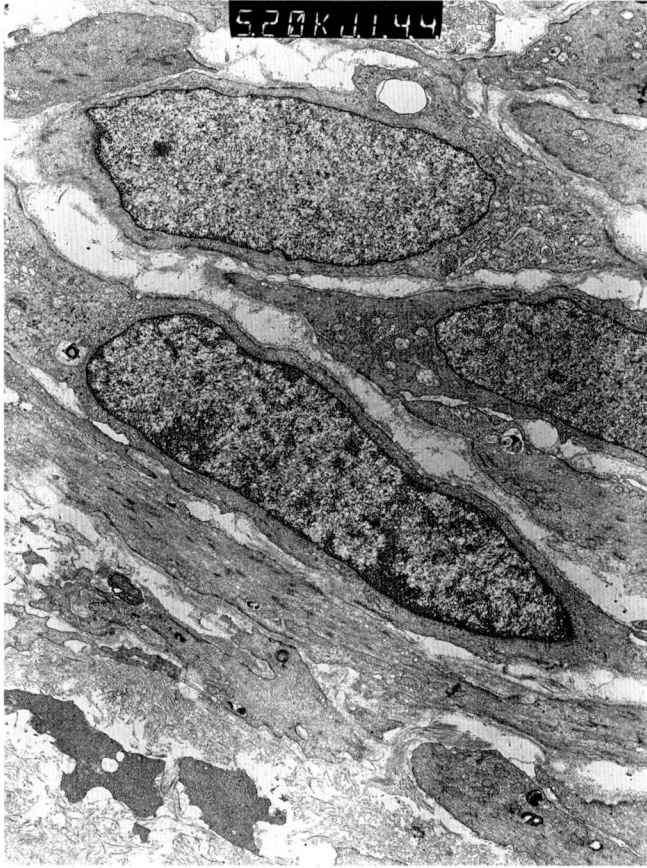

FIG 3.25 Ultrastructural features of an aspirate from leiomyosarcoma. Note the cytoplasmic filaments with densities.

necrotic lesions. As mentioned earlier, representative diagnostic areas may be difficult to sample adequately in cystic, necrotic, or hemorrhagic lesions. Vascular lesions often predominantly yield blood and only a few cells or tiny tissue fragments. Another difficulty with FNA is to dislodge a sufficient numbers of cells from lesions with an abundance of collagenous or hyalinized matrix.

Challenges in the diagnosis of aspiration smears and cores depend on the rarity of soft tissue lesions and on the specific problems connected to the interpretation of samples from some morphological subtypes of soft tissue lesions such as spindle cell neoplasms, pseudosarcomatous proliferations, and new entities in this area. Both cytologic and histologic diagnoses of benign and malignant spindle cell tumors of soft tissue may be difficult, as these lesions often share morphological and clinical characteristics with each other. For example, relatively common spindle cell lesions of fibroblasic and myofibroblastic origin share a cytomorphologic and occasionally an immunocytochemical profile with each other and with other entities such as smooth muscle and fibrohistiocytic neoplasms. In addition, the literature on the FNA of spindle cell tumors is still limited. An example of a difficulty in the interpretation of FNA smears from spindle cell neoplasms is schwannoma. Although most

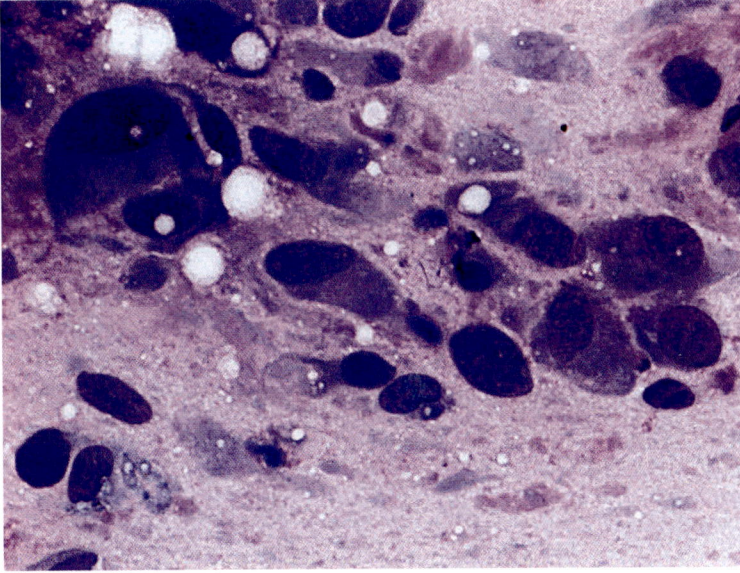

FIG 3.26   FNA of nodular fasciitis.

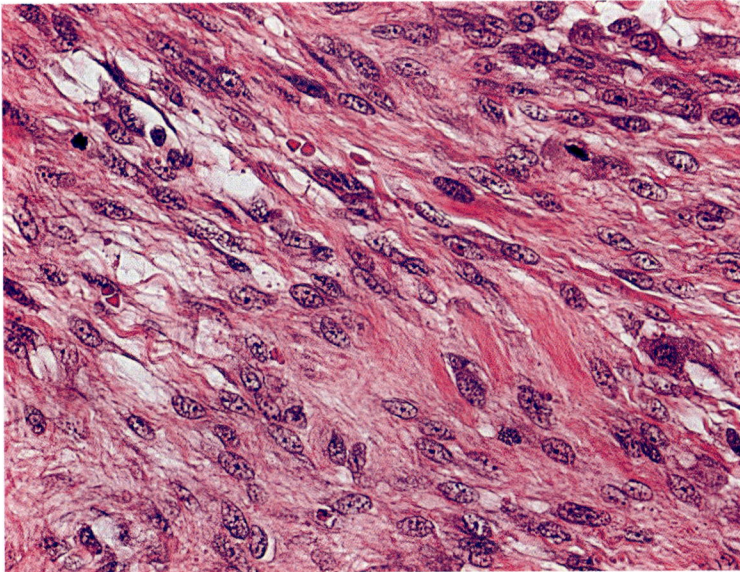

FIG 3.27   Histological section of nodular fasciitis corresponding to Fig 3.26.

schwannomas can be diagnosed by FNA because of their distinct cytomorphological features, smears that display predominantly Antoni A features and nuclear pleomorphism can be confused with other spindle cell tumors, including sarcomas [43]. Degenerative changes in FNA smears and CNB that contain atypical cells with anisocaryosis and hyperchromasia observed in ancient schwannomas can mimic sarcomas [44,45]. Patients with pseudosarcomatous proliferations in soft tissue such as nodular fasciitis, proliferative fasciitis, proliferative myositis, and pseudomalignant

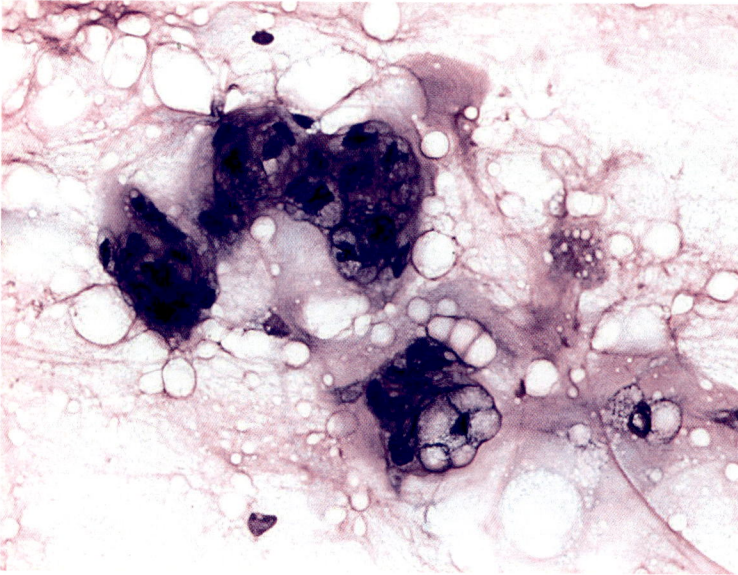

FIG 3.28 FNA smears from chondroid lipoma.

myositis ossificans benefit clearly from FNA and CNB. With a reliable diagnosis, conservative treatment can be a treatment option, as most cases regress spontaneously or greatly diminish some weeks after presentation [46,47]. Pseudosarcomatous proliferations of soft tissue, however, may be misdiagnosed as sarcoma. Both microscopic features of proliferating fibroblasts/myofibroblasts in FNA smears and histological sections may be worrisome (Figs 3.26 and 3.27).

Additional challenges in the FNA and CNB of soft tissue lesions are "new entities" in histopathologic diagnosis as well as rare soft tissue neoplasms. In such lesions, there is a lack of cytomorphologic criteria that permit accurate cytologic evaluation. In addition, not all pathologists/cytopathologists are experienced in the diagnosis of rare types of soft tissue neoplasms. Examples of rare tumors and new entities, hitherto difficult to diagnose correctly as benign or malignant, are chondroid lipoma (Fig 3.28), perineuroma, aggressive angiomyxoma, mixed tumor of soft tissue, spindle cell liposarcoma, and low-grade fibromyxoid sarcoma.

3.5 COMPLICATIONS OF FNA AND CNB OF SOFT TISSUE

The question of tumor cells spreading in the needle tract must be addressed. The incidence of this event in FNA examination is exceedingly low [36]. Nevertheless, in cases in which a deep-seated sarcoma is suspected, tattooing of the skin with sterile ink at the site of the thin or core needle insertion can be performed after aspiration (Fig 3.29). This procedure, applied to patients admitted for an examination of soft tissue lesions by FNA or CNB, helps the surgeon to remove the needle tract together with the excised tumor. Other complications of the aspiration procedure are minor and include small hematomas and localized tenderness. The author has never observed evidence of infection resulting from FNA or CNB procedures.

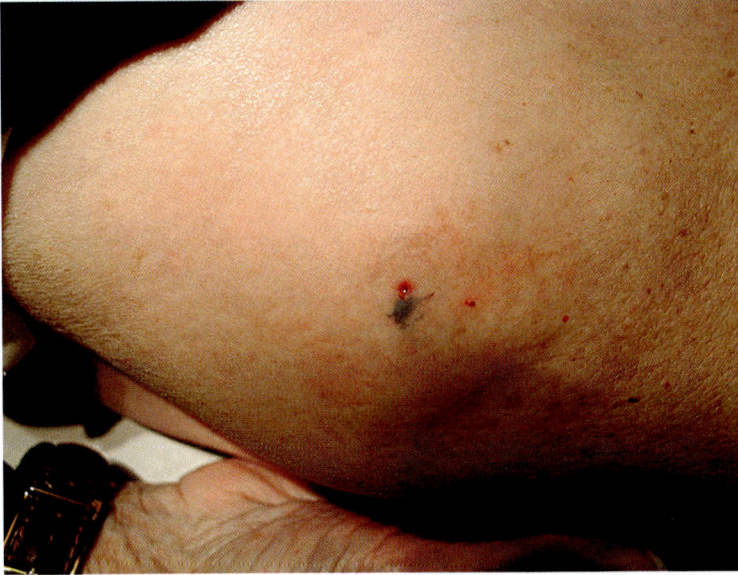

FIG 3.29 Tattoo of the skin at the site of thin or core needle insertion.

REFERENCES

1. Association of Directors of Anatomic and Surgical Pathology. Recommendations for the reporting of soft tissue sarcomas. Am J Clin Pathol 1999, 111: 594−598.

2. Nagira K, Yamamoto T, Akisue T, et al. Reliability of fine-needle aspiration biopsy in the initial diagnosis of soft-tissue lesions. Diagn Cytopathol 2002, 27: 354−361.

3. Åkerman M, Rydholm A. Aspiration cytology of soft-tissue tumors. The 10-year experience at an orthopaedic oncology center. Acta Orthop Scand 1983, 56: 407−412.

4. Rydholm A, Åkerman M, Idvall I, Persson BM. Aspiration cytology of soft tissue tumors. A prospective study of its influence on choice of surgical procedure. Int Orthop 1982, 6: 209−214.

5. Wakely P, Kneisl J. Soft tissue aspiration cytopathology. Diagnostic accuracy and limitations. Cancer 2000, 5: 292−298.

6. Åkerman M. Fine-needle aspiration cytology of soft tissue sarcoma: benefits and limitations. Sarcoma 1998, 155−161.

7. Kilpatrick SE, Geisinger KR. Soft tissue sarcomas: the usefulness and limitations of fine-needle aspiration biopsy. Am J Clin Pathol 1998, 110: 50−68.

8. Maitra A, Ashfaq R, Hossein Saboorian M, Lindberg G, Gokasian S. The role of fine-needle aspiration biopsy in the primary diagnosis of mesenchymal lesions. A community hospital-based experience. Cancer 2000, 3: 178−185.

9. Kilpatrick SE, Capellari JO, Bos GD, Gold SH, Ward WG. Is fine-needle aspiration biopsy a practical alternative to open biopsy for the primary diagnosis of sarcoma? Am J Clin Pathol 2001, 115: 59−68.

10. Welker JA, Henshaw RM, Jelinek J, Shmookler BM, Malawer MM. The percutaneous needle biopsy is safe and recommended in the diagnosis of Musculoskeletal masses. Outcomes analysis of 155 patients at a sarcoma referral center. Cancer 2000, 89: 2677−2686.

11. Ray-Coquard I, Ranchère-Vince D, Thiesse P, et al. Evaluation of core needle biopsy as a substitute to open biopsy in the diagnosis of soft-tissue masses. Eur J Cancer 2003, 39: 2021–2025.

12. Yao L, Nelson SD, Seeger LL, Eckardt JJ, Eilber FR. Primary musculoskeletal neoplasms: effectiveness of core-needle biopsy. Radiology 1999, 212: 682–686.

13. Mitsuyoshi G, Naito N, Kawai A, et al. Accurate diagnosis of musculoskeletal lesions by core needle biopsy. J Surg Oncol 2006, 94: 21–27.

14. Kilpatrick SE, Ward WG, Cappellari JO, Bos GD. Fine-needle aspiration biopsy of soft tissue sarcomas. A cytomorphologic analysis with emphasis on histologic subtyping, grading and therapeutic significance. Am J Clin Pathol 1999, 112: 179–188.

15. Costa MJ, Campman SC, Davis RL, Howell LP. Fine-needle aspiration cytology of sarcoma. Retrospective review of diagnostic utility and specificity. Diagn Cytopathol 1996, 15: 23–32.

16. Palmer HE, Mukunyadzi P, Culbreth W, Thomas JR. Subgrouping and grading of soft-tissue sarcomas by fie-needle aspiration cytology: a histopathologic correlation study. Diagn Cytopathol 2001, 24: 307–316.

17. Weir MM, Rosenberg AE, Bell DA. Grading of spindle cell sarcomas in fine needle aspiration biopsy specimens. Am J Clin Pathol 1999, 112: 784–790.

18. Jones C, Lju K, Hirschowitz S, Klipfel N, Layfield LJ. Concordance of histopathologic and cytologic grading in musculoskeletal sarcomas. Can grades obtained from analysis of fine-needle aspirates serve as the basis for therapeutic decisions? Cancer 2002, 96: 83–91.

19. Domanski HA, Åkerman M, Carlén B, Engellau J, Gustafson P, Jonsson K, Mertens F, Rydholm A. Core-needle biopsy performed by the cytopathologist: a technique to complement fine-needle aspiration of soft tissue and bone lesions. Cancer 2005, 105: 229–239.

20. Ayala AG, Ro JY, Fanning CV, Flores JP, Yasko AW. Core needle biopsy and fine-needle aspiration in the diagnosis of bone and soft-tissue lesions. Hematol Oncol Clin North Am 1995, 9: 633–651.

21. Bennert KW, Abdul-Karim FW. Fine needle aspiration cytology vs. needle core biopsy of soft tissue tumors. A comparison. Acta Cytol 1994, 38: 381–384.

22. Narvani AA, Tsiridis E, Saifuddin A, Briggs T, Cannon S. Does image guidance improve accuracy of core needle biopsy in diagnosis of soft tissue tumours? Acta Orthop Belg 2009, 75: 239–244.

23. Koenig CW, Duda SH, Truebenbach J, Schott UG, Maurer F, Claussen CD, Pereira PL. MR-guided biopsy of musculoskeletal lesions in a low-field system. J Magn Reson Imaging 2001, 13: 761–768.

24. Jenssen C, Siebert C, Bartho S. (Leiomyosarcoma of the inferior vena cava. Diagnosis using endoscopic ultrasound-guided fine-needle aspiration biopsy). Dtsch Med Wochenschr 2008, 133: 769–772.

25. Guiter GE, Gatscha RM, Zakowski MF. ThinPrep vs conventional smears in fine-needle aspirations of sarcomas: a morphological and immunocytochemical study. Diagn Cytopathol 1999, 21: 351–354.

26. Suthipintawong C, Leong AS-Y. Immunostaining of cell preparations: a comparative evaluation of common fixatives and protocols. Diagn Cytopathol 1996, 15:167–174.

27. Johnston WW, Szpak CA, Thor A, Simpson JF, Schlom J. Applications of immunocytochemistry to clinical cytology. Cancer Invest 1987, 5: 593–611.

28. Flens MJ, van der Valk P, Tadema TM, Huysmans AC, Risse EK, van Tol GA, Meijer CJ. The contribution of immunocytochemistry in diagnostic cytology. Comparison and evaluation with immunohistology. Cancer 1990, 65: 2704–2711.

29. Abendroth CS, Dabbs DJ. Immunocytochemical staining on unstained versus previously stained cytologic preparations. Acta Cytol 1995, 39: 379–386.

30. Kurtycz DFI, Logrono L, Leopando M, Slattery A, Inhorn SL. Immunocytochemistry controls using cell cultures. Diagn Cytopathol 1997, 17: 74–79.

31. Owens CL, Sharma R, Ali SZ. Deep fibromatosis (desmoid tumor): cytopathologic characteristics, clinicoradiologic features, and immunohistochemical findings on fine-needle aspiration. Cancer 2007, 111: 166–172.

32. Dabbs DJ, Wang X. Immunocytochemistry on cytologic specimens of limited quantity. Diagn Cytopathol 1998, 18: 166–169.

33. Bhatia P, Dey P, Uppal R, Shifa R, Srinivasan R, Nijhawan R.. Cell blocks from scraping of cytology smear: comparison with conventional cell block. Acta Cytol 2008, 52: 329–333.

34. Dabbs DJ, Abendroth CS, Grenko RT, Wang X, Radcliffe GE. Immunocytochemistry on the ThinPrep processor. Diagn Cytopathol 1997, 17: 388–392.

35. Leung SW, Bedard YC. Immunocytochemical staining on ThinPrep processed smears. Mod Pathol 1996, 9: 304–306.

36. Barth RJ Jr, Merino MJ, Solomon D, Yang JC, Baker AR. A prospective study of the value of core needle biopsy and fine needle aspiration in the diagnosis of soft tissue masses. Surgery 1992, 112: 536–543.

37. Carlen B. Diagnostic value of electron microscopy in rare malignant musculoskeletal tumors. Experience from an orthopedic tumor center. Ups J Med Sci 1996, 101: 69–85.

38. Nordgren H, Åkerman M. Electron microscopy of fine needle aspiration biopsy from soft tissue tumors. Acta Cytol 1982, 26: 179–188.

39. Kindblom LG, Walaas L, Widehn S. Ultrastructural studies in the preoperative cytologic diagnosis of soft tissue tumors. Semin Diagn Pathol 1986, 3: 317–344.

40. Åkerman M, Killander D, Rydholm A. Aspiration of musculoskeletal tumors for cytodiagnosis and DNA analysis. Acta Orthop Scand 1987, 58: 523–528.

41. Fernö M, Baldetorp B, Åkerman M. Flow cytometric DNA ploidy analysis of soft tissue sarcoma. A comparative study of preoperative fine needle aspirate and postoperative fresh tissue and archival material. Anal Quant Cytol Histol 1990, 12: 251–258.

42. Domanski HA. FNA cytology of soft tissue lesions: diagnostic challenges. Diagn Cytopathol. 2007, 35: 768–773.

43. Domanski HA, Åkerman M, Engellau J, Gustafson P, Mertens F, Rydholm A. Fine-needle aspiration of neurilemoma (Schwannoma). A clinicocytopathologic study of 116 patients. Diagn Cytopathol 2006, 34: 403–412.

44. Dahl I, Hagmar B, Idvall I. Benign solitary neurilemoma (Schwannoma). A correlative cytological and histological study of 28 cases. APMIS 1984, 92(A): 91–101.

45. Ryd W, Mugel S, Ayyash K. Ancient neurilemoma. A pitfall in the cytologic diagnosis of soft tissue tumors. Diagn Cytopathol 1988, 2: 244–247.

46. Dahl I, Åkerman M. Nodular fasciitis. A correlative cytologic and histologic study of 13 cases. Acta Cytol 1981, 25: 91–101.

47. Stanley M, Skoog L, Tani E, Horwitz C. Spontaneous resolution of nodular fasciitis following diagnosis by fine needle aspiration. Acta Cytol 1991, 35: 616–617.

Chapter *4*

Ancillary Techniques

Derived from the mesoderm layer of the embryonic stage, several non-epithelial cells constitute a supporting apparatus for tissues, organs, and systems. These include the vascular, the immunologic, and the supportive networks, which occur in benign tissues and in malignant neoplasms. Supportive networks are interconnected and provide systems of circulation, transport, communication, and defense among cells. This complex supportive function becomes specialized into mesoderm-derived tissues comprising of mesenchymal cells, such as blood vessels, lymphatics, cartilage, bone, muscle (smooth and striated), tendons, nerve, fat, bone marrow, and fibroconnective stroma. With progress in imaging techniques, such as ultrasounds, X-rays, computed tomography (CT) scans, and magnetic resonance imagings (MRIs), neoplasms of bone and soft tissues can be sampled via fine needle aspirates (FNAs) and core needle biopsies (CNBs). It thus becomes necessary to recognize mesenchymal cell neoplasms that can be undifferentiated completely or unresemble the various tissue types listed. It should be stressed, however, that these tumors no longer are believed to be derived from their respective parent tissue. Rather, one speaks of tumor differentiation into various subtypes of mesenchymal cell lineage, which clinically has less significance than the grade of the neoplasm being sampled.

The recognition of soft tissue tumor putative origins is a capital for diagnosis and proper patient management. Actually, pathologist may perform an accurate diagnosis on the basis of morphology and a combination of immunocytochemical, immunohistochemical and genomic results.

4.1 IMMUNOCYTOCHEMISTRY

Carlos Bedrossian, MD, PhD (Hon)

In contrast to epithelial neoplasms, there is a much smaller number of antibodies with restricted specificity that are useful in the recognition of distinct mesenchymal

Soft Tissue Tumors: A Multidisciplinary, Decisional Diagnostic Approach
Edited by Jerzy Klijanienko and Réal Lagacé
Copyright © 2011 John Wiley & Sons, Inc.

phenotypes. On the other hand, a greater number of translocations and other genetic alterations have been described in connection with the subtypes of soft tissue tumors. Once a benign, reactive process has been ruled out, it is useful to separate the proliferation according to its predominant cell population. A benign or malignant proliferation may contain cells with a readily recognizable direction of differentiation according to the products that they secrete. The proliferation may have immature cells without obvious phenotypic characteristics; in which case, they can be classified according to the predominant shape of the tumor cells, including 1) small round cells, 2) spindle cells, 3) epithelioid cells, and 4) pleomorphic large cells. Some of these tumor cells may be differentiated enough that they do not require immunohistochemistry for recognition and are defined by their typical morphology or distinctive intracellular products. They include fat in lipoma and well-differentiated liposarcoma, blood vessels in angiomas, smooth muscle in leiomyosarcoma, striated muscle in rhabdomyosarcoma, nerve tissue in neuroma, Verocay bodies in benign nerve sheath tumors, and a mixture of mesenchymal and epithelial elements in biphasic synovial sarcoma. The cytomorphology of soft tissue tumors may be limited in terms of individual cell morphology, but functionally, the same cell shape is shared by tumors that secrete numerous different extracellular substances, which are not easy to recognize in cytological specimens.

4.1.1 Tumors Defined by the Accumulation of Extracellular Substances

Among soft tissue tumors, the ones most difficult to recognize are neoplasms characterized not as much by their tumor cell population but as by the extracellular substances that they elaborate. Examples include collagen in fibrosarcoma, myxoid stroma in intramuscular myxoma, chondroid in cartilaginous tumors, osteoid in osseous tumors, and neurofibrils in neurofibromatosis. Although myxoid stroma can be recognized in a needle aspirate, the lack of pattern recognition precludes further characterization of the neoplasm. This lack of context makes it impossible to distinguish between an intramuscular myxoma and myxoid liposarcoma, for instance, or between these tumors and other myxoid neoplasms, including myxoid malignant fibrous histiocytoma (MFH)-like tumors and myxoid chondrosarcoma. Primitive mesenchymal cells express vimentin and are capable of differentiating into other subtypes that cannot be readily apparent by cytomorphology alone. Vimentin, therefore, is positive in virtually all mesenchymal tumors. As with carcinomas, certain sarcomas coexpress vimentin and keratin, notably epithelioid sarcoma, synovial sarcoma, and leiomyosarcoma.

4.1.2 Small Round Cell Tumors

This group of soft tissue neoplasms typically occurs in children and adolescents and shares the predominance of small, "blue" round cell tumors (SBRCTs) as their defining morphologic trait. Embryonal rhabdomyosarcoma expresses desmin, myogenin, MYO-D1, myoglobin, and HHF-35 (smooth muscle actin). Extraskeletal Ewing sarcoma and the peripheral neuroectodermal tumor are closely related neoplasms that share the t(11:22)(q21;q12) translocation. These tumors are positive for neurofilament, CD99 (Fig 4.1), CD-57 (Leu 7), S-100 protein neurone specific enolase (NSE), synaptophysin, PGP 9.5, and secretogranin II. Several primitive SBRCTs with characteristic clinical–pathological features have been grouped under the peripheral neuroectodermal tumor classification, including neuroblastoma, retinoblastoma,

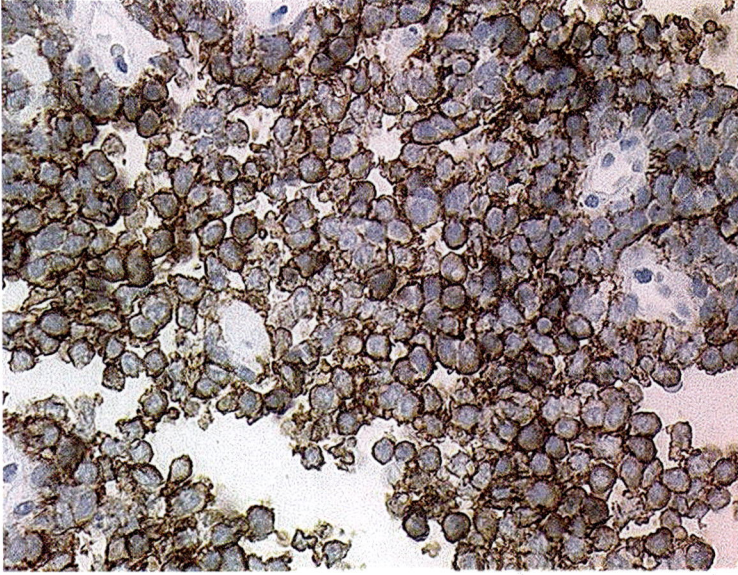

FIG 4.1 CD99 in a smear from Ewing sarcoma/peripheral neuroectodermal tumor.

medulloblastoma, ependymoblastoma, and pineoblastoma. Their immunoprofile overlaps closely with the peripheral neuroectodermal tumor so that their diagnosis depends heavily on clinical correlation. Of these, neuroblastoma may originate in the adrenal and elsewhere in the soft tissues. This tumor is positive for neurofilament, HISL-19, and NB-84 as well as for numerous neuroendocrine markers, including NSE, PGP 9.5, synaptophysin, chromogranin, and secretogranin. The desmoplastic small round cell tumor typically shows a reciprocal translocation t(11;22)(p13;q12) associated with the chimerical EWS-WT1 gene fusion transcript. The tumor is positive for vimentin, keratin (AE1/AE3), epithelial membrane antigen (EMA), desmin (dot pattern), WT1, and NSE. The Wilm's tumor, also known as nephroblastoma, can be monomorphous, comprising undifferentiated blastema. They are positive for WT-1, vimentin, and keratin, but they do not have any specific phenotypic markers. Other markers of SBRCT are helpful in excluding tumors with small blue cells, including lymphomas, which express the hematopoietic markers described. The diagnosis relies on clinicopathological correlation, pointing to the kidney as the primary site. In contrast, there are rare examples of polyphenotypic small, round cell tumors that are positive for various mesenchymal, epithelial, and myogenic markers and can express neuroectodermal determinants. They also may exhibit divergent cytomorphological features, including primitive areas and rudimentary gland formation, which may confuse the cytological diagnosis, particularly with limited cell samples.

4.1.3 Spindle Cell Tumors

Among spindle cell neoplasms, both leiomyosarcoma and rhabdomyosarcoma secrete desmin and muscle specific actin (MSA). Myoglobin, however, is positive only in rhabdomyosarcoma, although this antibody is not recommended in this case (see subsequent sections). Poorly differentiated liposarcoma with predominantly spindle cells contain rare lipoblasts but are positive with Sudan Black and Oil Red O lipid stains. Malignant peripheral nerve sheath tumors including schwannoma and neurofibroma are positive for the S-100 protein, CD-57 (Leu-7), collagen type IV, and laminin. Fibrosarcoma is a diagnosis of exclusion, relying on clinicopathological correlation, including the history of radiation. These tumors are positive for vimentin but little else. The association of tumor cells with collagen is not specific for this neoplasm or for others. Spindle cell angiosarcoma is positive for vascular markers CD-31 and CD-34 and expresses lectins of the Ulex europeus agglutinin (UEA-I) variety. The Kaposi sarcoma is positive for SMA, CD-31, and CD-34 but negative for UEA-I. Monophonic synovial sarcoma expresses keratin (CK-7, and CK-19, or both) CD-99, and EMA, as well as SMA and laminin. Some of these tumors also may express BCL-2 and the t(X:18) translocation by fluorescent in situ hybridization (FISH) analysis. Dermatofibrosarcoma protuberans is factor XIIIa negative and CD34 positive. Occasionally, dermatofibrosarcoma protuberans can show dedifferentiation with fibrosarcomatous areas. Originally considered of pericytic origin, hemangiopericytoma now is grouped with solitary fibrous tumor, a tumor of fibroblastic origin that occurs in the pleura and elsewhere in the soft tissues. Hemangiopericytoma shares a striking immunohistochemical overlap with solitary fibrous tumor. Markers frequently expressed in both entities include CD34 and CD99. SMA is only rarely positive. Immunohistochemistry is of limited value in reactive fibroblastic/myofibroblastic proliferations such as myositis ossificans, nodular fasciitis, and proliferative myositis. They uniformly express vimentin, sometimes SMA and HHF35, but desmin is usually negative.

4.1.4 Epithelioid Cell Tumors

Several soft tissue neoplasms comprising polygonal-shaped tumor cells have been recognized in the wake of epithelioid sarcoma, one of the first tumors in which the coexpression of vimentin and keratin was recognized. The first goal in the diagnosis of these neoplasms is to avoid confusion with metastatic carcinoma. The goal is to classify the sarcoma at hand that often is only cytomorphologically different than its spindle cell counterpart, with which they are histogenetically similar and share a nearly identical immunoprofile. Epithelioid sarcoma is a multinodular neoplasm with tumor cells positive for vimentin (perinuclear), keratin (AE1/AE3), EMA, CD-34, CD-31, and occasionally carcinoembryonic antigen (CEA). If the patient has a history of carcinoma elsewhere, then distinction from metastasis is impossible by immunohistochemistry alone and may depend on clinicopathological correlation. The tumor cells of epithelioid monophasic synovial sarcoma closely recapitulate the phenotype of the polygonal cell element in biphasic synovial sarcoma. As such, they are positive for CD-99 (MIC-1), EMA, keratin (AE1/AE3), CK-7, CK-8, CK-18, and CK-19, as well as for Ber-Ep4, E-cadherin, and calretinin, which renders the distinction between synovial sarcoma and malignant mesothelioma of the pleura a challenging prospect. Poorly differentiated epithelioid cells with a synovial phenotype may be difficult to recognize by immunohistochemistry alone. Cytogenetic demonstration of the t(x;18) (p11;q11) translocation and molecular detection of the typical SYT-SSX fusion may be needed to clinch the diagnosis of synovial sarcoma in these cases. Epithelioid angiosarcoma is a richly vascularized tumor, whose tumor cells are large, polygonal, and express EMA and keratin (AR|E1/AE3) along with a positive reaction for CD-31, CD-34, UEA-I, and factor VIII-RA. This tumor also may express the tumor-associated glycoprotein TAG-72, recognized by the D72.3. Epithelioid angiosarcoma must not be confused with another vascular lesion, the so-called neoplasm with perivascular epithelioid cell differentiation (PEComa), comprising hemosiderin-laden epithelioid tumor cells that react positively for SMA and HMB-45. Clear cell sarcoma of the soft tissues currently is considered the deep-seated counterpart of cutaneous melanoma. The tumor is positive for melanocytic markers S100 and HMB-45 and less consistently for melan-A (Mart-1). Other positive markers include vimentin, CD57, and NSE. Variable results occur with c-Kit (CD117). Other clear cell lesions that enter in the differential diagnosis of clear cell sarcoma can be excluded as follows: negativity for keratins and EMA excludes epithelioid sarcomas; SMA and desmin negativity rules out true epithelioid leiomyosarcoma; true epithelioid leiomyosarcoma is a term applied to a subset of leiomyosarcoma that either focally or as a predominant feature displays the presence of plump, vacuolated, polygonal-shaped epithelioid cells. This tumor previously was called leiomyoblastoma, but epithelioid leiomyosarcoma is the currently preferred nomenclature. This tumor is positive for desmin and/or SMA and is uniformly negative for epithelial and other markers of nonmyogenic phenotype. Howewer, most neoplasms previously classified as "epithelioid smooth muscle tumor" rather belong to the gastrointestinal stromal tumor (GIST) family. Alveolar soft part sarcoma consists of keratin-negative epithelioid tumor cells. Positivity for desmin, SMA, myosin, and Z-band protein suggests a myogenic pathway. However, this tumor often is negative for myogenin and MyoD1. A t(x;17) translocation resulting in a ASPL-TFE3 fusion gene has been linked to alveolar soft part sarcoma and can be detected immunohistochemically by the anti-TFE-3 antibody.

4.1.5 Pleomorphic Cell Tumors

This is a frequent pattern exhibited by soft tissue tumors, characterized by a mixed neoplastic cell population that includes small round cells, spindle cells, large epithelioid cells, and multinucleated giant cells. Paradoxically, the prototypical lesion of this group, the so-called MFH, is losing ground as a diagnostic category, because of refinements in recognizing the hystiocytic phenotype with better immunohistochemical precision. Tumor cells of so-called MFH bind peanut agglutinins and express several enzymes common in macrophages, such as alpha 1 antitrypsin (A1AT), alpha I anti chymo-trypsin (A1ACT), and ferritin. However, examples of this tumor often fail to express CD-68, a more reliable marker of histiocytic differentiation than the various enzymes used in the past. In addition, careful investigation of a putative MFH-like tumor may disclose further evidence of myogenic, neurogenic, or lipoblastic differentiation with lineage-specific markers, which negate the possible "myofibroblastic" or "fibrohistiocytic" nature of this neoplasm. Alveolar rhabdomyosarcoma combines immature small round cells with irregularly elongated "strap cells," whereas pleomorphic rhabdomyosarcoma displays a more variegated cell population, which mimics that of MFH-like tumors. Both of these tumors express myogenic markers such as desmin, MSA, Myo-D1, myogenin, and myoglobin. However, only alveolar rhabdomyosarcoma displays cytogenetic abnormalities, such as a consistent t(2;13)(q35;q14) translocation and a variant t(1;13)(p36;q14) translocation, by molecular biology studies. Pleomorphic liposarcoma also resembles an MFH-like tumor cytologically, which is compounded by the fact that they may show a strong reactivity with antibodies against proteolytic enzymes. Unlike MFH-like lesions, however, they may contain lipoblasts, may be positive for S-100, and only rarely express CD-68. Dedifferentiated liposarcomas resemble pleomorphic liposarcoma, except they are clinically preceded by a prior liposarcoma lacking clear-cut pleomorphic features. These lesions may show cytogenetic abnormalities present in a well-differentiated liposarcoma, including ring or giant marker chromosomes. Leiomyosarcoma, fibrosarcoma, and metastatic malignant melanoma are just a few additional tumors of the soft tissues that rarely can present with pleomorphic tumor cells, including multinucleated giant cells. Their differential diagnosis is achieved best by clinicalpathological correlation, including X-ray findings and cytomorphology aided by immunohistochemistry.

4.2 IMMUNOHISTOCHEMISTRY

Réal Lagacé, MD, FRCPC

Among the ancillary techniques useful to assess a soft tissue lesion correctly, immunohistochemistry has become a powerful tool, which also applies to histological study as fine needle aspirates (FNA). The main indications are to differentiate between pleomorphic sarcoma and anaplastic metastatic carcinoma or melanoma, as well as between pleomorphic sarcoma and primary large cell lymphoma of soft tissues. It is also of considerable value in distinguishing spindle cell low-grade sarcomas from pseudosarcomatous reactive processes, to name a few fasciitis and organ-based myofibroblastic proliferations. The use of antibodies to detect cellular, both cytoplasmic and nuclear markers that will help to precise the phenotype of a given tumor (either benign or malignant), is a routine procedure when dealing with a problematic soft tissue lesion in terms of precising its exact nature.

As any other procedure among the arsenal of cyto/histopathologists, immunohistochemistry has strengths and weaknesses. Most are related to the antibodies used in the technique and to the technical process itself (i.e., the analytic process). It is out of the scope of the present monography to discuss the methodologic components of the hardware of immunohistochemistry as well as the selection of a plethora of commercially available antibodies. We rather will focus on those antibodies relevant to the main indications mentioned previously and will try to determine how they will help to make an accurate diagnosis of a soft tissue tumor.

There are some "truisms" to remember when using immunohistochemistry for the diagnosis of a soft tissue tumor [1].

- Immunohistochemistry is an adjuncture to diagnosis, and it does not replace the routine cytological/histological stains; therefore never discart a classical morphologic diagnosis on the faith of a brown color.
- No antibody is totally specific of an organ and/or tissue.
- Among the numerous monoclonal and polyclonal antibodies for diagnostic purposes, only a small minority has proven to be of practical value.
- Although the expression of a class of antigens could be characteristic of some tumors, they could be expressed in different entities.

- The choice and the duration of fixation can influence numerous antigens, particularly the nuclear and the surface membrane antigens.
- Immunophenotype is an indication of tissue differentiation not of histogenesis.
- The frequent presence of tumor necrosis, especially in a high-grade soft tissue sarcoma, could influence and result in false-positive reactions.

So far, the use of antibodies/immunohistochemistry in the FNA of soft tissue tumors has not been evaluated yet in large series. This is true for our own large series of cases, of which only a few were studied by immunohistochemistry. Therefore, the present list of antibodies refers to literature reviews particularly dealing with conventional biopsy and surgical specimens of soft tissue tumor. However, numerous case reports and our own experience have demonstrated the utility of immunohistochemistry in the indications already mentioned.

Antibodies used to differentiate lesions of soft tissue could be put together in the following categories: nuclear markers, cytoplasmic markers, membrane markers, and stromal composants markers. However, for the purpose of the present review, we have referred to an exhaustive overview on the topic [2].

4.2.1 Antibodies Considered of Little Use

Some of these antibodies, although already considered specific, are not. To name a few, the so-called histiocytic markers lyzozyme, alpha 1-antitrypsin, and alpha 1-antichymotrypsin could be replaced advantageously by CD68. Myoglobin should be discarded from a selected panel of antibodies because it stains a lot of tissue components indistinguishable from true expression by striated muscle fibers whatever their stage of differentiation/development. It now is replaced successfully by antibodies of the MyoD family. Neurone-specific-enolase is of limited use given its nonspecificity.

In the early steps of immunohistochemistry, vimentin, a member of the class of intermediate filaments, was considered a good marker of mesenchymal cells. Additional studies have shown that it is expressed by almost all tumor types, namely tumors of epithelial cells. Later on, it also was used to confirm or to evaluate the quality of tissue fixation. Alpha 1-SMA and CD 34 largely are preferred to test the quality of immunostaining, adding to the fact that they could be good diagnostic markers.

4.2.2 Antibodies Useful for Soft Tissue Tumors Evaluation

According to the conventional morphology of a lesion, a limited number of useful antibodies could be used. Despite the numerous antibodies commercially available, either monoclonal or polyclonal, only a small subset have proved to be of practical value in the diagnosis of soft tissues neoplasms.

Epithelial markers such as pancytokeratin (AE1–AE3 and EMA) are an invaluable component of a basic panel of antibodies, particularly in cases of pleomorphic tumors, to distinguish sarcomatoid carcinoma from true sarcoma. It also is expressed by numerous soft tissue tumors, for instance, monophasic and poorly differentiated synovial sarcoma, epithelioid sarcoma, and myoepithelioma. The main pitfall to avoid is the aberrant/theoretically unexpected expression of epithelial markers by sarcomas (e.g., leiomyosarcoma, rhabdomyosarcoma, peripheral neuroectodermal tumor, and epithelioid angiosarcoma).

The S-100 protein when used in conjunction with other panels of antibodies is very useful, despite its poor specificity. Besides a strong and diffuse positivity by the benign peripheral nerve sheath tumors, it constantly is expressed in malignant melanoma and clear cell sarcoma of soft tissue. A focal and inconstant positivity is common in the malignant peripheral nerve sheath tumor, depending on the phenotype of the tumors. It also is expressed by other tumors, such as synovial sarcoma, extraskeletal myxoid chondrosarcoma, peripheral neuroectodermal tumor, myxoid, and round cell liposarcomas.

The muscular markers are tested frequently in soft tissue lesions either neoplasias or pseudotumors. A combination of desmin and SMA helps to identify some entities; rhabdomyosarcoma, for example, are desmin positive and SMA negative, and conversely, leiomyosarcomas are desmin weakly positive and SMA positive. Pseudoneoplasic proliferations, particularly the wide group of fasciitis and organ-based myofibroblastic proliferations, are SMA positive and usually desmin negative. One has to keep in mind that SMA can be expressed in a wide range of cells or lesions of a reactive nature. H-caldesmon (a high molecular weight isoform), which is a protein that regulates the cellular contraction combined with calmoduline, is considered to be specific for smooth muscle cells. Let us also recall that different types of actin isoforms react with different tissue components.

CD 34, despite ubiquitous expression, is a useful antibody. It gives positive reactions in a wide variety of soft tissue tumors including vascular tumors, dermatofibrosarcoma protuberans, gastrointestinal stromal tumor, spindle cell and pleomorphic lipomas, malignant peripheral nerve sheath tumor, epithelioid sarcoma, and solitary fibrous tumor. Needless to say that given a large spectrum of expression, it should be combined with other markers (e.g., CD 31) if one suspects a vascular tumor and CD 117 in a case of an expected gastrointestinal stromal tumor [Fig 4.2].

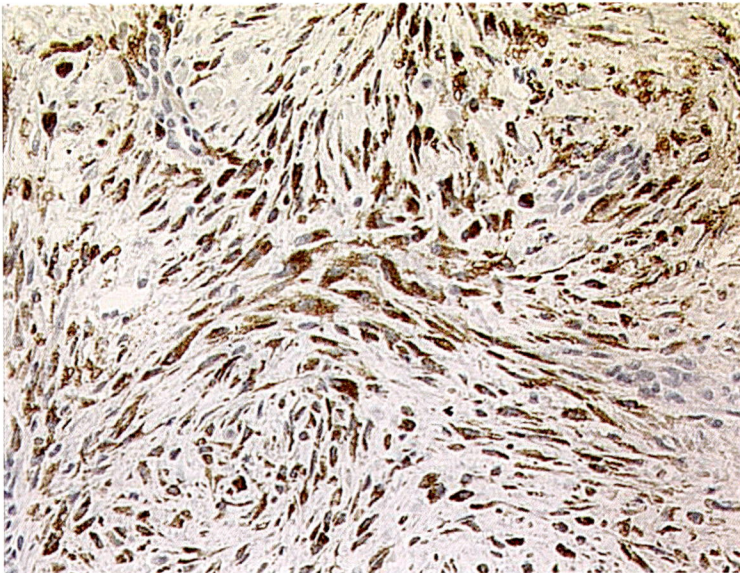

FIG 4.2   c-kit expression in a gastrointestinal stromal tumor.

A negative reaction for CD 34 combined with an expression of EMA, CK, CD 99, and Bcl2 will support a diagnosis of monophasic synovial sarcoma.

Originally considered specific of the peripheral neuroectodermal tumor, CD99 is a membrane marker expressed in a wide variety of entities; including peripheral neuroectodermal tumor, synovial sarcoma, solitary fibrous tumor, mesenchymal chondrosarcoma, neuroendocrine carcinoma, alveolar rhabdomyosarcoma, and lymphoblastic lymphoma.

4.2.3 Lymphoid Markers

Lymphoid markers such as CD45, CD3, CD20, and CD30 should be included in the panel of tested antibodies if one suspects a primary soft tissue large cell lymphoma and in some instances of round cell tumors.

4.2.4 Vascular Markers

CD34, CD31, and factor-VIII-related antigen are markers of endothelial differentiation. CD31 is the most sensitive and specific marker, which is not for CD34. Factor-VIII-related antigen is, in theory, absolutely specific for vascular tumors. However, because von Willebrand Factor is not produced only by endothelial cells, being a component in a circulating serum, it can be found in areas of hemorrhage and tumor necrosis. Let us recall that epithelial markers could be positive in vascular tumors, particularly epithelioid hemangioendothelioma and angiosarcoma.

4.2.5 Additional Markers

Immunohistochemistry is a relatively young and evolving science. New techniques and new markers are added to our diagnostic arsenal every year. For example, techniques of "antigen retrieval" (heat-induced epitope retrieval) and new detection systems allow the revision of already or previously recognized sensitivity and specificity of given markers. New classes of markers, given the heterogeneity of some soft tissue sarcoma, will impact their diagnostic accuracy and their biological comprehension. Thus, myogenin, a regulating protein of the transcription factors of the MyoD family, plays a critical role in the commitment of primitive mesenchymal cells toward the myogenic lineage, and therefore, these proteins are useful markers of rhabdomyoblastic differentiation before the expression of actin and desmin could be identified.

Mast cells, melanocytes, germ cells, some subsets of hematopoietic cells, and the interstitial cells of Cajal of the gastrointestinal tract normally express CD117, the c-Kit proto-oncongene product of a transmembrane receptor for a stem cell factor. CD117 is positive in numerous gastrointestinal stromal tumors (85–100%). One must be aware that CD117 gives positive results in cases of intraabdominal desmoid (fibromatosis), probably depending on the type of antibody used. A subset of other neoplasms are also positive for CD117 including seminoma, mast cell disease, rare cases of melanoma, angiosarcoma, and peripheral neuroectodermal tumor.

Human Herpes Virus type 8 (HHV8) is present invariably in Kaposi sarcoma, whatever its clinical variety. It can be detected either by methods of molecular biology (reverse transcript polymerase chain reaction [RT–PCR]), although the detection of the HHV8 latent antigen nuclear by immunohistochemistry on fixed paraffin-embedded specimens is also a sensitive and specific reaction to differentiate Kaposi sarcoma from other morphologically similar tumors.

The fusion transcript of the specific translocation t(11 ; 22) of tumors of Ewing sarcoma/peripheral neuroectodermal tumor spectrum can be revealed by immuno-histochemistry; the antibody reacts with the carboxy-terminal of the FLI 1 protein. It is positive in about 70% of cases and is more specific than CD99. However, positive reactions also have been reported with lymphoblastic lymphoma and in more than 95% of endothelial neoplasms of all types and degrees of malignancy.

Although immunohistochemistry has evolved since the early 1980s (new antibodies emergence—newer techniques of detection—evaluation of specificity and sensibility, etc.), the 1990s will pay testimony to additional methods of diagnosis, particularly molecular biology, which increasingly contributes to the accuracy of the diagnosis and the comprehension of the biology of tumors. Despite all the good news, there are and there always will be difficult cases (i.e., those tumors that "do not read the books"). Every pathologist/cytopathologist sometimes is frustrated with a particular tumor he has to sign out "pleomorphic malignant tumor, not otherwise specified (NOS), or immunohistochemical profile noncontributory." The typical examples of that "un-classified class" of neoplasms are some sarcomatoid carcinomas negative for epithelial markers and, conversely, sarcomas positive for the same markers. Moreover, molecular biology techniques have shown the continuing emergence of visceral mesenchymal tumors, including synovial sarcoma of the prostate and of the gastro-intestinal tract, for which the immunohistochemical profile did not contribute to the diagnosis. One can face similar problems with other neoplasic lesions, for example, epithelioid sarcomas, melanomas, and large cell anaplastic lymphomas.

In conclusion, immunohistochemistry is a powerful tool in the accuracy of diagnosis in soft tissue tumors. However, the reader must be aware of the limitation and the pitfalls inherent to the use of this ancillary technique. Careful and constant correlation with the orthopedic surgeon, the radiologist, and the cytopathologist must be emphasized, as wells as the integration of complementary information in the present and the future literature.

4.3 GENETIC TECHNIQUES

Jérôme Couturier, MD

Despite progress in the histopathological classification of soft tissue tumors in recent years, their accurate diagnosis often remains challenging because of overlapping features or poor differentiation, especially for round-cell tumors and undifferentiated sarcomas. Numerous soft tissue tumors types are characterized by recurrent chromosomal translocations related to the formation of specific fusion genes (Table 4.1). This specificity has made cytogenetic and molecular analyses an important part of the diagnostic process in soft tissue tumors [4,5]. Core-needle biopsies (CNBs) and FNAs are well suited for these techniques [6–8]. An advantage of FNA is that it permits collecting numerous tumor cells, with a low contamination of stroma, especially in round-cell tumors. Techniques currently used for detecting transloca-tions are karyotyping, in situ hybridization, and RT-PCR. A subset of soft tissue tumors is not associated with specific translocations, but exhibits characteristic

TABLE 4.1 **Specific chromosome translocations and gene fusions useful for diagnosis**

Entity	Chromosome translocations	Gene fusions
Ewing sarcoma/peripheral neuroectodermal tumor	t(11;22)(q24.3;q12.2) t(21;22)(q22.2;q12.2) t(7;22)(p21.2;q12.2) t(2;22)(q35;q12.2)	*EWSR1/FLI1, ERG, ETV1, FEV*
Desmoplastic small round cell tumor	t(11;22)(p13;q12.2)	*EWSR1/WT1*
Clear cell sarcoma	t(12;22)(q13.12;q12.2) t(2;22)(q33.3;q12.2)	*EWSR1/ATF1, CREB1*
Extraskeletal myxoid chondrosarcoma	t(9;22)(q22.33;q12.2) t(9;17)(q22.33;q12) t(9;15)(q22.33;q21.3)	*EWSR1, TAF15, TCF12/NR4A3*
Alveolar rhabdomyosarcoma	t(2;13)(q36.1;q14.11) t(1;13)(p36.13;q14.11)	*PAX3, PAX7/FOXO1*
Myxoid/round cell liposarcoma	t(12;16)(q13.3;p11.2) t(12;22)(q13.3;q12.2)	*FUS, EWSR1/DDIT3*
Angiomatoid fibrous histiocytoma	t(12;16)(q13.12;p11.2) t(12;22)(q13.12;q12.2) t(2;22)(q33.3; q12.2)	*FUS, EWSR1/ATF1 EWSR1/CREB1*
Low-grade fibromyxoid sarcoma	t(7;16)(q33;p11.2) t(11;16)(p11.2;p11.2)	*FUS/CREB3L2, CREB3L1*
Synovial sarcoma	t(X;18)(p11.22;q11.2)	*SS18/SSX1, SSX2, SSX4*
Dermatofibrosarcoma protuberans/Giant cell fibroblastoma	r, t(17;22)(q21.33;q13.1)	*COL1A1/PDGFB*
Infantile fibrosarcoma/Cellular mesoblastic nephroma	t(12;15)(p13.2;q25.3)	*ETV6/NTRK3*
Alveolar soft tissue sarcoma	der(17)t(X;17)(p11.23;q25.3)	*ASPSCR1/TFE3*

chromosome imbalances, losses, gains, or amplifications [9–11]. Profiles of these imbalances can be set up using tumor DNA hybridization on genome-wide micro-arrays comparative genome hybridization [CGH] or single nucleotide polymorphism [SNP] arrays [12]. Of course, other molecular assays currently not used as first-line diagnostic tests are used in translational research on soft tissue tumors, such as mutations and transcriptome analyses.

4.3.1 Karyotyping

Karyotype analysis is the classical method for identifying chromosome rearrangements in tumors, and almost all specific translocations known in soft tissue tumors have been detected using this method. Chromosome rearrangements known in soft tissue tumors are reported in Table 4.1. Karyotyping requires a short-term culture of fresh tumor cells after disaggregation. Soft tissue tumors can be divided roughly into the following types: round-cell tumors, mainly observed in children and young adults, and spindle-cell tumors, occurring more frequently in adults. Round-cell tumors, which are poorly cohesive, are submitted to mechanical dissociation with scalpels, grown in suspension, and harvested in 24–48 hours. Spindle-cell tumors require enzymatic disaggregation, usually by collagenase, and are grown as mono-layer cultures in plastic flasks. Cells usually are harvested for karyotyping 48 hours after the first splitting of the flask. The duration of culture is usually around 10–15 days and should not be extended beyond that time limit because of an overgrowth of normal fibroblasts from the stroma. Cytogenetic analysis requires relatively large samples (>0.5 cm^3); CNBs are not reliable samples for karyotyping, whereas FNAs can yield several million cells in round-cell tumors that are well suited for cultivation in suspension. After blockade of cells at the metaphase stage by colchicine, cultures are harvested and submitted to hypotonic treatment. Then, cells are fixed and spread on slides. Karyotypes are analyzed after G- or R-banding [13]. The analysis can be helped further by in situ hybridization. The main interest of karyotype analysis is that it is a genome-wide technique that does not require the knowledge of a suspected rearrangement. However, one must be aware of the fact that soft tissue tumors may not proliferate in vitro and, also, that false normal results can be obtained because of the mitotic activity of inflammatory or stromal cells.

4.3.2   In Situ Hybridization

This technique makes it possible to visualize specific DNA sequences (probes) and to detect their rearrangements on chromosomes or in interphase nuclei [14]. FISH uses probes labeled with fluorochromes, usually red and green, and chromosomes or nuclei are counterstained in blue by DAPI. It remains the gold standard of in situ hybridization techniques, even if chromogen-based methods now are emerging. The use of "break apart" dual color probes is the most reliable strategy for detecting translocations by FISH in soft tissue tumors (Fig 4.3). The DNA sequence of the gene of interest is covered by two probes, a proximal one labeled in red, for example, and a distal one labeled in green. The two probes are separated by a gap corresponding to the region of breakpoints. So a bicolor signal means a normal gene, and a split between the red and green signals means a translocation of the gene.

Other soft tissue tumors, such as well-differentiated liposarcoma, are character-ized by the presence of gene amplifications (e.g., *MDM2*, for well-differentiated liposarcoma). FISH is an appropriate technique for the detection of amplifications. Two probes labeled with different fluorochromes are cohybridized—a locus-specific probe of the gene of interest and a centromeric probe corresponding to the chromosome carrying the gene tested. The ratio of the copy number of the locus-specific probe over that of the centromeric probe is calculated, and an amplification exists if this ratio is >2. Multiple copies of the amplified gene often are grouped in clusters in interphase nuclei, corresponding to the presence of homogeneously staining regions (hsr), described in metaphase chromosomes.

FISH is a very fast and sensitive technique, and it has the advantage of being applicable to a variety of tumor materials, including sections from frozen or paraffin-embedded CNBs, FNAs, and cytogenetic preparations. On tissue sections, the FISH procedure preserves morphology, making it possible to focus the analysis on cells of interest. And also, as is shown in Table 4.1, a tumor can be characterized by a translocation of a pivot gene that can fuse to variant partners. This partner can be known or unknown; FISH has the advantage of being able to detect any transloca-tion of the gene of interest, whatever the partner.

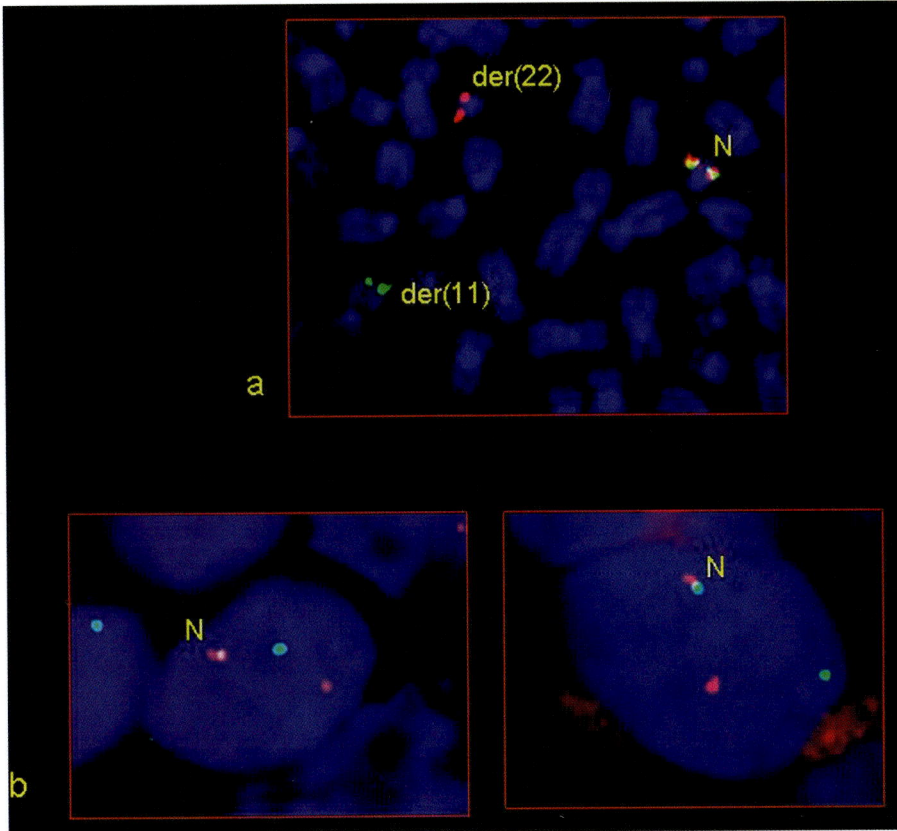

FIG 4.3 FISH with a EWSR1 dual-color breakapart probe on a Ewing tumor. The dual-color signal is split by the EWSR1 translocation. N: normal EWSR1 region on chromosome 22; der(22): derived chromosome 22 (red); der(11): derived chromosome 11 (green). (a) Metaphase chromosomes of the tumor. (b) Interphase nuclei on a section of paraffin-embedded tumor tissue.

4.3.3 RT-PCR

Fusion genes produce specific fusion transcripts that can be detected using RT-PCR assay [4,5]. It requires the knowledge of the potential variant fusions occurring in a given tumor type, and multiplex tests assaying several target sequences should be designed. Naturally, unknown variant fusions are missed by the test. RT-PCR can be used with frozen or paraffin-embedded CNBs and FNAs. Real-time RT-PCR has the advantage of high sensitivity, making it applicable on limited amounts of material, but it is dependent on the quality of the extracted RNA. Snap frozen tissue is the most reliable material for the technique, although some labs obtain satisfactory results from paraffin-embedded material, provided it had been fixed adequately. Attention should be paid to the risk of false positivity resulting from contamination in the pre-PCR step or from nonspecific annealing of the primers. Amplified fragments may be verified by sequencing. RT-PCR is a widely used test for the diagnosis of fusion transcripts in soft tissue sarcoma.

4.3.4 Genome-Wide Profiling

Some soft tissue tumors types are not characterized at present by specific translocations leading to gene fusions but by nonrandom imbalances of chromosome segments, losses, gains, or amplifications (Fig 4.4). Genome-wide profiles of these imbalances can be obtained using CGH or SNP arrays [12]. This technique is based on the hybridization of labeled tumor DNA on a whole-genome microarray (DNA chip), comprising from about 40×10^3 to more than 2×10^6 oligonucleotide probes. A resolution of $60-70 \times 10^3$ is, at present, sufficient for the detection of relevant copy number changes for a diagnostic purpose in soft tissue tumors at a reasonable cost. The tumor cell content in the sample should be $>50\%$. CGH or SNP arrays have the advantage of obtaining a high-resolution genome-wide profile from fresh or frozen CNBs and FNAs, with a resolution more than 100-fold higher than that of karyotyping and without eventual failures related to cell culture. However, balanced rearrangements remain undetected.

The microarray technology can be applied to transcriptome analysis, but this approach, if used in translational research, has not yet proven its utility in the clinical setting.

4.3.5 Collection and Management of the Samples

4.3.5.1 Core-Needle Biopsies. Biopsies intended for molecular analysis are collected in cryotubes and are frozen instantly in liquid nitrogen. A minimum of two biopsies put in separate tubes is recommended. Tubes are stored at $-80°C$ or in liquid nitrogen. They can be shipped in dry ice if necessary. Frozen sections can be prepared for FISH, or RNA or DNA can be extracted for performing RT-PCR or genome profiling. When a technique based on nucleic acids extraction is used, it is of good practice to check the tumor cell content on a frozen section of the fragment analyzed. CNBs usually are not suitable for karyotype analysis because of their limited volume. Fixed and paraffin-embedded CNBs are adequate for FISH, but the detection of fusion transcripts from this material may be difficult as a result of fragmentation of RNA by the fixation procedure.

4.3.5.2 Fine Needle Aspirates. FNAs can be collected directly in cryotubes— two separate tubes, when possible—and instantly frozen, but it is recommended to

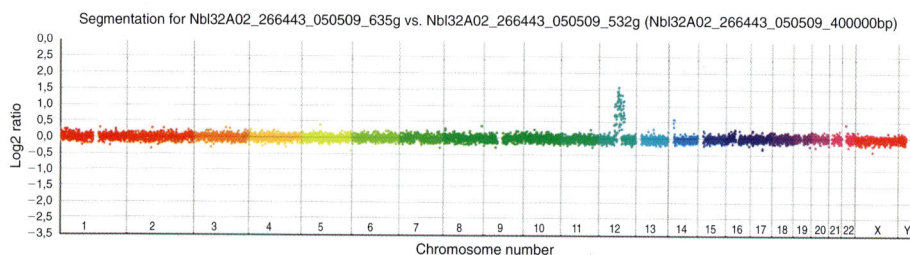

FIG 4.4 Genome profile of a well-differentiated liposarcoma obtained by CGH array on a NimbleGen 72K microarray. Presence of an amplification in the chromosome région 12q14-q15, including MDM2 and CDK4 genes.

evaluate the quality and the quantity of the sample and also to keep the possibility to perform, parallel with the RT-PCR assay, a karyotype analysis or a FISH test. In this case, the cytological sample is collected in 10-ml ethylene diamine tetra acetic acid (EDTA) Vacutainer^R type tubes filled with 7 ml of serumless RPMI culture medium, for example. Nucleated cells are enumerated quickly, and according to the available number of cells, the sample is split into several aliquotes for the various techniques that may be indicated and for storage. Fine-needle aspiration is especially helpful for round-cell tumors in which it often yields a high number of cells with a low contamination by the stroma. The cells obtained have intact nuclei and are well suited for FISH analysis.

4.3.6 Diagnostic and Molecular Classification of Soft Tissue Tumors

4.3.6.1 Diagnosis of Malignancy. The diagnosis of malignancy is usually the first objective of a FNA or a CNB. The observation of genomic alterations, even unbalanced, by karyotype or a CGH analysis is not a criterion of malignancy, and several types of soft tissue benign tumors bear chromosome abnormalities. The diagnosis will be made based on the specific rearrangements observed. For example, the differential diagnosis between lipoma and well-differentiated liposarcoma may be challenging, but the latter displays a characteristic amplification of the *MDM2* gene [9]. Another example is the low-grade fibromyxoid sarcoma, a malignant tumor with bland histologic features, with a characteristic t(7;16) translocation leading to a fusion *FUS/CREB3L2*.

4.3.6.2 Molecular Classification. Soft tissue tumors can be divided into the following main groups based on their genetics: those with simple or relatively simple recurrent chromosome rearrangements, (i.e., translocations resulting in gene fusions or amplifications, occurring in about 40% of sarcomas, and representing about 20 different sarcomas types [3−5,11], and those with complex rearrangements, which concern mainly pleomorphic sarcomas [9,10].

Typically, sarcoma-associated translocations lead to the fusion of transcription factors or of tyrosine kinase genes, which leads to their deregulation. The identification of specific rearrangements has refined the classification of soft tissue tumors considerably since the past two decades and these molecular markers have been taken into account in the latest World Health Organization (WHO) classification [15,16]. Based on an identical translocation, histologically distinct tumors have been grouped in a single tumor type, such as Ewing's sarcoma and peripheral neuroectodermal tumor or myxoid and round cell liposarcoma. Conversely, tumor types sometimes difficult to differentiate based on their histological features, such as solid-alveolar and poorly differentiated embryonal rhabdomyosarcoma, can be characterized reliably by the presence or absence of a specific gene fusion.

Well-differentiated liposarcoma, which may raise a difficult differential diagnosis with lipoma, is also a tumor with relatively simple cytogenetics, with ring chromosomes in excess carrying amplifications of the *MDM2* and, less frequently, *CDK4* genes mapping to chromosome bands 12q14-q15 [11]. The diagnosis is performed easily by FISH on tissue sections.

About 60% of soft tissue tumors, mainly adult spindle-cell and pleomorphic sarcomas, and so-called MFH lack a specific translocation and show complex rearrangements. However, the analysis of several of these tumors by CGH array has shown that approximately 20% of them show an amplification of *MDM2* and often *CDK4* and, therefore, are dedifferentiated liposarcoma [10,16,17]. In these cases, an additional amplification occurs of either *JUN* or *MAP3K5*, mapping to 1p32 and 6q23, respectively [18,19]. Genome-wide profiling is the test of choice for detecting potential multiple amplifications.

The identification of specific chromosome rearrangements has made molecular techniques helpful ancillary tools for the precise diagnosis of soft tissue tumors. In practice, the molecular diagnosis strategy must be adapted according to the suspected type of tumor. RT-PCR or FISH usually are used as first-line techniques for translocation tumors when fresh or frozen material is available. FISH is used preferentially for paraffin-embedded material. FISH is also the appropriate technique for the detection of *MDM2/CDK4* amplification for the diagnosis of well-differentiated liposarcoma. The CGH array is well suited for the analysis of coamplifications characteristic of dedifferentiated liposarcoma. Interpreted in conjunction with cytologic and histologic data, results of all these techniques will contribute to an accurate diagnosis, which is a prerequisite for an effective treatment of patients, particularly for targeted therapy eligibility.

Because pediatric oncology is among the poles of excellence at Institut Curie, considerable attention has been paid and much emphasis have been focused on the routine use of FNA biopsy and genetics in terms of diagnosis, prognosis, and targeted therapies of solid tumors. Entities like Ewing/peripheral neuroectomermic tumor and desmoplastic small round cell tumor will be discussed and enhanced in later chapters and will demonstrate how these ancillary procedures, combined with adequate immunohistochemistry, are mandatory adjuvants in the management of pediatric neoplasms.

4.4 GRADING OF SOFT TISSUE TUMORS

Réal Lagacé, MD, FRCPC

The histological type of soft tissue sarcoma does not always provide sufficient information to predict its clinical course and therefore to plan therapy. It is widely recognized that grading is the most important prognostic factor and the best indicator of metastasis risk in adult soft tissue sarcoma. Grading based on histological parameters only evaluates the malignant potential of a given tumor and the probability for development of distant metastases. On the other hand, staging based on both clinical and histological parameters provides information on the extension of the tumor.

Several grading systems, most relying on various histological parameters, have been proposed and therefore tested and have proved to correlate with prognosis. The most controversial point is the respective values of histologic typing and grading [20,21]. The mitotic index and the importance of tumor necrosis seem to be the two most important parameters to predict the outcome/biologic behavior of soft tissue sarcoma. Presently, there is a large consensus among pathologists to use two different systems, the National Cancer Institute (NCI) and the Fédération Nationale des Centres de Lutte contre le Cancer (FNCLCC).

The NCI system relies on the histological type, the pleomorphism, and the mitotic index of a sarcoma. The parameters account for sarcomas grades I and III. The rest of the tumors are either grades II or III according to the percentage of tumor necrosis, with a threshold of 15% to separate sarcomas of grades II and III.

The FNCLCC system also evaluates three parameters selected after a multivariate analysis of several histological features, tumor differentiation, mitotic rate, and percentage of tumor necrosis. A score is attributed independently to each parameter (tumor differentiation 1 to 3, tumor necrosis 1 or 2 according to less than or more than 50% of tumor necrosis, mitosis 1 to 3, according to 1 to 9, 9 to 19, and 20 and more mitoses / 10 HPF), and the grade is obtained by adding the three attributed scores [22]. The most controversial point is the respective values of histological typing and grading. This system was found useful in more them 90% of adult sarcomas and later on has been adapted to pediatric nonrhabdomyosarcomatous sarcomas [23]. It has been stated that the system was not suitable for core needle biopsies.

A comparative study [24] of both systems was done in a series of 410 patients by univariate analysis. The prognostic value was good for the two systems, although 34% grade II discrepancies were discovered. Using the NCI system, there were more grade II sarcomas. A better correlation was noted with overall prognosis and metastase-free survival with the FNCLCC system.

Given the limitations and the pitfalls of grading, it is very important to respect the following rules to obtain the highest performance and reproducibility of the systems. Grading is used only for untreated primary soft tissue tumors. It should be applied on representative and well-processed materiel. Grading is not a substitute for histological diagnosis and does not differentiate benign and malignant lesions, and therefore, before grading, one must be sure that one is dealing with a true sarcoma and not a pseudosarcoma. Grading is not applicable to all types of soft tissue sarcoma; the significance of the histological parameters differs for various sarcomas. Therefore, grade is of no prognostic value for some histological types such as malignant peripheral nerve sheath tumor. It is not recommended for entities like angiosarcoma, extraskeletal myxoid chondrosarcoma, low-grade fibromyxoid sarcoma, alveolar soft port sarcoma, clear cell sarcoma, epithelioid sarcoma, and dedifferentiated liposarcoma. On the other hand, a recent study [25] has shown that the FNCLCC system has the most predictive factor of metastasis for pleomorphic sarcoma and synovial sarcomas and has the second and third independent factor for leiomyosarcoma and liposarcoma.The parameters of grading must be evaluated carefully particularly for mitosis counting, which should be done rigorously.

There are numerous controversies in the literature regarding the tentative of grading with aspirates and core needle biopsy specimens. As a rule, one can state that FNA cytology of soft tissue tumors generally is limited best to centers with a high case volume and a well-integrated multidisciplinary team because careful clinico-pathologic correlation and considerable experience are required to make an accurate diagnosis. Moreover, one has to take into consideration the problems of unavoidable limited sampling, which has an impact on the diagnostic accuracy and the access to materiel for ancillary procedures.

A limited number of studies have attempted to determine the degree of reliability of FNA in the initial diagnosis of soft tissue lesions. In a retrospective study of 301 soft tissue lesions of the extremities and trunk [26], sensitivity and specificity for diagnosising of a malignant lesion were 92% and 97% respectively. More specifically, subgrouping and grading of soft tissue tumors by FNA gave contradictory results. Whereas sarcomas were recognized adequately in 92% of cases, subtype was identified in only 14%. Discrepancies in grading were observed among different types of sarcoma. A correlative cytological/histological review showed that the assigned cytologic grade accurately reflected the histologic grade in 90% of sarcomas, when segregated into high and low grades [27]. Pleomorphic, small round cell, and epithelioid/polygonal subgroups corresponded to high-grade sarcomas in all cases with only minor noncorrelations. Major grading miscorrelations occurred in 50% of myxoid and 90% of spindle cell sarcomas. Another study dealing with the grading of spindle cell sarcomas in FNA specimens applying the histological parameters of grading was done in a limited series of 36 specimens [28], without knowledge of the sarcoma subtype. Three grades were assigned according to the following: grade I was assigned for minimal nuclear atypia and overlap, absence of necrosis, and mitotic figures; grade II was characterized by moderate nuclear atypia, at least a moderate overlap, appreciable mitotic figures, and necrosis; severe nuclear atypia distinguished grade III from grade II. One major noncorrelation between FNA and histologic grade was defined as misclassifications of grade I versus grades II or III. A major noncorrelation resulted from a probable FNA interpretation error. In 15 of 16 FNA, specimens of grades II or III sarcomas lacking mitoses, necrosis, or both, the degree of nuclear atypia reflected the grade. In the remaining case, the degree of nuclear overlap and necrosis determined the grade. The authors concluded that the histologic grading of sarcoma could be applied accurately to most FNA specimens of spindle cell sarcomas without knowledge of the sarcoma subtype.

A review [29] of a series of 54 cases of histologically documented spindle cell sarcomas attempted to determine the accuracy of cytological grading of spindle cell sarcomas. The FNA specimens were graded according to a three-tier system proposed for FNA smears, whereas the histological sections were graded using the FNLCLCC system; hence, the cytological grading was correlated with the histological grade. The overall cytologic and histologic concordance was 40/54 (74%) cases for each grade, the respective concordance was 9/13 (69%) for grade I, 19/25 (76%) for grade II, and 17/16 (75%) for grade III cases. Major noncorrelation was noted in 10/54 (18.5%) cases, and minor correlation was noted in 4/54 (7.4%) cases, hence the statement that "it is possible to accurately predict the grade in 74% of cases of spindle cell sarcomas." Cytological and histological concordance was better (75%) for high grades (grade II and III) as compared with grade I sarcomas (60%). Sampling error caused by morphologic heterogeneity in sarcomas could cause noncorrelation in a few cases.

Another study [30] investigated the ability of FNA to subtype and grade accurately a series of 107 primary sarcomas of the musculoskeletal system. Corresponding surgical material was available for 77 cases. The surgical material was rereviewed for accuracy of diagnosis and for assignment of grade independently of the cytologic examination. The correlation of cytologic with the histopathologic grade was made and analyzed by the kappa test. Correlation between cytological and surgical grades was significant for all three observers (p < .001). Only the nuclear grade showed a consistent correlation in the predicted final surgical grade. Cellularity, mitotic rate, and the presence of necrosis were not statistically significant for predicting histopathologic grade. Accurate exact subtyping by cytologic examination was achieved in +/−55% of cases. The prediction of histopathological subtype by cytologic analysis was most successful when stroma was present or when high-grade features indicative of MFH were observed. There was little agreement in relation to the histopathologic type as predicted by cytology for low-grade spindle cell sarcoma. Although this study showed a statistically significant correlation between the cytologically assigned grade and the final histopathological grade, statistical analysis revealed only a moderate correlation between the two. Cytological analysis tended to undergrade in comparison with final histopathological grading. Only analysis of nuclear atypia showed a good correlation with the final surgical grade. FNA was only moderately successful at predicting the subtype for musculoskeletal sarcomas in this series.

Previous correlative cytological/histological studies realized in our institution from a selection of 2378 soft tissue tumor, benign, intermediary, and malignant neoplasms will be emphasized in the forthcoming chapters.

4.5 FUTURE INVESTIGATIONS OF ANCILLARY TECHNIQUES

Stamatios Theocharis, MD, PhD,

4.5.1 The Omics Technologies in Soft Tissue Tumors Detection, Classification, and Treatment

Soft tissue sarcomas define a group of histologically and genetically diverse tumors that account for approximately 1% of all adult malignancies with an annual incidence in the United States of approximately 9000 cases with more than 50 histologic subtypes [31,32]. Soft tissue sarcoma subtypes are diagnosed by morphological findings, immunophenotyping, and karyotyping assisted by molecular analysis of specific-gene rearrangements. Because of the rarity of the disease and the pleomorphic features, soft tissue sarcoma misdiagnosis remains a common pitfall and may result in treatment delay or in the inadvertent use of ineffective, highly toxic therapies [33,34].

The molecular classification of soft tissue sarcomas includes two major categories based on the following: 1) a single recurrent genetic alteration, such as chromosomal translocations or activating mutation, and 2) nonrecurrent genetic aberrations, which form part of a complex abnormal karyotype [35]. On the other hand, the therapeutic options remain limited for soft tissue sarcoma patients for whom frontline chemotherapy regimens fails [36]. For these reasons, a better understanding of soft tissue tumor biology is of critical importance to improve current diagnostic and prognostic markers and to enhance therapeutic interventions. The advantages occurring from the application of the "Omics" technologies (genomics, proteomics, and metabolomics), are of crucial importance in the discovery of new biomarkers and the underline pathways. These technologies recently have been applied for cancer diagnosis, prognosis, and response to treatment. The data available so far on Omics technologies application in soft tissue sarcomas are included in the following sections.

4.5.2 Genomics

Genomics is related to the study of an organism's entire genome. Post-DNA sequencing [37], the dramatic improvement of related technology, and the establishment of specific microarrays enable us to assess, simultaneously, the expression levels of thousands of genes in the same sample. In such microarray analysis, it is important to profile as many tumor specimens as possible, covering a spectrum of conventionally determined diagnoses. These results can identify genes that discriminate subsets within a diagnostic entity and can reveal discordances between conventional diagnoses and gene expression patterns. If clinical data are available, then genes that correlate with clinically relevant end points such as stage, therapeutic response, and metastasis also can be identified. From these analyses, the investigator compiles lists of genes that are relatively disease specific and may relate to a diagnostic subset analysis or clinical correlates. These lists then can be mined to identify potentially useful diagnostic markers and genes that might participate in growth-regulatory pathways [38]. Although cancer diagnosis relied primarily on histopathological and/or cytological criteria, the genomic expression patterns provided a novel concept for diagnosis, especially when the malignancy distinction is difficult to achieve with standard methods (clinical, radiological, specimen microscopic, or immunohistochemical examination). Additionally, the discovery of multigene predictive disease models for specific tumor types allowed clinicians to identify high-risk individuals who where deemed to have early stage disease by the current staging techniques. Such an approach enables both an early diagnosis and subsequent therapeutic intervention [39].

In recent years, different gene expression studies on sarcoma have been conducted, but the small sample size was a limiting factor for many of them [40]. Genomic profiling of soft tissue sarcoma subtypes reveals a propensity for tumors of less karyotypic diversity to segregate from the more pleomorphic subtypes. Certain statistical methods can distinguish pleomorphic subgroups from other sarcomas. One of the initial studies analyzed 41 soft tissue sarcoma samples by cDNA microarray of 5520 genes [41]. In this study, synovial sarcoma and GIST samples formed distinct groups. Interestingly, almost half the leiomyosarcoma samples formed a clustering group, whereas the remaining leiomyosarcoma samples clustered with that of malignant fibrous histiocytoma and liposarcomas. Peripheral nerve sheath tumors formed the last distinct group. In the same study, the GIST samples clustered by their own set of 125 genes. The GIST samples presented a different gene expression than the leiomyosarcoma group, also providing evidence for the origin of cells responsible for these tumors [41]. More recently, Price et al. presented a sensitive and specific two-gene classifier capable of distinguishing GIST from leiomyosarcoma with a top-scoring pair analysis [42].

Another important study was conducted on 51 soft tissue sarcoma cases, representing different histological subtypes [43]. The study focused on high-grade lesions, which usually pose a diagnostic challenge and potentially would benefit from molecular-based classification. Statistical tests were performed on experimental groups identified by cluster analysis to find discriminating genes that subsequently could be applied in a support vector machine algorithm [43,44]. Synovial sarcomas, round cell/myxoid liposarcomas, clear cell sarcomas, and GISTs displayed remarkably distinct and homogenous gene expression profiles, whereas pleomorphic tumors proved heterogeneous. A subset of malignant fibrous histiocytomas, a controversial histological subtype, was identified as a distinct genomic group. The support vector machine algorithm supported a genomic basis for a diagnosis presenting high sensitivity and specificity [43,44]. In another study of genomic profiling of sarcomas, 181 tumor specimens representing 16 classes of soft tissue sarcomas and osteosarcomas were characterized for biomarker analysis, gene ontology, and gene/pathway discovery. The results of the study proposed a different profile in tyrosine kinases and receptor tyrosine kinases associated with each sarcoma subtype [45].

A novel approach for the detection of subclinical disease in Ewing family tumors using gene expression profiles recently was reported by Cheung et al. [46]. A set of genes identified by microarray analysis provided prognostic information and served as a more sensitive and specific means to detect subclinical disease than the standard fusion protein with prognostic implications [46].

Previous sarcoma gene expression profiling studies reported that liposarcomas tended to cluster with malignant fibrous histiocytoma and leiomyosarcoma. However, cases with specific liposarcoma subtypes were extremely limited in these studies, making clear distinction impossible between specific subtypes [41,43]. A liposarcoma-specific RNA expression profiling study compared eight pleomorphic with eight dedifferentiated liposarcomas and reported no correlation between the expression data and the histopathologic subtype [47]. Another liposarcoma-specific microarray study of 28 liposarcomas (11 well differentiated, 3 dedifferentiated, 7 myxoid, and 7 round cell) and eight lipomas found by hierarchical clustering analysis that the dedifferentiated tumors formed a cluster with the myxoid/round cell subtype and that the well-differentiated liposarcomas clustered with lipoma [48]. According to the previous study, it was impossible to distinguish well-differentiated liposarcoma from lipoma based on gene expression profiles, and the incorrect grouping of dedifferentiated samples with myxoid/round cell tumors was most likely because of the limited sample numbers analyzed in the study. Another problem of such studies enrolling a limited number of cases per subgroup was that the same data set was used for both gene signature discovery and model validation. In a more recent study, a 142-gene predictor of tissue class was derived to determine automatically the class of an independent validation set of lipomatous samples and showed the feasibility of liposarcoma classification based entirely on gene expression monitoring. Differentially expressed genes for each liposarcoma subtype compared with normal fat were used to identify histology-specific candidate genes with an indepth analysis of signaling pathways that are important to liposarcoma pathogenesis and to progression in the well-differentiated/dedifferentiated subset [49].

The activation of cell cycle and checkpoint pathways in well-differentiated/dedifferentiated liposarcoma also provided several possible novel therapeutic strategies with *MDM2* serving as a particularly promising target. It also was shown that Nutlin 3a, an *MDM2* antagonist, preferentially induced apoptosis and growth arrest in dedifferentiated liposarcoma cells compared with normal adipocytes. Such results support the development of a clinical trial with *MDM2* antagonists for liposarcoma subtypes that overexpress *MDM2* and show the promise of using this expression data set for a new drug discovery in liposarcoma [19]. Widely used histopathologic and clinical criteria, such as liposarcoma subtype, location, age, and size, can be incorporated into liposarcoma-specific nomograms and used to estimate patient outcome [50].

4.5.3 Proteomics

Recent development in cancer biology has been the study of global protein expression, an approach known as proteomics. The discordance between specific mRNA and protein expression makes this platform much more useful. Additionally, as the findings at the protein level are more applicable to subsequent immunohistochemical studies, the results can be validated using routinely processed paraffin-embedded tissues and clinical information [51,52]. Proteomic technologies have been used to develop novel molecular subclassifications and diagnostic biomarkers for different malignancies. A two-dimensional difference gel electrophoresis (2D-DIGE) was used to generate the global protein expression profiles of 80 soft tissue sarcoma samples with seven different histopathological backgrounds. Sixty-seven protein spots distinguished the subtypes of soft tissue sarcoma. Hierarchical clustering with these 67 protein spots resulted in the grouping of all 80 sarcoma samples corresponding to histological classification. The expression pattern of tropomyosin isoforms was different in conventional and pleomorphic leiomyosarcoma. Different proteins, including alpha 1 antitrypsin, alpha actinin 1, HSP 27, and elongation factor 2, were identified that could differentiate between malignant fibrous histiocytomas and leiomyosarcoma in grade II into low- and high-risk patients' groups, which differed significantly with respect to survival rates. Such results established proteomics as a powerful tool to develop novel biomarkers for the diagnosis and molecular classification of soft tissue sarcomas. The identification of proteins associated with survival in a grade-III sarcoma will allow delineation of a high-risk group that may benefit from adjuvant therapy and the exclusion of low-risk patients in whom additional therapies are unlikely to exhibit clinical benefit [53]. Using 2D-DIGE and mass spectrometry, global protein expression studies also were performed on bone and soft tissue sarcomas to develop novel diagnostic and therapeutic biomarkers and allow molecular classification of the tumors. Among 1500 protein variants identified in the 2D-DIGE, 67 proteins correctly distinguished the eight subtypes of 99 histologically classified soft tissue sarcomas. Hierarchical clustering demonstrated leiomyosarcoma, and malignant fibrous histiocytomas shared a similar protein expression profile; clear cell sarcoma, synovial sarcoma, and malignant peripheral nerve sheath tumor could be grouped according to their protein expression patterns. Pleomorphic leiomyosarcoma and malignant fibrous histiocytomas presented similar tropomyosin isoform expression patterns. Patients with GIST expressing pfetin protein presented better survival rates than those whose tumors lacked it. Several protein spots associated with chemosensitivity of osteosarcoma to preoperative chemotherapy were identified and could serve as diagnostic and prognostic markers for osteosarcoma and new therapeutic targets for the disease [54]. Proteomic analysis using 2D-DIGE provides novel information on the biology of bone and soft tissue sarcomas that could be used for both the diagnosis and the treatment of these tumors.

4.5.4 Metabolomics

Metabolomics (or metabonomics) is the comprehensive analysis of the low-molecular-weight molecules, or metabolites, which are the intermediates and products of metabolism study of a global metabolite profile in a system (cell, tissue, or organism) under a given set of conditions [55,56]. Metabolites, on the one hand, result from the interaction of the system's genome with its environment; they are not merely the end product of gene expression, but they form part of the regulatory system in an integrated manner [57]. On the other hand, the metabolic fingerprint for each individual varies considerably as a consequence of diet, lifestyle, environment, and genetic effects. Disease states and drug treatments also can alter the metabolic phenotype of an individual, which has been one of the difficulties limitations for the use of metabolomics in clinical medicine [58]. No report on the use of metabolomics in soft tissue sarcomas diagnosis and treatment has been referred up to now; nevertheless, this technology could be of some importance in examining the patients' response to therapy and disease recurrences in this type of malignancy.

4.6 CONCLUSIONS

Transcriptional profiling is a powerful tool for analyzing the relationships between tumors, discovering new tumor subgroups, assigning tumors to predefined classes, and predicting disease outcome. A more systematic approach to the classification of soft tissue tumors based on gene expression analysis using microarrays should be of great importance. Continued progress on further adapting the rapidly evolving technologies of genomics and proteomics and, to a lesser extent, of metabonomics in multicenter, coordinated trials should be of critical importance for accurate diagnosis of and the most rapid reductions in morbidity and mortality from soft tissue tumors.

REFERENCES

1. Fletcher CDM, personnal communication. 1997. Meeting of the British division of the IAP.
2. Coindre JM. Immunohistochemistry in the diagnosis of soft tissue tumours. Histopathology 2003, 43: 1–16.
3. Antonescu CR. The role of genetic testing in soft tissue sarcoma. Histopathology 2006, 48: 13–21.
4. Lazar A, Abruzzo LV, Pollock RE, Lee S, Czerniak B. Molecular diagnosis of sarcomas: chromosomal translocations in sarcomas. Arch Pathol Lab Med 2006, 130: 1199–1207.
5. Gulley ML, Kaiser-Rogers KA. A rational approach to genetic testing for sarcoma. Diagn Mol Pathol 2009, 18: 1–10.
6. Kilpatrick SE, Bergman S, Pettenati MJ, Gulley ML. The usefulness of cytogenetic analysis in fine needle aspirates for the histologic subtyping of sarcomas. Mod Pathol 2006, 19: 815–819.
7. Krishnamurthy S. Applications of molecular techniques to fine-needle aspiration biopsy. Cancer 2007, 111: 106–122.
8. Barroca H. Fine needle biopsy and genetics, two allied weapons in the diagnosis, prognosis, and target therapeutics of solid pediatric tumors. Diagn Cytopathol 2008, 36: 678–684.
9. Dei Tos AP. Classification of pleomorphic sarcomas: where are we now? Histopathology 2006, 48: 51–62.
10. Guillou L, Aurias A. Soft tissue sarcomas with complex genomic profiles. Virchows Arch 2009, 456: 201–217.
11. Coindre JM, Pédeutour F, Aurias A. Well-differentiated and dedifferentiated liposarcomas. Virchows Arch 2010, 456: 167–179.
12. Dutt A, Beroukhim R. Single nucleotide polymorphism array analysis of cancer. Curr Opin Oncol 2007, 19: 43–49.

13. Shaffer LG, Tommerup N. ISCN 2009: An international system for human cytogenetic nomenclature. Basel, Switzerland: Karger, 2009.

14. Tanas MR, Goldblum JR. Fluorescence in situ hybridization in the diagnosis of soft tissue neoplasms: a review. Adv Anat Pathol 2009, 16: 383–391.

15. Fletcher CDM, Unni KK, Mertens F, World Health Organisation classification of tumours. Pathology and genetics of tumours of soft tissue and bone. editors. Lyon, France: IARC Press; 2002.

16. Fletcher CD. The evolving classification of soft tissue tumours: an update based on the new WHO classification. Histopathology 2006, 48: 3–12.

17. Idbaih A, Coindre JM, Derré J, et al. Myxoid malignant fibrous histiocytoma and pleomorphic liposarcoma share very similar genomic imbalances. Lab Invest 2005, 85: 176–181.

18. Mariani O, Brennetot C, Coindre JM, et al. JUN oncogene amplification and over-expression block adipocytic differentiation in highly aggressive sarcomas. Cancer Cell 2007, 11: 361–374.

19. Chibon F, Mariani O, Derré J, et al. ASK1 (MAP3K5) as a potential therapeutic target in malignant fibrous histiocytomas with 12q14-q15 and 6q23 amplifications. Genes Chromosomes Cancer 2004, 40: 32–37.

20. Brown FM, Fletcher CD. Problems in grading soft tissue sarcomas. Am J Clin Pathol 2000, 114: S82-S89.

21. Coindre JM. Grading of soft tissue sarcomas: a review and update. Arch Pathol Lab Med 2006, 130: 1448–1453.

22. Trojani M, Contesso G, Coindre JM, et al. Soft-tissue sarcomas of adults; study of pathological prognostic variables and definition of a histopathological grading system. Int J Cancer 1984, 33: 37–42.

23. Parham DM, Webber BL, Jenkins JJ 3rd, Cantor AB, Maurer HM. Nonrhabdomyosarcomatous soft tissue sarcomas of childhood: formulation of a simplified system for grading. Mod Pathol 1995, 8: 705–710.

24. Guillou L, Coindre JM, Bonichon F, et al. Comparative study of the National Cancer Institute and French Federation of Cancer Centers Sarcoma Group grading systems in a population of 410 adult patients with soft tissue sarcoma. J Clin Oncol 1997, 15: 350–362.

25. Coindre JM, Terrier P, Guillou L, et al. Predictive value of grade for metastasis development in the main histologic types of adult soft tissue sarcomas: a study of 1240 patients from the French Federation of Cancer Centers Sarcoma Group. Cancer 2001, 91: 1914–1926.

26. Nagira K, Yamamoto T, Akisue T, et al. Reliability of fine-needle aspiration biopsy in the initial diagnosis of soft-tissue lesions. Diagn Cytopathol 2002, 27: 354–361.

27. Palmer HE, Mukunyadzi P, Culbreth W, Thomas JR. Subgrouping and grading of soft-tissue sarcomas by fine-needle aspiration cytology: a histopathologic correlation study. Diagn Cytopathol 2001, 24: 307–316.

28. Weir MM, Rosenberg AE, Bell DA. Grading of spindle cell sarcomas in fine-needle aspiration biopsy specimens. Am J Clin Pathol 1999, 112: 784–790.

29. Mathur S, Kapila K, Verma K. Accuracy of cytological grading of spindle-cell sarcomas. Diagn Cytopathol 2003, 29: 79–83.

30. Jones C, Liu K, Hirschowitz S, Klipfel N, Layfield LJ. Concordance of histopathologic and cytologic grading in musculoskeletal sarcomas: can grades obtained from analysis of the fine-needle aspirates serve as the basis for therapeutic decisions? Cancer 2002, 96: 83–91.

31. Jemal A, Siegel R, Ward E, Murray T, Xu J, Thun MJ. Cancer statistics 2007. CA Cancer J Clin 2007, 57: 43–46.

32. Fletcher CDM, Unni KK, Mertens F, editors. Pathology of tumours of soft tissue and bone. In: World Health Organization classification of tumours. Lyon, France: IARC Press; 2002, p. 5.

33. Hasegawa T, Yamamoto S, Nojima T, Hirose T, Nikaido T, Yamashiro K, Matsuno Y. Validity and reproducibility of histologic diagnosis and grading for adult soft-tissue sarcomas. Human Pathol 2002, 33: 111–115.

34. Brennan M, Alektiar K, Maki R. Sarcomas of soft tissue and bone: soft tissue sarcoma. Cancer: principles and practice of oncology. Philadelphia, PA: Williams and Wilkins; 2001.

35. Mertens F, Fletcher CD, Dal Cin P, et al. Cytogenetic analysis of 46 pleomorphic soft tissue sarcomas and correlation with morphologic and clinical features: a report of the CHAMP study group: chromosomes and morphology. Genes Chromosomes Cancer 1998, 22: 16–25.

36. Bramwell VH. Adjuvant chemotherapy for adult soft tissue sarcoma: is there a standard of care. J Clin Oncol 2001, 19: 1235–1237.

37. Sanger F, Nicklen S, Coulson AR. DNA sequencing with chain-terminating inhibitors. Proc Natl Acad Sci U S A 1977, 74: 5463–5467.

38. Borden EC, Baker LH, Bell RS, et al. Soft tissue sarcomas of adults: state of the translational science. Clin Cancer Res 2003, 9: 1941–1956.

39. Conley AP, Trent J, Zhang W. Recent progress in the genomics of soft tissue sarcomas. Curr Opin Oncol 2008, 20: 395–399.

40. Tschoep K, Kohlmann A, Schlemmer M, Haferlach T, Issels RD. Gene expression profiling in sarcomas. Crit Rev Oncol Hematol 2007, 63: 111–124.

41. Nielson TO, West RB, Linn SC, et al. Molecular characterization of soft tissue tumors: a gene expression study. Lancet 2002, 359: 1301–1307.

42. Price ND, Trent J, El-Naggar AK, et al. Highly accurate two-gene classifier for differentiating gastrointestinal stromal tumors and leiomyosarcomas. Proc Natl Acad Sci U S A 2007, 104: 3414–3419.

43. Segal NH, Pavlidis P, Antonescu CR, et al. Classification and subtype prediction of adult soft tissue sarcoma by functional genomics. Am J Pathol 2003, 163: 691–700.

44. Furey TS, Christanini N, Duffy N, Bednarski DW, Schummer M, Haussier D. Support vector machine classification and validation of cancer tissue samples using microarray expression data. Bioinformatics 2000, 16: 906–914.

45. Baird K, Davies S, Antonescu CR, et al. Gene expression profiling of human sarcomas: inshights into sarcoma biology. Cancer Res 2005, 65: 9226–9235.

46. Cheung IY, Feng Y, Danis K, Shukla N, Meyers P, Ladanyi M, Cheung NK. Novel markers of subclinical disease for Ewing family tumors from gene expression profiling. Clin Cancer Res 2007, 13: 6978–6983.

47. Fritz B, Schubert F, Wrobel G, et al. Microarray-based copy number and expression profiling in dedifferentiated and pleomorphic liposarcoma. Cancer Res 2002, 62: 2993–2998.

48. Shimoji T, Kanda H, Kitagawa T, et al. Clinicomolecular study of dedifferentiation in well-differentiated liposarcoma. Biochem Biophys Res Commun 2004, 314: 1133–1140.

49. Singer S, Socci ND, Ambrosini G, et al. Gene expression profiling of liposarcoma identifies distinct biological types/subtypes and potential therapeutic targets in well differentiated and dedifferentiated liposarcoma. Cancer Res 2007, 67: 6626–6636.

50. Dalal KM, Kattan MW, Antonescu CR, Brennan MF, Singer S. Subtype specific prognostic nomogram for patients with primary liposarcoma of the retroperitoneum, extremity, or trunk. Ann Surg 2006, 244: 381–391.

51. Chen G, Gharib TG, Wang H, et al. Protein profiles associated with survival in lung adenocarcinoma. Proc Natl Acad Sci U S A 2003, 100: 13537–13542.

52. Yanagisawa K, Shyr Y, Xu BJ, et al. Proteomic pattern of tumour subsets in non-small-cell lung cancer. Lancet 2003, 362: 433–439.

53. Suehara Y, Kondo T, Fujii K, et al. Proteomic signatures corresponding to histological classification and grading of soft-tissue sarcomas. Proteomics 2006, 6: 4402–4409.

54. Kawai A, Kondo T, Suehara Y, Kikuta K, Hirohashi S. Global protein expression analysis of bone and soft tissue sarcomas. Clin Orthop Relat Res 2008, 466: 2099–2106.

55. Nicholson JK, Lindon JC, Holmes E. Metabonomics: understanding the metabolic responses of living systems to pathophysiological stimuli via multivariate statistical analysis of biological NMR spectroscopic data. Xenobiotica 1999, 29: 1181–1189.

56. Goodacre R, Vaidyanathan S, Dunn WB, Harrigan GG, Kell DB. Metabolomics by numbers: acquiring and understanding global metabolite data. Trends Biotechnol 2004, 22: 245–252.

57. Di Leo A, Claudino W, Colangiuli D, Bessi S, Pestin M, Binganzoli L. New strategies to identify molecular markers predicting chemotherapy activity and toxicity in breast cancer. Ann Oncol 2007, 18(Suppl 12): xii8-xii14.

58. Bollard ME, Stanley EG, Lindon JC, Nicholson JK, Holmes E. NMR based metabonomic approaches for evaluating physiological influences on biofluid composition. NMR Biomed 2005, 18: 143–162.

Chapter 5

Principal Aspects in Fine Needle Aspiration and Core Needle Biopsies

Jerzy Klijanienko, MD, PhD MIAC and Réal Lagacé, MD, FRCPC

Knowledge of normal mesenchymal tissue is essential to avoid pitfalls or misinterpretation of soft tissue lesions. Usually, aspiration using a fine needle is selective and smears comprise mostly tumor cells. From experience, fragments of normal tissue are limited and in small amounts in fine needle aspiration (FNA) specimens with the exception of adipose tissue particularly for biopsies from some anatomical sites, including the breast, the retroperitoneum, and the soft tissues of limbs and trunk. Also, one must keep in mind that some tumors do have a component of normal supporting tissue and could be rich in inflammatory cells. Desmoplastic reactions in different types of tumors can be stroma-rich or stroma-poor.

5.1 NORMAL TISSUE

5.1.1 Adipose Tissue

Adult fat is generally hypocellular with cells devoid of lipid droplets in an alcohol-fixed material. Our aspiration technique (see subsequent sections) allows obtaining fragments of adipose tissue characterized by clusters of grape-like, optically clear adipocytes with distinct cytoplasmic membranes and small dark peripheral nuclei. Collagen fibers, rare fibroblasts, and vessels of capillary size could be present in small amounts. These three-dimensional aggregates have been compared with soap bubbles.

Soft Tissue Tumors: A Multidisciplinary, Decisional Diagnostic Approach
Edited by Jerzy Klijanienko and Réal Lagacé
Copyright © 2011 John Wiley & Sons, Inc.

5.1.2 Fibers

With deep lesions, smears contain fragments of striated muscle whose fibers are disrupted and irregularly arranged. The number of peripheral nuclei could be variable, with the normal muscle fibers harboring fewer nuclei than the degenerated ones. Beware of large non-neoplastic myofibers with multiple nuclei, which are observed in infiltrating lesions such as desmoid tumors and inflammatory and/or degenerative processes. Stromal conjonctive tissue usually is present in larger fragments with collagen fibers and fibroblasts (see subsequent section). In a wide variety of organs and in the stromal soft tissues, aggregates of smooth muscle cells can be present in the aspirates. Often, smooth muscle cells of vascular walls can complicate the cytologic interpretation.

5.1.3 Cellular and Stromal Components

Connective tissue is the basic framework of organs and forms an important component of normal soft tissues as well as the supportive environment of soft tissue lesions. Therefore, elements of connective tissue are frequently parts of FNA and core needle biopsy (CNB) aspirates. The three structural components are ground substance, fibers, and cells.

Air-dried smears stained by one of the Giemsa-based methods should be preferred to the Papanicolaou technique to demonstrate ground substance. The matrix stains from a pale blue to a deep -red purple color according to the amount of acid mucopolysaccarides (i.e., if it is stroma-rich or stroma-poor).

Normal fibroblasts (resting fibroblasts) and activated fibroblasts (myofibroblasts) are the principal cellular components of the connective tissue, although myofibroblasts rarely are observed, as they are a constituent of reactive inflammatory processes and/or pseudoneoplastic conditions (see subsequent section). Fibroblasts are spindle-shaped cells with slender bipolar cytoplasm. They could be modified by the trauma of aspiration and appear more oval and short and devoid of cytoplasmic processes in comparison with nontraumatized fibroblasts. Nuclei are roundish, ovoid, or fusiform, and are placed centrally with uniform chromatin and small nucleoli, if present. They are observed to be either dissociated single cells or in small clusters of loosely attached cells. Myofibroblasts are larger cells with plump nuclei, have finely granular chromatin and harboring one or two prominent nucleoli, and occasionally showing an indented nuclear membrane. Cytoplasm is abundant, has shorter cytoplasmic processes, and lacks the wispy cytoplasmic characteristic of resting fibroblasts.

5.1.4 Giant Cells

Giant cells are not a normal cell component of mesenchymal soft tissues. Benign or reactive giant cells of histiocytic type do show greater amounts of cytoplasm devoid of cytoplasmic processes, have multiple nuclei arranged in different fashions, and show morphologic characteristics similar to mononuclear histiocytes. In fact, the latter, if present in smears, are large round or polygonal cells with variable amounts of granular or foamy cytoplasm and whose nuclei sometimes have a deep indentation with a kidney shape. Pending on the type of tumor, the cytoplasm could contain vacuoles of various size and/or pigments.

5.2 CYTOLOGIC CLASSIFICATION OF SOFT TISSUE TUMORS BASED ON THE PRINCIPAL PATTERNS

Instead of classifying soft tissue tumors according to their histogenesis/phenotype, the cytological classification into five different groups was used for diagnosis and comments. The five cytology dominant patterns were individualized as follow: spindle cell, the most frequent pattern in adult soft tissue tumors and pleomorphic, epithelioid, myxoid, and small round/ovoid cell patterns, but keep in mind that overlap between those different patterns may be present in the same specimen. For example, a rhabdoid tumor may be classified as well as an epithelioid or a round cell tumor. Similarly, angiosarcoma could fit in a spindle cell diagnosis, and epithelioid leiomyosarcoma may be classified into spindle cell, polymorphous cell, epithelioid cell, and more in a myxoid group [1–3].

5.2.1 Spindle-Cell Pattern

The spindle cell pattern may be divided into two distinctive groups of specimens: "low-grade spindle cell pattern" and "malignant spindle cell pattern." The "low-grade spindle cell pattern" malignancy only could be suspected morphologically, whereas the "malignant spindle cell pattern" is more evident. Aspirates in "low-grade spindle cell pattern" are poorly and moderately to highly cellular (Figs 5.1 and 5.2). The principal characteristic is the predominance of sheets and fascicles of elongated

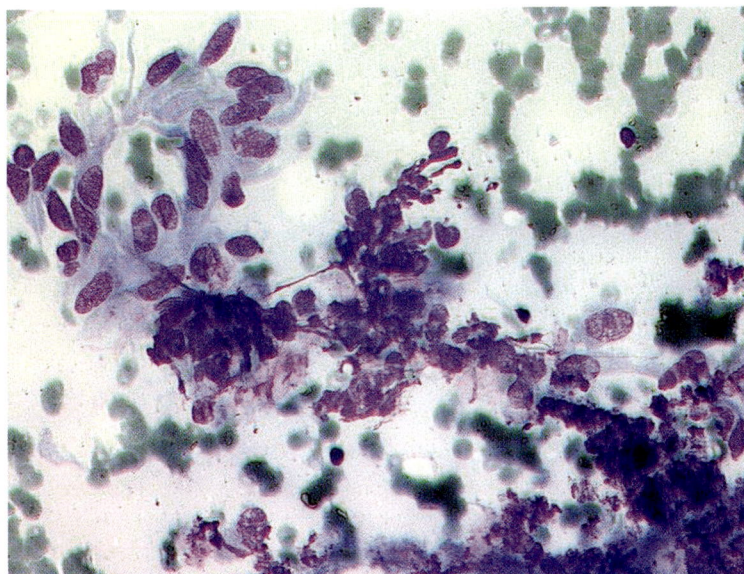

FIG 5.1 Desmoid tumor. Spindle-shaped, benign-looking cells, and nonspecific collagen debris.

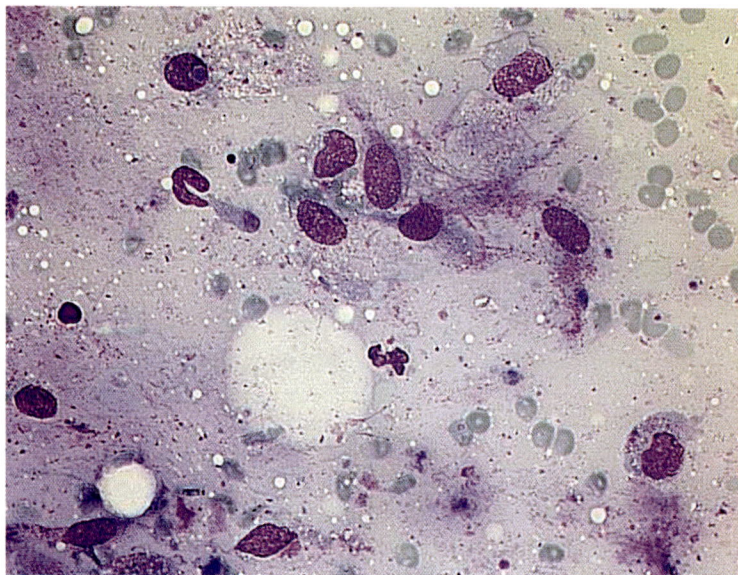

FIG 5.2 Benign fibrous histiocytoma. Spindle cells with "dirty" cytoplasm resembling macrophages.

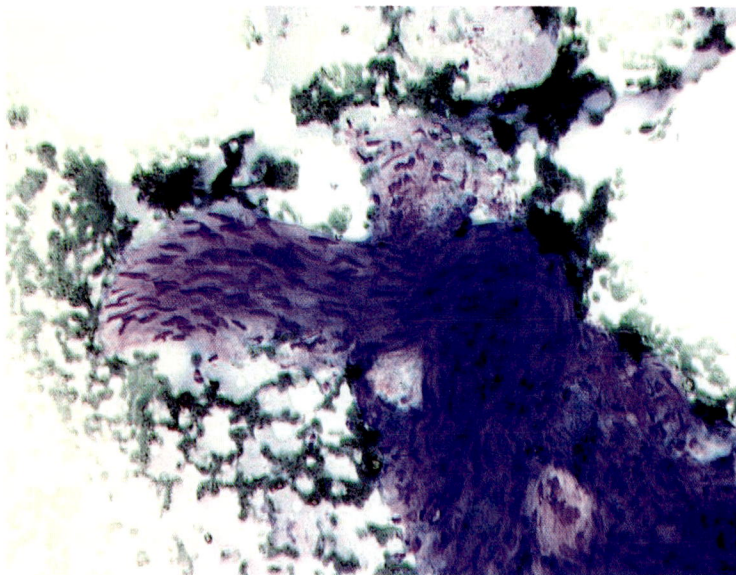

FIG 5.3 Neurofibroma. Bland spindle cells in cohesive clusters resembling normal nerve.

cells with spindle nuclei that parallel the cell shape (Fig 5.3). The frequent bipolar cytoplasm is observed readily. Often, the tumor cells are dissociated, although the degree of intercellular cohesion may be variable and influenced by the morphologic type of spindle cell tumor. The greatest diagnostic difficulty encountered is distinguishing between benign and low-grade malignant tumors, hence the occurence of

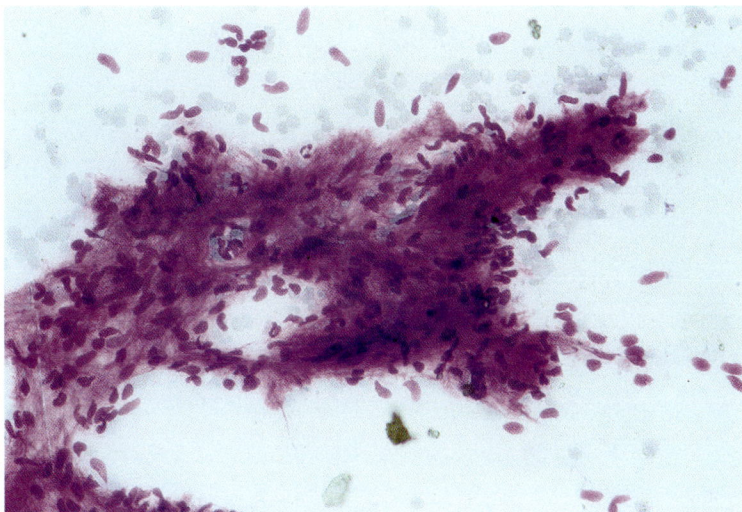

FIG 5.4 Dermatofibrosarcoma protuberans. Small and regular cells within collagen fibers.

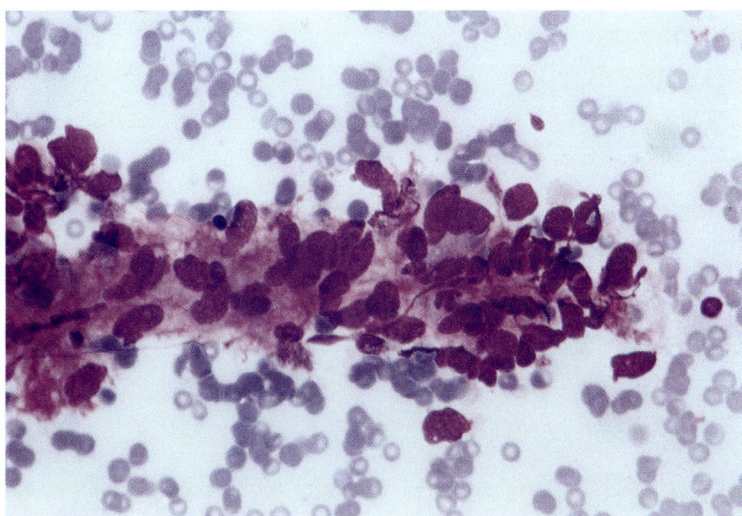

FIG 5.5 Dermatofibrosarcoma protuberans. Small and roundish cells within collagen fibers.

false-positive and false-negative results in comparison with high-grade tumors (Figs 5.4–5.8). By cytomorphologic examination, distinguishing various phenotypes of spindle cell sarcomas is challenging. However, subtle clues can help to determine accurately the tumoral subtype (see subsequent section). In "malignant spindle cell pattern," the smears are always cell-rich and show cells with cytonuclear atypia, huge nucleoli, and well-preserved cytoplasms (Figs 5.9 to 5.11). Occasionally, mitotic figures also are observed.

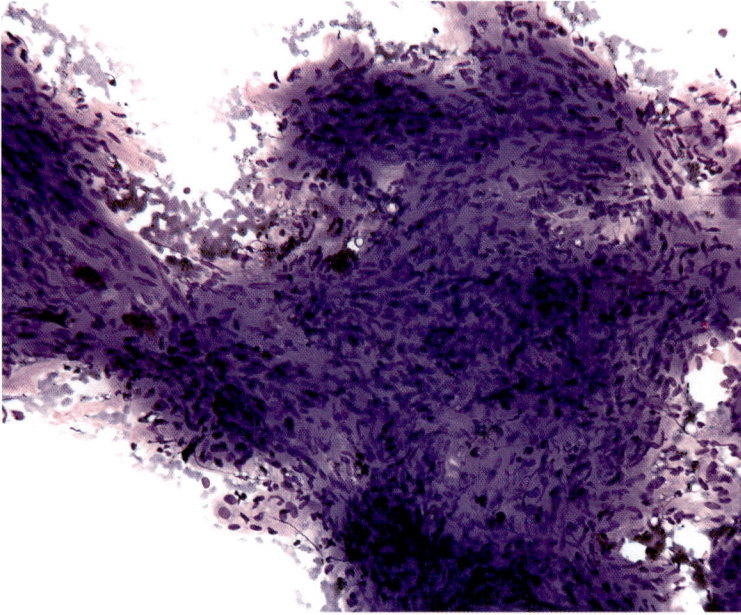

FIG 5.6 Low-grade malignant peripheral nerve sheath tumor. Cohesive spindle cells in "nerve-like" clusters. Compare with Fig 5.3.

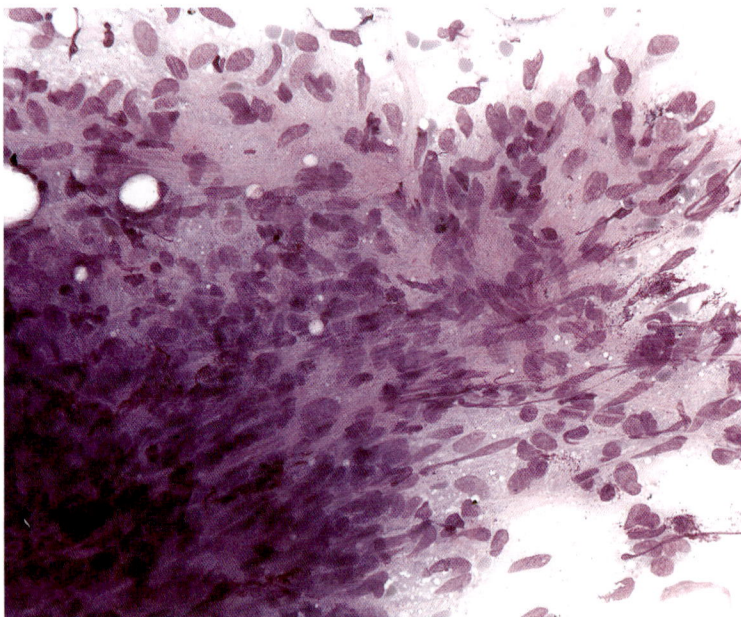

FIG 5.7 Low-grade malignant peripheral nerve sheath tumor. Spindle cells with slight cytonuclear atypia.

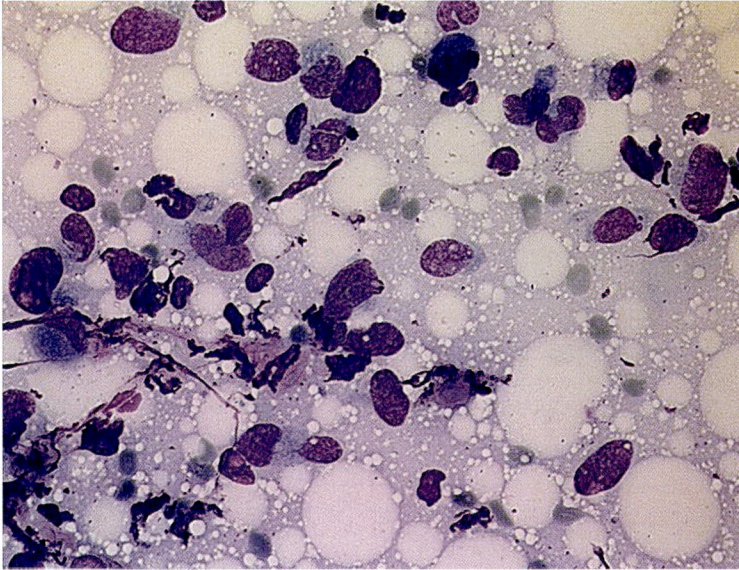

FIG 5.8 Infantile fibrosarcoma. Nonspecific spindle and roundish cells.

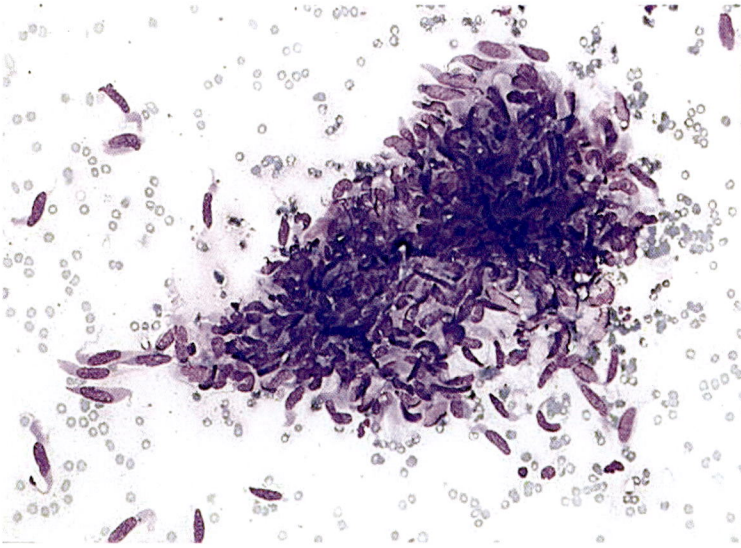

FIG 5.9 Low-grade leiomyosarcoma. Regular isolated and clustered spindle cells with "cigar-like" nuclei.

5.2.2 Myxoid Pattern

Several soft tissue tumors or pseudotumors could be included in that category of patterns (Figs 5.12–5.17). Depending on the tumor type and/or the site from which the specimen is biopsied, the stroma is partly myxoid in entities like a myxoid variant of dermatofibrosarcoma protuberans, paucicellular areas of myxoid malignant

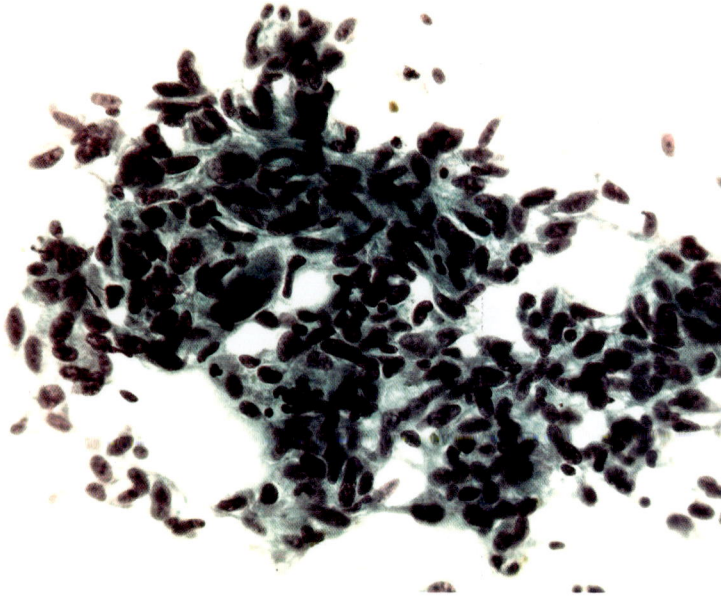

FIG 5.10 Low-grade leiomyosarcoma. Atypical spindle cells.

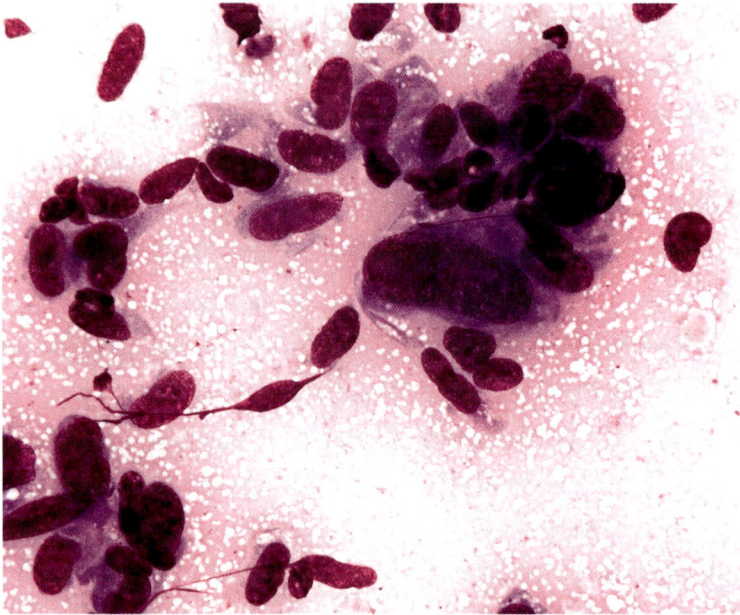

FIG 5.11 Low-grade leiomyosarcoma. Atypical spindle cells.

fibrous histiocytoma, or diffusely myxoid-like myxoma and well-differentiated myxoid liposarcoma [4]. The appearance of the myxoid matrix is similar and the tinctorial affinities vary according to the quantity of acid mucopolysaccharides. At first glance, when the aspirated material is smeared on the glass slide, a typical appearance of a thick, viscous, glue-like, and more or less hemorrhagic fluid is

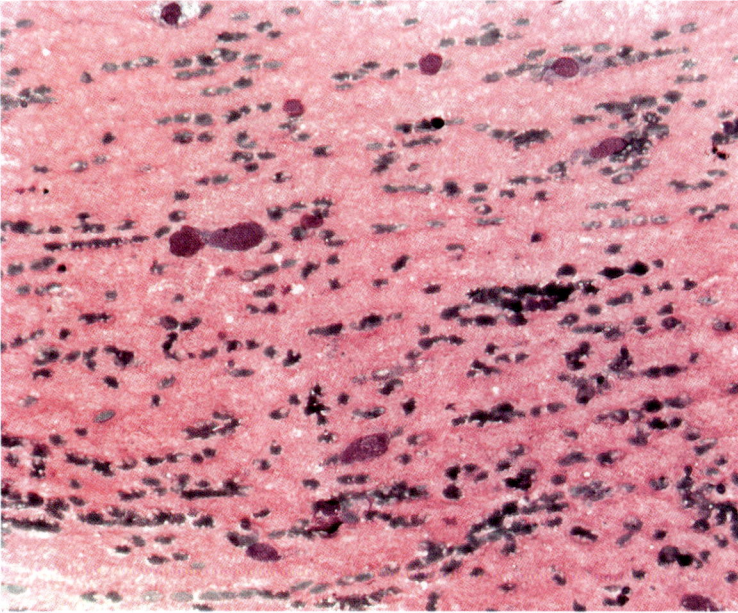

FIG 5.12 Myxoid leiomyosarcoma. Abundant myxoid matrix and rare spindle/roundish cells. This aspect may be misinterpreted as myxoma.

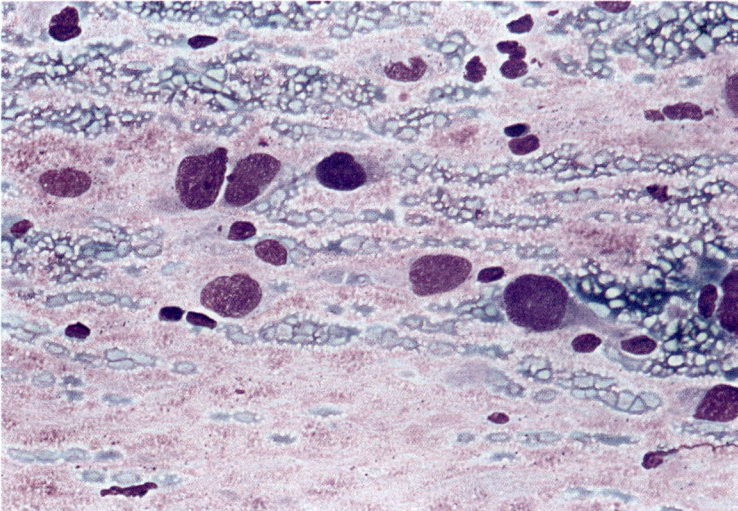

FIG 5.13 Myxoid leiomyosarcoma. Malignant cells. This aspect may be observed in other malignant myxoid tumors.

observed. Depending on the amount of extracellular matrix material, one observes irregularly shaped fragments of moderate size embedding a variable quantity of tumor cells (e.g., paucicellular in intramuscular myxoma) that are more cellular in myxoid leiomyosarcoma and round cell liposarcoma. This myxoid matrix varies from fibrillar to homogeneous in appearance. It is metachromatic especially in

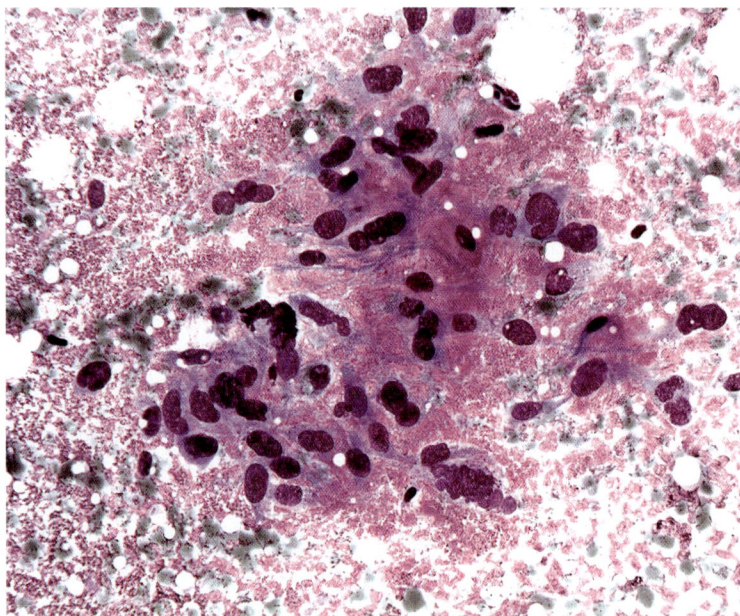

FIG 5.14 Myxoid leiomyosarcoma. Malignant cells. This aspect may be observed in other malignant myxoid tumors.

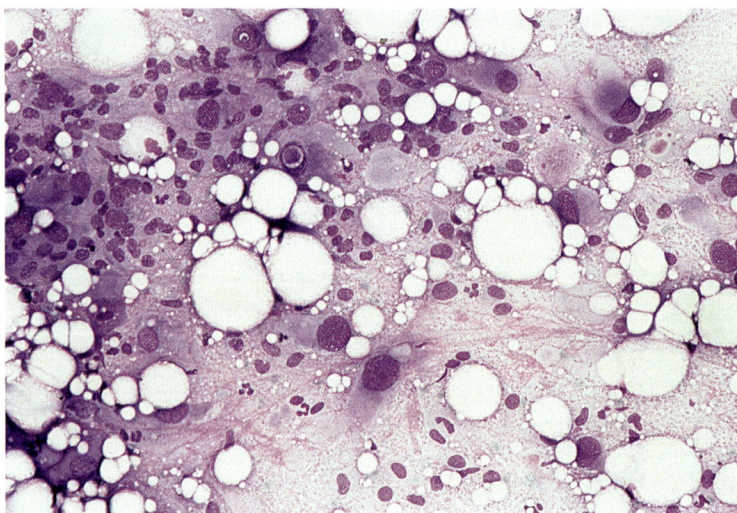

FIG 5.15 Myxoid liposarcoma. Polymorphous atypical and regular roundish cells within myxoid matrix. The differential diagnosis between lipoblasts and pseudolipoblasts may be difficult.

myxoid chondrosarcoma because of the presence of acid mucopolysaccharides with sulfated radicals (proteoglycans and glucoamineglycans). Some pitfalls are to be avoided in the interpretation of myxoid sarcomas. These include benign soft tissue lesions like intramuscular myxoma, schwannoma, particularly those rich in Antoni B

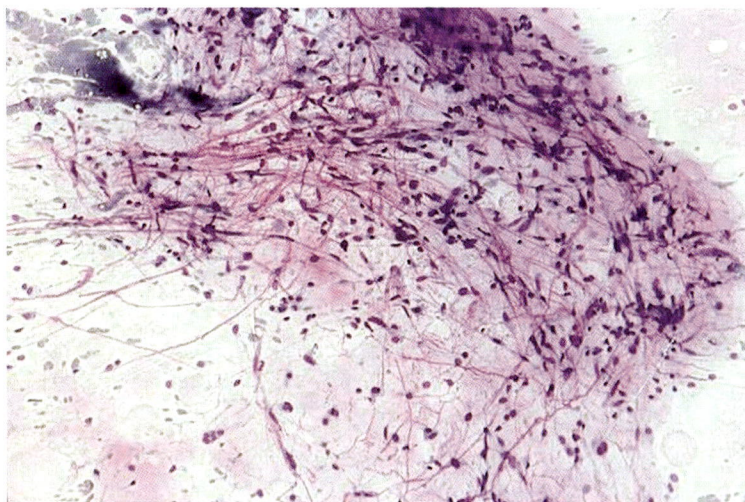

FIG 5.16 Myxoid malignant fibrous histiocytoma. Abundant myxoid and scant regular spindle cells.

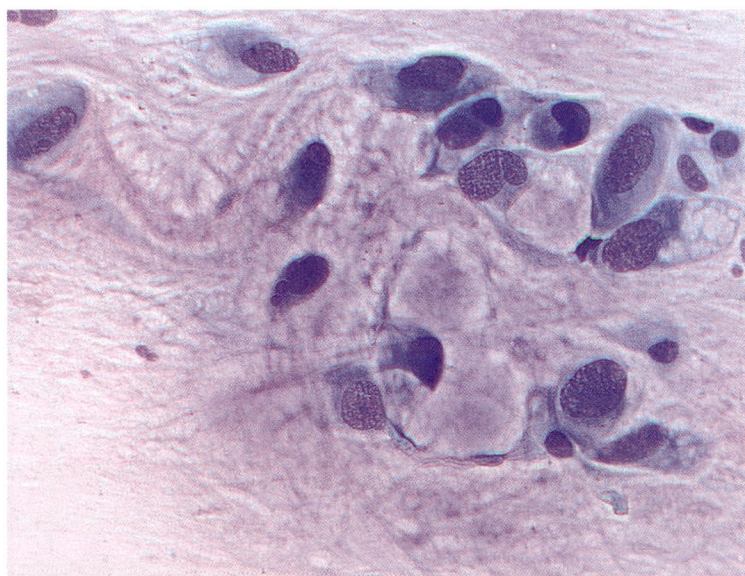

FIG 5.17 Fibromyxosarcoma. Myxoid background and malignant spindle cells.

areas and so on, and frequent pseudoneoplastic lesions of which various forms exist of fasciitis (nodular-proliferative-decubitus etc.) and nonmesenchymal/nonsarcomatous malignancies. Let us recall that once we have the conviction that a myxoid mesenchymal neoplasm is identified as a sarcoma, the determination of its subtyping may be difficult with the exception of some entities (e.g., myxoid liposarcoma, which is recognized readily by its typical arborized, chicken-wire vasculature). Clinical presentation and ancillary techniques could help to precise the diagnosis for distinguishing a chordoma from an extraskeletal myxoid chondrosarcoma.

5.2.3 Pleomorphic Pattern

Smears in this group of sarcomas are always cell-rich. Experienced pathologists/ cytopathologists agree that precising the phenotype of a pleomorphic sarcoma, even with the use of ancillary techniques, is a frustrating, time-consuming, futile, and wastefull exercise. However, one cannot stress enough the importance of separating pleomorphic sarcomas from other pleomorphic malignancies such as mainly sarcomatoid carcinoma, malignant melanoma, and large cell anaplastic lymphoma, as well as benign entities like pleomorphic lipoma and fasciitis with atypical and monstrous cells.

Pleomorphic lesions are identified readily on smears at first glance at low magnification microscopic examination (Figs 5.18–5.23). They are cellular with a typical variation of cellular and nuclear size and volume. There is a marked nuclear pleomophism as well as numerous atypical multinucleated tumor cells. An admixture of small round cells with a high nuclear/cytoplasmic ratio with large spindle cells could be observed in the same microscopic field. Necrotic debris are identified frequently. Pleomorphic malignant fibrous histiocytoma (MFH) and pleomorphic liposarcoma are the chief candidates of that cytologic cellular pattern. Clues that help in the differential diagnosis are discussed in detail subsequently.

5.2.4 Epithelioid Pattern

The FNA epithelioid cell pattern—also called polygonal cell—is the less frequent category of soft tissue sarcoma (Figs 5.24–5.28). Entities such as epitheliod sarcoma, rhabdoid tumor, and epitheliod angiosarcoma belong to this cytological subgroup. Gastrointestinal stromal tumor (GIST)—formerly epithelioid leiomyoma/leiomyosarcoma— is also a member of this group and it will be discussed after. Tumor cells are round or polygonal and have abundant cytoplasm and well-defined cytoplasmic borders. Nuclei are prominent and often eccentrically positioned, containing vesicular chromatin and large

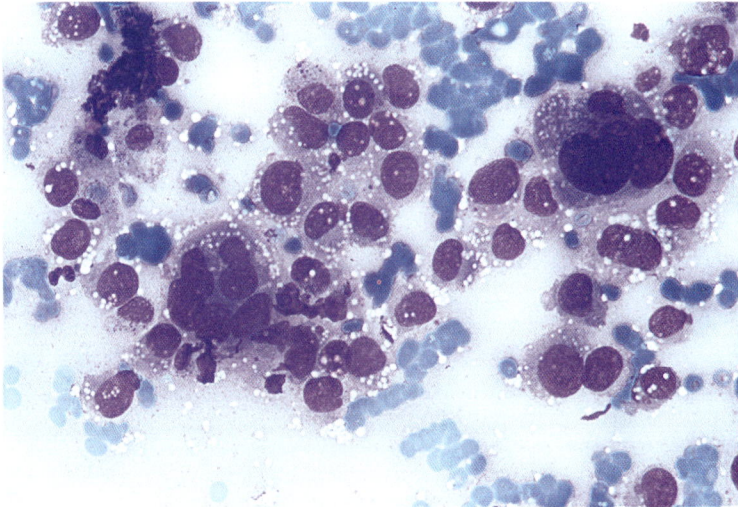

FIG 5.18 Pleomorphic liposarcoma. Polymorphous malignant cells and lipoblasts.

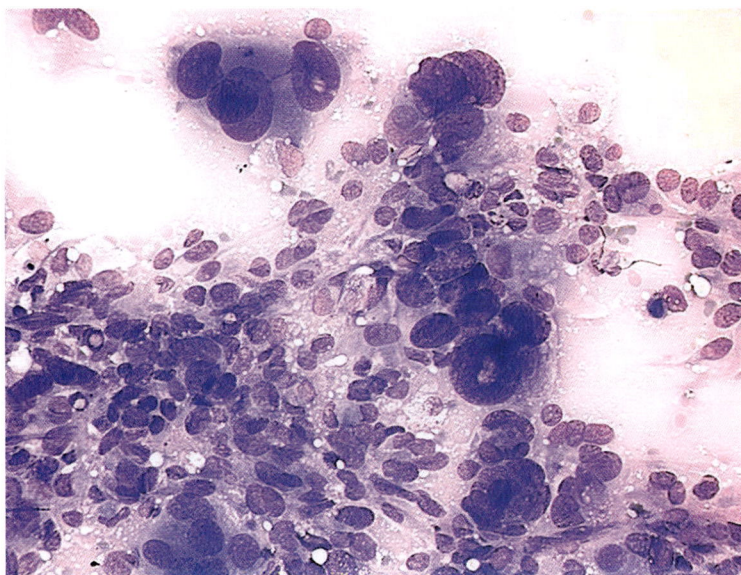

FIG 5.19 Pleomorphic leiomyosarcoma. Polymorphous malignant spindle and roundish cells.

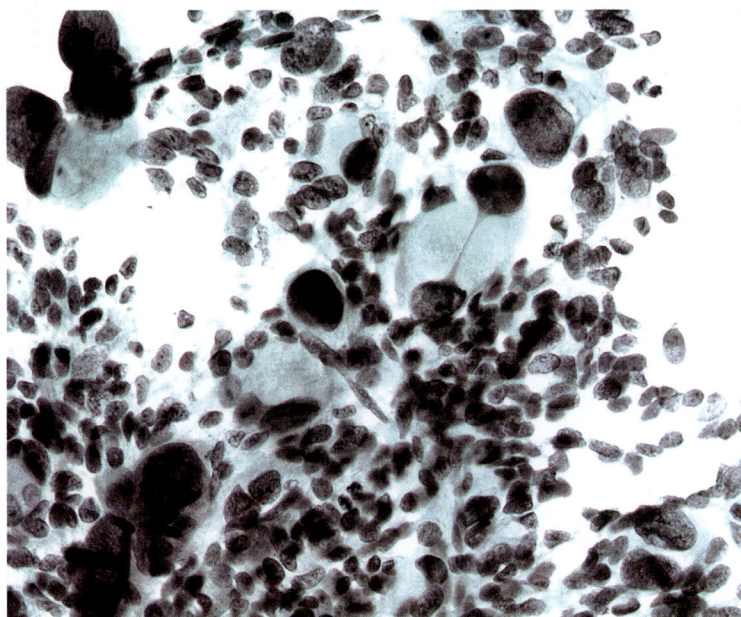

FIG 5.20 Pleomorphic leiomyosarcoma. Polymorphous malignant spindle and roundish cells.

nucleoli. Binucleated and multinucleated cells are not rare. Aspirates from these tumors are generally moderately to highly cellular and low-magnification examination shows dissociated tumor cells and small aggregates or clusters of cells. Like other cytologic subtypes of cellular components, knowledge of clinical data, medical history, and imaging

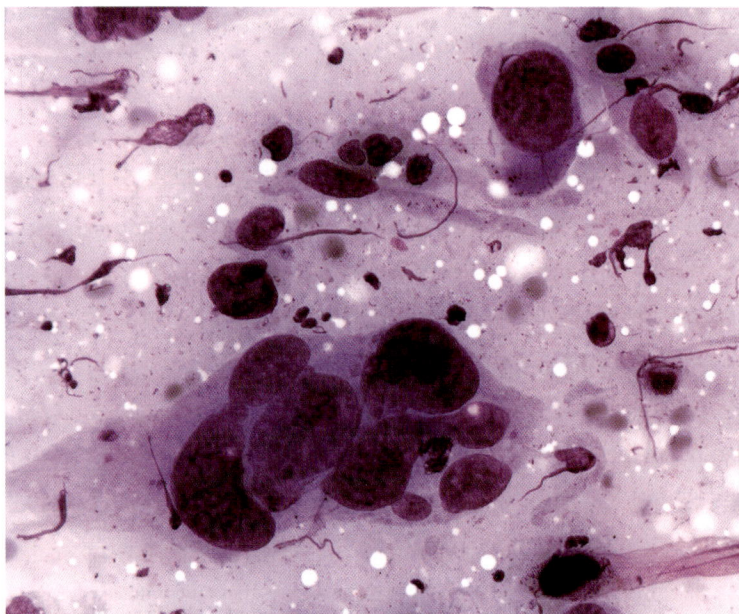

FIG 5.21 Pleomorphic malignant peripheral nerve sheath tumor. Malignant spindle cells. Compare with Fig 5.19 to realize the difficulty in the differential diagnosis.

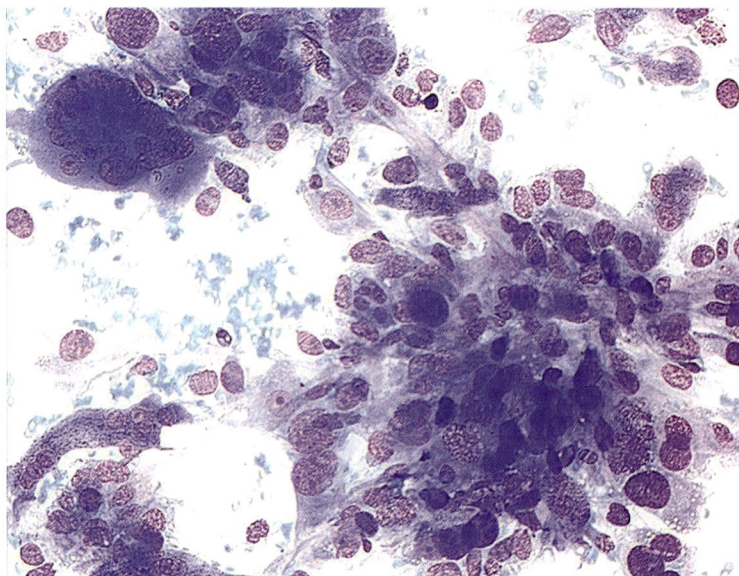

FIG 5.22 Extraskeletal osteosarcoma. Polymorphous morphology comprising of malignant roundish, spindle, and multinucleated cells.

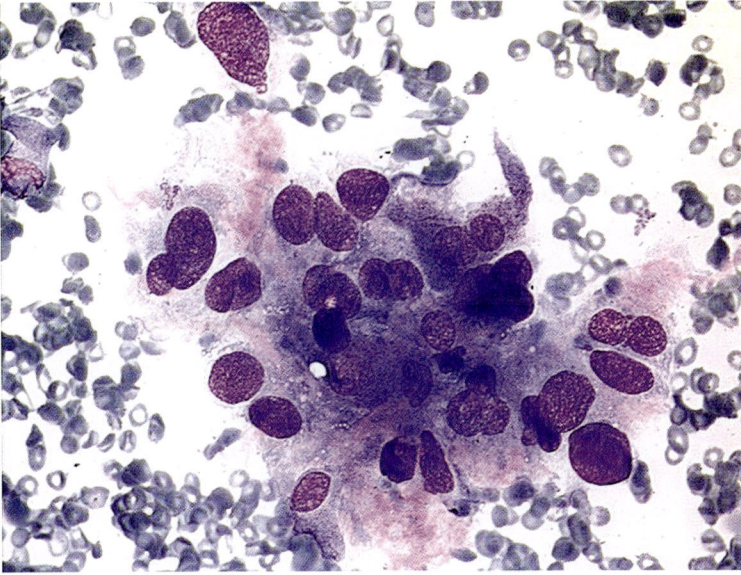

FIG 5.23 Extraskeletal osteosarcoma. Polymorphous morphology comprising of malignant roundish, spindle, and multinucleated cells. Note the presence of eosinophilic osteoid, allowing the accurate diagnosis.

Library
College of Physicians & Surgeons of B.C.
300 - 669 Howe St.
Vancouver, BC V6C 0B4

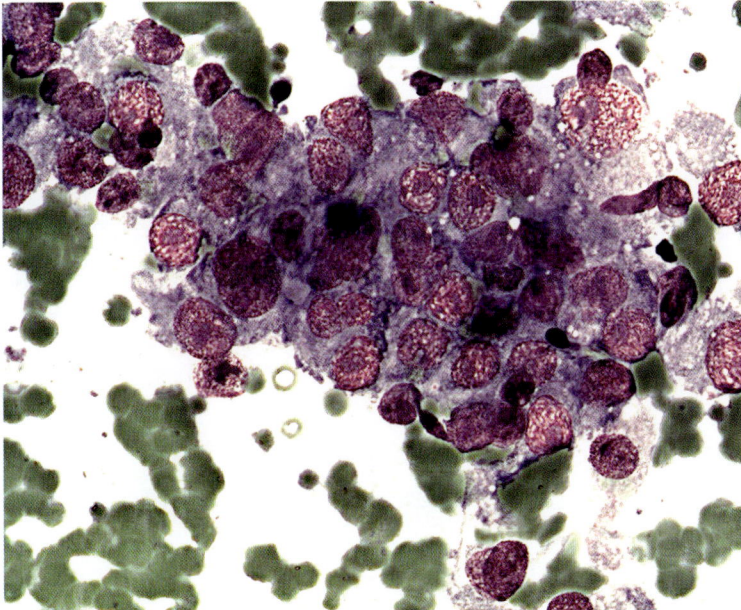

FIG 5.24 Rhabdoid tumor. Cohesive epithelial-like cells in clusters. Nuclei are irregular and nucleolated.

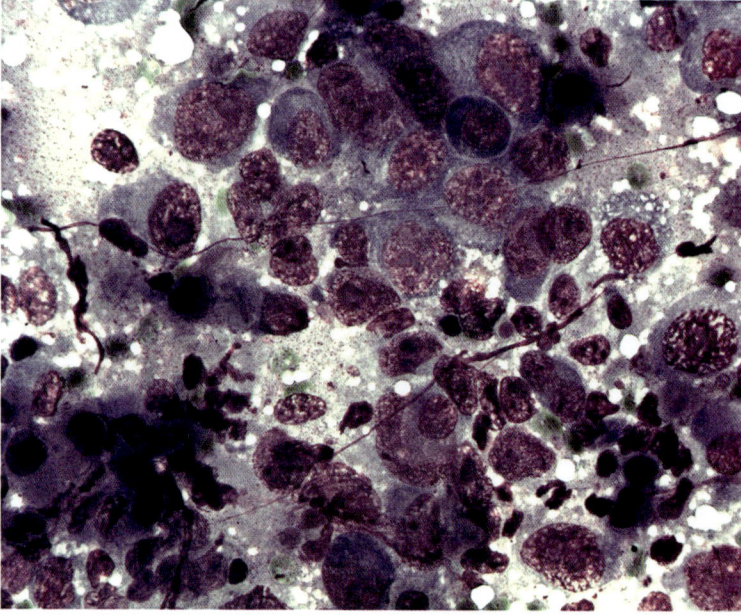

FIG 5.25 Epithelioid sarcoma. Cells have large cytoplasm, which mimics carcinoma. Compare with Fig 5.24.

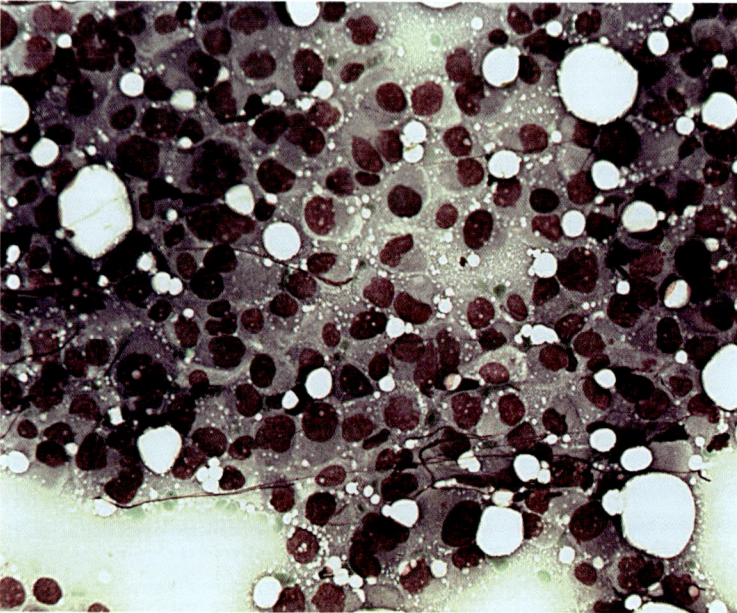

FIG 5.26 Alveolar sarcoma resembling lobular breast carcinoma.

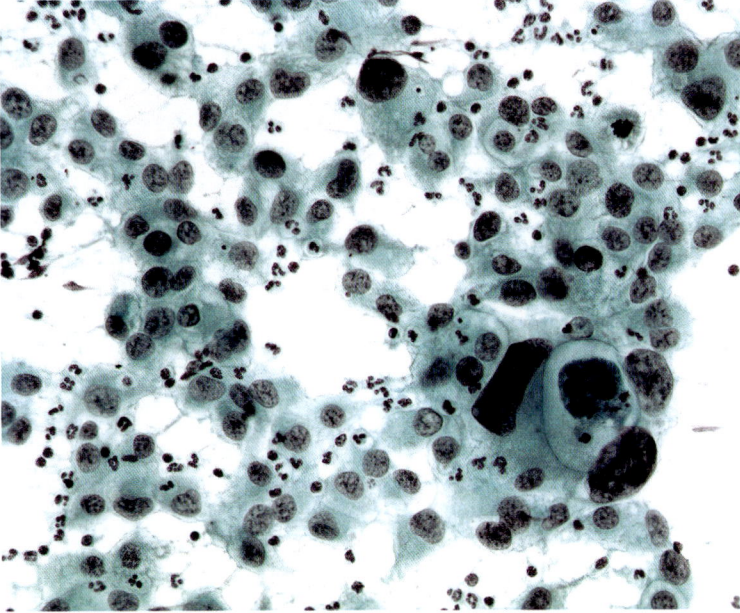

FIG 5.27 Epithelioid leiomyosarcoma. Cohesive, epithelial-like cells.

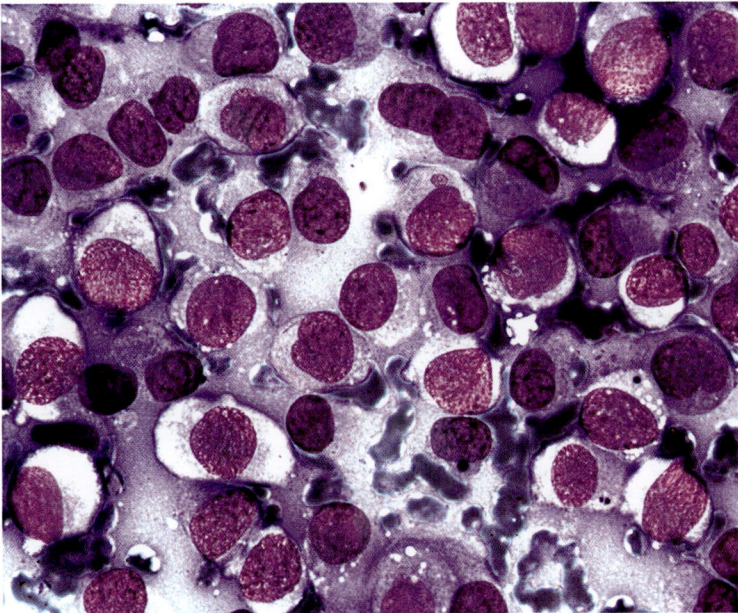

FIG 5.28 Epithelioid clear cell sarcoma. Epithelioid cells similar to cells of epithelioid malignant melanoma.

pictures are essential for diagnosis. The main diagnostic pitfalls are metastatic carcinomas and melanoma.

Some soft tissue tumors do not fit into any of these described classes of FNA aspirates. Entities like benign tumors of adipose tissue and well-differentiated liposarcoma fall into those categories. The diagnosis of liposarcoma typically relies on the presence of lipoblasts, and it is well known that they are rare in several well-differentiated liposarcomas. Therefore, in such instances, the overall picture and the cellular components of the tumor are preferred indicators for diagnosis.

5.2.5 Small Round/Ovoid Cell Pattern

Most round cell sarcomas are observed in the pediatric population, with adults being affected in a minority of cases. Typically, smears obtained by FNA and CNB of these tumors are cell-rich. They consist of small, homogeneous round cells whose cytoplasm is present in variable amounts (Figs 5.29–5.34). Nuclei are rounded to ovoid, bland with small nucleoli, and rarely prominent like in cases of atypical large cell Ewing sarcoma/ peripheral neuroectodermal tumor. Obviously, the appearance depends on the subtype of the soft tissue tumor (e.g., embryonal and alveolar rhabdomyosarcoma consist of cells with different degrees of maturation, so-called early or late-rhabdomyoblasts). In contrast, aspirates from typical Ewing sarcoma/ peripheral neuroectodermal tumor demonstrate a more homogeneous cytologic picture with characteristic double cell population—larger cells and darker cells. Entities including metastatic small cell carcinoma, non-Hodgkin lymphoma, and the rare variety of small cell melanoma are to be considered in the differential diagnosis with knowledge of the clinical setting.

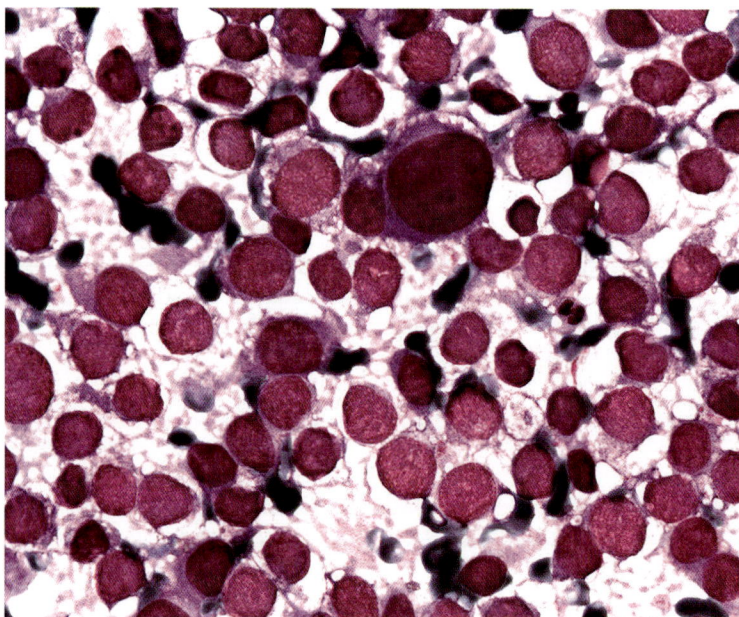

FIG 5.29 Ewing sarcoma. Roundish and monomorphic area.

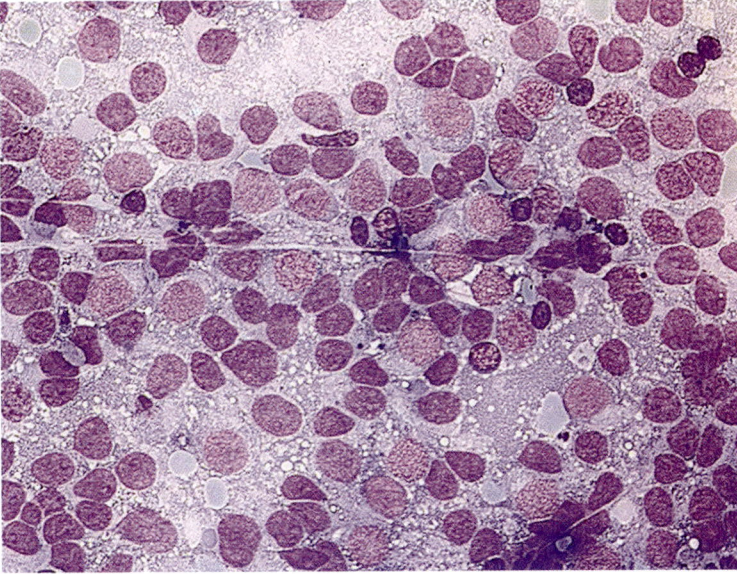

FIG 5.30 Ewing sarcoma. Typical double population of roundish cells.

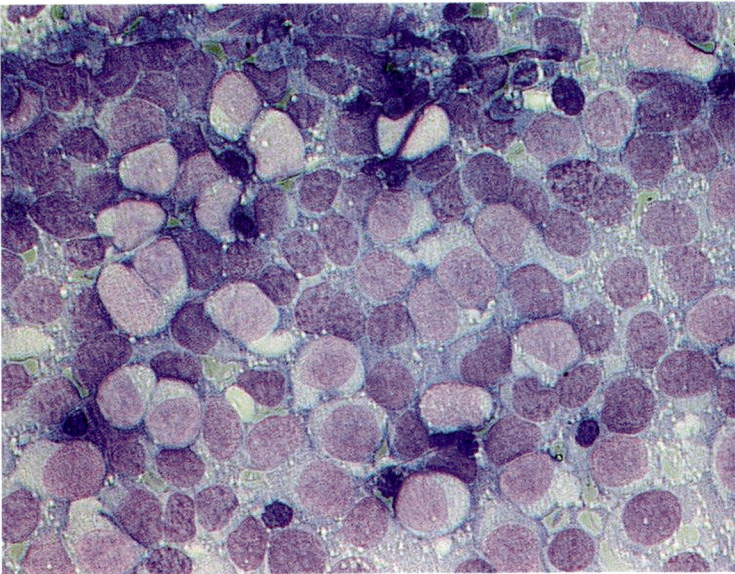

FIG 5.31 Ewing sarcoma. Typical double population with clearer cells.

5.2.6 Exclusive Patterns by FNA and CNB

The five different groups of the aforementioned cytological patterns do not correspond entirely to patterns observed by histology. For example, the following neoplasms preferably would be included in a histological alveolar group: alveolar

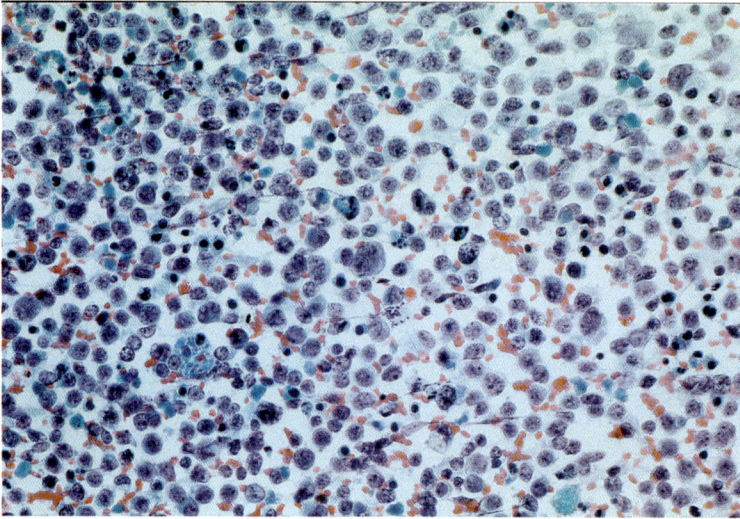

FIG 5.32 Alveolar rhabdomyosarcoma. Round and polymorphous cells. Some are binucleated or have eccentric cytoplasm. The diagnosis of rhabdomyosarcoma is evident using only morphologic criteria.

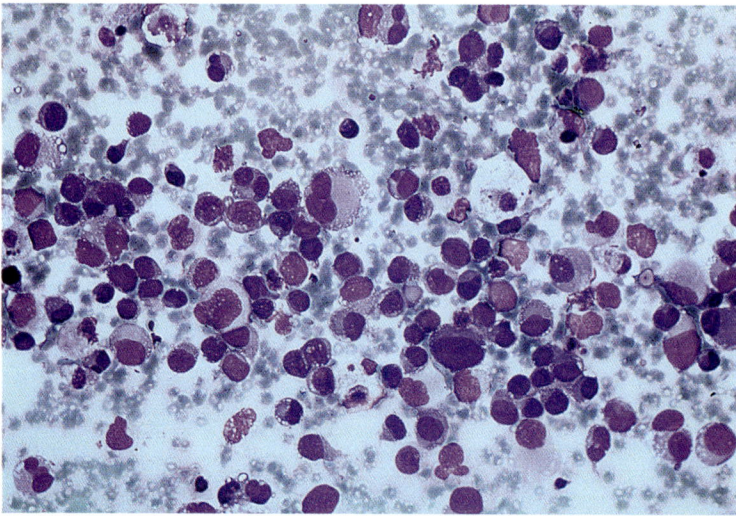

FIG 5.33 Alveolar rhabdomyosarcoma. Round and polymorphous cells. Some are binucleated or have eccentric or microvacuolated cytoplasm.

soft part sarcoma, clear cell sarcoma of tendon and aponeurosis, alveolar rhabomyo-sarcoma, paraganglioma, and cases of metastatic renal cell carcinoma. For the purpose of this monograph, some of these entities are included either in the epithelioid or the round cell variants. The pericytoma-like pattern also is not observed by FNA/CNB. It includes tumors depicting the following pattern either focally or diffusely: solitary fibrous tumor, synovial sarcoma (particularly the monophasic variant), extraskeletal

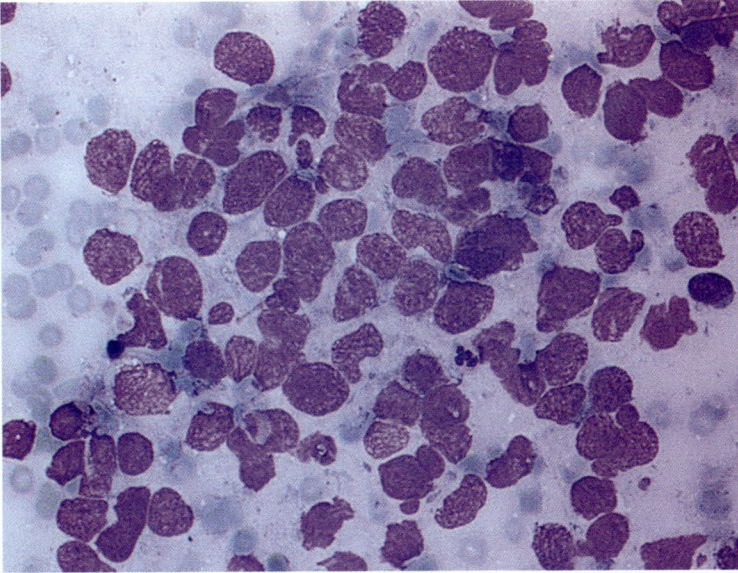

FIG 5.34 Desmoplastic small round cell tumor. Poorly differentiated round cells resembling neuroblastoma.

mesenchymal chondrosarcoma, and the great "imitator" metastatic renal cell carcinoma. True hemangiopericytoma is an entity of debatable nosology and remains a diagnosis of exclusion. The so-called malignant hemangiopericytoma represents a morphologic modulation in round cell sarcoma of a recognized phenotype, and the term should be avoided. The plethora of benign and intermediate vascular tumors also does not fit in any of the cytological patterns, whereas the malignant ones are discussed in the spindle cell and epithelioid groups.

5.3 DIAGNOSTIC ACCURACY OF FNA IN SOFT TISSUE TUMORS

A retrospective survey of the cytopathology files of the Institut Curie from 1954 to December 2009, which included more than 340,000 cases, allowed retrieving more than 2600 mesenchymal tumors. All available clinical charts were reviewed and the cytology and corresponding histological sections were identified and confirmed. The pathology samples were reviewed and reclassified according to the most recent characterizations [3,5]. A detailed morphologic analysis and the contents of a series of entities have been discussed in the literature in the last decade.

5.3.1 Spindle Cell-Tumors Including Pleomorphic, Epithelioid, and Myxoid Patterns

Eight-hundred-eighty-five tumors in 728 patients presenting spindle cell tumors were sampled cytologically. Six-hundred-twenty-three tumors in 479 patients were malignant, and 262 tumors in 249 patients were benign. The FNA technique was used as an initial method of diagnosis without previous histological examination (primary tumors) in 529 cases (59.8%) and was recurrent (the initial histologic diagnosis was known) in 216 (24.4%) cases and metastatic (from a known and histologically studied primary site) in 140 (15.8%) cases.

In the group of 623 spindle cell sarcomas (Table 5.1), the review of original cytology diagnosis showed that 265 (42.5%) tumors were diagnosed accurately, diagnosed as another type of sarcoma in 301 (48.3%) cases, rendered suspicious in 29 (4.7%) cases, and were misdiagnosed as a benign connective tumor (false negative) in 15 (2.4%) cases. Thirteen (2.1%) samples were unsatisfactory for cytodiagnosis. When the FNA technique was used as an initial diagnostic method in 293 tumors, the review showed that 90 (30.7%) cases were diagnosed accurately, 165 (53.3%) cases were diagnosed as another type of sarcoma, 18 (6.1%) case were rendered suspicious, and 11 (3.8%) cases were a false negative. Nine (3.1%) samples were unsatisfactory for diagnosis.

In the group of 262 spindle cell benign tumors (Table 5.2), the review of original cytology diagnosis showed that 106 (40.5%) tumors were diagnosed accurately, 100 (38.2%) tumors were diagnosed as another type of benignancy (usually as "benign connective tumor"), 13 (4.9%) tumors were misdiagnosed as sarcoma (false positive), and 19 (7.2%) tumors samples were rendered suspicious. Twenty four (9.1%) cases were unsatisfactory for diagnosis. When the FNA technique was used as an initial diagnostic method in 236 tumors, the review showed that 101 (42.8%) cases were diagnosed accurately, 88 (37.3%) cases were diagnosed as another type of benignancy (usually as a "benign connective tumor"), 8 (3.4%) cases were misdiagnosed as sarcoma (false positive), and 17 (7.2%) cases samples were rendered suspicious. Twenty-two (9.3%) cases were unsatisfactory for diagnosis. Statistical analysis showed that for all lesions, sensitivity was 97.5 and specificity was 86.6%. When only primary tumors were analyzed, sensitivity was 96.1 and specificity was 88.3%. It is interesting to state that the cytological diagnosis of a "benign connective tumor" does not always lead to histological verification (a typical example is lipoma or desmoid). Consequently, FNA is a powerful method for diagnosis, probably much higher than is shown in the statistics.

5.3.2 Round Cell Sarcomas

We have analyzed 256 round cell sarcomas in 176 patients (selected entities are shown in Table 5.3). One hundred twenty three were primary with 35 recurrences and 88 metastases. In this group, the review of the original cytology diagnosis showed that 215 (84%) tumors were diagnosed accurately, 37 (14.4%) cases were diagnosed as other type of sarcoma, 3 (0.8%) cases were rendered suspicious, and 1 (0.8%) case was unsatisfactory for cytodiagnosis. No case was misdiagnosed as a false negative. When the FNA technique was used as an initial diagnostic method in 123 tumors, the review showed that 95 (77.2%) cases were diagnosed accurately, 27 (22%) cases were diagnosed as another type of sarcoma, and 1 (0.8%) case was rendered suspicious. No case was rendered false negative or was unsatisfactory for diagnosis.

The collective review of the literature shows that FNA is a powerful diagnostic method in other centers (Table 5.4). Sensitivity and specificity of FNA ranges from 88.5% to 97.5% and from 81.5% to 100%, respectively.

TABLE 5.1 Cytohistological correlations in selected non-round-cell sarcomas according to primary and nonprimary tumor nature (based on our previous publications [6–13])

Tumor type #tu/#pts #P/#R/#M	Accurate	Malignant	Suspicious	Subtotal malignant and suspicious	False negative	Unsatisfactory
Synovial sarcoma 74 tu/48 pts 28 P/27 R/19 M						
All	29 (39.2)	41 (55.4)	2 (2.7)	72 (97.3)	0	2 (2.7)
Primary	11 (39.3)	14 (50)	2 (7.1)	27 (96.4)	0	1 (3.6)
MFH 113 tu/92 pts 49 P/49 R/15 M						
All	29 (25.6)	78 (69)	1 (0.9)	108 (95.5)	2 (1.8)	3 (2.7)
Primary	6 (12.2)	41 (83.8)	1 (2)	48 (97.4)	0	1 (2)
Leiomyosarcoma 132 tu/100 pts 73 P/30 R/29 M						
All	50 (38.9)	74 (56)	4 (2.5)	128 (97.4)	1 (0.1)	3 (2.5)
Primary	16 (21.9)	50 (68.5)	4 (5.5)	70 (95.9)	0	3 (4.1)
MPNST 37 tu/28 pts 18 P/13 R/6 M						
All	6 (16.2)	31 (83.8)	0	37 (100)	0	0
Primary	1 (5.6)	17 (94.4)	0	18 (100)	0	0
Liposarcoma 89 tu/58 pts 25 P/36 R/28 M						
All	57 (64)	24 (27)	4 (4.5)	85 (95.5)	0	4 (4.5)
Primary	14 (56)	7 (28)	1 (4)	22 (88)	0	3 (12)
Dermatofibrosarcoma protuberans 14 tu/13 pts 10 P/4 R/0 M						
All	1	6	0	7 (50)	6	1
Primary	0	5	0	5 (50)	4	1
Angiosarcoma 34 tu/28 pts 18 P/7 R/9 M						
All	22 (64.7)	9 (26.5)	3 (8.8)	34 (100)	0	0
Primary	8 (44.4)	8 (44.4)	2 (11.2)	18 (100)	0	0
Fibromyxosarcoma 16 tu/12 pts 7 P/7 R/2 M						
All	9	6	1	16 (100)	0	0
Primary	3	4	0	7 (100)	0	0

(*Continued*)

TABLE 5.1 (Continued)

Tumor type #tu/#pts #P/#R/#M	Accurate	Malignant	Suspicious	Subtotal malignant and suspicious	False negative	Unsatisfactory
GIST 11 tu/9 pts 3 P/3 R/5 M						
All	0	9	2	11 (100)	0	0
Primary	0	3	0	3 (100)	0	0
Malignant hemangioendothelioma 6 tu/2 pts 3 P/1 R/2 M						
All	1	2	3	6 (100)	0	0
Primary	1	2	0	3 (100)	0	0
Other sarcomas 96 tu/88 pts 57 P/13 R/25 M						
All	61 (63.5)	21 (22)	9 (0.9)	91 (85.6)	5 (4.4)	0
Primary	30 (52.6)	14 (24.6)	8 (14)	52 (91.2)	5 (8.8)	0
Low-grade fibromyxosarcoma 1 tu/1 pt 1 P/0 R/0 M						
All	0	0	0	0 (0)	1	0
Primary	0	0	0	0 (0)	0	0
Total 623 tu/479 pts 293 P/190 R/140 M						
All	265 (42.5)	301 (48.3)	29 (4.7)	595 (95.5)	15 (2.4)	13 (2.1)
Primary	90 (30.7)	165 (53.3)	18 (6.1)	273 (93.1)	11 (3.8)	9 (3.1)

Tu; tumor, pts; patients, P; primary, R; recurrent, M; metastatic, MFH; malignant fibrous histiocytoma, MPNST; malignant peripheral nerve sheath tumor, Mal; Malignant, NOS; not otherwise specified, LG; low-grade.

5.4 SMEAR COMPOSITION AND THE DIFFERENTIAL DIAGNOSIS OF SOFT TISSUE TUMORS

The cytological analysis and differential diagnosis are based on the following criteria

- Cellulartity
- Cell pattern
- Stroma pattern
- Balance of cells/stroma quantity
- Architecture
- Secretions

5.4.1 Cellularity on Smears

Cellularity depends on the tumor histology and the quality of the sample. Smears from round cell sarcomas are cell-rich, which parallels the histologic component.

TABLE 5.2 **Cytohistological correlations in selected spindle cell benign tumors according to primary and recurrent nature (based on our previous publications [14,15])**

Tumor type #tu/#pts #P/#R	Accurate	Benign	Subtotal accutate and benign	False positive and suspicious	Unsatisfactory
Benign fibrous histiocytoma 36 tu/35 pts 33 P/3 R					
All	22 (61.1)	11 (30.6)	33 (91.7)	3 (8.3)	0
Primary	21 (63.6)	10 (30.3)	31 (93.9)	2 (6.1)	0
Schwannoma 34 tu/ 34 pts 34 P					
All primaries	13 (38.2)	15 (44.2)	28 (82.4)	3 (8.8)	3 (8.8)
(Lymph)angioma 54 tu/52 pts 52 P/2 R					
All	24 (44.4)	9 (16.7)	33 (61.1)	8 (14.8)	13 (24.1)
Primary	24 (46.1)	9 (17.4)	32 (63.5)	7 (13.4)	12 (23.1)
Desmoid 44 tu/39 pts 32 P/12 R					
All	8 (18.2)	34 (77.2)	42 (95.4)	1 (2.3)	1 (2.3)
Primary	5 (15.6)	25 (78.1)	30 (93.7)	2 (6.3)	0
Nodular Fasciitis 7 tu/7 pts 7 P					
All primaries	1	2	3	3	1
Benign GIST 7 tu/7 pts 7 P					
All primaries	0	4	4	2	1
Leiomyoma 12 tu/12 pts 12 P					
All primaries	1	7	8	1	3
Spindle-cell lipoma 4 tu/4 pts 4 P					
All primaries	2	1	3	1	0
Neurofibroma 11 tu/9 pts 9 P/2 R					
All	6	3	9	1	
Primary	5	3	8	0	1

(Continued)

TABLE 5.2   (Continued)

Tumor type #tu/#pts #P/#R	Accurate	Benign	Subtotal accutate and benign	False positive and suspicious	Unsatisfactory
Neuroma 11 tu/11 pts 11 P All primaries	5	5	10	0	1
Hemangiopericytoma 3 tu/3 pts 2 P/1 R All	1	2	3	0	0
Primary	1	1	2	0	0
Inflammatory tumor 13 tu/12 pts 9 P/4 R All	5	3	8	5	0
Primary	5	2	7	2	0
Solitary fibrous tumor 2 tu/2 pts 2 P All primaries	0	2	2	0	0
Other benign tumors 11 tu/11 pt All primaries	5	2	7	4	0
Benign NOS 13 tu/13 pts 13 P All primaries	13	0	13	0	0
Total 262 tu/249 pts 236 P/26 R All	106 (40.5)	100 (38.2)	206 (78.7)	32 (12.2)	24 (9.1)
Primary	101 (42.8)	88 (37.3)	189 (80.1)	25 (10.6)	22 (9.3)

Smears of spindle cell low-grade sarcomas (like dermatofibrosarcoma protuberans, infantile fibrosarcoma, etc.) are generally of low cellularity compared with corresponding surgical sections. Smears of pleomorphic sarcomas or high-grade spindle-cell sarcomas are usually highly cellular. Smears of predominantly fibrous tumors or mature adipocytes are usually cell-poor (like desmoids or lipomas).

5.4.2 Cell Pattern

Cells may show a great morphologic variability going from spindle-shaped, to roundish, epithelioid-like, and pleomorphic. Giant multinucleated malignant-looking or benign-looking tumors are also a precious indication. Some entities show naked nuclei, binucleation, and malignant mulinucleated giant cells. A detailed analysis of the nuclei, nucleoli, and mitotic figures should be done. Cytoplasms may be anhistic, granulated, microvacuolated, or striated.

5.4.3 Stroma Pattern

Stroma is characterized by the connective tissue components, which are fibrillary, or myxoid with chondroid/osteoid differentiation. A detailed analysis of stroma is often strongly indicative of tumor origin. Stroma is evaluated better with the May-Grunwald-Giemsa (MGG) stain and eventually the Papanicolaou stain. In some laboratories, the Diff-Quik (DQ) stain may replace MGG because it is a variant of MGG. MGG and DQ stains allow a better analysis of stroma than the Papanicolaou stain, whereas the Papanicolaou stain reveals better nuclear definition.

5.4.4 Balance Cells/Stroma Quantity

Smears from soft tissue tumors show stromal and cellular components. Their relationship and their quantity are indicative of their histological architecture and component. Depending on the tumor histology, the smear may be cell-rich, or cell-poor and stroma-rich or stroma-poor.

5.4.5 Architecture

The demonstration of a given architecture on smears is very informative about the architecture. The architecture is an important factor. The observation of cells streams, rosettes, Verocay bodies, dispersed patterns, and so on are also indicative for diagnosis.

5.4.6 Secretions

An important clue in diagnosis is the observation of necrosis and secretions like mucin in biphasic synovial sarcoma. Similarly, intercytoplasmic osteoid is observed in well-differentiated osteoblasts.

5.4.7 Differential Diagnosis

From a practical point of view, smears in soft tissue tumors may be classified according to a predominant cytologic pattern. The differential diagnosis is discussed in concordance with clinicoradiological data.

Superficial tumors comprising spindle-shaped cells without cytonuclear atypia, scant connective fragments, and numerous naked nuclei are representative of a "low-grade mesenchymal tumor" because this diagnosis of a benign condition leads to surgery. The nonrecognition of a tumor low-grade of malignancy, such as derma-tofibrosarcoma, is not dramatic from a clinical point of view, and a definitive diagnosis will be made on a surgical specimen. Inversely, several benign conditions, such as nodular fasciitis, can contain pleomorphic cells that are misdiagnosed as malignancy.

Usually, the diagnosis of high-grade sarcoma does not raise major difficulties. Pleomorphic morphology with atypical cells, mitotic figures, necrosis, and an

TABLE 5.3   Cytohistological correlations in selected round cell sarcomas according to primary and nonprimary tumor nature, (based on our previous publications [16,17])

Tumor type #tu/#pts #P/#R/#M	Accurate	Malignant	Suspicious	Subtotal malignant and suspicious	False negative	Unsatisfactory
Rhabdomyosarcoma 180 tu/109 pts 58 P/34 R/88 M						
All	155 (86.1)	21 (11.7)	3 (1.7)	179 (99.5)	0	1 (0.5)
Primary	43 (74.1)	14 (24.2)	1 (1.7)	58 (100)	0	0
Rhabdoid tumor 19 tu/12 pts 11P/1 R/7 M						
All	14 (74)	5 (26)	0	19 (100)	0	0
Primary	6 (55)	5 (45)	0	11 (100)	0	0
Ewing sarcoma/ peripheral neuroectodermal tumor 50 tu/50 pts						
Only primary	46 (92)	4 (8)	0	50 (100)	0	0
Desmoplastic small round cell tumor 7 tu/5 pts 4 P/3 M						
All	0	7 (100)	0	7 (100)	0	0
Primary	0	4 (100)	0	4 (100)	0	0
Total 256 tu/176 pts 123 P/35 R/98 M						
All	215 (84)	37 (14.4)	3 (0.8)	255 (99.2)	0	1 (0.8)
Primary	95 (77.2)	27 (22)	1 (0.8)	123 (100)	0	0

TABLE 5.4   Selected cytology literature data dealing with soft tissue tumors*

Entity	# cases	Sensitivity	Specificity	Reference
Spindle cell tumors—primary	98			18
Spindle cell tumors—primary	117			19
Spindle cell tumors—primary	7			20
Spindle cell tumors—primary	72	89	87	21
Myxoid sarcomas, all	18			22
Spindle cell tumors—all	77			23
Spindle cell tumors—primary	53	88.5	81.5	24
Sarcoma—primary	96			25
Spindle cell tumors—primary				26
− Deep lesions	166	92	97	
− Superficial lesions	113	90	98	
Bone and soft tissue lesions	1114	96	98	27
All	885	97.5	86.6	Institut Curie
Primary	529	96.1	88.3	

*Some reports include several pseudotumoral lesions and bone or round cell sarcomas.

inflammatory background lead to the diagnosis of a high-grade pleomorphic sarcoma. This group includes a large spectrum of entities such as pleomorphic malignant fibrous histiocytoma, pleomorphic liposarcoma, pleomorphic leiomyosarcoma, high-grade malignant peripheral nerve sheath tumor, and so on. If the nonseparation between entities is not possible with cytology, then the accurate diagnosis can be reached on histological sections with the use of ancillary techniques, although a limited number of cases is unclassifiable. The presence of lipoblasts is suggestive of pleomorphic liposarcoma. Scant osteoid could be representative of extraskeletal pleomorphic osteosarcoma. The following morphologic criteria suggest synovial sarcoma: solid areas of spindle-shaped cells with pseudopapillary clusters, a biphasic component with epithelial cells, a vascularization, and an occasional presence of squamous or mucin-secreting cells.

Tumors comprising spindle-shaped cells associated with a fibrillary stroma are representative of neural origin. The observation of whorls of cells and Verocay bodies is diagnostic of schwannoma or "atypical" schwannoma. A similar tumor exhibiting a polymorphous pattern with cytonuclear atypia and multinucleated giant cells are more often malignant peripheral nerve sheath tumors. Tumors comprising of epithelioid cells with a characteristic pseudocarcinomateous pattern should raise the suspicion of an angiosarcoma and an epithelioid sarcoma as well as clear cell sarcoma, alveolar soft part sarcoma, and epithelioid sarcoma.

Round cell sarcomas are, by definition, of high grade. Rhabdomyosarcomas show rhabdomyoblasts, binucleated cells, and abundant cytoplasms. The alveolar component of rhabdomyosarcomas may depict an alveolar architecture, sometimes observed at low magnification. The association of pleomorphism with spindle-shaped cells is in favor of embryonal rhabdomyosarcoma. Rhabdoid tumors may show a rhabdomyoblastic morphology, but cells are more pleomorphic, and have irregular nuclei and well-visible nucleoli. Frequently, cytoplasms contain perinuclear condensations corresponding to intermediate filaments. Desmoplastic round cell sarcoma also may be composed of roundish cells, but cells usually are preserved poorly with irregular nuclei, and scant connective fragments are observed clearly in the background. Extraskeletal Ewing sarcoma/peripheral neuroectodermal tumors consist of regular, roundish cells which usually present characteristic double cell population, darker/smaller, and clearer/larger cells. Spindle-shaped cells also may be observed occasionally. The rosette formations are strongly in favor of a diagnosis of the Ewing sarcoma/peripheral neuroectodermic tumor family.

The wide chapter of myxoid soft tissue tumors raises diagnostic problems. Among low-grade myxoid tumors, the presence of lipoblasts suggests a diagnosis of myxoid liposarcoma. The observation of a significant number of round or spindle-shaped cells is suggested of round cell variant of myxoid liposarcoma. Some other benign or malignant entities exhibit a myxoid background, including myxoid histiocytoma, myxoid malignant fibrous histiocytoma, myxoid peripheral nerve sheath tumor. A definitive diagnosis often is reached on histological sections. The morphological approach in fine needle aspiration smears to differentiate soft tissue tumors is presented in Table 5.5.

In summary, FNA may be a good tool in the diagnosis of soft tissue tumors. It always should be correlated with the clinical and radiological data and in some cases other ancillary techniques (e.g., infantile fibrosarcoma, Ewing sarcoma/peripheral neuroectodermal tumor, alveolar rhabdomyosarcoma, synovial sarcoma etc.).

TABLE 5.5 Morphological approach in fine needle aspiration smears to differentiate soft tissue tumors

Patten	Possibility of diagnosis	What to do
Low-grade spindle cell tumors — Spindle and oval cells without prominent cytonuclear atypia — Mitotic figures are scant or absent — Connective debris — Naked nuclei — No necrosis — Inflammatory cells — Variable cellularity	1. Fibromatoses or desmoids 2. Nodular fasciitis 3. Dermatofibrosarcoma protuberans 4. Benign fibrous histiocytoma (cellular and atypical variants)	— Clinical and radiological informations are important — Larger and superficial tumors may be dermatofibrosarcomas protuberans — Benign fibrous histiocytoma may contain myxoid or atypical cells. Angiomatoid variant may be misinterpreted as malignant melanoma (quality of pigment) — Some cells exhibit histiocytic morphology in benign fibrous histiocytoma
Tumors with fibrillary stroma — Spindle and oval cells — Slight to marked cytonuclear atypia — Mitotic figures are scant or absent — Fibrillary stroma — Parallel alignment — Connective fragments simulating normal nerve — Comma-like nuclei — No necrosis — Usually high cellularity	1. Benign peripheral nerve sheath tumor (schwannoma, ancient schwannoma, or neurofibroma) 2. Malignant peripheral nerve sheath tumor (low grade)	— Schwannomas and neurofibromas may have similar morphology — If cytonuclear atypia is present, differentiate between ancient schwannoma and low-grade malignant peripheral nerve sheath tumor
Malignant spindle cell tumors — Spindle cells — Possibility of oval cells — Marked cytonuclear atypia — Mitotic figures are present — Connective fragments — Possibility of necrosis — Usually extremely high cellularity	1. Leiomyosarcoma 2. Synovial sarcoma 3. Fibrosarcoma 4. Malignant fibrous histiocytoma, storiform pattern 5. Spindle cell malignant peripheral nerve sheath tumor 6. Spindle cell angiosarcoma 7. Kaposi sarcoma	— Usually there is no problem diagnosing malignancy — Accurate typing may be difficult — Search for cigar-like nuclei, pseudopapillary patterns, epithelial cells, and fibrillary stroma
Myxoid tumors — Spindle or oval cells — Moderate cytonuclear atypia — Mitotic figures are scant	1. Myxoid liposarcoma (with round and spindle cells variants) 2. Myxofibrosarcoma	— Chondroid material may be detected — In myxoid tumors, search for lipoblasts and anastomosing

(Continued)

TABLE 5.5 (Continued)

Patten	Possibility of diagnosis	What to do
— Abundant myxoid background — Usually moderate cellularity	3. Myxoid leiomyosarcoma 4. Myxoma and cellular myxoma 5. Chordoma 6. Extraskeletal myxoid chondrosarcoma	or curvilinear vessels or chicken- wire vessels — Low-grade fibromyxoid sarcoma are low-grade tumors with spindle cells and scant (sometimes undetectable) myxoid — In liposarcoma, search for round or spindle cells — Myxomas may consist only of myxoid and cells may be absent — Chordoma is characterized by strongly magenta myxoid and physaliphorous cells. Compare with clinical and radiological data
Atypical Lipomateous Tumors — Well-differentiated lipoblasts — Moderate cytonuclear atypia — Mitotic figures are scant or absent — Usually moderate cellularity	1. Well-differentiated liposarcoma/Atypical lipoma 2. Spindle cell/Pleomorphic lipoma	— The distinction may be difficult. Search for cytological evidence of malignancy — Clinical presentation
Epithelioid tumors — Roundish cells — Possibility of spindle cells — Cohesive clusters — Various cytonuclear atypia — Mitotic figures are present — Possibility of necrosis — Usually extremely high cellularity	1. Epithelioid sarcoma 2. Epithelioid leiomyosarcoma (GIST) 3. Epithelioid angiosarcoma 4. Granular cell tumor 5. Rhabdoid tumor 6. Alveolar soft part sarcoma 7. Clear cell sarcoma 8. Malignant melanoma	— Angiosarcomas may have pseudocarcinomatous morphology. Search for spindle cells with grayish cytoplasms — Granular cell tumors exhibit characteristic granulomatous cytoplasms, mitoses are absent — Rhabdoid tumors present frequently as highly atypical and polymorphous cells — Alveolar sarcoma and clear cell sarcoma have a characteristic morphology
Pleomorphic sarcomas — Polymorphous, clearly malignant cells — Marked cytonuclear atypia — Numerous mitotic figures — Necrosis is present	1. Pleomorphic malignant fibrous histiocytoma 2. Pleomorphic liposarcoma 3. Pleomorphic leiomyosarcoma and rhabdomyosarcoma 4. Extraskeletal osteosarcoma	— The diagnosis of malignancy is usually accurate — Search for lipoblasts and osteoid/cartilage or fibrillary stroma

(Continued)

TABLE 5.5 (Continued)

Patten	Possibility of diagnosis	What to do
– Usually inflammatory background – Usually extremely high cellularity	5. Pleomorphic malignant peripheral nerve sheath tumor	– The distinction between these entities may be not possible and is not necessary
Round cell sarcomas – Roundish, clearly malignant cells – Moderate cytonuclear atypia – Numerous mitotic figures – Necrosis may be present – Usually extremely high cellularity	1. Embryonnal and alveolar rhabdomyosarcoma 2. Ewing sarcoma/peripheral neuroectodermal tumor 3. Desmoplastic small round cell tumor 4. Extraskeletal mesenchymal chondrosarcoma 5. Poorly differentiated synovial sarcoma	– Clinical and radiological informations are important – Search for rhabdomyoblasts, binucleation, rosettes, and double cell population – Chondroid is usually well detected – Poorly differentiated synovial sarcoma may mimick Ewing sarcoma/peripheral neuroectodermal tumor, search for rosettes and double cell population

REFERENCES

1. Layfield LJ. Cytopathology of bone and soft tissue tumors. New York: Oxford University Press; 2002.

2. Åkerman M, Domanski HA. The cytological features of soft tissue tumours in fine needle aspiration smears classified according to histiotype. In: Orell SR, editor. Monographs in Clinical Cytology. Volume 16. The Cytology of Soft Tissue Tumours. Basel, Kargel; Switzerland: 2003, pp. 17–84.

3. Geisinger K, Abdul-Karim FW. Fine needle aspiration biopsy of soft tissue tumors. In: Strauss M, editor. Enzinger and Weiss's soft tissue tumors. 5th edition. St. Louis, MO: Mosby; 2008, pp. 103–117.

4. Graadt van Roggen JF, Hogendoorn PC, Fletcher CDM. Myxoid tumours of soft tissue. Histopathology 1999, 35: 291–312.

5. Fletcher CDM, Unni KK, Mertens F, editors, World Health Organization classification of tumours. Pathology and genetics. Tumours of soft tissue and bone. Lyon, France: IARC Press; 2002.

6. Klijanienko J, Caillaud JM, Lagacé R, Vielh P. Cytohistologic correlations in 56 synovial sarcomas in 36 patients. The Institut Curie experience. Diagn Cytopathol 2002, 27: 96–102.

7. Klijanienko J, Caillaud JM, Lagacé R, Vielh P. Comparative fine-needle aspiration and pathologic study in malignant fibrous histiocytoma. Cytodiagnostic features of 95 tumors in 71 patients. Diagn Cytopathol 2003, 29: 320–326.

8. Klijanienko J, Caillaud JM, Lagacé R, Vielh P. Fine-needle aspiration of leiomyosarcoma. A correlative cytohistopathological study of 96 tumors in 68 patients. Diagn Cytopathol 2003, 28: 119–125.

9. Klijanienko J, Caillaud JM, Lagacé R, Vielh P. Cytohistologic correlations of 24 malignant peripheral nerve sheath tumors (MPNST) in 17 patients. The Institut Curie experience. Diagn Cytopathol 2002, 27: 103–108.

10. Klijanienko J, Caillaud JM, Lagacé L. Fine-needle aspiration in liposarcoma. Cyto - histologic correlative study including well-differentiated, myxoid, and pleomorphic variants. Diagn Cytopathol 2004, 30: 307–312.

11. Klijanienko J, Caillaud JM, Lagacé R. Fine-needle aspiration of primary and recurrent dermatofibrosarcoma protuberans. Diagn Cytopathol 2004, 30: 261–265.

12. Klijanienko J, Caillaud JM, Lagacé R, Vielh P. Cytology in angiosarcoma including classic and epithelioid variants. Institut Curie's experience. Diagn Cytopathol 2003, 29: 140–145.

13. Colin P, Lagacé R, Caillaud JM, Sastre-Garau X, Klijanienko J. Fine-needle aspiration in myxofibrosarcoma. Institut Curie experience. Diagn Cytopathol, 2010, 38: 343–346.

14. Klijanienko J, Caillaud JM, Lagacé R. Fine-needle aspiration in primary and recurrent benign fibrous histiocytoma (classic, myxoid and angiomatoid variants). Diagn Cytopathol 2004, 31: 387–391.

15. Klijanienko J, Caillaud JM, Lagacé R. Cytohistologic correlations in schwannomas (neurilemmomas) including "ancient," cellular and epithelioid variants. Diagn Cytopathol 2006, 33: 517–522.

16. Klijanienko J, Caillaud JM, Orbach D, et al. Cyto-histological correlations in primary, recurrent and metastatic rhabdomyosarcoma: the institut Curie's experience. Diagn Cytopathol 2007, 35: 482–487.

17. Klijanienko J, Couturier J, Bourdeaut F, et al. Fine-needle aspiration as a diagnostic technique in 50 cases of primary Ewing sarcoma/peripheral neuroectodermal tumor (ES/ PNET). Institut Curie's experience. Diagn Cytopathol, in press.

18. Gonzáles-Cámpora R, Muñoz-Arias G, Otal-Salaveri C, et al. Fine needle aspiration cytology of primary soft tissue tumors. Morphologic analysis of the most frequent types. Acta Cytol. 1992, 36: 905–917.

19. Bennert KW, Abdul-Karim FW. Fine needle aspiration cytology vs. needle core biopsy of soft tissue tumors. A comparison. Acta Cytol 1994, 38: 381–384.

20. Powers CN, Berardo MD, Frable WJ. Fine-needle aspiration biopsy: pitfalls in the diagnosis of spindle-cell lesions. Diagn Cytopathol 1994, 10: 232–241.

21. Maitra A, Ashfaq R, Saboorian MH, Lindberg G, Gokaslan ST. The role of fine-needle aspiration biopsy in the primary diagnosis of mesenchymal lesions. A community-based experience. Cancer 2000, 90: 178–185.

22. Kilpatrick SE, Ward WG, Bos GD. The value of fine-needle aspiration biopsy in the differential diagnosis of adult myxoid sarcoma. Cancer 2000, 90: 167–177.

23. Palmer HE, Mukunyadzi P, Culbreth W, Thomas JR. Subgruping and grading of soft-tissue sarcomas by fine-needle aspiration cytology: a histopathologic correlation study. Diagn Cytopathol 2001, 24: 307–316.

24. Bezabih M. Cytological diagnosis of soft tissue tumours. Cytopathology 2001, 12: 177–183.

25. Kilpatrick SE, Capellari JO, Bos GD, Gold SH, Ward WG. Is fine-needle aspiration biopsy a practical alternative to open biopsy for the primary diagnosis of sarcoma? Am J Clin Pathol 2001, 115: 59–68.

26. Nagira K, Yamamoto T, Akisue T, et al. Reliability of fine-needle aspiration biopsy in the initial diagnosis of soft-tissue lesions. Diagn Cytopathol 2002, 27: 354–361.

27. Khalbuss WE, Teot LA, Monaco SE. Diagnostic accuracy and limitations of fine-needle aspiration cytology of bone and soft tissue lesions. Cancer 2010, 118: 24–32.

Chapter 6

Particular Aspects

Jerzy Klijanienko MD, PhD, MIAC and

Réal Lagacé MD, FRCPC

6.1 LOW-GRADE SPINDLE CELL TUMORS

Benign and malignant low-grade spindle cell lesions of soft tissue include a wide variety of entities, some of which easily can be confused with high-grade malignant tumors. Over the last 30–40 years, new lesions have been described and their clinicopathologic setting has been well identified, (e.g., nodular fasciitis and its clinicomorphologic variants). Older lesions like the group of fibromatoses have been reclassified based on better defined diagnostic criteria, immunohistochemistry, and genetic profiles. Identification of the translocation t(17;22) has become a useful tool for an accurate diagnosis of dermatofibrosarcoma protuberans when the basic conventional morphology is not totally representative of the entity.

We have selected for this review entities prone to represent problems in the histological/cytological interpretation that could simulate malignant tumors; fibromatoses, nodular fasciitis, and dermatofibrosarcomas protuberans will be analyzed in more detail. Two morphologic variants of benign fibrous histiocytoma deserve comments because their morphology easily is confused with malignancies.

It is important to recall that some entities of this group present serious limitations for the use of fine needle aspiration (FNA) and core needle biopsy (CNB) for diagnosis. For example, maturating fasciitis and fibromatoses are difficult to distinguish even at the histopathological level. Moreover, being stroma-rich in dense collagen fibers, cytological aspirates are frequently cell-poor and consequently rendered insufficient for diagnosis. Therefore, it seems that fine needle aspiration and core needle biopsy diagnoses in low-grade spindle cell tumors should be limited to "low-grade spindle cell tumor of uncertain malignant potential" and should be compared with radiologic imaging and require histopathologic evaluation.

Soft Tissue Tumors: A Multidisciplinary, Decisional Diagnostic Approach
Edited by Jerzy Klijanienko and Réal Lagacé
Copyright © 2011 John Wiley & Sons, Inc.

The diagnosis of benignancy in fibromatoses and desmoids should be concluded after the exclusion of sarcoma in accordance with radiology imaging and clinical presentation. However, an accurate cytological diagnosis is possible in the case of nodular fasciitis and benign fibrous histiocytoma, whereas dermatofibrosarcomas protuberans are characterized by a high false-negative rate [1].

6.1.1   Fibromatoses and Desmoids

Fibromatoses/desmoids is the general term used for a group of benign fibrous tissue proliferations of similar microscopic appearance. These are locally aggressive neoplasms, that are locally infiltrative with tissue destruction but, unlike sarcomas, never metastasize. Excluded from this category are nonspecific reactive tissue proliferations associated with the inflammatory process or are secondary to injury [2]. Their nomenclature is complex, particularly regarding the fibromatoses of infancy and childhood, which will not be discussed in the present review, and are different in morphology as well as in their clinical settings.

For practical purposes, adult fibromatoses are subdivided into fibromatoses of Dupuytren type (including Ledderhose disease, Peyronie's disease, and knuckle pads), also called superficial fibromatoses because they seem to develop from the overlying superficial fascia or aponeurosis, whereas deep fibromatosis are called musculoaponeurotic or desmoid type. In terms of cytological approach, only the deep-seated fibromatosis are the most frequently aspirated; whatever the clinical setting of adult fibromatoses—extraabdominal, abdominal, and intraabdominal— their morphological composition at the microscopic level is similar. They differ by their localization and a predominance to occur mostly in females. However, most occur between the second and the fourth decades. Most are sporadic lesions, whereas some cases are familial, as is common with mesenteric fibromatoses. As already stated, they are locally aggressive and destructive lesions, can be very harmful and are dependent on the area of the body affected, (e.g., head and neck and popliteal desmoids present much more serious management surgical problems in comparison with the abdominal wall and soft tissues of a limb). The ratio of recurrence is high, ranging in the literature from as low as 19% [3–5] to as high as 76%. Spontaneous regressions of desmoids have been reported in sporadic cases.

Abdominal fibromatosis, although similar in morphology and by its infiltrative character, deserves special consideration because of its clinical profile (characteristic localization with involvement of the muscle rectus abdominis, and a tendency to occur in women of childbearing age during or after pregnancy). Intraabdominal fibromatosis refers to a group of related lesions rather than a single entity. It encompasses pelvic fibromatoses, mesenteric fibromatoses, and fibromatoses of Gardner syndrome; the latter is inherited as an autosomal dominant trait occurring in approximately 50% of children of the affected parents.

6.1.1.1   Histopathology. The histologic picture of fibromatoses is constant with minimal variations from case to case. The infiltrating and destructive character already has been emphasized. The tumor consists of a proliferation of elongated, slender, spindle-shaped cells separated by abundant collagen with little or no cell-to-cell contact (Fig 6.1). The cellular density is variable from tumor to tumor, with some being hypocellular and others showing more compact areas of tumor cells (Figs 6.2

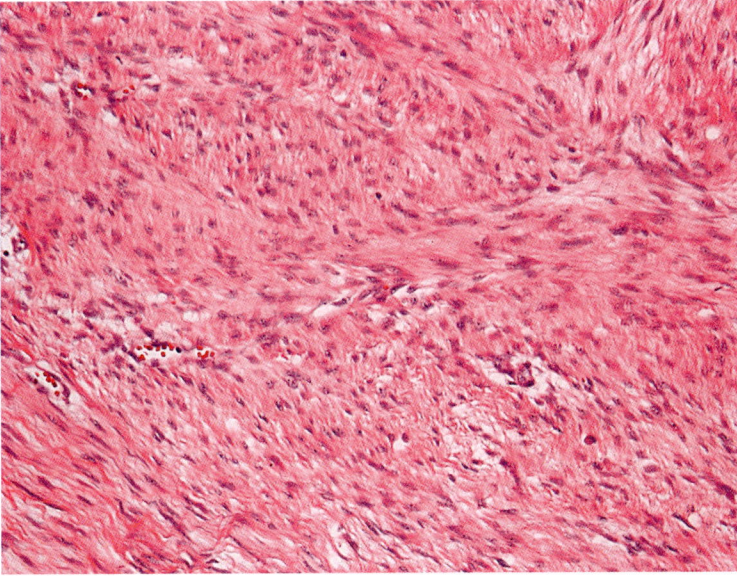

FIG 6.1 Desmoid tumor, area of abundant collagenous stroma.

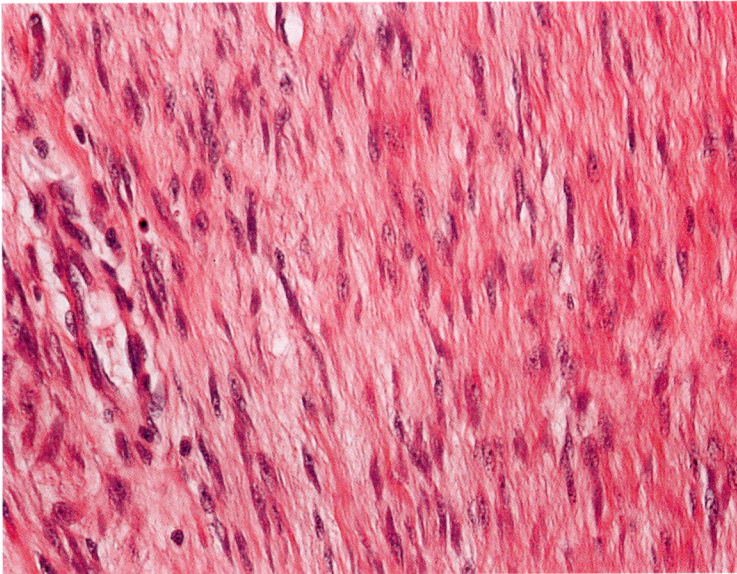

FIG 6.2 Higher magnification in a desmoid tumor showing a population on spindle monotonous cells.

and 6.3). Frequently, at the periphery of the tumor, one observes entrapped myofibers undergoing degenerative changes with the formation of giant multi-nucleated cells (Fig 6.4). The density of stroma is variable ranging from loosely collagenic fibers in a myxoid background to densely hyalinized collagen (Fig 6.5).

Distinguishing fibromatoses from low-grade fibrosarcoma could be difficult. Paradoxically, low-grade fibrosarcomas are better-demarcated tumors with increasing

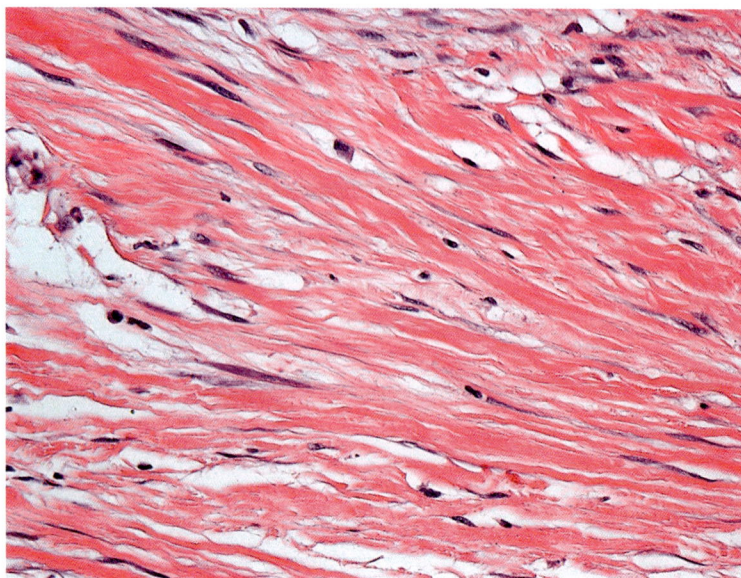

FIG 6.3   Desmoid tumor, hypocellular area.

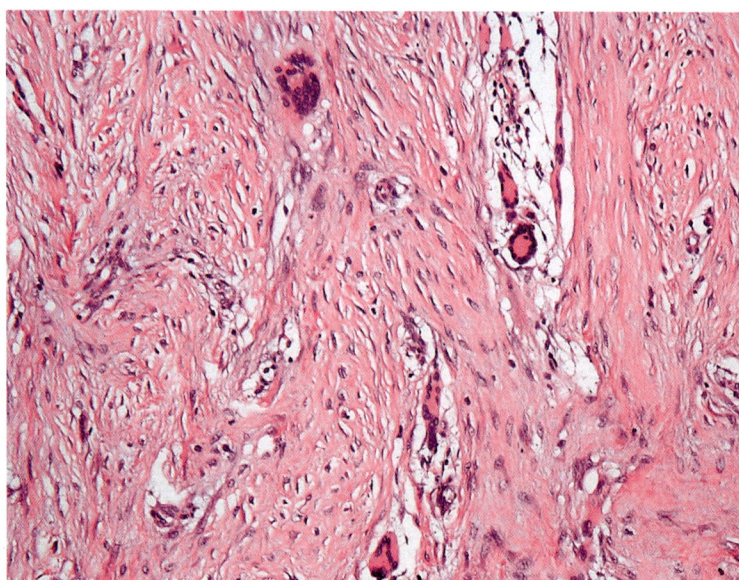

FIG 6.4   Desmoid tumor, entrapped myofibers with degenerative striated muscle cells.

cellularity and mitosis. In addition, nuclei of fibromatoses are bland in comparison with mild-to-moderate atypia in grade I fibrosarcoma.

An immunohistochemical profile is helpful to precise the diagnosis; fibroblasts of desmoids are smooth muscle actin positive, rarely desmin positive, and occasionally estrogen and progesteron receptors positive. Positivity for CD117 and beta-catenin

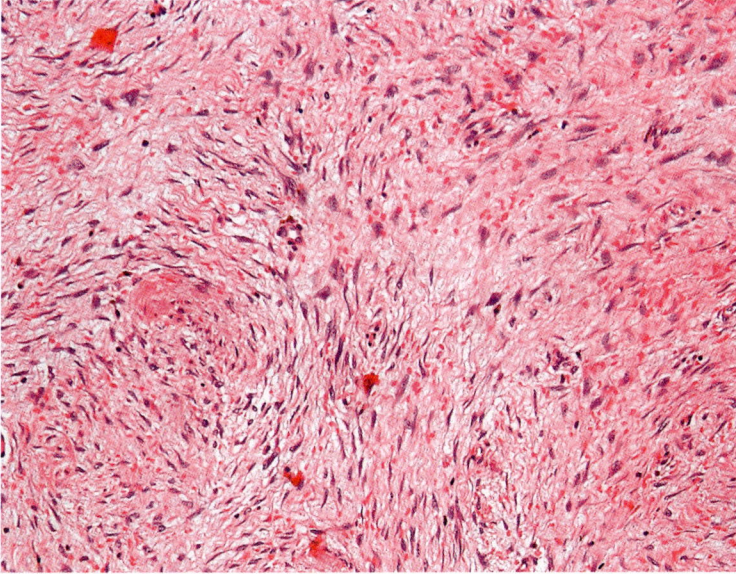

FIG 6.5 Desmoid tumor, loose collagen fibers in a myxoid background.

also has been reported, but it seems that it is antibody-dependant. The immunohistochemical profile of fibrosarcoma is deceptive, depicting only vimentin positivity.

6.1.1.2 Cytopathology. Cytology smears are usually cell-poor and stroma-poor. Cellular material frequently is reduced to benign, spindle-shaped cells with elongated nuclei and eosinophilic ground substance (Figs 6.6 and 6.7). Some cells may be roundish (Fig 6.8). Spindle-shaped cells may exhibit tapering cytoplasmic processes (Fig 6.9). Predominantly bland spindle cells with long, fusiform nuclei and metachromatic matrix material is present in most tumors (Figs 6.10 and 6.11). The tumor cells are present both singly and as fragments embedded in the matrix (Fig 6.12). No cytonuclear atypia or mitosis usually is observed, but cell-rich and irregular cells also are described (Fig 6.13). There are also occasionnal multinucleated cells consistent with degenerating skeletal muscle fibers and adipocytes. In the background, inflammatory cells may be observed.

6.1.1.3 Differential Diagnosis. The following are key features of fibromatoses and desmoids.

- Dermatofibrosarcoma protuberans (DFSP)
- Benign fibrous histiocytoma
- Nodular fasciitis
- Low-grade spindle cell sarcoma

Fine needle aspiration is a useful procedure for the initial and recurrent diagnosis of fibromatoses and in the separation of fibromatoses from other benign and malignant soft tissue lesions. The main cytologic differential diagnosis includes nodular fasciitis, dermatofibrosarcoma protuberans, and low-grade spindle cell sarcomas. The smears in nodular fasciitis are cell-rich and stroma-poor. The presence

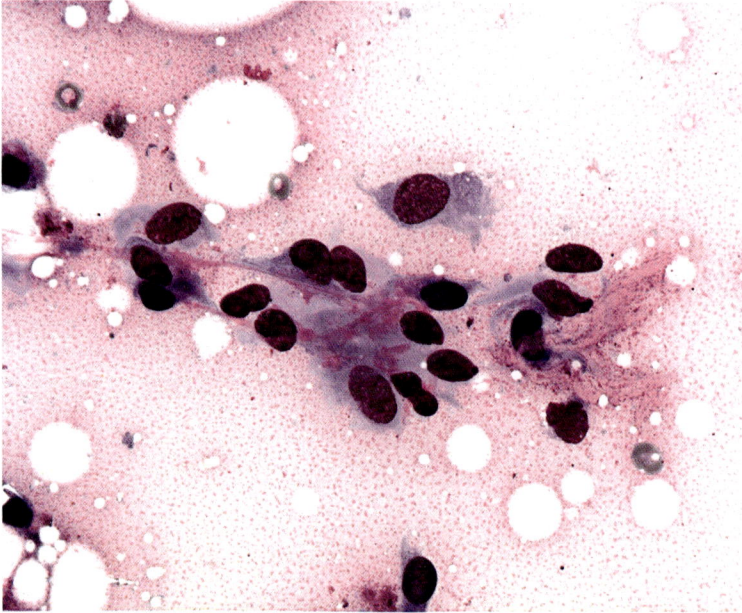

FIG 6.6 Desmoid tumor, benign, spindle-shaped cells with elongated nuclei and eosinophilic ground substance.

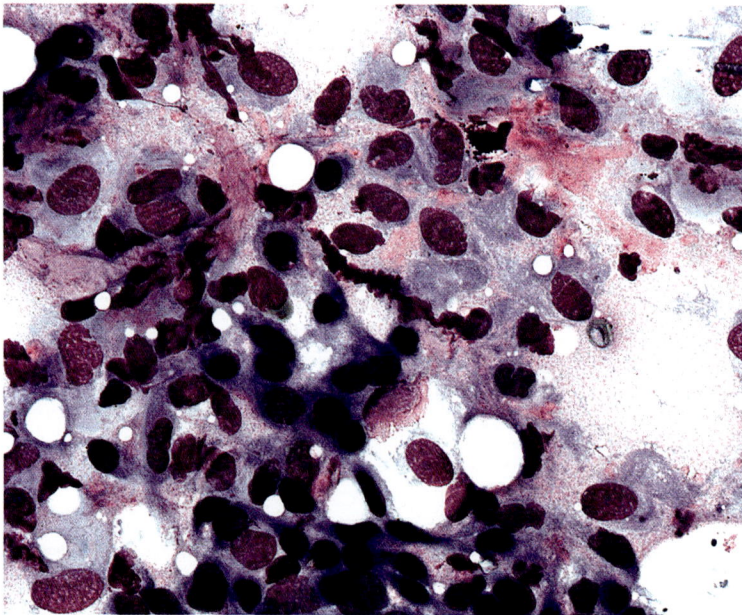

FIG 6.7 Desmoid tumor, benign, spindle-shaped cells with elongated nuclei and eosinophilic ground substance of higher cellularity.

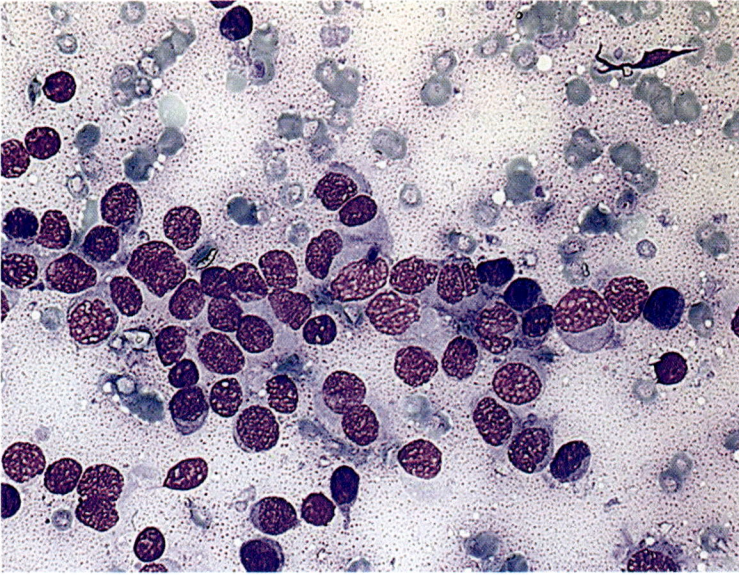

FIG 6.8 Desmoid tumor, roundish cells.

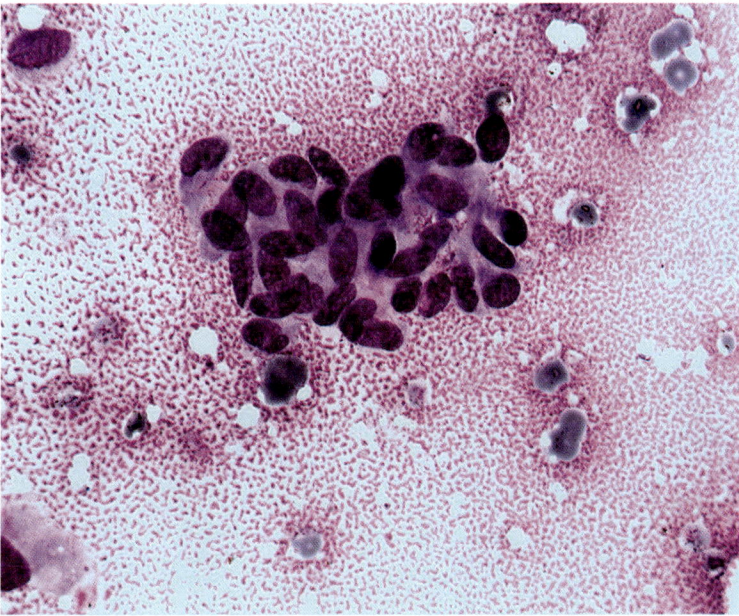

FIG 6.9 Desmoid tumor, spindle-shaped cells with tapering cytoplasmic processes.

of spindle-shaped fibroblasts with moderate cytonuclear atypia and the presence of multinucleated cells within a myxoid background are strongly in favor of this diagnosis. Inversely, fibromatoses / desmoids are cell-poor and contain moderate amounts of regular fibroblasts. Hypercellularity, cytonuclear atypia, and mitotic figures are rather suggestive of malignancy (Table 6.1).

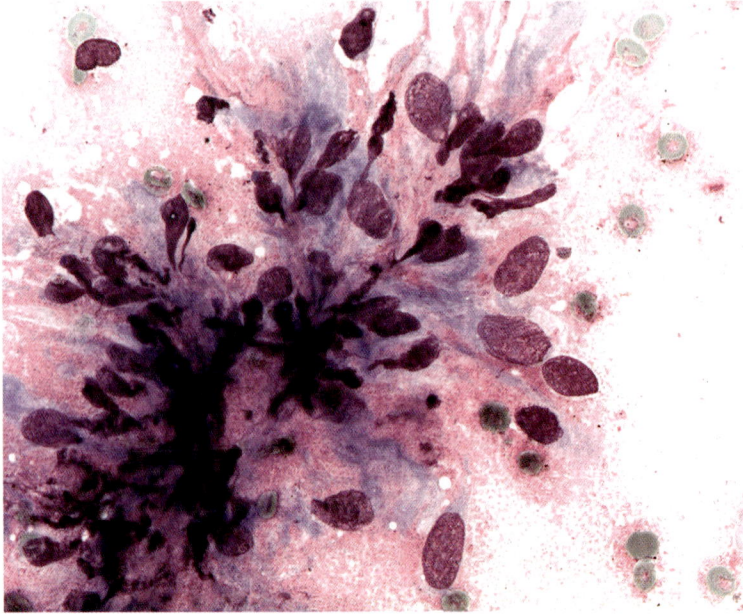

FIG 6.10 Desmoid tumor, metachromatic matrix.

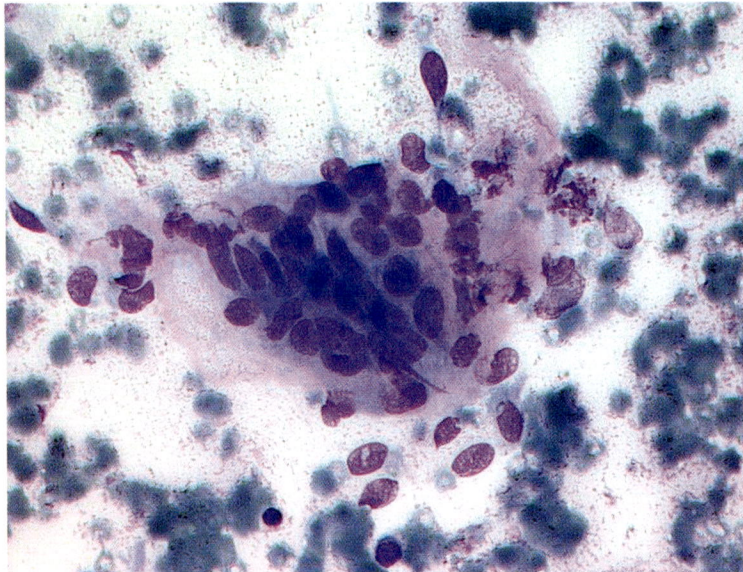

FIG 6.11 Desmoid tumor, polymorphous cells within connective eosinophilic background.

6.1.1.4 Comments. There is a limited number of cytology studies of fibromatoses / desmoids [6—10]. A concensus persists that "negative for malignancy fine needle aspiration diagnosis" allows eliminating spindle cell sarcoma rather then performing an accurate diagnosis. Because of the infiltrative nature of desmoids, the radiographic

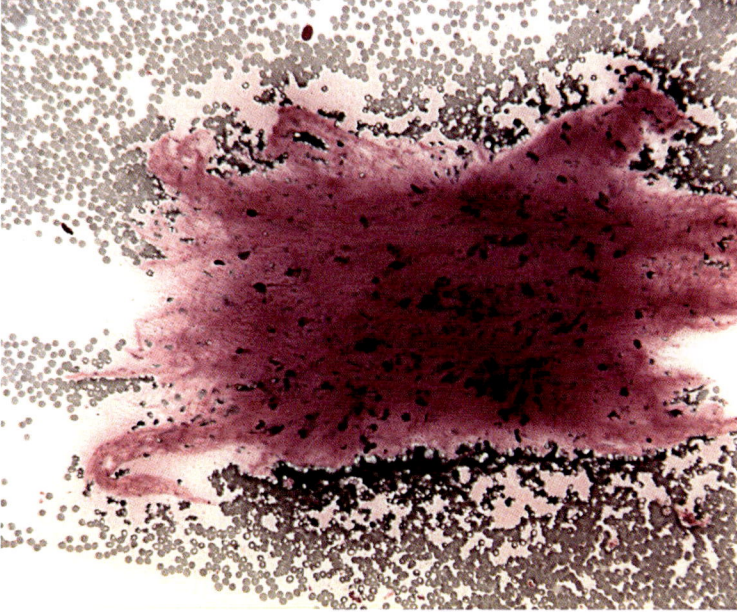

FIG 6.12 Desmoid tumor, single cells embedded in the matrix. Note the low cellularity.

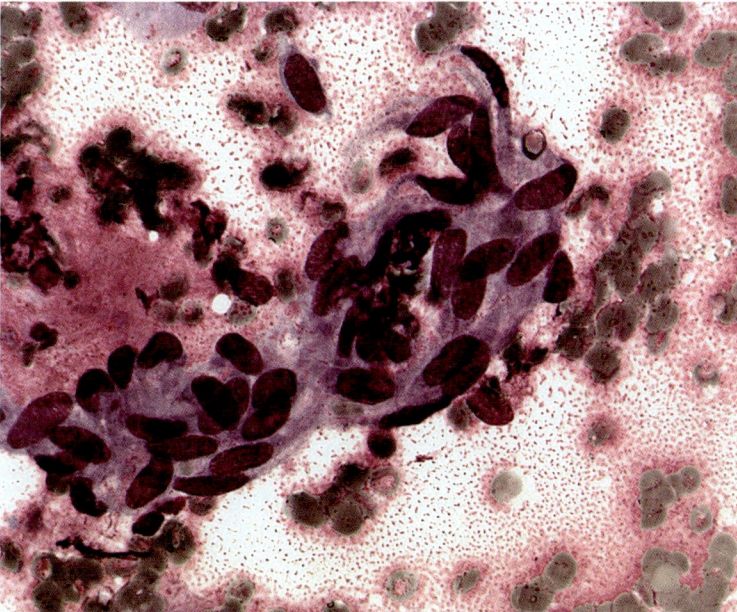

FIG 6.13 Desmoid tumor, irregular cells. Compare with Fig 5.9.

impression is frequently suspicious for malignancy. The diagnostic accuracy of fine needle aspiration and core needle biopsy in 69 and 26 patients, respectively, who have had surgical resections for desmoids / fibromatosis has been evaluated [8]. Cytology-based diagnoses of desmoid / fibromatosis were rendered in 35 of 69 cases, with other

TABLE 6.1 Cytologic differential diagnosis of fibromatoses/desmoid

	Fibromatosis / desmoid	Nodular fasciitis	Low-grade spindle cell sarcoma	DFSP
Hypercellularity	−	++	++	+
Cytonuclear atypia	+/−	+	+	+/−
Giant cells	+/−	+	+	−
Mitotic figures	−	++	++	+/−
Myxoid	−	+	Depending tumor type	+/−

++; frequent, +; rare, +/−; occasionally observed, −; absent.

benign spindle cell proliferations in 26 cases and spindle cell sarcoma in the remaining 4 cases. Cytology was shown fairly reliable for recognizing the benign nature of desmoids. Another study [6] showed that the aspirates of fibromatoses consisted of groups of loosely cohesive, bland-appearing, spindle-shaped cells with oval to elongated nuclei and cytoplasmic tags. Individual spindle cells and rare inflammatory cells also were present. The authors concluded that fine needle aspiration was a useful procedure for the initial and recurrent diagnosis of fibromatoses and in the separation of fibromatoses from other benign and malignant soft tissue lesions.

6.1.1.5 Clinical and Fine Needle Aspiration Key Features. The following are in favor of the diagnosis:

— Poorly cellular material comprising spindle-shaped regular cells
— Hyalinized tissue fragments
— Characteristic clinical and radiological presentations

The following is a difficulty in the diagnosis:

— Some smears may be rich with a mixture of fibroblasts/myofibroblasts

The following is evidence against the diagnosis:

— Atypical cells, numerous mitotic figures

6.1.2 Nodular Fasciitis

Tumor-like lesions, often reactive processes, form a diverse group of distinct entities that are different in their clinical behavior. This category includes nodular fasciitis and its clinicomorphologic variants such as proliferative fasciitis, proliferative myositis, and ischemic fasciitis (atypical decubital fibroplasia). Another recently identified sub-group now is termed "organ-associated pseudosarcomatous myofi-broblastic proliferations." Most of these lesions are reactive processes clinically characterized by a rapid increase in volume of a tender, sometimes painful, superficial or deep soft tissue nodule. They occur at any age but are more common in young adults between 20 and 40 years of age. With rare exceptions, they are small lesions whose sites of predilection are the limbs, although they can be observed in any part of the body (e.g., the special variant of cranial fasciitis which affects mostly infants during the first year of life and involves the soft tissues of the scalp and the underlying skull). Proliferative faciitis and its deeper muscular counterpart, proliferative myositis, tend to affect older patients (mean 54 years) and is similar to nodular fasciitis in terms of a clinical rapid-growing mass and sites affected. If nodular fasciitis is a relatively well-circumscribed lesion, hence the designation "nodular," then deeper lesions of the proliferative variety are poorly circumscribed with infiltrating borders. In fact, low-magnification microscopic examination of proliferative myositis gives an architectural "checker-board" pattern because of its infiltrating character. Myxoid or fibrous stroma and cellularity, according to the stage of the lesion, give different gross aspects. Ischemic fasciitis predominantly involves soft tissue over bony prominences and occurs in elderly and physically debilited and immobilized patients bedridden or wheelchair-bound. All these lesions are self-limited, benign, and are the consequence of fascial/muscular injury. Their morphologic composition is analogous to the fibrovascular phasis of inflammatory reaction, characterized by the abundance of activated fibroblasts/myofibroblasts.

6.1.2.1 *Histopathology.*
The main histologic characteristics of nodular fasciitis are unencapsulated proliferation of spindle-shaped cells with plumped nuclei (Fig 6.14), distinct nucleoli, and abundant basophilic cytoplasm with distinct borders (Fig 6.15). In early stages, cells resemble "fibroblasts in tissue culture" (Fig 6.16). Mitoses are frequent and typical. Secondary changes are variable according to the stage of the lesion which includes microcysts (Fig 6.17), erythrocyte extravasation, myxoid loose stroma, and delicate thin-walled capillaries. Some lesions may countain a limited number of multinucleate giant cells resembling osteoclasts. Maturating fasciitis show a more densely collagenous stroma that could simulate fibromatoses.

The morphologic hallmark of proliferative fasciitis is the presence of numerous so-called "ganglioid cells"; these cells are large, round, or polygonal with abundant

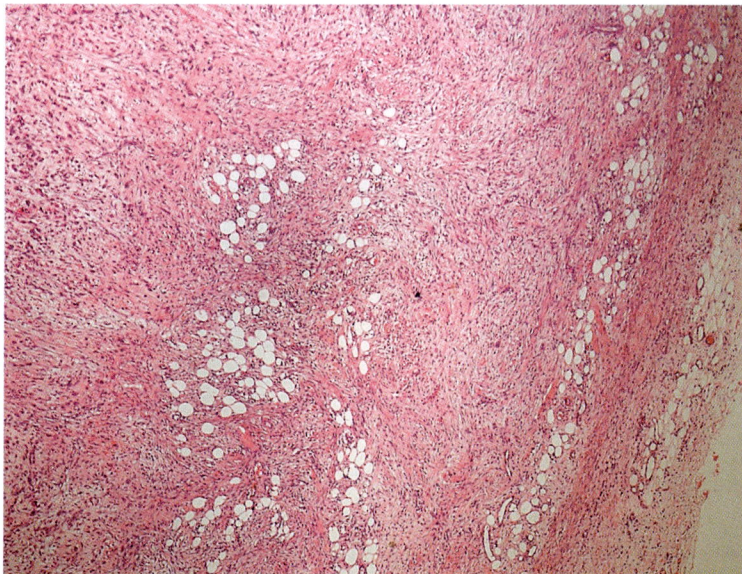

FIG 6.14 Nodular fasciitis, unencapsulated lesion in the vicinity of a fascia.

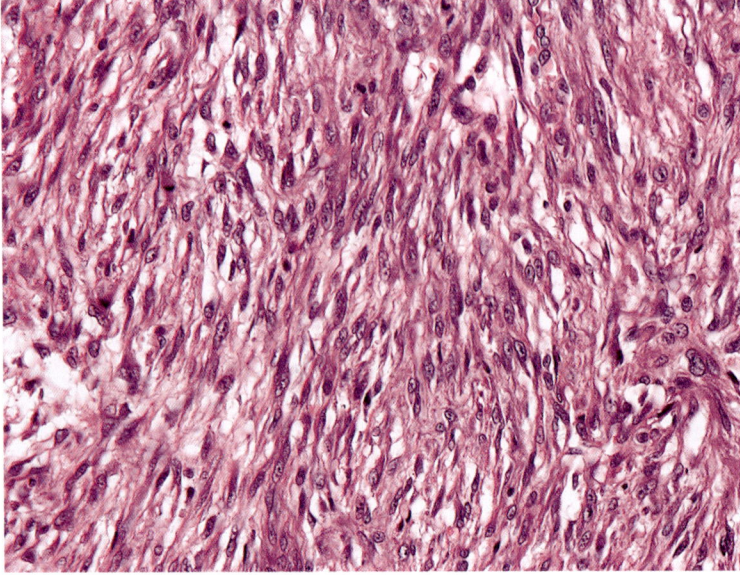

FIG 6.15   Nodular fasciitis, spindle-shaped cells with plumped nuclei and basophilic cytoplasm.

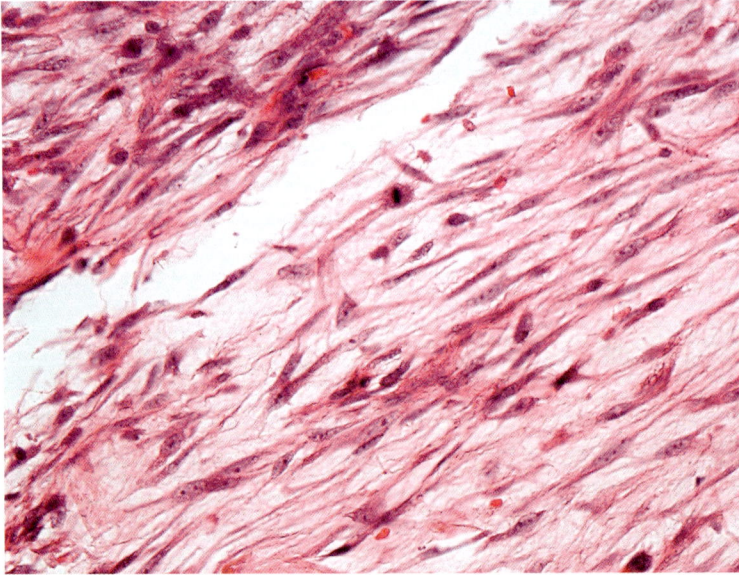

FIG 6.16   Nodular fasciitis, spindle cells mimicking fibroblasts in tissue culture.

basophilic cytoplasm and well-defined borders (Fig 6.18). Nuclei are large and vesicular with prominent nucleoli. Such cells have been misinterpreted in the past as rhabdomyo-blasts, malignant ganglion cells, hence, false-positive diagnosis as sarcomas. Ganglioid cells are intermixed with fibroblasts and foci of acute inflammation. It is not unusual that the center of lesions contain a fibrin network. As already stated, proliferative fasciitis are deeper infiltrating lesions extending along the interlobular septa of the subcutaneous

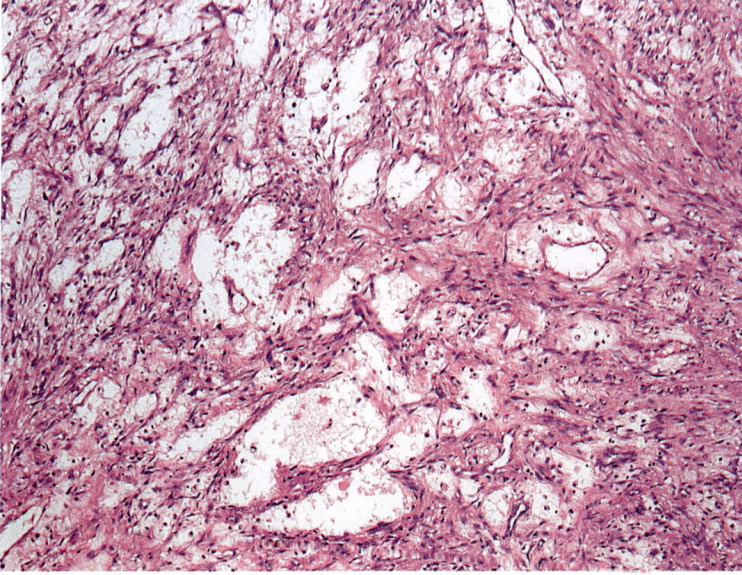

FIG 6.17 Nodular fasciitis, microcysts.

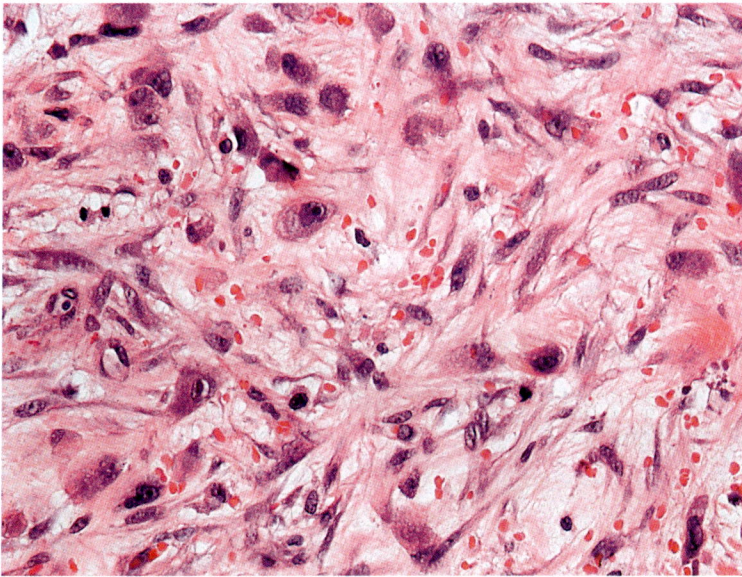

FIG 6.18 Proliferative fasciitis with so-called ganglioid cells.

tissue or between individual myofibers for the muscular variant. They also tend to be more mitosis-rich. A typical immunohistochemical profile of nodular fasciitis is characterized by the expression of alpha smooth muscle actin, which is the hallmark of activated fibroblasts/myofibroblasts.

Organ-associated pseudosarcomatous proliferations have been identified relatively recently and originally were termed "postoperative spindle cell nodules,"

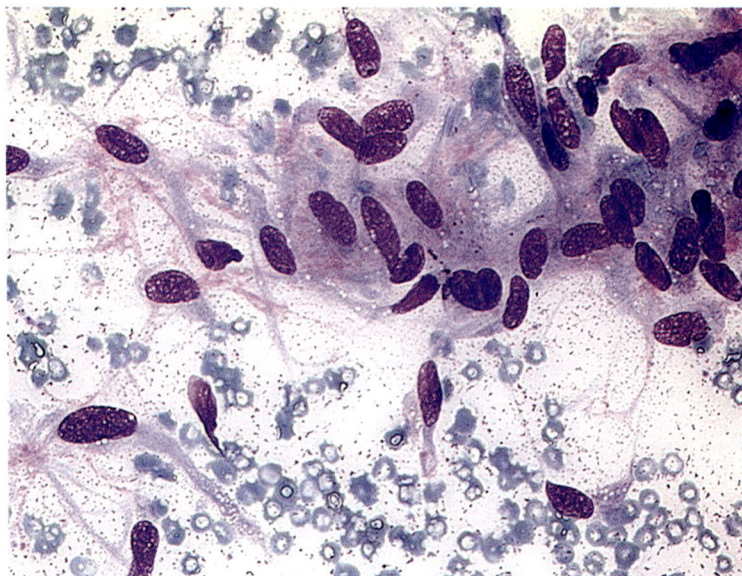

FIG 6.19 Nodular fasciitis, isolated spindle-shaped cells.

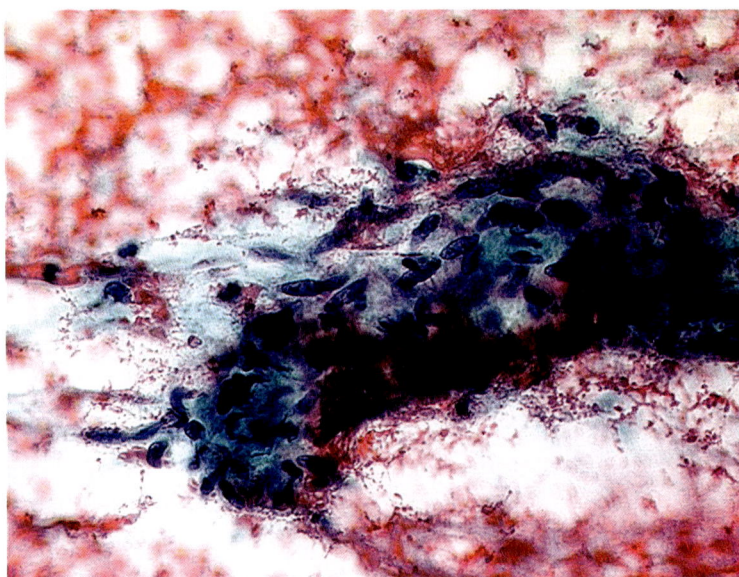

FIG 6.20 Nodular fasciitis, clustered spindle-shaped cells.

although they do not all occur after previous biopsies or surgical procedures. The original descriptions focused on lesions of the genitourinary tract; they are in fact more frequent in those settings. These tissues are exophytic nodular/polypoid lesions that may infiltrate the affected organs deeply. At microscopic examination, the lesion is similar to nodular fasciitis and is reminiscent of the fibrovascular phases of inflammatory reaction. The immunohistochemical profile resembles a reactive

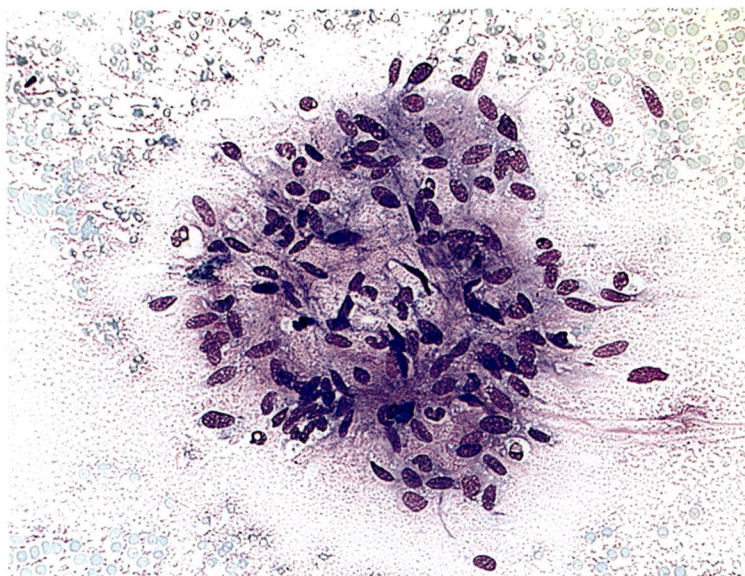

FIG 6.21 Nodular fasciitis, isolated or clustered spindle-shaped cells.

process. The identification of epithelial markers raised concerns about sarcomatoid carcinoma. Evidence suggests that it represents a non-neoplastic reparation process.

6.1.2.2 Cytopathology. Cytological smears are consistently hypercellular and stroma-poor. They consist of an admixture of plump, isolated, or clustered spindle-shaped cells (Figs 6.19 to 6.21), rare giant and/or multinucleated cells of histiocytic origin (Fig 6.22). Cytoplasms may be well delimited and granular. Mitotic activity is detectable but not atypical. Some cases may show a myxoid background (Fig 6.23) as well as inflammatory cells.

6.1.2.3 Differential Diagnosis. The following are key features of nodular fasciitis.

- Desmoids
- Low-grade spindle cell sarcoma
- Dermatofibrosarcoma protuberans
- Benign fibrous histiocytoma
- Benign peripheral nerve sheath tumor (nevroma, schwannoma)

Nodular fasciitis should be distinguished from a benign peripheral nerve sheath tumor and from low-grade spindle-cell sarcoma. Benign peripheral nerve sheath tumors exhibit typical fibrillary connective tissue and may show Verocay bodies. Some schwannomas also may exhibit a myxoid background, which appears more finely fibrillar. However, cell clusters are noted for alternating areas of hypercellularity and hypocellularity.

The differentiation from low-grade spindle-cell sarcoma is based on the presence of atypical mitotic figures. The differential diagnosis is presented in Table 6.1.

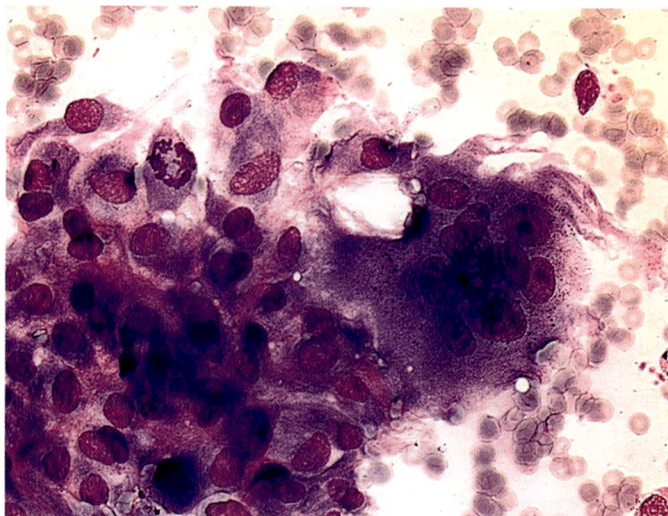

FIG 6.22   Nodular fasciitis, multinucleated cells of histiocytic origin. Note the presence of mitosis (upper left).

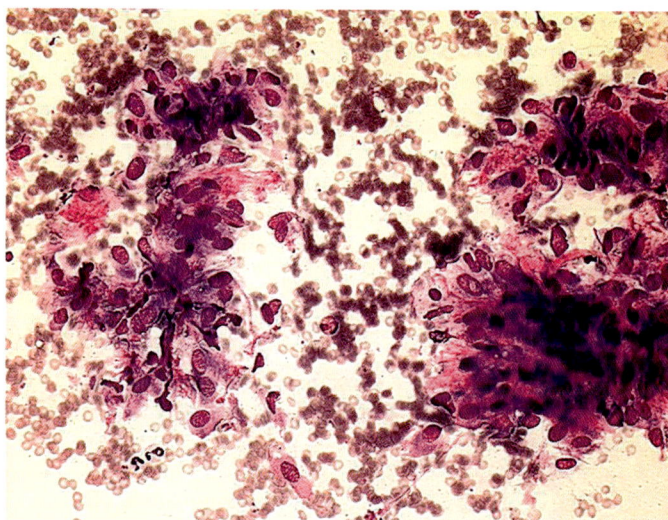

FIG 6.23   Nodular fasciitis, myxoid background.

6.1.2.4   Comments. Usually, smears of nodular fasciitis are hypercellular with overlapping, relatively isomorphic spindle cells that may be mistaken cytologically for sarcoma. They show a mixture of spindle cells showing occasional long cytoplasmic process and cells with abundant cytoplasm with round-to-oval eccentric nuclei mimicking myoepithelial cells. Aggregates of spindle cells also may be embedded in a myxoid background with occasional small tufts of a fibrillar myxoid stroma. At least 40 cases of cytology of nodular fasciitis have been published in the literature [11–15]. An accurate cytologic diagnosis of nodular fasciitis is important because it obviates the need for surgical excision.

6.1.2.5 FNA Key Features. The following are in favor of the diagnosis:

- Hypercellular smears showing mononuclear cells with eccentric, regular nuclei
- Multinucleated giant cells
- Macrophages or inflammatory background

The following are difficulties in making a diagnosis:

- Mitotic figures
- Myxoid background.

The following is evidence against a diagnosis:

- Necrosis, important cytonuclear atypia, atypical mitoses

6.1.3 Dermatofibrosarcoma Protuberans

Dermatofibrosarcoma protuberans now is best classified as a cutaneous fibroblastic neoplasm of intermediate malignancy. Although it can occur at any site, the trunk and proximal extremities are sites of predilection. Dermatofibrosarcoma protuberans is a slowly growing, infiltrating, and locally aggressive tumor that recurs in about 50% of the effected patients. The fibrosarcomatous variety of dermatofibrosarcoma protuberans, more recently described, persues a more aggressive clinical course resulting in metastatic disease. Howewer, subsequent studies [16] seem to show that behavior can be favorable following a wide local excision to extend that its biological behavior shows little increased risk of metastases over conventional dermatofibrosarcoma protuberans. They probably represent a phenomena of tumor progression/dedifferentiation.

6.1.3.1 Histopathology. Apart its exophytic sometimes polypoid and protuberans appearance, dermatofibrosarcoma protuberans is characterized by a diffuse infiltrative pattern of growth of the dermis and subcutis (Fig 6.24). Hyperplasia of the overlying epidermis is absent. The tumor could expend deeply between the septa of subcutaneous tissue creating a lace-like or honeycombing effect. Frequently, cutaneous adnexae and preexisting nerve bundles and vessels are engulfed by the cellular proliferation. The main histologic composition is characterized by a proliferation of monotonous spindle cells of fibroblast type grouped in a storiform or cartwheel pattern (Fig 6.25). The cells are admixed with an inconspicuous vasculature. They show remarkable monomorphism and rarely a low mitotic activity (Fig 6.26). This uniformity of cell composition is a first step to differentiate dermatofibrosarcoma protuberans from fibrohistiocytic neoplasms. The presence of so-called "myoid balls" is observed in some cases (Fig 6.27). Secondary changes are rare. Myxoid variants of dermatofibrosarcoma protuberans have been described as well as a pigmented variant (Bednar tumor) when pigmented melanocytes are dispersed in the tumor. The distinction of dermatofibrosarcoma protuberans from a peripheral nerve tumor must be considered, particularly the diffuse form of neurofibroma, which shares an infiltrative pattern with dermatofibrosarcoma protuberans as well as a bland spindle cell component. By immunohistochemistry, neurofibroma is

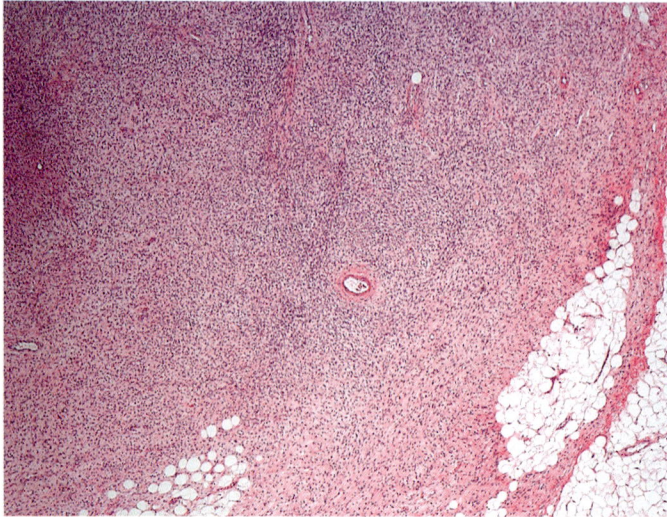

FIG 6.24 Dermatofibrosarcoma protuberans, infiltrative pattern of growth.

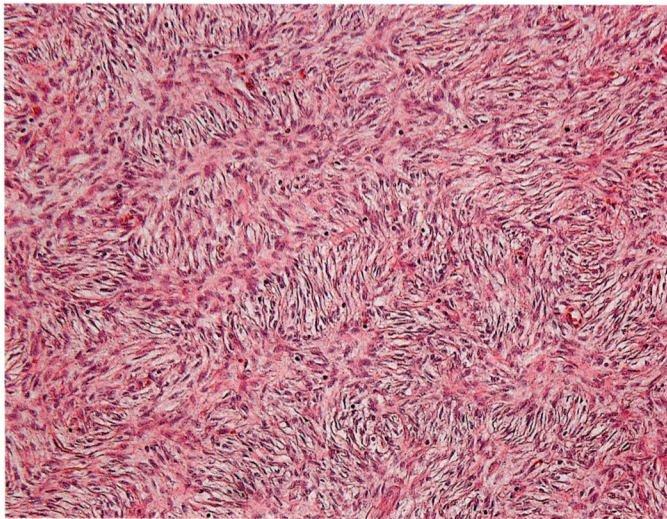

FIG 6.25 Dermatofibrosarcoma protuberans, characteristic storiform pattern.

diffusely positive for S-100 protein, whereas dermatofibrosarcoma protuberans is S-100 negative.

6.1.3.2 Cytopathology.

Fine needle aspiration smears are usually hypercellular and stroma-poor. They are homogenous. They include a storiform pattern within stromal fragments (Figs 6.28–6.31), isolated spindle cells, naked nuclei, and slight-to-moderate cytonuclear atypia (Figs 6.32 and 6.33). Mitotic figures, fibrillary stromal fragments, and a myxoid background may be observed occasionally (Fig 6.34). Giant cells, necrosis, or marked cytonuclear atypia are not observed.

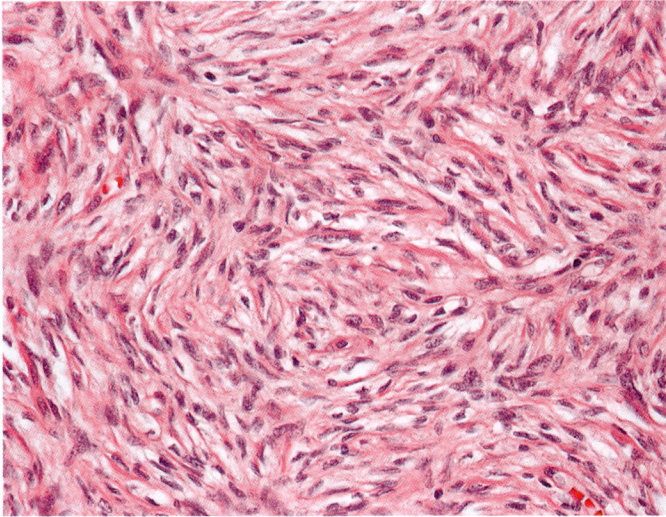

FIG 6.26 Dermatofibrosarcoma protuberans, monotonous spindle cells of fibroblastic type.

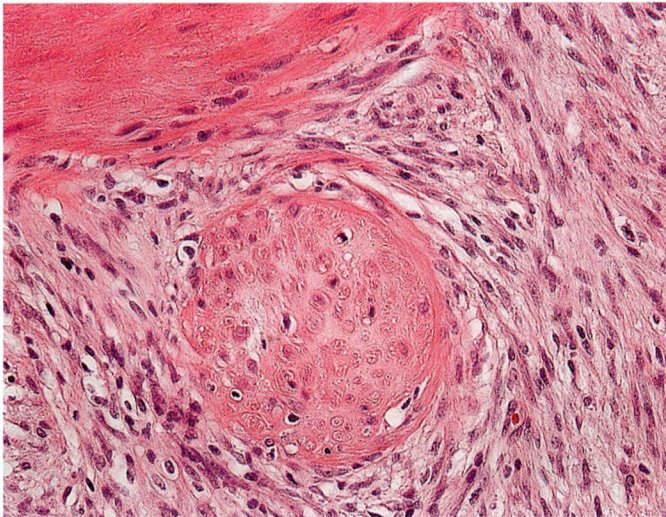

FIG 6.27 Dermatofibrosarcoma protuberans, so-called "myoid ball."

6.1.3.3 Differential Diagnosis. The following entities should be differentiated with dermatofibrosarcoma protuberans:

- Desmoids
- Low-grade spindle cell sarcoma
- Low-grade malignant peripheral nerve sheath tumor
- Nodular fasciitis
- Benign fibrous histiocytoma

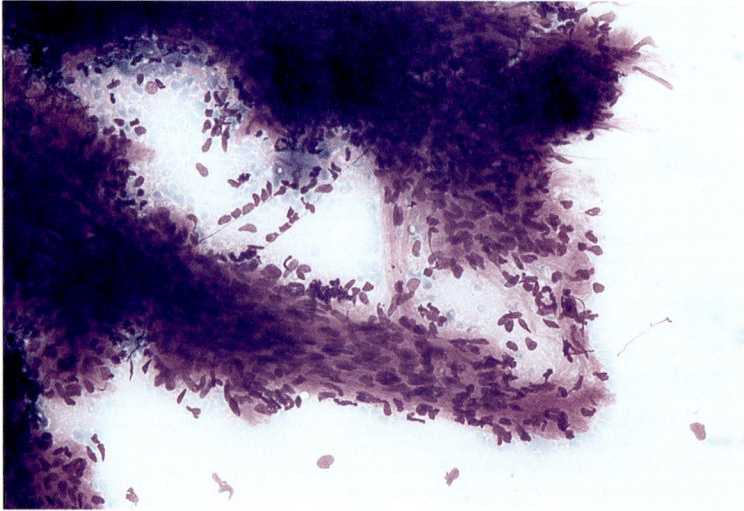

FIG 6.28 Dermatofibrosarcoma protuberans, storiform pattern within stromal fragments.

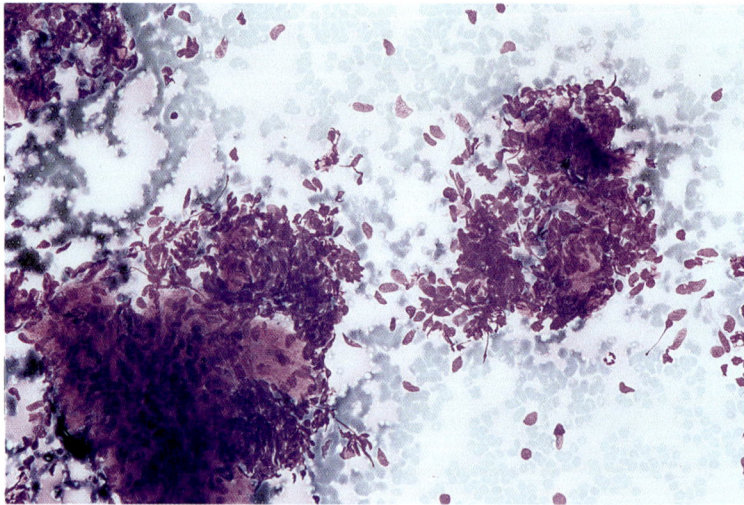

FIG 6.29 Dermatofibrosarcoma protuberans, isolated cells.

Dermatofibrosarcoma protuberans could raise difficulties in differential diagnosis with low-grade fibrosarcoma, fibromatosis, and fibrohistiocytic tumors. Besides some of its histologic characteristics, the immunohistochemical profile is characteristic showing a diffuse CD34 immunoreactivity that allows an accurate diagnosis. The distinction between benign fibrous histiocytoma occasionally proves difficult, particularly with superficial biopsies. Once again, CD34 is expressed rarely and focally by benign fibrous histiocytoma. The knowledge of the clinical setting, the size, and the configuration of the lesion could suggest the diagnosis.

Cytogenetic analyzes as well as molecular biology are useful adjuncts. The former depicts a supernumerary ring of chromosome 11 and amplification sequences of

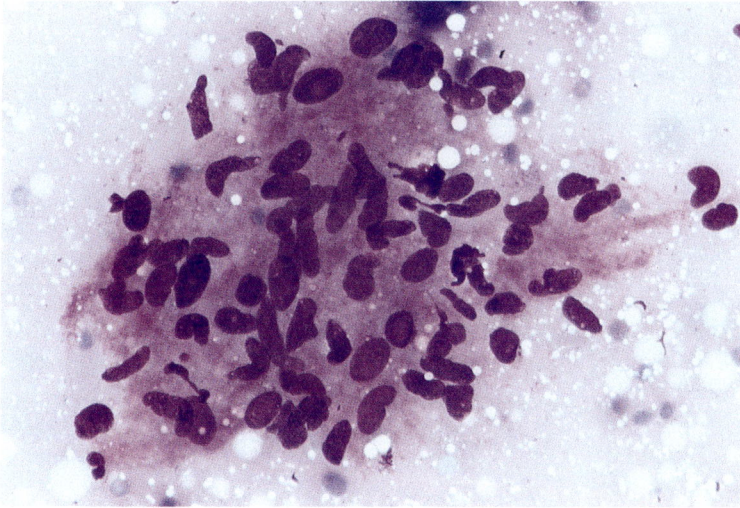

FIG 6.30 Dermatofibrosarcoma protuberans, storiform pattern within stromal fragments.

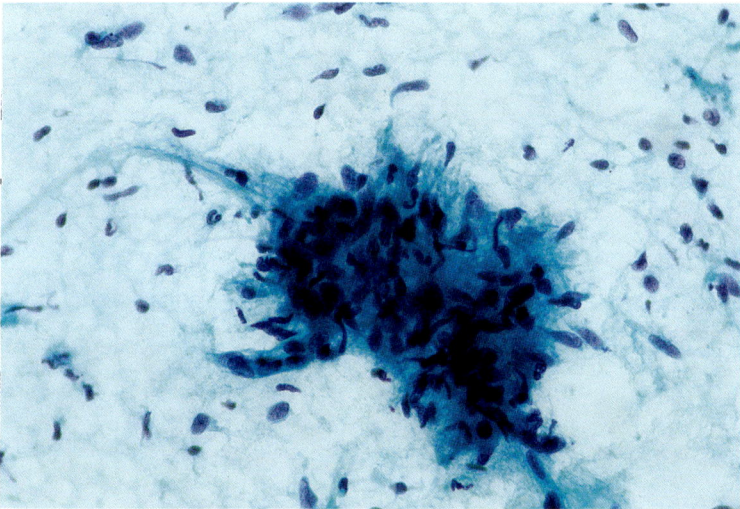

FIG 6.31 Dermatofibrosarcoma protuberans, same case as Fig 6.30, Papanicolaou.

chromosome 17 and 22. The fusion transcript COL1A1-PDGF beta of the translocation t(17;22)(q21;q13) can be revealed by reverse transcript polymerase chain reaction (RT-PCR) or florescent in situ hybridization (FISH). The demonstration of similar changes in giant cell fibroblastoma allows ascertaining that this tumor is the juvenile counterpart of dermatofibrosarcoma protuberans.

Dermatofibrosarcoma protuberans should be differentiated from other benign, low- and intermediate-grade spindle cell neoplasms such as low-grade fibrosarcoma, myxofibrosarcoma, low-grade malignant peripheral nerve sheath tumor, benign

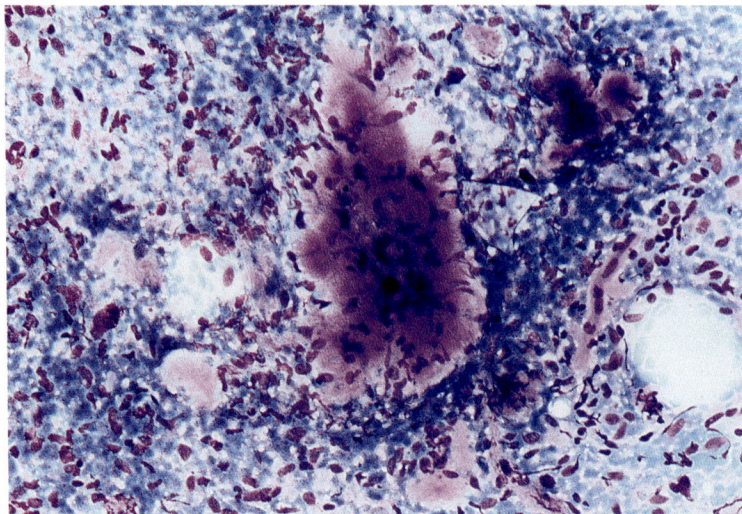

FIG 6.32 Dermatofibrosarcoma protuberans, isolated spindle cells, naked nuclei, and connective fragments.

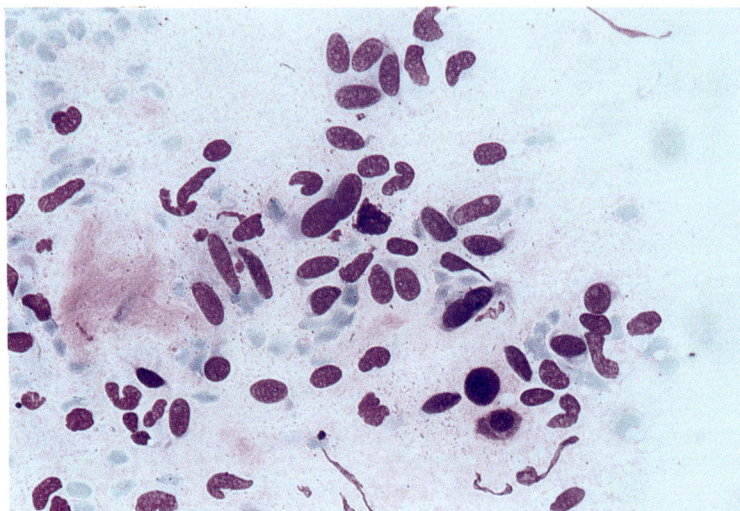

FIG 6.33 Dermatofibrosarcoma protuberans, isolated spindle cells, naked nuclei, and slight-to-moderate cytonuclear atypia.

peripheral nerve sheath tumor, nodular fasciitis, benign fibrous histiocytoma, and low-grade fibromyxoid sarcoma [17] (Table 6.2). The main diagnostic criterion supporting a diagnosis of sarcoma is the presence of pleomorphic spindle cells [18]. Fibrosarcomas, fibromyxosarcomas, and malignant peripheral nerve sheath tumor (depending on histological grade) may share similar cytonuclear atypia. Fibrosarcomas occur in deep soft tissues and usually are characterized by atypical

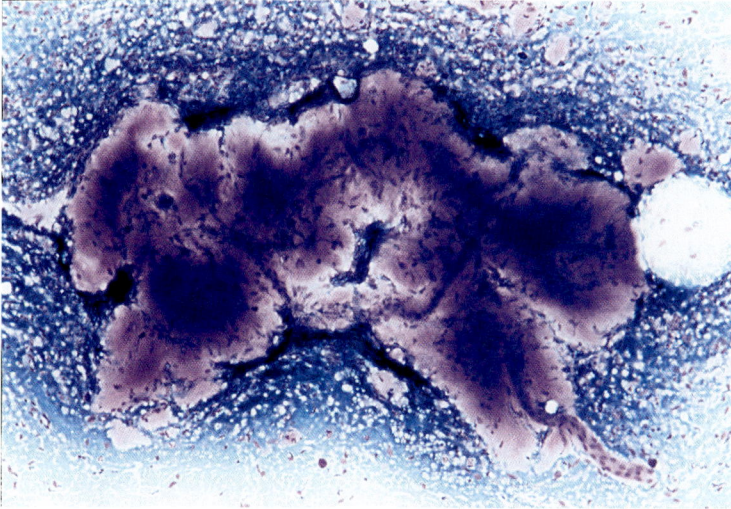

FIG 6.34 Dermatofibrosarcoma protuberans, myxoid background.

TABLE 6.2 Cytological differential diagnosis of dermatofibrosarcoma protuberans

	Dermatofibrosarcoma protuberans	Benign peripheral nerve sheath tumor	Benign fibrous histiocytoma
Spindle cells	++	++	++
Giant cells	−	−	+
Histiocytic cells	−	−	++
Cytonuclear atypia	+/−	+/−	+/−
Mitotic figures	−	+/−	−

++; frequent, +; rare, +/−; occasionally seen, −; absent.

and isolated spindle cells. Cellular fascicles, stromal fragments, and occasionally, a myxoid background could be observed [19]. Myxofibrosarcomas are also tumors of subcutaneous tissue like dermatofibrosarcoma protuberans. However, their cellular component consists of variably pleomorphic spindle cells, isolated or aggregates, admixed with an abundant myxoid matrix [20]. Low-grade malignant peripheral nerve sheath tumors frequently are associated with a known history of neurofi-bromatosis 1 or a preexisting neurofibroma. Smears in low-grade malignant peripheral nerve sheath tumor consist of spindle-shaped cells with wavy nuclei, comma-shaped naked nuclei, and polymorphous oval-to-rounded cells in various proportions. The most reliable morphological characteristic of well-differentiated tumors is the presence of typical comma-shaped cells, occasionally arranged in palisades, in conjunction with twisted or wavy nuclei [21]. Moreover, conventional and myxoid dermatofibrosarcoma protuberans are diffusely CD34 positive and smooth muscle actin negative, which is helpful in the differential diagnosis [21–23]. Fibrosarcomateous variants of dermatofibrosarcoma protuberans tend to lose CD34 expression.

Cytologically, benign nerve sheath tumors are characterized by loose tissue fragments with a fibrillar background and variable numbers of cellular clusters of spindle cells representative of Verocay bodies [24]. Vascular arcades, fishhook nuclei, and epithelioid cells also are reported [25]. Nodular fasciitis [26] may be indistinguishable from dermatofibrosarcoma protuberans. A history of a rapidly growing mass or nodule often present for only 1−2 weeks, and a diffuse expression of smooth muscle actin by the cells are strongly suggestive of a nodular fasciitis diagnosis. A background of erythocytes and round mononuclear inflammatory cells are also indicative of fasciitis.

The cellular component of fibrous histiocytoma is more polymorphous; smears consist of an admixture of histiocytes, which may be epithelioid, multinucleated giant, and regular spindle cells. Cytonuclear atypia is usually mild or absent [27].

6.1.3.4 *Comments.*

When correlating the cytohistological findings, all smears show a similar morphology, whatever the histological subtype. Smears constantly consist of slightly atypical spindle cells, a delicate fibrillary stroma, naked nuclei, and a storiform pattern. Mitotic figures, a myxoid background, mast cells, and lipocytes rarely were present. According to Layfield, the following cytological characteristics could be observed in dermatofibrosarcoma protuberans [17]: smears of moderate cellularity containing single cells and cells entrapped within tissue fragments (frequently with a storiform pattern) stromal fragments with a fibrillar character, plump oval-to-spindle isolated cells with bland nuclear features and a fine chromatine pattern, a moderate amount of cytoplasm with a pale finely granular appearance, and rare mitotic figures. Similar observations were also reported by others [18,22,28,29].

A review of the literature displays only 47 cases of dermatofibrosarcoma protuberans studied by cytological methods [1,18,22,30−38), and among those, only two studies [18,38] describe the cytohistological correlations in detail. However, as the number of primary tumors investigated is limited, the characterization of cytological representative findings for an accurate diagnosis prior to the surgery is not well established.

Among the wide variety of proposed diagnoses are low-grade spindle sarcoma, fibrosarcoma, sarcoma "not otherwise specified," benign connective tissue, spindle cell tumor, fibromatosis, nodular fasciitis, and schwannoma. An accurate cytological diagnosis of recurrent or metastatic dermatofibrosarcoma protuberans is influenced strongly by the knowledge of a previous history [18,29,31,39].

6.1.3.5 *FNA Key Features.*

The following are in favor of the diagnosis:

- Smears rich in spindle cells isolated or clustered
- Discrete cytonuclear atypia.

The following are difficulties in making a diagnosis:

- Rare mitotic figures

The following are evidence against a diagnosis:

— Numerous mitotic figures
— Giant multinucleated cells, histiocytic cells
— Fibrillary stroma

6.1.4 Benign Fibrous Histiocytoma (Cellular and Atypical Variants)

The following different histologic subtypes have been described: classical benign fibrous histiocytoma, aneurysmal, epithelioid, cellular, and atypical (pseudosarcomatous) variants. The last two types could generate an overdiagnosis and be confused with sarcomas.

Cellular benign fibrous histiocytoma is a distinctive variant. About 25% of the lesions may reccur [40]. They can occur at any anatomical localization, although they are observed more frequently in the upper and lower limbs and in the head and neck regions. Atypical benign fibrous histiocytoma has been characterized morphologically among a series of 59 cases that included all variants [41]. Atypical benign fibrous histiocytoma, also called pseudosarcomatous, is a rare variant of benign fibrous histiocytoma. As indicated by its appellation, it differs from conventional benign fibrous histiocytoma by its cellular composition. Clinically, atypical benign fibrous histiocytomas are solitary lesions, occurring mainly in lower and upper extremities, trunk, and head and neck, which is similar to other forms of benign fibrous histiocytoma. Local reccurences and rare cases of metastases have been documented. It has been suggested that atypical benign fibrous histiocytoma has a broader clinicopathlogic spectrum than previously revealed. Complete excision is the treatment of choice to avoid recurrences. As a rule, a benign outcome is to be expected in most cases. Practically, this histologic variant of benign fibrous histiocytoma shows a higher tendency to recur locally than conventional forms.

6.1.4.1 Histopathology. Histologically, cellular benign fibrous histiocytoma differs from the conventional variant by some histologic features, namely a fascicular nonstoriform pattern (Fig 6.35), moderate mitotic rate (Fig 6.36), and frequent extension into the subcutaneous fat (Fig 6.37). Other features not commonly observed in these tumors are focal cytologic polymorphism, epidermal alterations of usual benign fibrous histiocytoma (Fig. 6.38), and foci of necrosis. The immunohistochemical profile shows positivity for vimentin and alpha smooth muscle actin. These lesions are to be distinguished from dermatofibrosarcoma protuberans and leiomyosarcoma, with which they initially have been confused.

Most atypical benign fibrous histiocytoma are localized in the dermis with a superficial involvement of the subcutis. The presence of scattered bizarre pleomorphic cells, sometimes multinucleated (Fig 6.39), is the main feature of these lesions. Tumor cells can be spindle and/or polyhedral, depicting irregular, hyperchromatic, and large nuclei in a background of classic benign fibrous histiocytoma (Fig 6.40). The degree of pleomorphism is variable, ranging from focal and minimal to marked. Some cells have vesicular nuclei with prominent acidophilic nucleoli mimicking Hodgkin's cells. Atypical mitoses are noted in several lesions. Among other worrisome features different from classical benign fibrous histiocytoma are

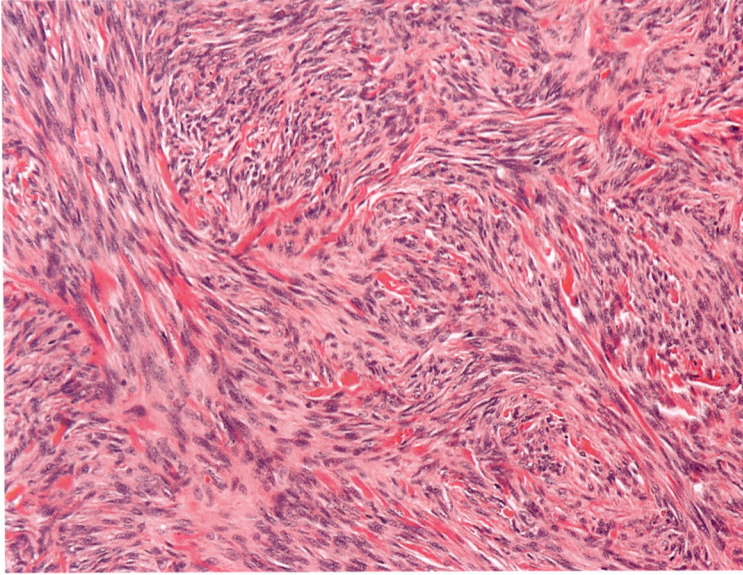

FIG 6.35 Benign fibrous histiocytoma, cellular variant, fascicular nonstoriform pattern of growth.

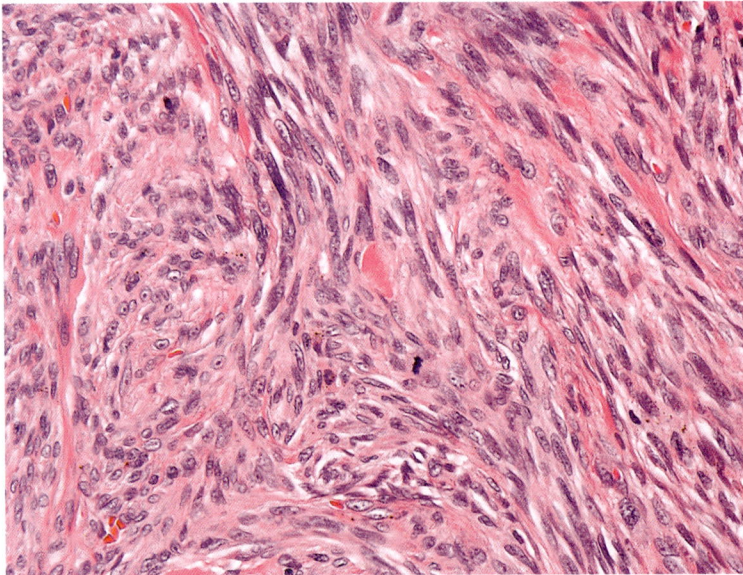

FIG 6.36 Benign fibrous histiocytoma, cellular variant, moderate mitotic rate.

large size (diameter >2 cm), extension to subcutis, and geographic necrosis. The immunohistochemical profile shows positivity for CD34 and focal alpha smooth muscle actin. Usual fibrohistiocytic markers like CD68 and FXIIIa are positive. A potential pitfall for overdiagnosis is pleomorphic sarcoma.

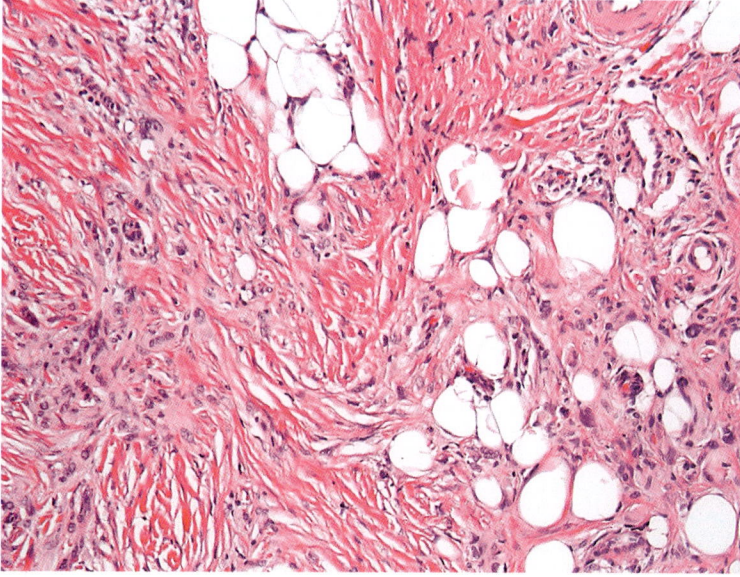

FIG 6.37 Benign fibrous histiocytoma, cellular variant, extension into the subcutaneous tissue.

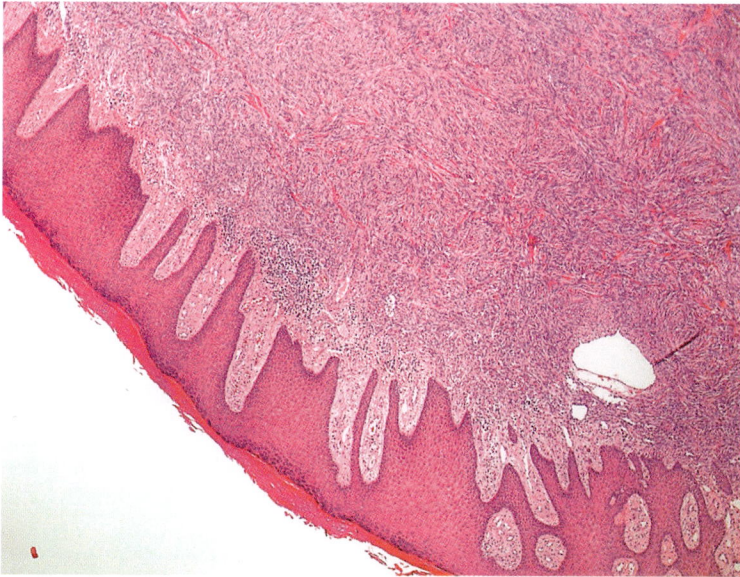

FIG 6.38 Benign fibrous histiocytoma, cellular variant, epidermal induction common to most benign fibrous histiocytoma.

6.1.4.2 *Cytopathology.* In cellular and atypical variants of benign fibrous histiocytoma, cytopathology samples are usually hypercellular (Fig 6.41). Smears are surprisingly homogenous and consist of roundish or polygonal histiocytic cells with finely vacuolated cytoplasm (Figs 6.42–6.44) and/or of small regular spindle cells

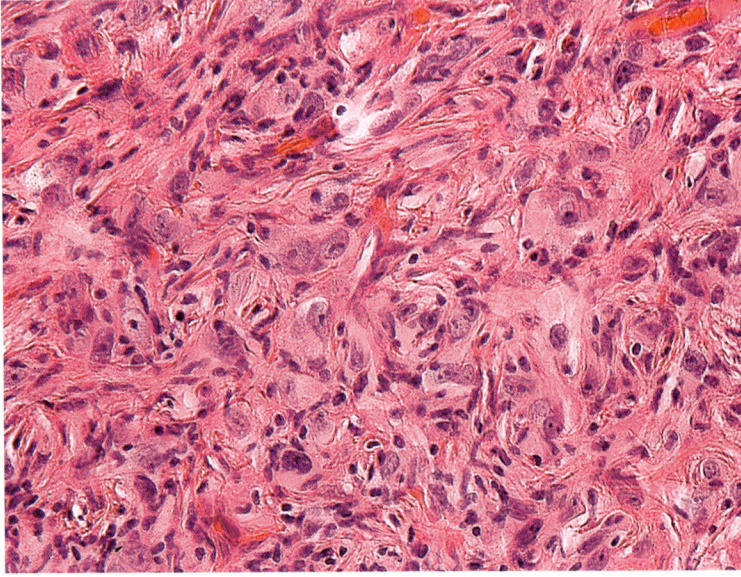

FIG 6.39 Benign fibrous histiocytoma, atypical variant, showing bizarre pleomorphic cells with large hyperchromatic nuclei.

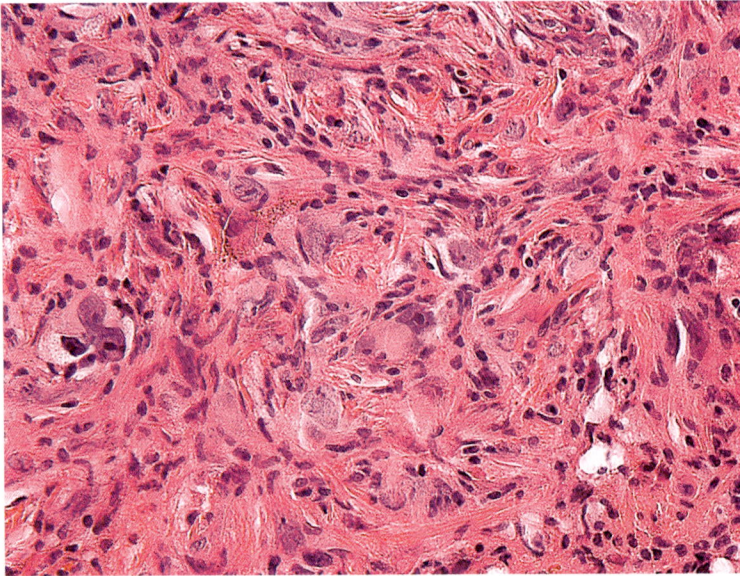

FIG 6.40 Benign fibrous histiocytoma, same case as Fig 6.39. Bizzare cells in a background of classical fibrous histiocytoma.

attached to vascular structures (Figs 6.45 and 6.46). Multinucleated Touton-like cells also may be present (Fig 6.47). Important cytonuclear atypia is observed occasionally in an atypical variant. In aneurysmal variants, numerous siderophages usually are present (Fig 6.48). A scant myxoid background may be observed in myxoid benign

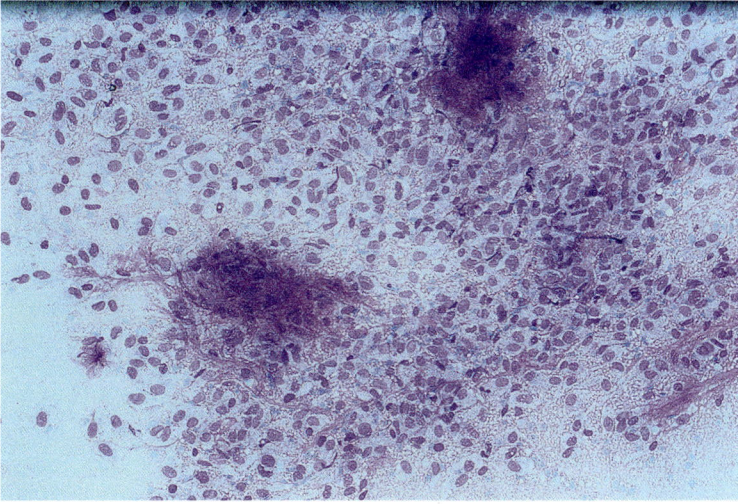

FIG 6.41 Benign fibrous histiocytoma, roundish or polygonal pseudohistiocytic cells.

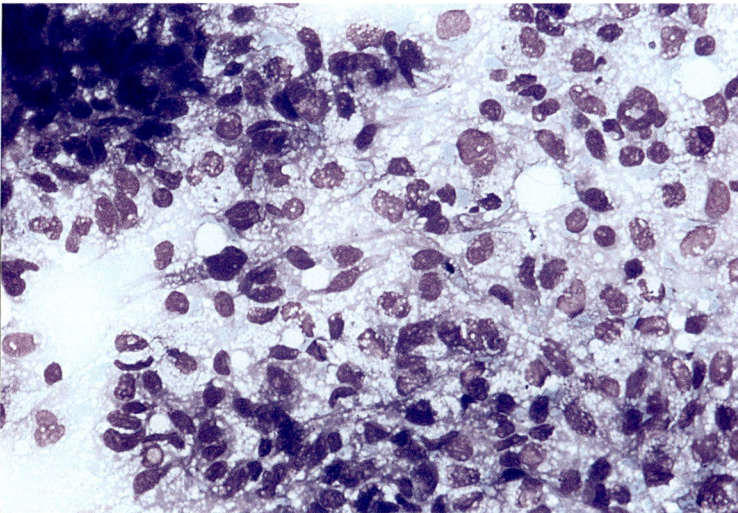

FIG 6.42 Benign fibrous histiocytoma, pseudohistiocytic cells with finely vacuolated cytoplasm.

fibrous histiocytoma. Inversely, storiform pattern, round cells, prominent atypia, necrosis, or mitotic figures are never observed.

6.1.4.3 *Differential Diagnosis.* Cytologically, benign fibrous histiocytoma should be differentiated from other benign, low- and intermediate-grade spindle neoplasms such as low-grade fibrosarcoma, dermatofibrosarcoma protuberans [42,43], nodular fasciitis [44], and monophasic synovial sarcoma [45] (Table 6.3). An aneurysmal variant will be differentiated from malignant melanoma. Fibrosarcomas are deep-seated

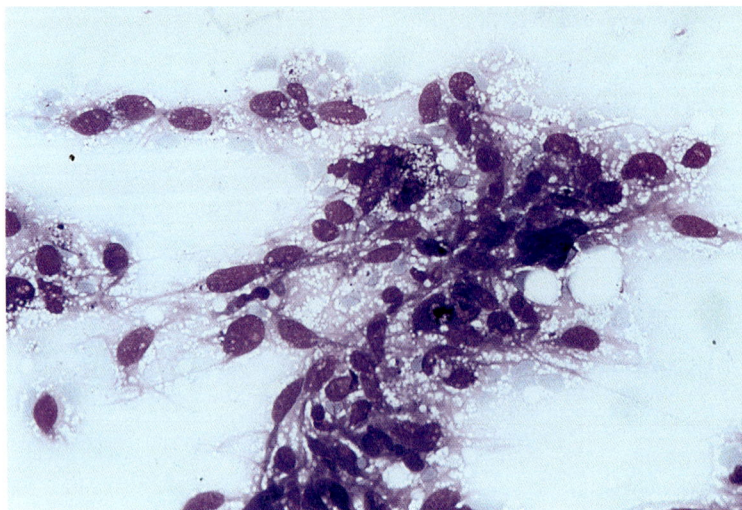

FIG 6.43 Benign fibrous histiocytoma, polymorphous pseudohistiocytic cells.

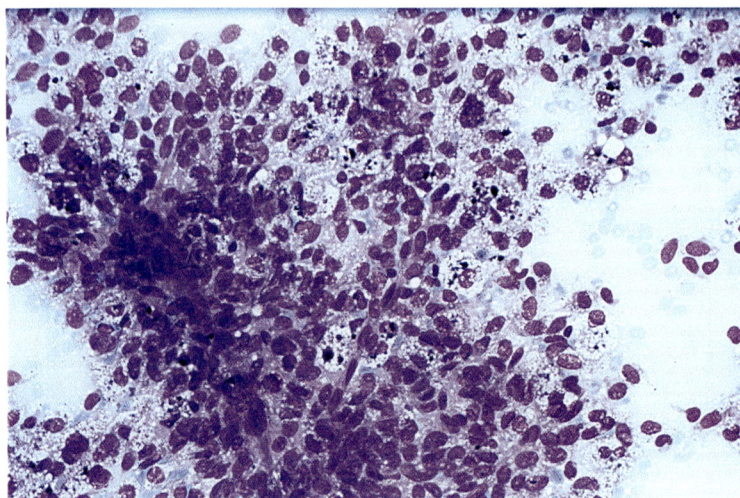

FIG 6.44 Benign fibrous histiocytoma, roundish or polygonal histiocytic cells. Dirty background.

neoplasms, and cytological findings usually show atypical and isolated spindle cells. Cellular fascicles, stromal fragments, and occasionally, myxoid background may be observed [46].

The smears in dermatofibrosarcoma protuberans consist of isolated spindle cells, connective fragments with storiform and/or fibrillary pattern, and naked nuclei. Giant cells, or marked cytonuclear atypia are exceptional [42,43]. Moreover, dermatofibrosarcoma protuberans are CD34 positive and smooth muscle actin negative, a feature that may help considerably in the differential diagnosis.

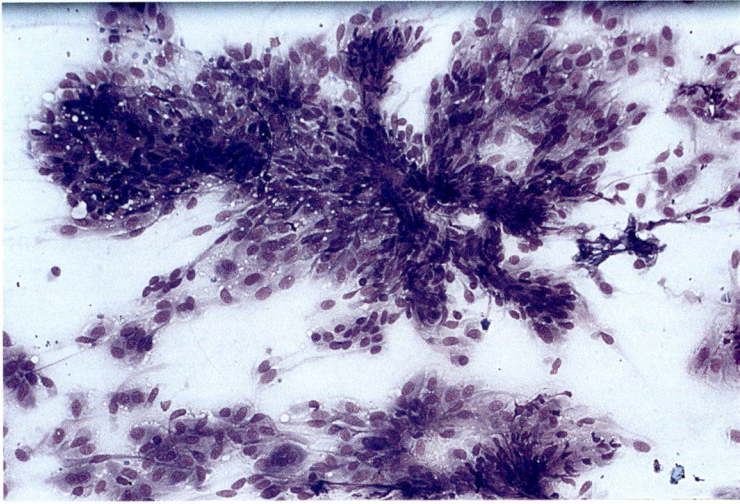

FIG 6.45 Benign fibrous histiocytoma, regular spindle cells attached to vascular structures.

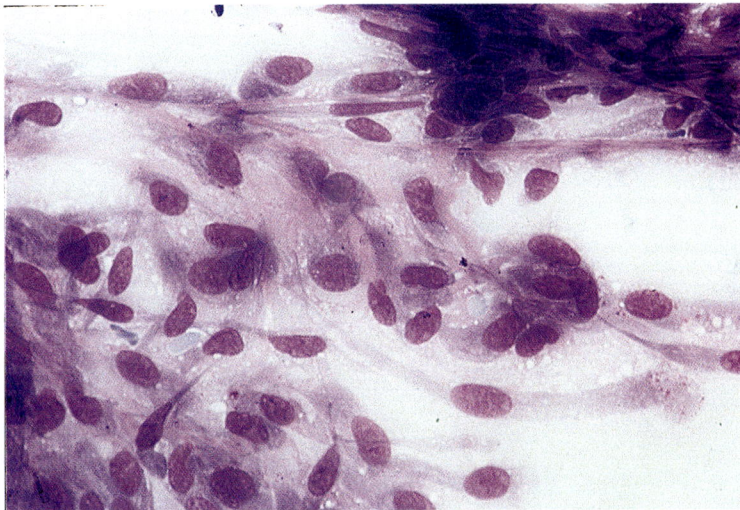

FIG 6.46 Benign fibrous histiocytoma, regular spindle cells.

Nodular fasciitis [44] may be difficult to distinguish from benign fibrous histiocytoma. However, smears may show the presence of roundish, polygonal, triangular, and ganglioid cells, the latter particularly in the proliferative variant of fasciitis. Clinical evolution and immunohistochemistry may help in the differential diagnosis because its cellular component is usually strongly positive for alpha smooth muscle actin.

Smears in synovial sarcoma are cell-rich, stroma-poor, of striking uniformity lacking nuclear pleomorphism, and mostly consist of ovoid-to-rounded tumor cells with scant tapering cytoplasm. Branching papillary-like tumor tissue fragments with

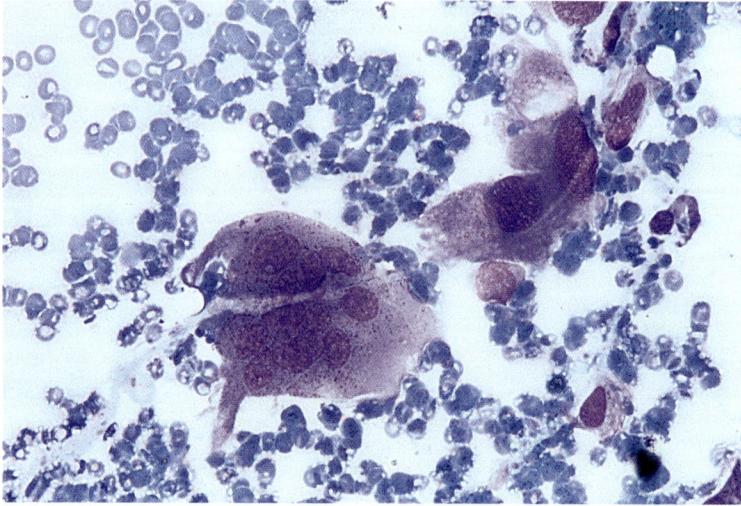

FIG 6.47 Benign fibrous histiocytoma, multinucleated, Touton-like cells.

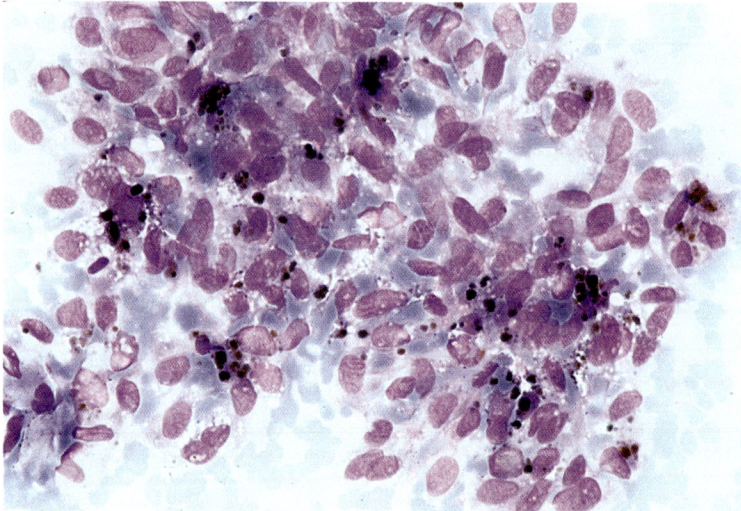

FIG 6.48 Benign fibrous histiocytoma, aneurysmal variants, numerous siderophages. This pattern should be differentiated from malignant melanoma.

TABLE 6.3 Cytological differential diagnosis of benign fibrous histiocytoma

	Benign fibrous histiocytoma		MFH	Low-grade fibrosarcoma	DFSP	Nodular fasciitis	Monophasic synovial sarcoma
	Cellular	Atypical					
Spindle cells	++	++	++	+	++	++	+
Giant cells	+	+/−	++	−	−	+	−
Histiocytic cells	++	++	−	−	−	−	−
Atypia	+/−	+	++	+	+/−	+/−	+
Mitotic figures	−	+/−	+	+	−	−	+

MFH; Mlignant fibrous histiocytoma, ++; frequent, +; rare, +/−; occasionally seen, −; absent.

vascular structures and comma-like nuclei are also characteristic of both monophasic and biphasic variants [45].

6.1.4.4 *Comments.* Comparing the cytology components with histological diagnoses, there is no difference in smears composition between cellular and atypical variants. Benign fibrous histiocytoma is an entity whose clinical presentation is rather characteristic as are its cellular components of histiocyte-like cells, polymorphic macrophages, small regular spindle cells, and Touton-like cells. When those findings are associated with the presence of atypical cells, one has to consider the possibility of other neoplasms, especially with cases of recurrent tumors or in patients with a past history of cancer, hence the indication and the usefulness of fine needle aspiration cytology in those situations.

Cytologic literature describing benign fibrous histiocytoma is limited [27,46–48]. Fiedman et al. [46] described one case localized in the breast. Bezabih [47] reported three cases, and all of them were confirmed as benign fibrous histiocytoma by histology and accurately were diagnosed cytologically. Akerman et al. [48] and Layfield [49] have delineated cytologic criteria diagnostic of benign fibrous histiocytoma. Other large series [27] described 36 tumors and a false-positive rate of 8.3% of cases. In all instances, similar observations were made: tumors consisted of ovoid-to-stellate cells with short cytoplasmic processes, eosinophilic, finely granular or vacuolated cytoplasm, indistinct cell borders, ovoid or kidney-like nuclei and finely granular chromatin, and small or indistinct nuclei. Anisokaryosis was mild. In addition, giant cells of Touton-like type and siderophages also were observed. Cellularity was scant to abundant depending on the degree of sclerosis.

6.1.4.5 *FNA Key Features.* The following are in favor of the diagnosis:

- Numerous spindle-shaped and histiocytic cells
- Giant multinucleated cells

The following are difficulties in making a diagnosis:

- Discrete cytonuclear atypia
- Siderophages
- Myxoid background

The following is evidence against a diagnosis:

- Mitotic figures, prominent cytonuclear atypia

6.1.5 Solitary Fibrous Tumor

Solitary fibrous tumor is an uncommon mesenchymal tumor of probable fibroblastic type. First described in the pleura [50], the entity has come to be recognized as ubiquitous [51,52], affecting middle-aged adults, although rare cases have been described in children. Much attention has been focussed on solitary fibrous tumor by virtue of its resemblance to classical hemangiopericytoma, depicting the characteristic prominent hemangiopericytoma-like vascular pattern. Indeed, many reported cases of hemangiopericytoma rather belong to those categories of neoplasms that now are grouped under the hemangiopericytoma/solitary fibrous tumor. Both entities share several clinical and morphologic characteristics as well as a similar immunohistochemical profile [53]. Abnormality of the long arm of chromosome 12 has been reported in classical hemangiopericytoma, whereas a trisomy 21 is apparented to solitary fibrous tumor [54]. Most hemangiopericytomas and solitary fibrous tumors are histologically benign, although rare cases depict atypical features. Malignant neoplasms are evaluated according to similar parameters as hemangiopericytoma and are defined by increased cellularity, more than four mitotic figures/10 high power field necrosis, and hemorrhage [55].

6.1.5.1 *Histopathology.*

6.1.5.1 *Histopathology.* Hemangiopericytoma/solitary fibrous tumors are deep-seated circumscribed soft tissue neoplasms or exophytic masses when occurring on the serosal surfaces. Their histological picture is variable in appearance, depending on the proportion of tumor cells and fibrous stroma (Figs 6.49 and 6.50). It is said that "the cellular end of the spectrum" could correspond to the classical hemangiopericytoma, whereas the predominantly hyalinized tumors represent the end of "classical solitary fibrous tumor." Considerable overlapping is observed from case to case. Cellular areas composed of solid sheets of patternless or short ill-defined fascicles of spindle cells arranged around a prominent vasculature that typically depict a "staghorn" or "swamp-like" pattern (Fig 6.51). Secondary changes such as myxoid areas, interstitial hyalinization, and coarse-walled vessels are frequent (Fig 6.52).

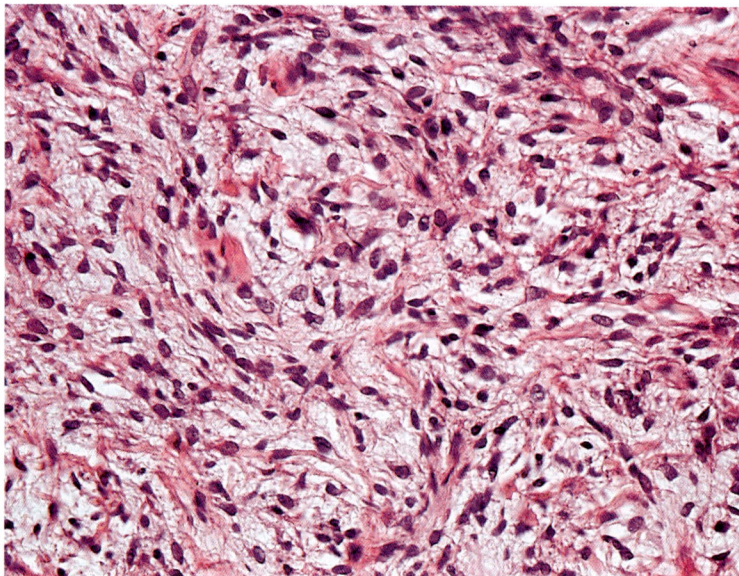

FIG 6.49 Solitary fibrous tumor, cellular area within a loose collagenous stroma.

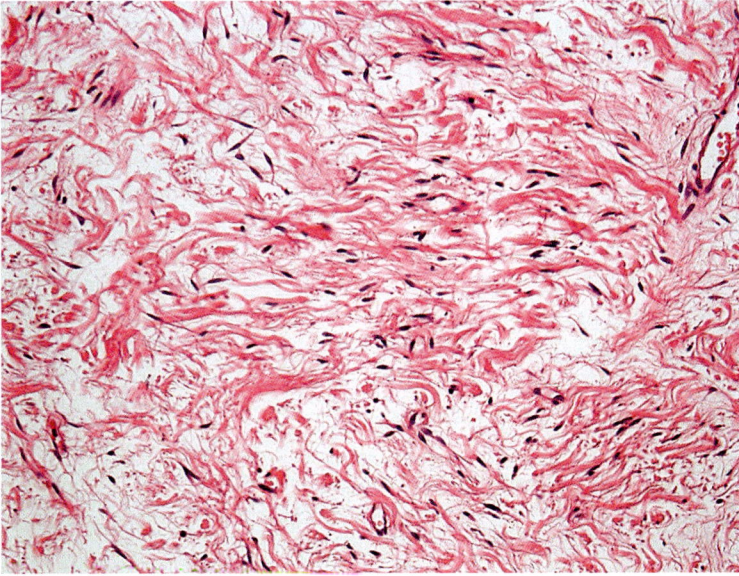

FIG 6.50 Solitary fibrous tumor, hypocellular component in a predominatly fibrous stroma.

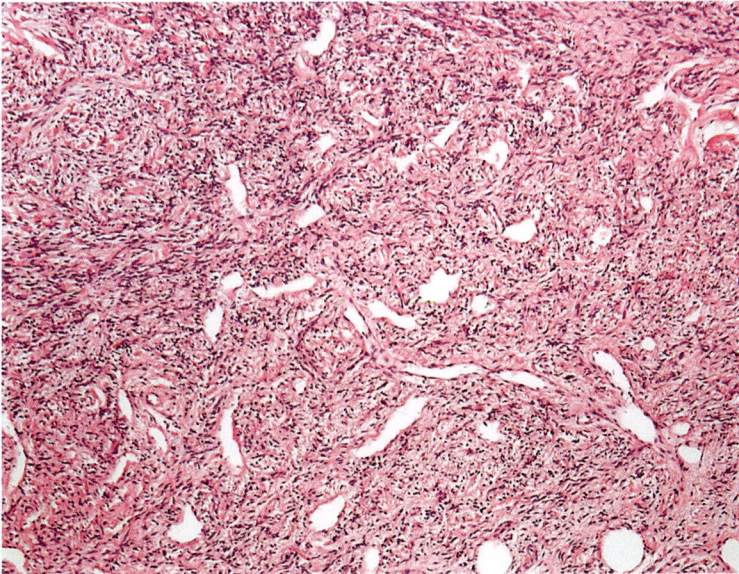

FIG 6.51 Solitary fibrous tumor, hemangiopericytoma-like vascular pattern with solid sheets of patternless short ill-defined fascicles of spindle cells.

Immunohistochemically, CD34 is expressed in most cases of solitary fibrous tumor (80–90%). Other useful markers are CD99, bcl2, and epithelial membrane antigen (EMA). Classical hemangiopericytomas are also positive for CD34, although less frequently. The high sensitivity for CD34 expression by solitary fibrous tumor

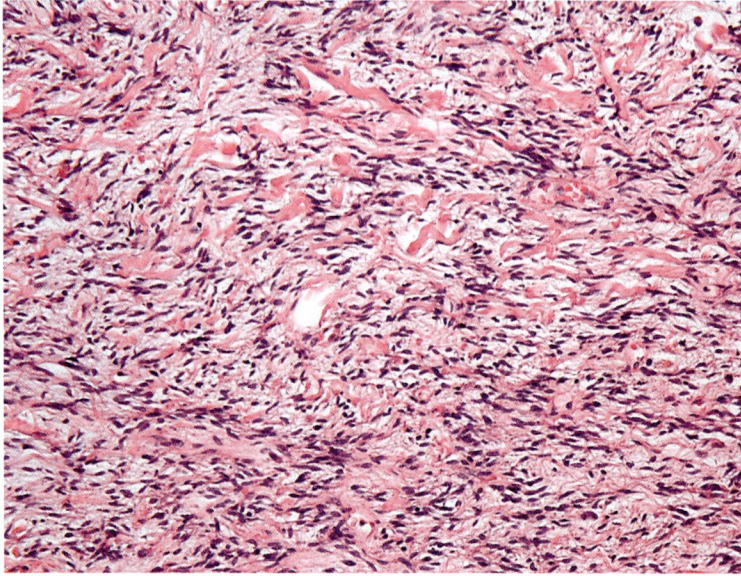

FIG 6.52 Solitary fibrous tumor, interstitial hyalinization

accounts for the increasing number of extrapleural tumors and the decreasing diagnosis of classical hemangiopericytoma.

6.1.5.2 Cytopathology. Smears in solitary fibrous tumor vary in cellularity, going from scant to hypercellular. They show predominantly discohesive spindle-shaped or roundish cells, with ovoid nuclei, evenly distributed chromatin, inconspicuous nucleoli, and scant-to-moderate cytoplasm with focally wispy, collagenous inter-cellular material. Moderate pleomorphism is common. No mitotic activity is detected. The background never shows chondromyxoid matrix, inflammatory cells, or necrosis, but it may contain fragments of collagenized stromal tissue (Figs 6.53 and 6.54). There is no evidence of a myoepithelial differentiation.

6.1.5.3 Differential Diagnosis. The following entities should be differentiated with solitary fibrous tumor:

— Benign fibrous histiocytoma
— Synovial sarcoma
— Extraskeletal mesenchymal chondrosarcoma
— Low-grade spindle cell sarcoma

Because solitary fibrous tumors show isolated spindle-shaped cells with moderate atypia and a clear background, they should be differentiated from other spindle cell tumors, especially from benign fibrous histiocytoma and monophasic synovial sarcoma. Benign fibrous histiocytoma usually shows benign cells with histiocytic morphology. However, its superficial localization is characteristic. Inversely, synovial

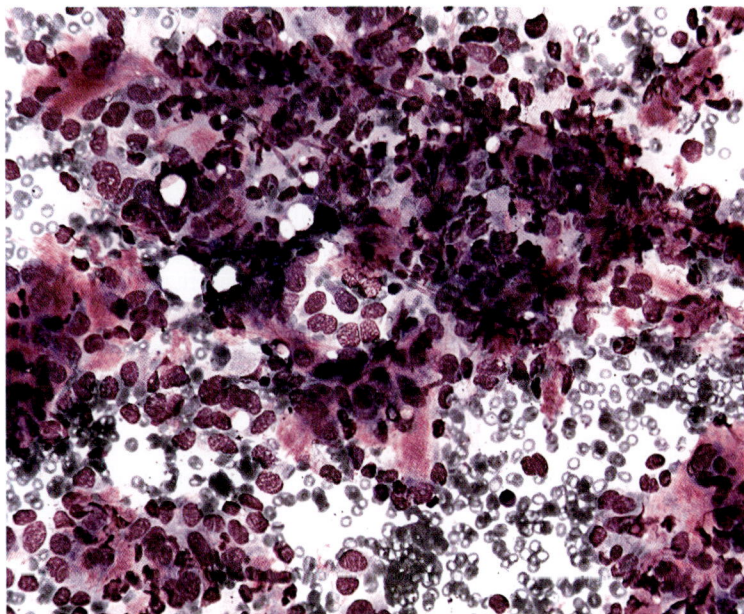

FIG 6.53 Solitary fibrous tumor, roundish and spindle cells without cytonuclear atypia. Scant collagenized stromal tissue.

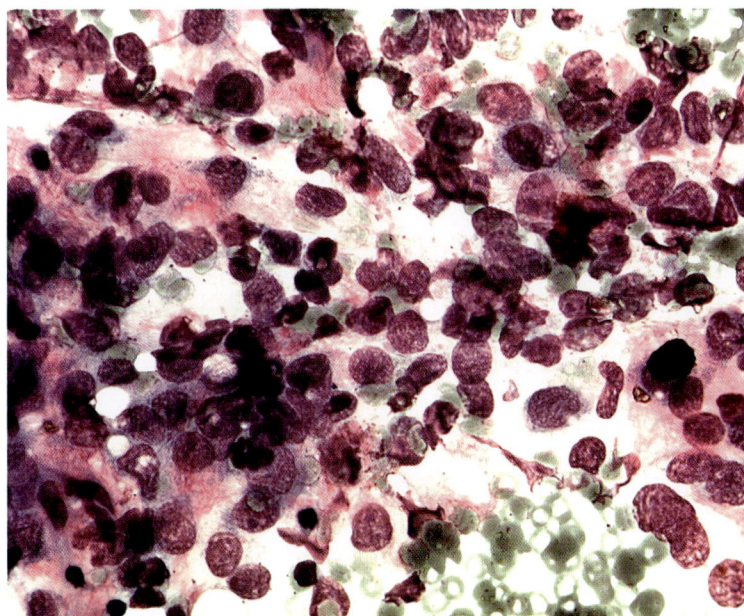

FIG 6.54 Solitary fibrous tumor. Same case as Fig 6.53, higher magnification.

sarcoma may occur in the anatomical sites of solitary fibrous tumor. Its hypercellularity and pseudopapillary growth favor this diagnosis.

6.1.5.4 Comments. Morphological variants of hemangiopericytoma/solitary fibrous tumor have been described. The lipomatous hemangiopericytoma/solitary fibrous tumor is a rare variant showing variable amount of mature fat tissue [56]. Meningeal hemangiopericytoma is morphologically similar to hemangiopericytoma/ solitary fibrous tumor and consequently is no longer considered a variant of meningioma [57]. The entity originally described under the appellation of "giant cell angiofibroma" of the orbit [58] and later on of the extraorbital soft tissue [59] belongs by virtue of its morphology and immunohistochemical profile to the hemangiopericytoma/solitary fibrous tumor family.

Although solitary fibrous tumors usually are found in the pleura, they can occur in various other locations, such as the orbit, nasal cavity, paranasal sinuses, mediastinum, breast, vagina, meninges, salivary glands, soft tissues, and are a target for fine needle aspiration. Cytological reports are limited in number and only case reports or small series have been published [60–64]. Tumors usually were diagnosed as "benign connective lesions." We have observed only two examples of pleural solitary tumor, both diagnosed accurately.

6.2 TUMORS WITH FIBRILLARY STROMA

Benign tumors of peripheral nerves are somewhat different from other mesenchymal tumors by virtue of tissue components from which they develop, hence a variety of features that parallel their lineage of origin (i.e., Schwann cells and perineural cells). Either of superficial or deep localization, they are prone to minimal repeated traumatisms/compression resulting in secondary changes like in "ancient schwannoma." They also constitute a unique and important group of benign soft tissue tumors whose malignant transformation is a well-recognized biological outcome, particularly when they originate in association with neurofibromatosis type 1.

In terms of cytological approach, we will concentrate on three entities that could result in difficulties in histological and cytological diagnosis, mainly benign schwannoma/ancient schwannoma, neurofibroma, and low-grade nerve sheath sarcoma whose debates on nosology and terminology resulted in the designation of malignant peripheral nerve sheath tumor for those sarcomas.

6.2.1 Benign Peripheral Nerve Sheath Tumors (Schwannoma, Ancient Schwannoma and Neurofibroma)

Benign tumors of peripheral nerves account for the second most frequent soft tissue tumor, outnumbered only by lipoma if one excludes benign conventional fibrous histiocytoma. Superficial tumors are candidates to diagnosis by cytology, although most primarily will be diagnosed and treated by simple surgical excision. Schwannoma (formerly neurilemmoma) recapitulates more or less the morphology of normal well-differentiated Schwann cells. Ancient schwannoma, by virtue of their more or less long-standing evolution, will display degenerative changes, some of which are related to the cellular cytologic patterns described earlier, myxoid changes and atypical cells, and foamy or granular histiocytes. On the other hand, neurofibroma will display a more polymorphic cellular composition ranging from typical Schwann cells to spindle cells of fibroblast lineage. Both groups of tumors share some similar morphologic constituents; they differ in growth pattern, the cellular composition (as already indicated), the syndromes to which they are associated, and finally, their cytogenetic alterations. In this review, pseudotumors of peripheral nerves such as Morton's neuroma, traumatic neuroma, and "myxoma"of nerve sheath/ganglion are excluded.

6.2.1.1 *Histopathology.* Most of schwannomas are solitary nodules surrounded by a thin fibrous capsule containing portions of residual nerve fibers. Neurites are observed within the tumor. The main histologic characteristics are the presence of areas of high and low cellularity known as patterns of Antoni A an B. The relative composition of both components is variable among neoplasms. An Antoni A pattern is characterized architecturally by nuclear palisading, whorling of the cells like in meningiomas (Fig 6.55). Schwann cells are grouped in compact clusters with distinct cytoplasmic borders arranged in bundles or interlacing fascicles. They have twisted nuclei. Verocay bodies are formed by two compact rows of well-aligned nuclei separated by fibrillary cell processes, which also are demonstrated on cytological smears. An Antoni B pattern is "patternless" (i.e., relatively hypocellular and not well organized [Fig 6.56]). Microcystic changes and delicate collagen fibers are observed within a loose matrix, and irregularly distributed and more prominent long vessels are representative of this pattern.

Ancient schwannomas—also called schwannomas with degenerative changes—are usually larger and deeper tumors whose main histologic characteristics are the presence of cells with marked nuclear atypias of degenerative type, microcyts, calcifications, hemorrhage, and hyalinization of vessels walls (Figs 6.57–6.59).

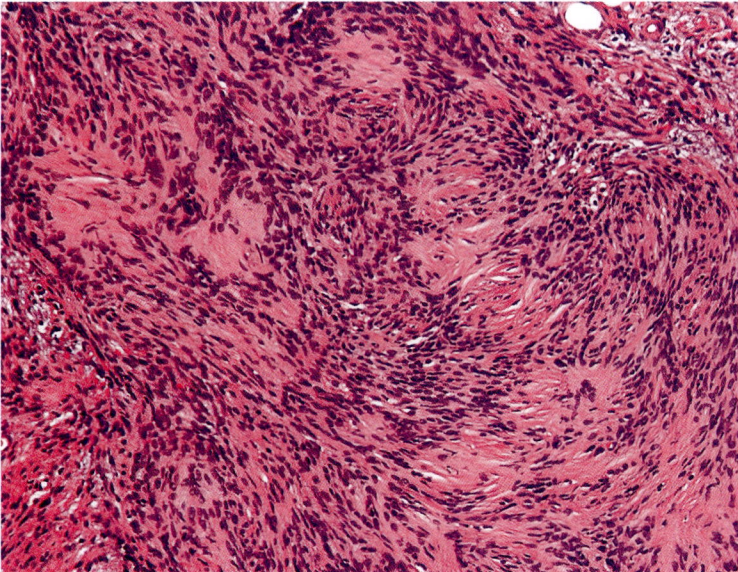

FIG 6.55 Schwannoma, typical Antoni A pattern.

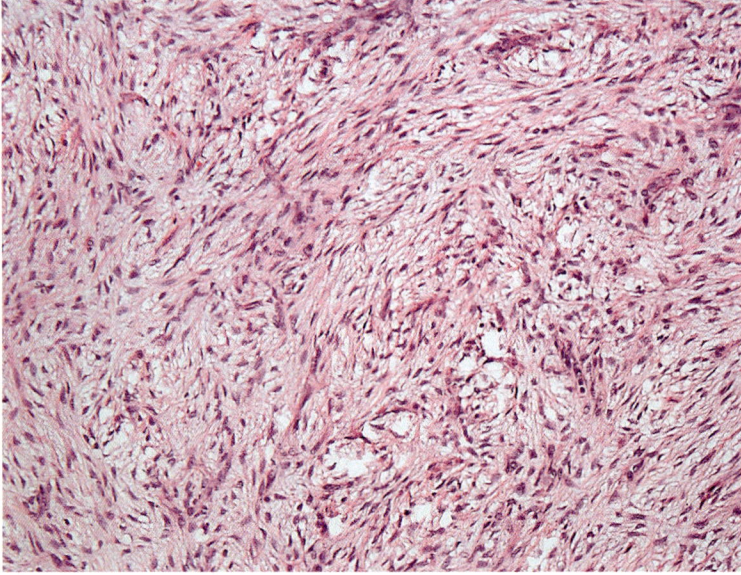

FIG 6.56 Schwannoma, Antoni B pattern depicting a relatively hypocellular and not well-organized pattern.

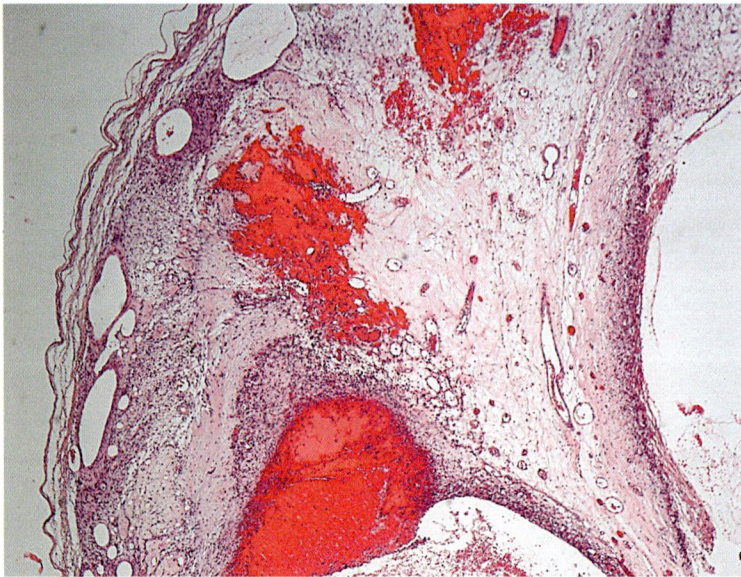

FIG 6.57 Ancient schwannoma: main histologic features are microcysts-hemorrhage-hyalinized stroma and atypical Schwann cells.

A pitfall in the differential diagnosis is obviously the degree of nuclear atypia observed; Schwann cell nuclei are large, hyperchromatic, and often multinucleated, but they are devoid of mitoses. The overall morphologic picture, as stated previously, helps in the diagnosis.

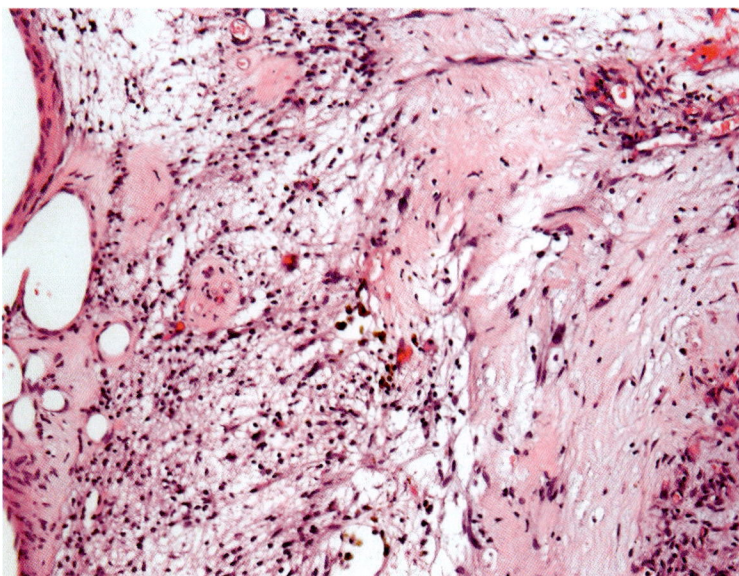

FIG 6.58 Ancient schwannoma: Higher magnification from Fig 6.57. Main histologic features are microcysts-hemorrhage-hyalinized stroma and atypical Schwann cells.

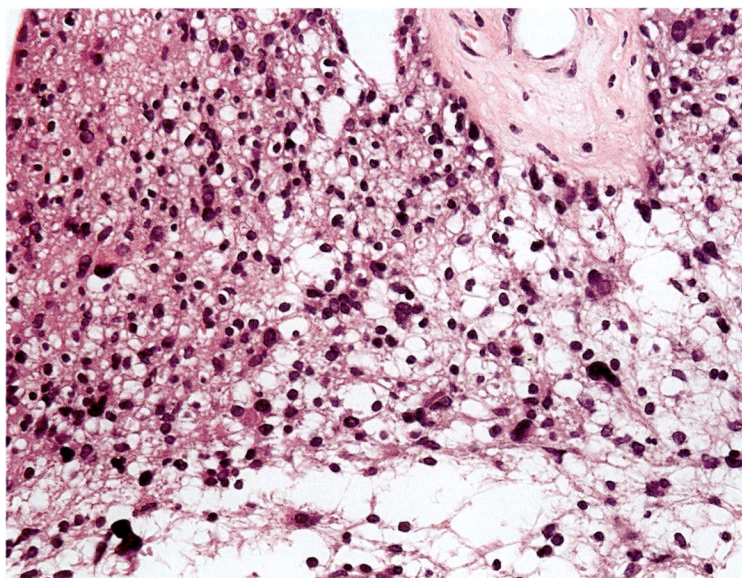

FIG 6.59 Ancient schwannoma: atypical round cells with poorly defined cytoplasmic margins and hyalinized vessel wall.

The composition of neurofibroma is more variable in function of its content of cells, collagen and myxoid stroma. They are solitary or multiple lesions localized or diffuse, although most tumors are solitary localized neoplasms whose typical clinical presentation are skin nodules or polypoid lesions. Several variants have been

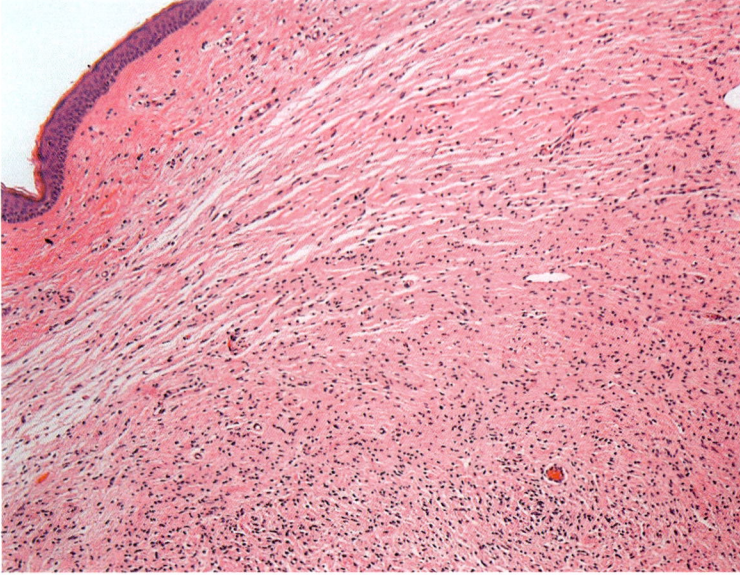

FIG 6.60 Neurofibroma, unencapsulated cutaneous mass.

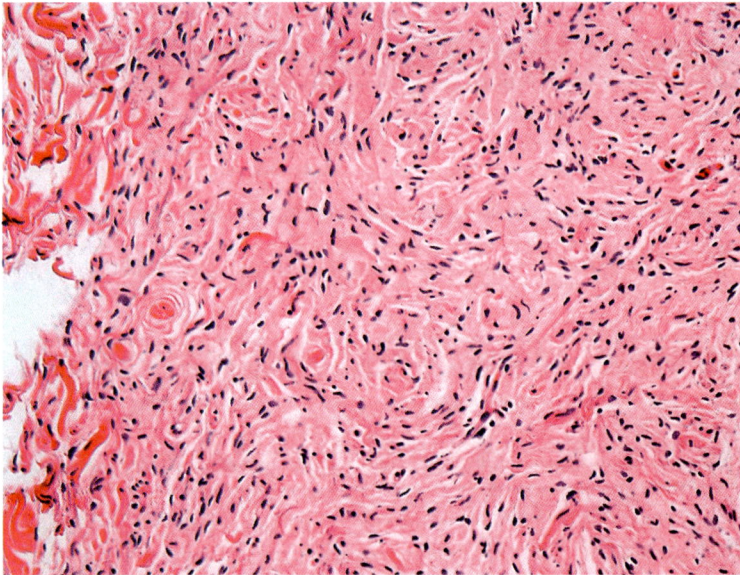

FIG 6.61 Neurofibroma. Higher magnification showing spindle cells whose cytoplasm is confounded with the extracellular matrix.

described—epitheliod, granular cell, but are rather rare and are not discussed in the present review. Typically, the neurofibromas are well circumscribed but unencapsulated neoplasms with ill-defined margins (Fig 6.60). Tumor cells are elongated spindle cells with comma-shaped nuclei, and the poorly defined cytoplasm is confounded with the extracellular matrix (Fig 6.61). A second cellular component is made of

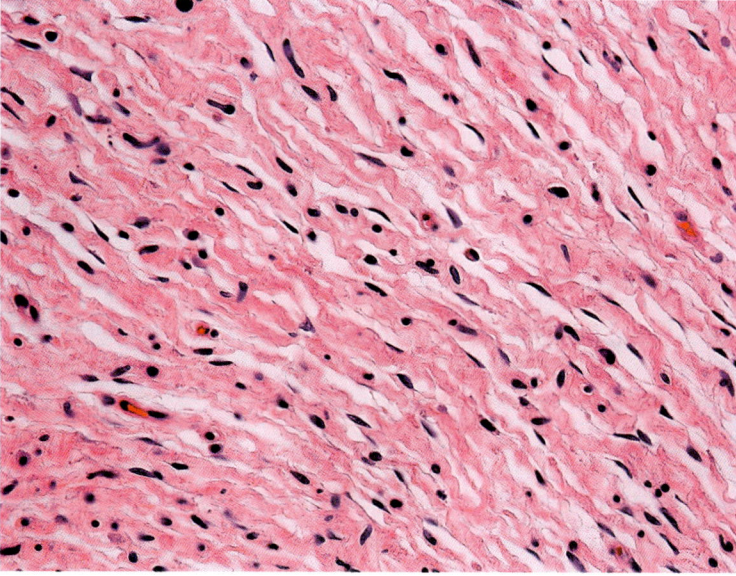

FIG 6.62 Neurofibroma, fibrous stroma with spindle- and comma-shaped nuclei.

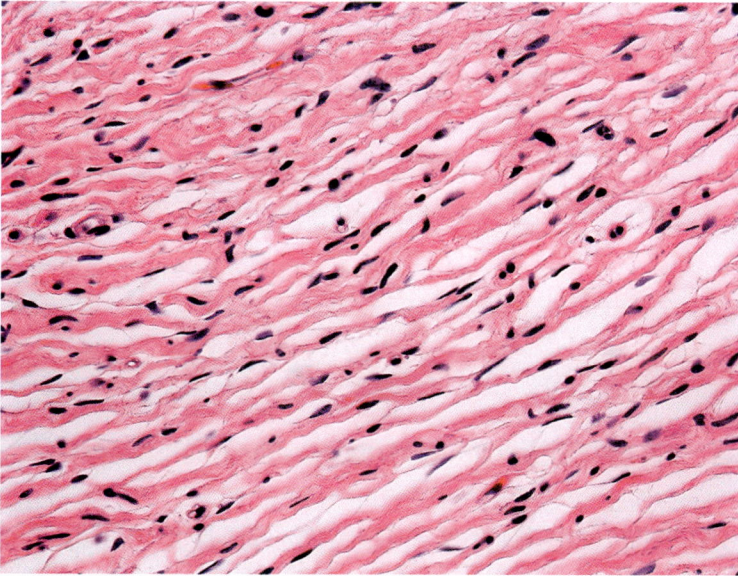

FIG 6.63 Neurofibroma, comma-shaped nuclei interspersed within a densely hyalinized stroma.

short spindle cells. Other constituents include numerous mast cells, fibromyxoid stroma sometimes densely hyalinized (Figs 6.62 and 6.63). Mitoses are absent. One mitosis could be a "case for concern" (see later). Cellular areas of neurofibroma simulate an Antoni A pattern of schwannoma, although there is not a clear partition between the two zones.

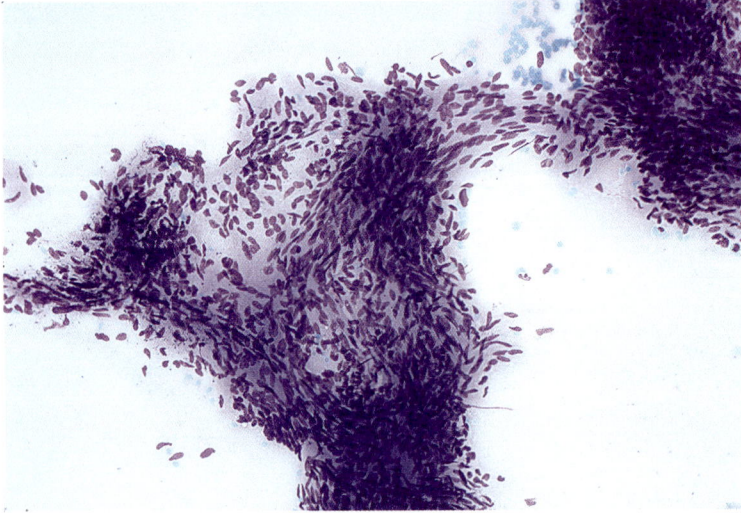

FIG 6.64 Schwannoma, various proportions of cohesive scant spindle or round cells.

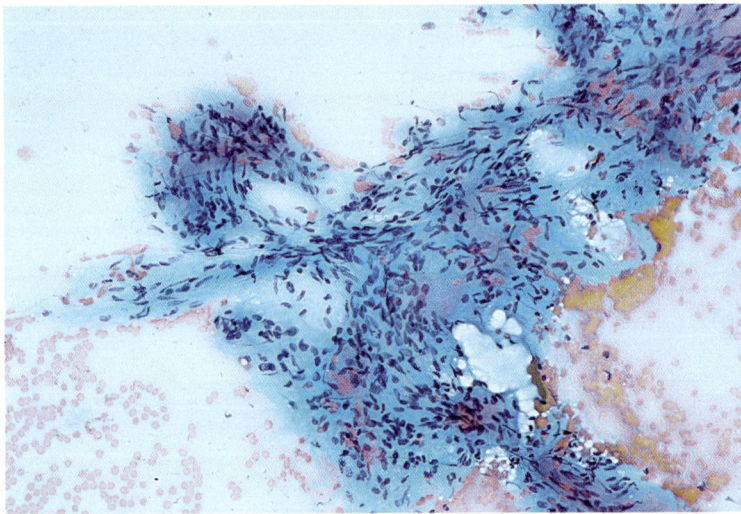

FIG 6.65 Schwannoma, same case as in Fig 6.64, Papanicolaou.

6.2.1.2 Cytopathology. Schwannomas are cytologically characteristic and consist of various proportions of cohesive scant spindle or round cells (Figs 6.64–6.66) within connective tissue fragments (Verocay bodies) (Figs 6.67–6.70), fishhook naked nuclei (Fig 6.71), isolated regular spindle cells, and/or round cells with nuclear inclusions arranged in palisades and delicate fibrillary stroma (Fig 6.72). Occasionally, a myxoid background may be present (Fig 6.73) as well as mast cells. Cells whose cytoplasm contains melanin pigment occasionally are observed in certain variants. Neurofibroma has a similar cytomorphology (Figs 6.74 and 6.75), but Verocay bodies are absent. Usually, neurofibromas show large clusters of fibrillary stroma containing parallel, regular, and wavy cells resembling normal nerve.

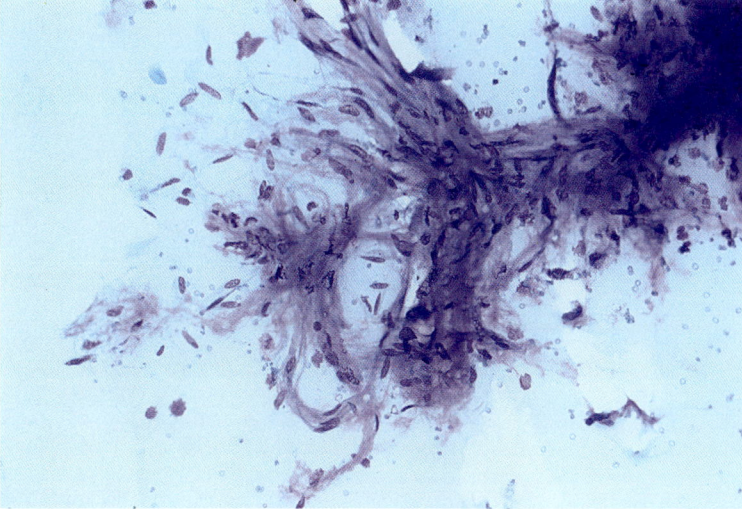

FIG 6.66 Schwannoma, spindle cells.

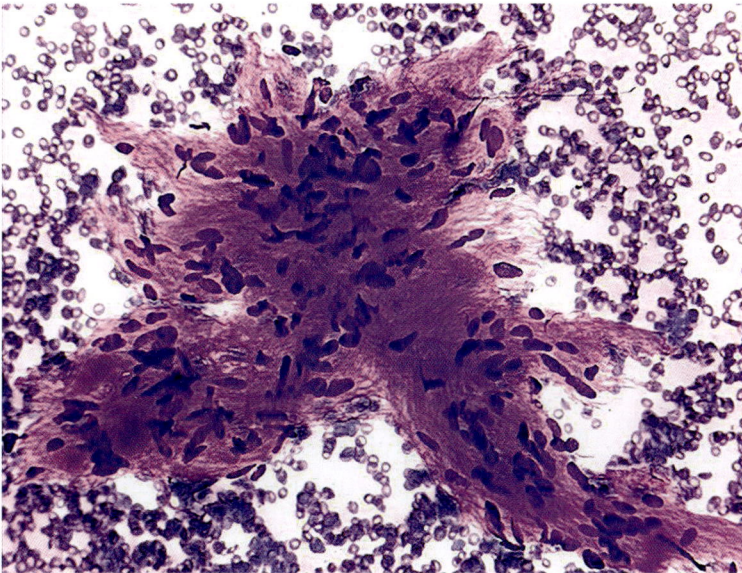

FIG 6.67 Schwannoma, connective tissue fragments.

6.2.1.3 *Differential Diagnosis.* The following entities should be differentiated:

— Schwannoma
— Neurofibroma
— Low-grade malignant peripheral nerve sheath tumor

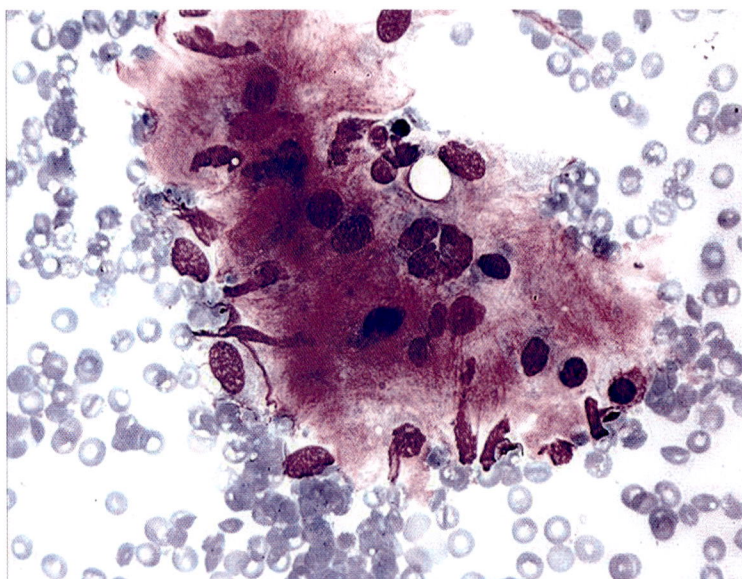

FIG 6.68 Schwannoma, connective tissue fragments and well-differentiated Verocay bodies.

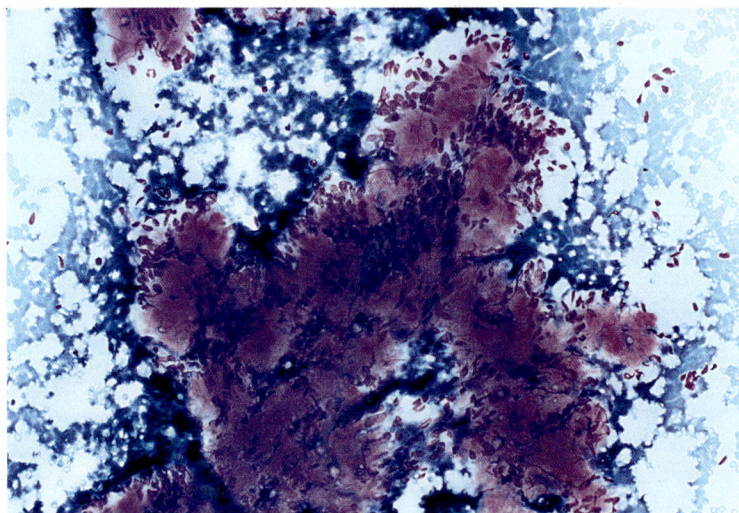

FIG 6.69 Schwannoma, low magnification, Verocay bodies.

Among the principal entities to consider in the differential diagnosis, well-differentiated malignant peripheral nerve sheath tumor may pose serious difficulties, especially when dealing with highly cellular variants of schwannoma or schwannoma with cytonuclear atypias ("ancient" schwannoma) (Table 6.4). In well-differentiated malignant peripheral nerve sheath tumor, smears consist of various proportions of spindle-shaped cells with wavy nuclei, comma-shaped naked nuclei, polymorphous

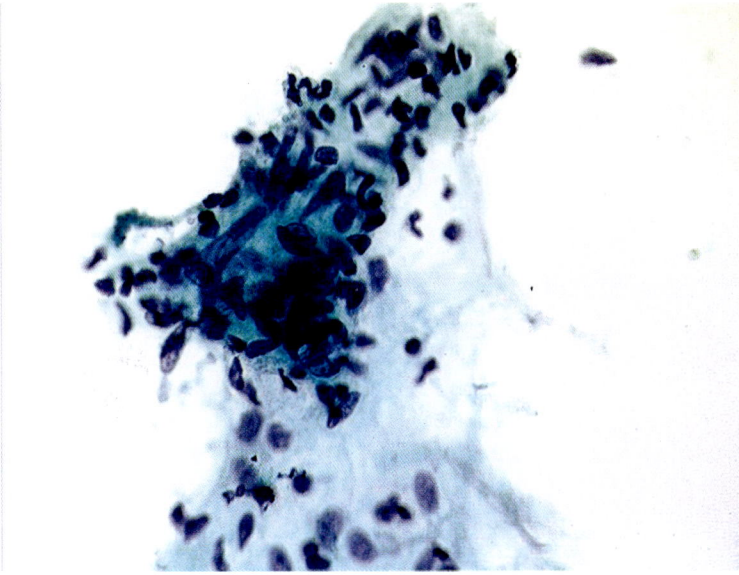

FIG 6.70 Schwannoma, connective tissue fragments and well-differentiated Verocay bodies, Papanicolaou.

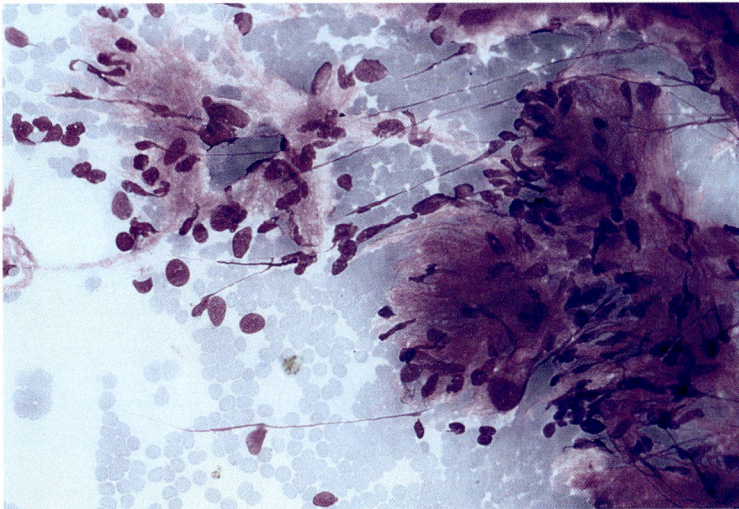

FIG 6.71 Schwannoma, fishhook naked nuclei.

oval-to-rounded cells, and anaplastic multinucleated cells with geographical-like nuclei. A recent review of spindle cell malignant peripheral nerve sheath tumors [65] have shown that the most reliable morphological characteristic is the presence of typical comma-shaped cells, occasionally arranged in palisades, in conjunction with highly characteristic twisted or wavy nuclei. Principal discriminative morphological differences rely on the presence of mitotic figures and on the absence of Verocay bodies.

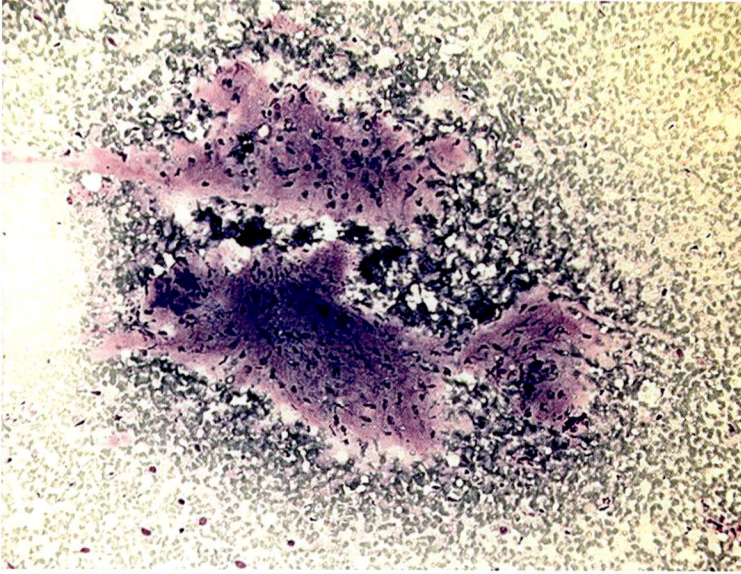

FIG 6.72 Schwannoma, delicate fibrillary stroma.

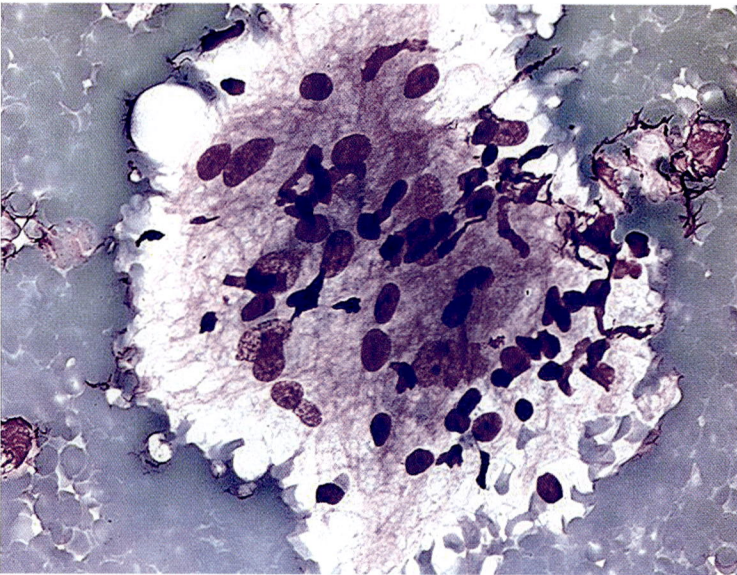

FIG 6.73 Schwannoma, myxoid background.

Immunocytochemistry is of help in the diagnosis. S-100 protein positivity does not distinguish between schwannoma and low-grade malignant peripheral nerve sheath tumor, but it does indicate a peripheral nerve sheath differentiation [66,67]. S-100 combined with desmin and/or smooth muscle actin positivity indicates smooth muscle tumors [67].

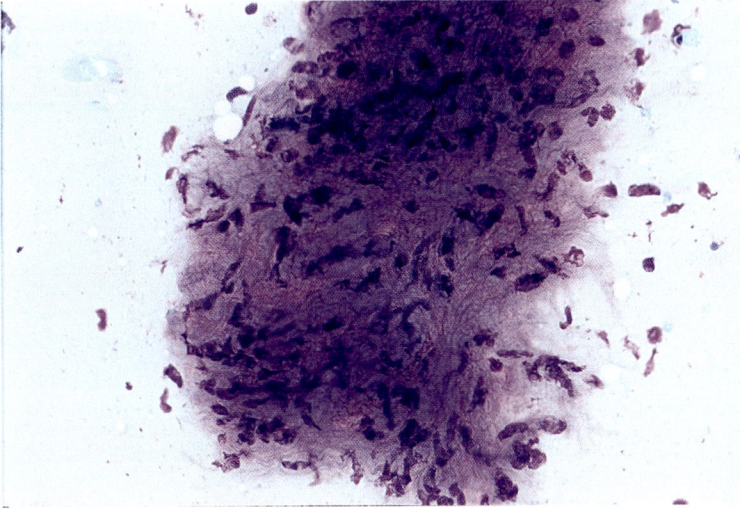

FIG 6.74 Neurofibroma, similar morphology to schwannoma, but Verocay bodies are absent.

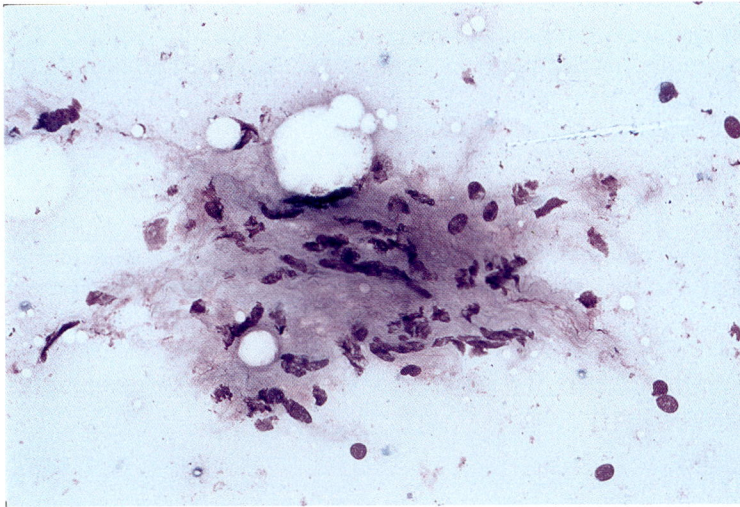

FIG 6.75 Neurofibroma, fibrillary background.

6.2.1.4 Comments. There were no major cytomorphologic differences in cell and stromal components among classical, ancient, cellular, and epithelioid variants. Myxoid stroma, mast cells, and intranuclear inclusions are limited to the classical subtype. Moderate cytonuclear atypia is more frequent in "ancient schwannoma" than in other subtypes. Round cells may be observed in classic and epithelioid schwannoma.

A small cytology series of schwannomas has been published in the last few decades [68–75]. A collective analysis, including case reports, of the 132 cases therein reported shows that an accurate diagnosis of benign schwannoma is made in 57%

TABLE 6.4 Cytological differential diagnosis of schwannoma and neurofibroma

	Schwannoma	Neurofibroma	Low-grade malignant peripheral nerve sheath tumor
Verocay bodies	++	−	−
Fishhook naked nuclei	++	+	++
Fibrillary stroma	++	+	++
Cytonuclear atypia	+/−	−	++
Palisading	+/−	−	+/−
Isolated spindle cells	+/−	+/−	++
Mitotic figures	−	−	++
Myxoid	+/−	+/−	+/−
Mast cells	+/−	+/−	+/−
Intranuclear inclusions	+/−	−	−

++; Frequent, +; rare, +/− occasionally seen, −; absent.

of cases. Diagnosis of other benign conditions was reported in 33%, suspicious/false-positive was reported in 8%, and unsatisfactory diagnosis as reported in 2% of cases.

"Ancient" and cellular variants of schwannomas could be responsible for generating diagnostic problems. This entity usually displays cellular degenerative changes, including moderate cytonuclear atypia and pleomorphism, along with a tendency to nuclear palisading [65, 76]. Similar findings added to atypical morphology with hypercellularity, deep location, and markedly fascicular growth pattern are representative of cellular schwannomas [77,78]. A reported example of an epitheliod schwannoma [79] was characterized by numerous groups of plump epithelioid cells along with multinucleated cells. Our example of epithelioid schwannoma [68] was unremarkable and consisted of Verocay bodies and numerous fishhook naked nuclei, therefore being not distinctive from classical schwannoma.

Smears of neurofibroma (benign nerve sheath tumors) [73] are characterized by scant cellularity, with loose tissue fragments depicting a fibrillar background and a greater number of clusters of closely packed spindle cells. Neither mitotic activity nor significant nuclear atypia are found [68].

6.2.1.5 FNA Key Features. The following are in favor of the diagnosis:

— Cell and stroma rich smears
— Spindle-shaped cells with wavy nuclei
— Comma-shaped naked nuclei
— Delicate fibrillary matrix
— Verocay bodies

The following are difficulties in making a diagnosis:

— Myxoid substance
— Moderate cytonuclear atypia in "ancient schwannoma"

The following are evidence against a diagnosis:

— Polymorphous cells with prominent cyto-nuclear atypia
— Anaplastic multinucleated cells with geographical-like nuclei
— Mitotic figures

6.2.2 Low-Grade Malignant Peripheral Nerve Sheath Tumor

The diagnosis of malignant peripheral nerve sheath tumor traditionally has been one of the most difficult and elusive among soft tissue tumors because of the lack of standardized diagnostic criteria [80]. Its incidence is variable according to the series that appeared in the literature. Diagnostic criteria for tumors developing outside a peripheral nerve and not associated with a neurofibromatosis 1 were not well defined until recently. The term malignant peripheral nerve sheath tumor has come to be accepted for all those malignant tumors resulting from the peripheral nerve or sharing a line of differentiation among the elements of the nerve sheath as mentioned earlier (i.e., Schwann cells, perineural, and fibroblasts). This accounts for the heterogeneity of phenotype of malignant peripheral nerve sheath tumors ranging from tumors that recapitulate the composition of neurofibroma toward pleomorphic sarcomas of malignant fibrous histiocytoma type, heterologous differentiation like rhabdomyoblastic (Triton tumor), glandular, angiosarcomatous, epithelioid, bone, and cartilage. In the present chapter, we will focus only on criteria of differential diagnosis of tumors with fibrillary stroma (i.e., the well-differentiated malignant peripheral nerves sheath tumor).

6.2.2.1 Histopathology. Most malignant peripheral nerve sheath tumors are large tumors, more than 5–10 cm in maximum diameter, and they are localized in deep soft tissues. Originating within a major peripheral nerve or in a preexisting neurofibroma, gross appearance is similar to other soft tissue tumors. As already stated, one mitosis is a case for concern, although it is not sufficient for a sarcoma. Low-grade malignant peripheral nerve sheath tumor tends to recapitulate the cellular composition of neurofibroma. Typical tumors consist of spindle cells with a more or less fascicular appearance with a transition between high and low cellular myxoid areas (Figs 6.76 and 6.77). Single cells are elongated, with poorly defined cytoplasm with a wispy appearance similar to cells of benign neurofibroma (Fig 6.78). Cell nuclei frequently depict a comma-shaped deformation. They can be more or less hyperchromatic with a variable degree of pleomorphism. In all cases, mitotic figures must be demonstrated (Fig 6.79). Heterologous elements are rare in these better differentiated tumors.

As a rule, malignant peripheral nerve sheath tumors otherwise would resemble fibrosarcomas in their overall architecture.

Some subtle features are described in more specialized textbooks, being not totally specific and will not be emphasized. Recall that the better differentiated low-grade malignant peripheral nerve sheath tumors are found in Von Recklinghausen disease, hence the appellation of "malignant neurofibroma." These tumors therefore have to fulfill recognized criteria of malignancy of malignant peripheral nerve sheath tumor.

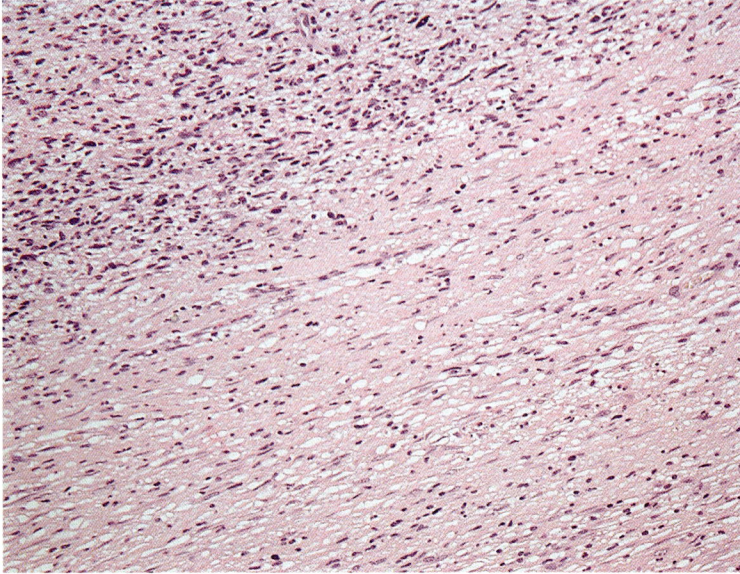

FIG 6.76 Low-grade malignant peripheral nerve sheath tumor, transition between areas of low-and high-grade sarcoma.

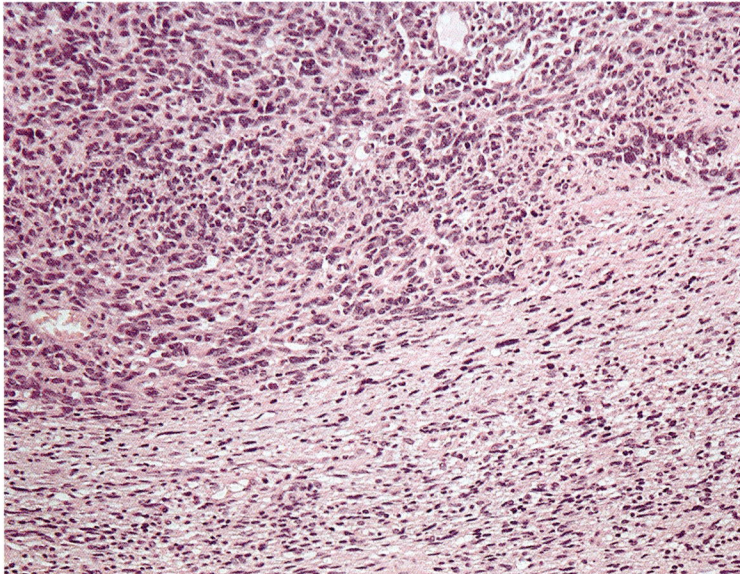

FIG 6.77 Low-grade malignant peripheral nerve sheath tumor, transition between areas of low-and high-grade sarcoma. Higher magnification from 6.76.

6.2.2.2 Cytopathology. Smears in low-grade malignant peripheral nerve sheath tumor consist of spindle-shaped cells with wavy nuclei (Fig 6.80), comma-shaped naked nuclei, and polymorphous oval-to-rounded cells (Fig 6.81). When anaplastic multinucleated cells with geographical-like nuclei are present in various proportions,

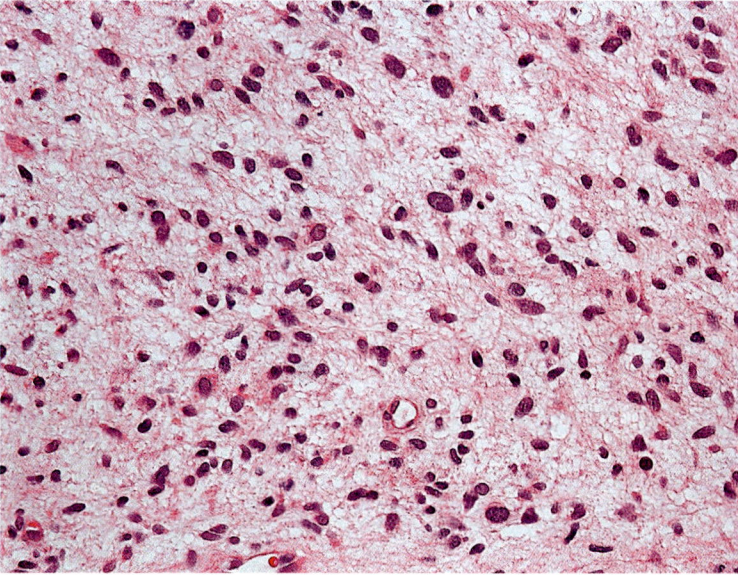

FIG 6.78   Low-grade malignant peripheral nerve sheath tumor, dispersed spindle cells with rare atypical nuclei in a fibrillary stroma.

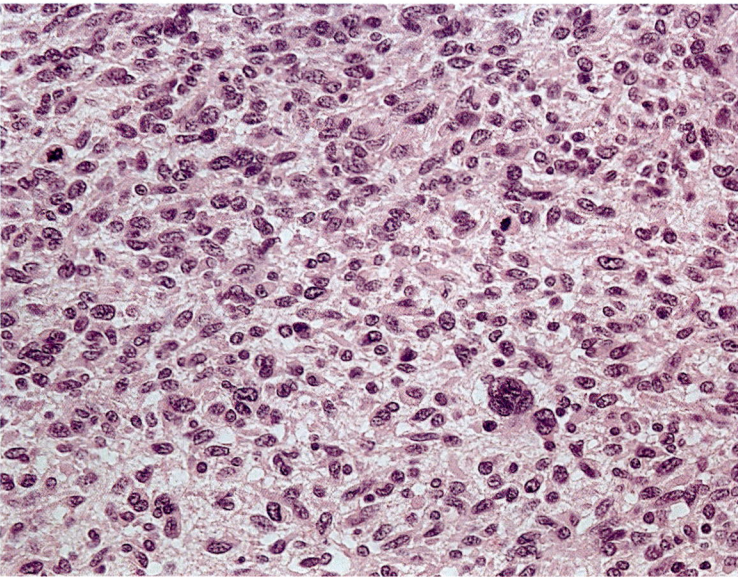

FIG 6.79   Low-grade malignant peripheral nerve sheath tumor, with the same tumor showing more or less hyperchromatic nuclei and variable pleomorphism. Mitosis is present.

the diagnosis of high-grade malignant peripheral nerve sheath tumor should be evocated. Cells are both dispersed and in clusters. Nuclear chromatin is bland, and nucleoli are inconspicious in all cases. Mitotic figures frequently are observed. Palisading is never observed. There is a stromal background material of nonspecific

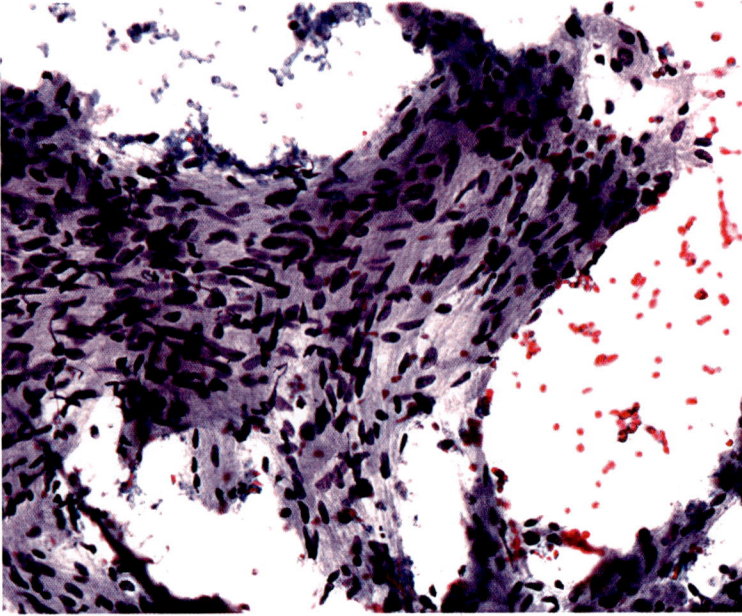

FIG 6.80 Low-grade malignant peripheral nerve sheath tumor, spindle-shaped cells with wavy nuclei.

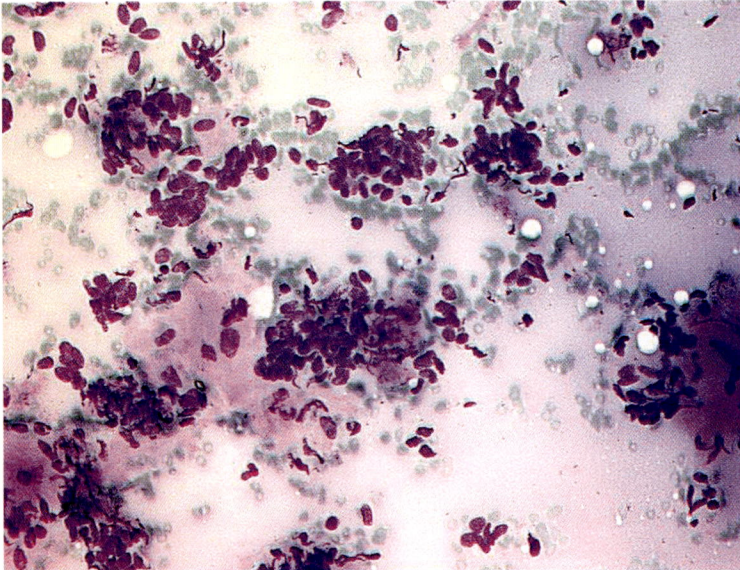

FIG 6.81 Low-grade malignant peripheral nerve sheath tumor, comma-shaped naked nuclei, and polymorphous oval-to-rounded cells. Note the presence of fibrillary stroma. Malignant nature is evident.

fragments of dense connective tissue, delicate fibrillary matrix, or myxoid substance. Necrosis is scant. Occasionally, intranuclear inclusions are observed.

6.2.2.3 Differential Diagnosis. The following entities should be differentiated from low-grade malignant peripheral nerve sheath tumor:

— Synovial sarcoma
— Leiomyosarcoma
— "Ancient" schwannoma

The differential diagnosis of low-grade malignant peripheral nerve sheath tumor includes benign forms of nerve sheath tumors and other types of spindle cell sarcoma, principally synovial sarcoma, fibrosarcoma, and low-grade leiomyosarcoma [76,81–86] (Table 6.5).

The benign nerve sheath tumors are characterized by loose tissue fragments with a fibrillar background and by more cellular clusters of spindle cells representative of Verocay bodies [68, 77]. However, vascular arcades, fishhook nuclei, and epithelioid cells also were reported. Given its morphological diversity and the lack of standardized diagnostic criteria, the cytological diagnosis of low-grade malignant peripheral nerve sheath tumor may be difficult. The correlation between the described cytological features and the clinical information—origin of the tumor from a nerve trunk, a preexisting neurofibroma, and patients with known history of neurofibromatosis 1—could be indicative of the malignant peripheral nerve sheath tumor diagnosis.

The entity called "ancient shwannoma" usually displays degenerative changes, including nuclear atypia and pleomorphism, along with a tendency to nuclear palisading. This pattern is indicative of schwannian differentiation but is an uncommon finding in malignant peripheral nerve sheath tumor [82].

TABLE 6.5 Cytological differential diagnosis in low-grade malignant peripheral nerve sheath tumor

	Malignant peripheral nerve sheath tumor	Synovial sarcoma	Leiomyosarcoma	"Ancient" schwannoma
Spindle cells	++	++	++	++
Round cells	−	+	++	+
Giant cells	+	+/−	+/−	−
Blunt-ends	−	−	+/−	−
Binucleated	+/−	−	+/−	−
Mitotic figures	+	+	+/−	−
Fibrous stroma	−	+	+/−	+
Myxoid stroma	+	+/−	in myxoid ++	−
Inflammation	−	+/−	+/−	−
Necrosis	+	+/−	+/−	−
Calcifications, metaplastic bone	+/−	+	−	−

++; Frequent, +; rare, +/− occasionally seen, −; absent.

Synovial sarcoma [87] consists of a mixture of dispersed monotonous cells and small clusters of cells with bland chromatin, inconspicuous nucleoli, oval-to-spindle-shaped cytoplasm, branching tumor tissue fragments, vessel stalks, pseudopapillary structures, and scant background mucin. Cohesive epithelial cells, poorly differentiated monotonous round cells, mast cells, necrosis, secretory mucin, and rosette-like structures occasionally may be observed and are strongly suggestive of synovial sarcoma. Howewer, some examples of synovial sarcoma may exhibit comma-like nuclei, marked nuclear atypia, and scarce connective stromal fragments, which resemble malignant peripheral nerve sheath tumor. In malignant peripheral nerve sheath tumor, a wavy appearance, elongated and slender nuclei, focally prononced nuclear atypia, bizarre giant multinucleated cells, and fibrillary metachromic stroma are indicative of the diagnosis. However, other features such as vicinity to a nerve or a history of neuroma or neurifibromatosis 1 are helpful in the differential diagnosis. Differential, immunocytochemical studies may be inconclusive [80], although t(x;18) translocation is strongly in favor of synovial sarcoma [87].

Low-grade leiomyosarcomas may show tissue fragments with a fascicular or storiform pattern and a rhythmic arrangement of nuclei closely resembling nerve sheath tumor palisades [88]. Nevertheless, the cytonuclear morphology of malignant peripheral nerve sheath tumor strongly differs from that of leiomyosarcoma, in which the fibrillar eosinophilic cytoplasm is arranged symmetrically around blunt-ended nuclei [89].

6.2.2.4 Comments. Similar to the features of malignant peripheral nerve sheath tumor observed in tissue sections [80], cytologic aspirates can consist of spindle-shaped, epithelioid, and rhabdomyoblastic (in malignant Triton tumor) cells. The group of spinde cell tumors also may be divided into two groups: those exhibiting recognizable neurogenic differentiation that are histologically well-differentiated tumors and those showing anaplastic pleomorphic features that are histologically anaplastic [81].

A review of the reported data concerning spindle cell malignant peripheral nerve sheath tumor reveals that the most reliable morphological characteristic of well-differentiated tumors is the presence of typical comma-shaped cells, occasionally arranged in palisades, in conjunction with highly characteristic twisted or wavy nuclei [89]. Molina et al. [85] and Jiménez-Heffernan et al. [81] reported that neurogenic differentiation was recognizable in all of their cases: the smears showed spindle-shaped cells with elongated, slender, and often wavy nuclei as well as a delicate, fibrillary metachromatic stroma in the background. In our previous study [65] well-differentiated malignant peripheral nerve sheath tumors consisted of small spindle cells, wavy nuclei, comma-like naked nuclei with few pleomorphic cells, and a fibrillary matrix.

Despite numerous reports, the cytomorphological patterns of malignant peripheral nerve sheath tumor are documented insufficiently in the literature. In consonance with the wide histopathological diversity, cytologic correlations, except for one [81], are limited to single case reports or small series. The cytologic criteria of malignant peripheral nerve sheath tumor have been described in a series of studies including 55 tumors in 49 patients [82–85, 89]. Preexisting neurofibroma or a history of neurofibromatosis 1 was noted in nine patients [81, 89–93]. Of 29 cases of primary and 24 cases of recurrent/metastatic listed in the literature, 45 tumors were correlated with histology and 22 were well-differentiated, 5 were anaplastic [81,93], 4 were epithelioid [81, 92], 1 was a malignant Triton tumor [81], and 2 were alignant melanotic shwannomas [94].

A collective analysis of these series and of our cases shows that malignant peripheral nerve sheath tumor (including high-grade) could be diagnosed accurately in 32 (40.5%) out of 79 specified cases, whereas 41 (51.9%) cases were diagnosed as other types of sarcoma. The remaining three (3.8%) cases were classified as suspicious [84], and three (3.8%) cases were classified as false negative [65,76,84,95].

6.2.2.5 *Clinical and FNA Key Features.* The following are in favor of the diagnosis:

— Nerve localization
— Cell and stroma-rich smears
— Spindle-shaped cells with wavy nuclei
— Comma-shaped naked nuclei
— Polymorphous oval-to-round cells
— Atypical multinucleated cells with geographical-like nuclei
— Delicate fibrillary matrix

The following are difficulties in making a diagnosis:

— Myxoid substance
— Palisading absent

The following are evidence against a diagnosis:

— Verocay bodies
— Lack of nuclear atypia

6.3 MALIGNANT SPINDLE CELL TUMORS

Among the different groups of mesenchymal malignancies, spindle cell sarcomas are well known to generate problems in differential diagnosis in terms of precising their phenotype. As emphasized before, distinguishing benign and low-grade tumors is difficult and constitutes a potential to generate false-positive and false-negative results with FNA and CNB techniques. Because of a large group of entities whose spindle cells are the main characteristic component (e.g., leiomyosarcoma, synovial sarcoma, fibrosarcoma, malignant peripheral nerve sheath tumor, Kaposi sarcoma, angiosarcoma, and malignant fibrous histiocytoma), the determination of a tumor phenotype in fine needle aspiration material is both challenging and decieving. With the exception of fibrosarcoma, these varieties of spindle cell sarcomas have been studied in details in the recent years, and consequently, these findings will form the basis of the present review. The exclusion of classical fibrosarcoma from these studies was justified by the marked decrease incidence of that tumor as a result of better immunohistochemical, genetic, and molecular biology characteristics, principally in synovial sarcoma and malignant peripheral nerve sheath tumor. Practically, fibrosarcoma has become a diagnosis of exclusion, with no precise immunohistochemical profile nor genetic or molecular biology profile. However, variants of fibrosarcoma have been identified and better characterized, for instance, myxofibrosarcoma, low-grade fibromyxoid sarcoma, and sclerosing epithelioid fibrosarcoma.

The overall general architectural and cytological patterns of spindle cell soft tissue tumors have been described earlier in Chapter 5.

6.3.1 Leiomyosarcoma

Leiomyosarcoma develops in four different clinical settings: retroperitoneum, cutaneous and subcutaneous, deep-seated, and of vascular origin. Leiomyosarcoma accounts for 5–10% of soft tissue sarcomas and are largely tumors of adult individuals, occuring most often in the retroperitoneum and axial soft tissue structures. Occasionally, leiomyosarcoma may originate in parenchymatous organs such as the prostate, orbit, breast, pancreas, liver, kidney, bone, uterus, lung, ovary, urinary bladder, portal vein, and oral cavity. They also affect the immunocompromised patients. First observed as a complication of renal transplantation and immunosuppression [96] in the early 1970s, they have been associated with acquired immunodeficiency syndrome (AIDS), particularly among children, involving parenchymal organs [97].

Leiomyosarcoma of soft tissue originates principally in the retroperitoneal space and the abdominal cavity with a distinct female predominance (70%). They are large tumors and often nonsurgically resectable. Given better characterization of gastrointestinal stromal tumors (GISTs), its incidence has decreased, and now it is mandatory to consider this entity in the differential diagnosis of spindle cell/epitheliod neoplasms of those cavities. Cutaneous leiomyosarcoma refers to small tumors developing in the dermis, sometimes extending into the subcutis. There is general agreement among pathologists to use the denomination of "atypical smooth muscle tumor" for those lesions limited to the dermis that have no metastatic potential, although they can recur, which is different if the tumor extends into the subcutis. These are small nodules (<2 cm), frequently excised at the first medical visit and hence limited fine needle aspiration material. Indeed, leiomyosarcoma of vascular origin are rare entities, with only a few hundred cases reported in the literature. Most originate in the inferior vena cava and some originate in the arteries, principally the pulmonary artery. They are life-threatening because of their localization that precludes surgical resection. In the past, leiomyosarcoma of the extremities/limbs were considered uncommon. Molecular genetics and biology techniques presently show a tendancy to reverse this incidence. Tissue microarrays of leiomyosarcoma tend to delineate two different gene profiles of leiomyosarcoma according to their site of origin and the degree of differentiation [98].

Whatever their clinical setting, leiomyosarcomas, either cutaneous or deep-seated, are investigated frequently with the fine needle aspiration technique. Correlative cytological/histological review [99] has allowed distinguishing several features of leiomyosarcoma according to their cytological grades.

6.3.1.1 *Histopathology.* According to their grade of differentiation, there are some variable features. The best-differentiated tumors consist of fascicles of spindle cells with eosinophilic cytoplasm (Fig 6.82). Elongated, cigar-shaped (truncated ends) (Fig 6.83) or rounded nuclei, nuclear segmentation, and paranuclear vacuoles

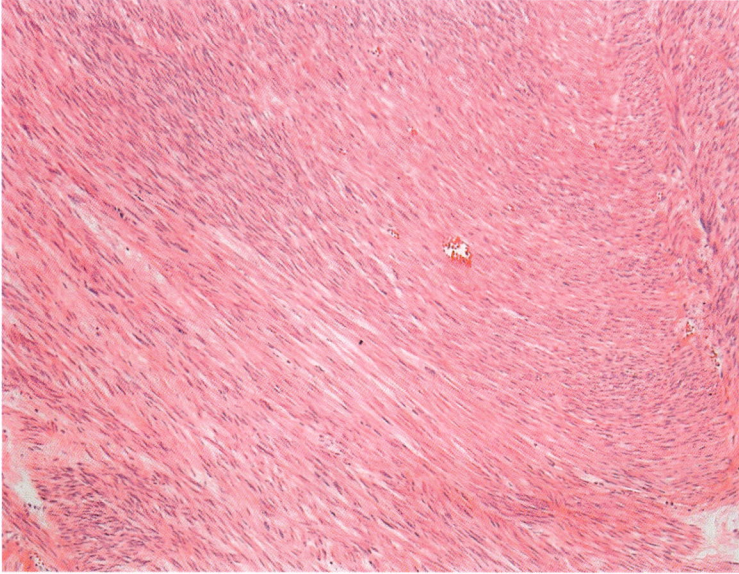

FIG 6.82 Leiomyosarcoma, long fascicles of closely packed spindle cells with eosinophilic cytoplasm.

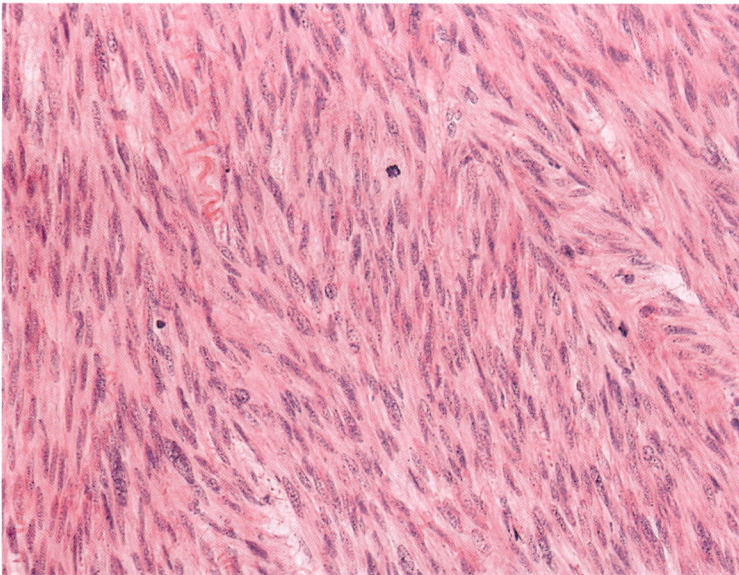

FIG 6.83 Leiomyosarcoma, elongated cigar-shaped nuclei with occasional nuclear segmentation.

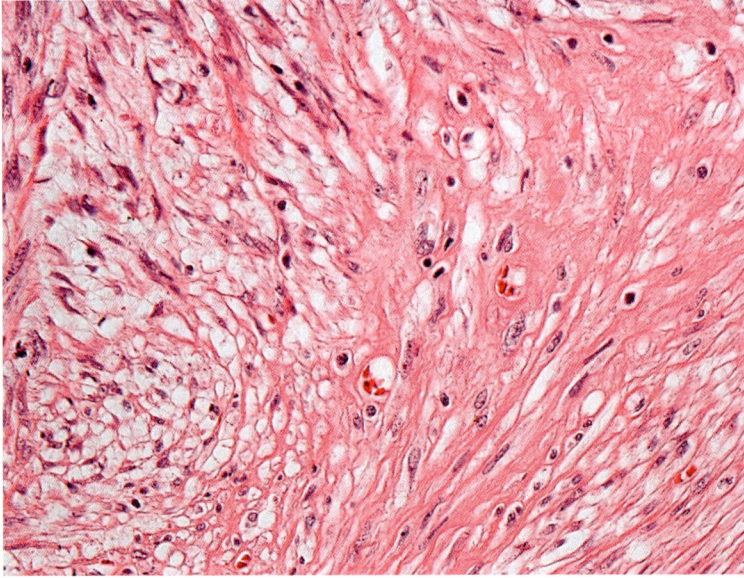

FIG 6.84 Leiomyosarcoma, paranuclear vacuoles within a low-grade area.

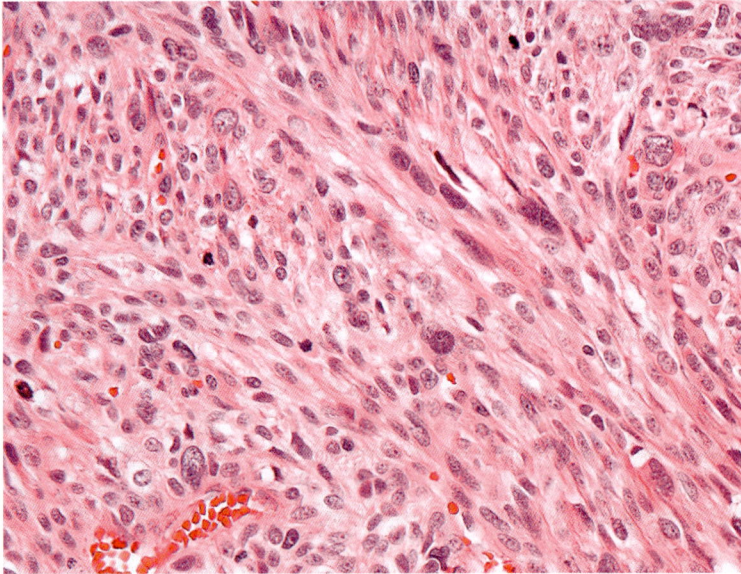

FIG 6.85 Leiomyosarcoma, numerous pleomorphic nuclei in a relatively hypercellular area.

commonly are observed (Fig 6.84). The mitotic index varies considerably from tumor to tumor as well as the atypical features and pleomorphism (Fig 6.85). Because of the large volume of some tumors, the quality of the stroma is variable: myxoid changes, hyalinization, and foci of necrosis could be present. A myxoid variant of leiomyosarcoma has been described [100] (Fig 6.86).

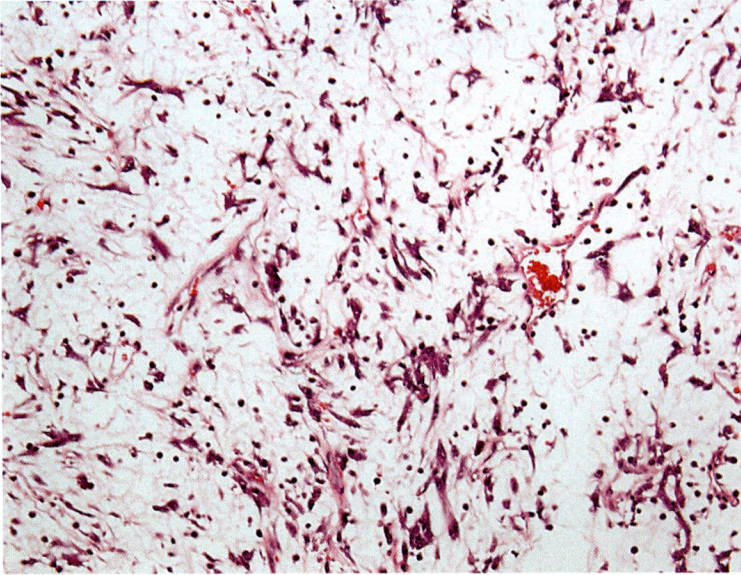

FIG 6.86 Leiomyosarcoma, atypical spindle cells in a myxoid background.

6.3.1.2 Cytopathology.
In classical, low-grade (well-differentiated) leiomyosarcomas, tumor cells occur singly, in loose groupings, or also are packed closely in cohesive groupings (Figs 6.87–6.89). Most tumor cells are elongated, but sometimes they are rounded or oval (Fig 6.90). A few multinucleated giant cells with irregular and atypical nuclei may be observed. Nuclei are ovoid, spindle-shaped, or elongated, and some of which have blunted ends (Fig 6.91). They depict a finely or slightly coarsely granular chromatin pattern as well as nuclear segmentation and are often in parallel arrangements [101,102]. The cytoplasm is scanty and ill defined, and some of them appear as irregular nuclei (Fig 6.92). The cellular and nuclear atypia are variable but minimal. Mitotic figures and necrosis are rare. Scattered naked nuclei are common. Background material is generally scant. The presence of abundant fibrillar or collagenous material and blood vessels within tumor fragments or cell clusters have beed described [103].

In contrast, high-grade (poorly differentiated) pleomorphic leiomyosarcomas show the large spindle-shaped cells more frequently as well as round, giant, and binucleated cells. However, cells may have finely eosinophilic intracytoplasmic granulations, blunt-ended nuclei (cigar-like), intranuclear inclusions, and smears may contain fibrotic dense connective tissue. Usually both spindle-shaped and pleomorphic cells may be found in the same aspiration.

6.3.1.3 Differential Diagnosis.
The following entities should be differentiated from leiomyosarcoma:

 — Leiomyoma
 — Low-grade malignant peripheral nerves sheath tumor
 — Synovial sarcoma
 — Benign fibrous histiocytoma
 — Dermatofibrosarcoma protuberans
 — GIST

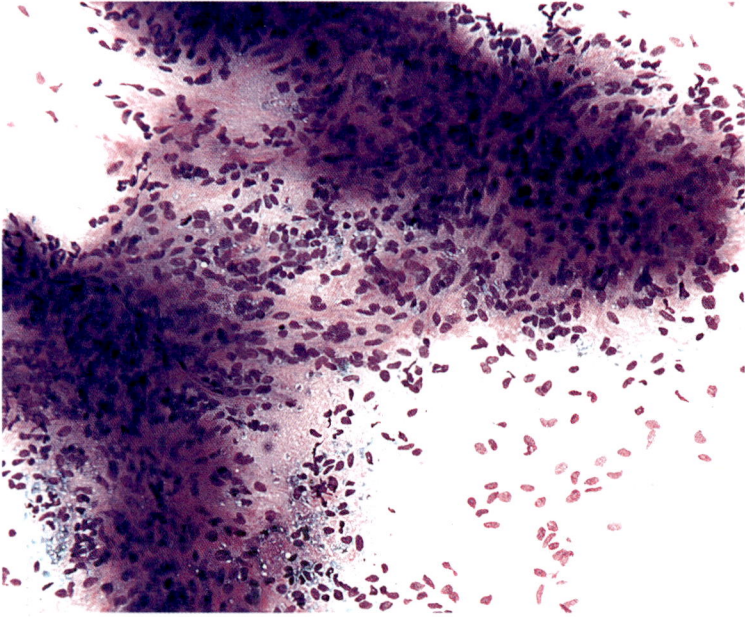

FIG 6.87 Leiomyosarcoma, various proportions of spindle-shaped, cohesive, and small- or large-sized cells. Malignant character is evident.

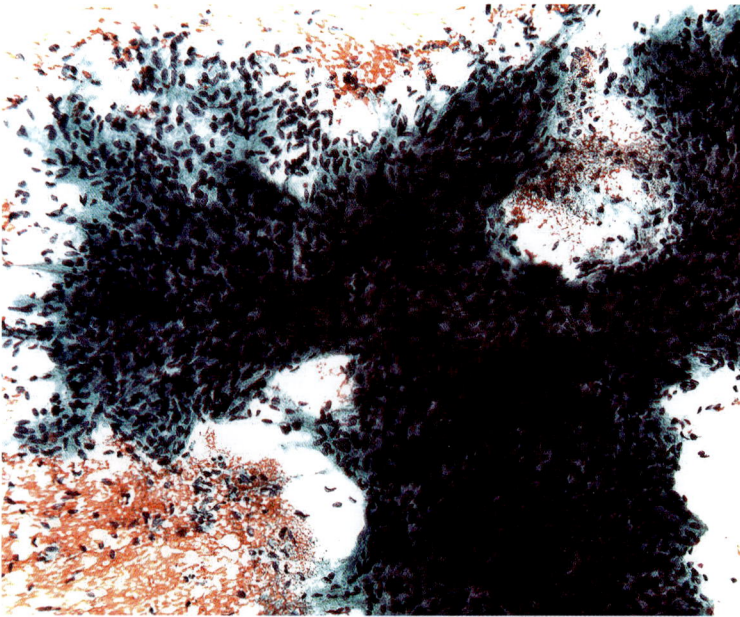

FIG 6.88 Leiomyosarcoma, same aspect that on Fig 6.87 seen in Papanicolaou.

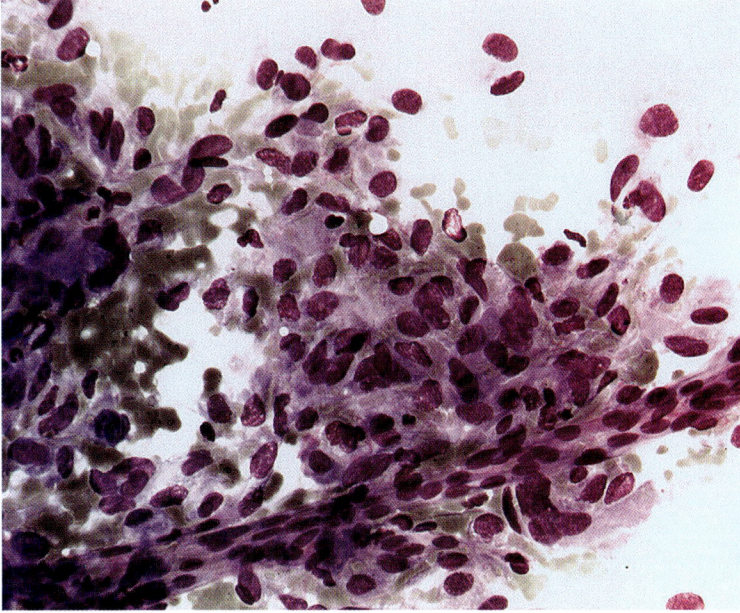

FIG 6.89 Leiomyosarcoma, loose clusters of tumor cells.

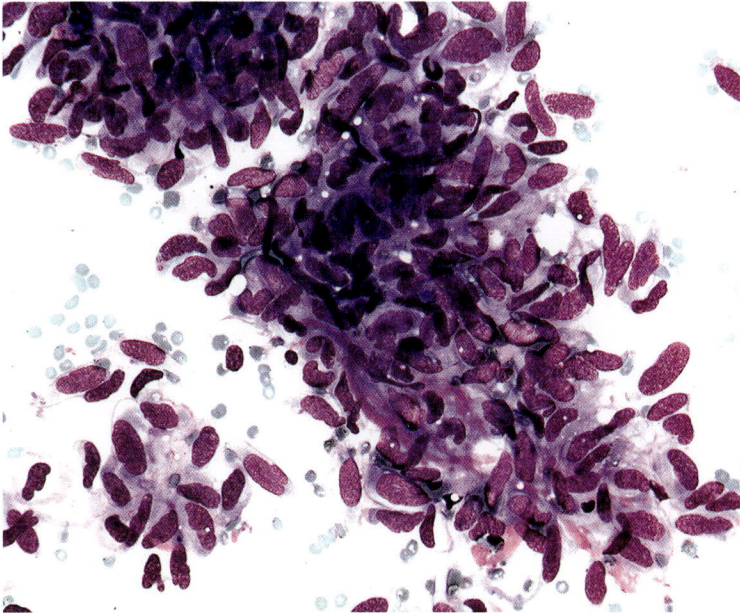

FIG 6.90 Leiomyosarcoma, elongated or rounded cells.

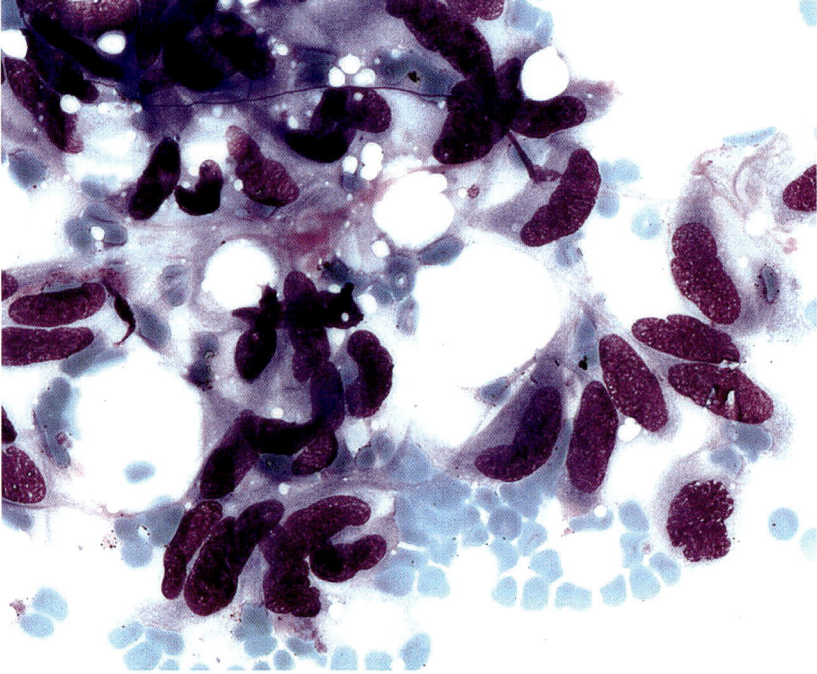

FIG 6.91 Leiomyosarcoma, elongated nuclei with blunted ends.

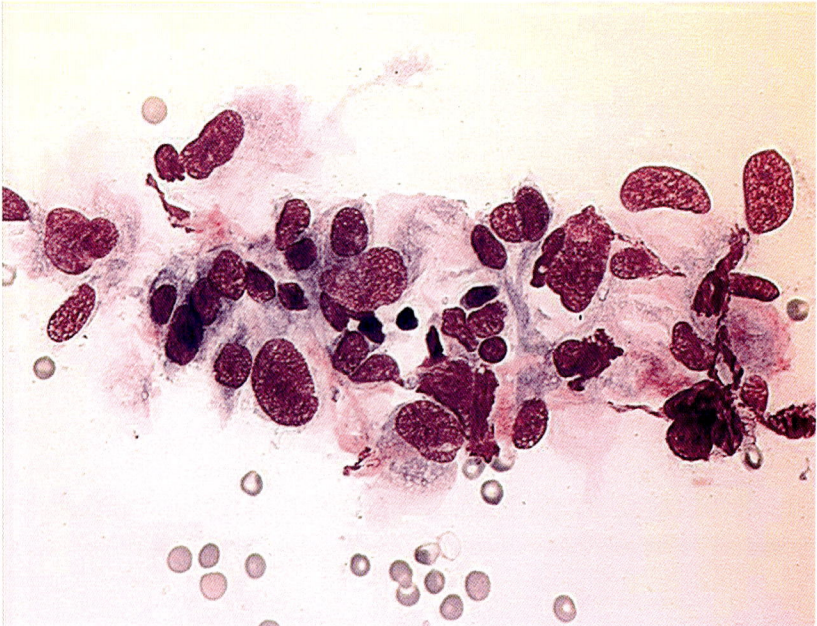

FIG 6.92 Leiomyosarcoma, irregular nuclei.

Principal entities to consider in the differential diagnosis are all other spindle cell lesions including, for the cutaneous variety, benign fibrous histiocytoma, dermatofibrosarcoma protuberans, and spindle cell melanoma (Table 6.6), all of which can be differentiated by an appropriate panel of antibodies, including CD34, CD117, smooth muscle actin, desmin, caldesmon, MelanA, HMB45, and S-100. For deeper and retroperitoneal tumors, gastrointestinal stromal tumor is the principal candidate followed by fibromatosis and other rare mesenchymal neoplasms in these cavities.

The cytological spectrum of the differential diagnosis of low-grade leiomyosarcoma includes entities such as leiomyoma, low-grade malignant peripheral nerves sheath tumor, and monophasic synovial sarcoma. Leiomyomas mainly consist of cohesive groups of cells with loosely and irregurarly arranged nuclei, exhibiting a syncytial appearance. The presence of closely packed tumor cells with elongated nuclei in a parallel, side-by-side arrangement strongly supports the diagnosis of leiomyosarcoma [101]. Scattered, solitary tumor cells with cigar-shaped nuclei, blunt ends, and scanty, ill-defined cytoplasm appearing as naked nuclei are also findings strongly suggestive of the diagnosis [103].

Spindle-shaped cells and variable nuclear pleomorphism in malignant peripheral nerve sheath tumor may mimic leiomyosarcoma [104], but the wavy, elongated, and slender nuclei, focally prononced nuclear atypia, occasional giant multinucleated cells, and fibrillary stroma are rather suggestive of malignant peripheral nerve sheath tumor. However, other features such as the knowledge of the vicinity to a nerve, a history of neuroma or neurofibromatosis 1, positive immunostaining for S-100 protein, and negative staining for muscle-specific actin or desmin (in non-Triton tumors) are helpful ancillary studies. A mixture of dispersed, monotonous cells and small clusters of cells with oval-to-spindle-shaped cytoplasm, branching tumor tissue

TABLE 6.6 Cytological differential diagnosis of low-grade leiomyosarcoma

	Low-grade leiomyosarcoma		Leiomyoma	Low-grade malignant peripheral nerve sheath tumor	Synovial sarcoma
	Classic	Epithelioid			
Spindle cells	++	++	++	++	+/−
Round cells	+	++	−	−	+
Giant cells	+	+/−	−	−	−
Granular cytoplasms	+/−	−	−	−	−
Blunt-ends	++	−	+	−	−
Binucleated	−	+	−	+/−	−
Mitotic figures	+	−	−	+	+
Fibrous stroma	+/−	−	+	−	−
Myxoid stroma	−	−	−	+/−	−
Inflammation	+/−	+/−	−	−	+/−
Necrosis	−	−	−	−	+/−

++; frequent, +; common, +/−; occasionally seen, −; absent.

fragments, scant background mucin, and rarely cohesive epithelial cells are strongly suggestive of synovial sarcoma [105].

6.3.1.4   *Comments.* Several cytological studies of leiomyosarcoma with a total of 229 cases have been reported, of which only 7 [99,101,103,106,107] included more than 5 cases. A comprehensive assessment of the cytological findings representative of this entity is therefore difficult given the heterogeneity of the material and the variability of the criteria used for classifying leiomyosarcoma. A quick overview of these reports shows that all subtypes (i.e., classical, epithelioid [99,105,108], and myxoid [99,107,109,110] are identified.

Low-grade (grades I and II) tumors manifest certain morphological differences in comparison with grade III tumors. Low-grade leiomyosarcoma showed more small, spindle-shaped cells in parallel alignment, more large, spindle-shaped cells, and more cells with blunt-ended nuclei than tumors of grade III (pleomorphic leiomyosarcoma). Cells with granular cytoplasm and scant fibrous stroma are observed exclusively in low-grade tumors. Inversely, background necrosis was much more frequent (68%) in high-grade than in low-grade tumors. Other morphological parameters such as round, giant, and binucleated cells, intranuclear inclusions, mitotic figures, myxoid matrix; and an inflammatory background, were distributed equally in all histological grades.

In general, low-grade leiomyosarcoma is more difficult to diagnose than tumors of high grade. In our previous analysis of 96 leiomyosarcomas [99] including all grades, the review of original cytology reports showed that 23 (24%) tumors were diagnosed accurately and specifically as leiomyosarcoma, 44 (45.8%) were diagnosed as sarcoma not otherwise specified, 13 (13.6%) were diagnosed as fibrosarcoma, 5 (5.3%) were diagnosed as myxofibrosarcoma, 3 (3.1%) were diagnosed as malignant fibrous histiocytoma, and 1 (1%) case was diagnosed each as liposarcoma, malignant peripheral nerve sheath tumor, angiosarcoma, and rhabdomyosarcoma. Two (2.1%) samples were considered suspicious for sarcoma not otherwise specified and two (2.1%) samples were unsatisfactory. A separate analysis of those tumors for which fine needle aspiration was used as the initial diagnostic procedure gave the following results: only 10 tumors (18.6%) were diagnosed accurately and specifically as leiomyosarcoma, 40 (74%) were diagnosed as other types of sarcomas, 2 (3.7%) were considered suspicious for malignancy, and 2 (3.7%) other aspirates were unsatisfactory.

6.3.1.5   *FNA Key Features.* The following are in favor of the diagnosis:

- Various proportions of spindle-shaped, cohesive, and small- or large-sized cells
- Parallel alignments
- Ovoid, spindle-shaped, or elongated nuclei with blunted ends
- Naked nuclei

The following are difficulties in making a diagnosis:

- Mitotic activity, necrosis, slight pleomorphism

The following are evidence against a diagnosis:

− Marked pleomorphism
− Fibrillary stroma
− Psudopapillary structures
− Epithelial cells

6.3.2 Synovial Sarcoma

Synovial sarcoma, both biphasic and monophasic variants, belongs to the category of spindle cell sarcomas. Obviously poorly differentiated synovial sarcoma, is excluded from that group whose cytologic and histologic cellular composition is closer to the round cell pattern (see chapter 6.8). Inclusion of the biphasic variety into this group is mandatory because a proportion of those tumors are predominantly spindle cell-rich with a minimal portion of epithelial component. Most of synovial sarcoma recognized morphologically are of the monophasic type given the better histologic identified features, the routine use of a selected panel of antibodies, and the demonstration by molecular biology of both transcripts SSX-1 and SSX-2 of the translocation t(x;18) [111]. On cytological grounds, synovial sarcoma obeys the same morphologic criteria as other members of the group.

Despite the term synovial sarcoma and its morphologic resemblance to developing synovial membrane, so far, no evidence has indicated that synovial sarcoma originates from synovial membrane, and therefore, most current literature classes synovial sarcoma as a malignant soft tissue tumor of uncertain origin, although we have observed rare cases originating within the synovial membrane (see chapter 6.8.5). By contrast, it is an entity that is well defined both clinically and morphologically and moreover is substantiated by cytogenetic and molecular biology findings. Synovial sarcoma is more prevalent in adolescents and young adults (15−45 years of age), with a slight male predominance. There is a wide anatomic distribution, with most occurring in the lower limbs followed by the upper extremities, head and neck, and trunk. Molecular biology techniques allowed substantiating additional cases in unexpected sites such as the prostate, the lung, and the gastrointestinal tract. X-rays are helpful in the diagnosis. Calcification and even ossification are demonstrated in several cases.

6.3.2.1 Histopathology. In its spindle cell composition, synovial sarcoma shows similar features to other mesenchymal neoplasms, hence the indication to confirm the diagnosis, even if classical patterns are obvious, by adding cytogenetics and molecular studies as indicated. It responds to similar cytological/histological criteria of the spindle cell sarcomas, which will not be repeated. However, several particular histologic findings are helpful for the precision of the diagnosis. If one excepts the typical cases of biphasic type and the rare monophasic epithelial variant, then the basic morphology of monophasic fibrous synovial sarcoma consists of a component of spindle-shaped cells grouped in compact sheets (Fig 6.93) totally indistinguishable from fibrosarcoma save for the absence of the herringbone pattern (Fig 6.94). Generally, the mitotic index is low and rarely outnumbered 10/50 HPF, with the exception of the poorly differentiated forms. The cellular portion alternates with stromal changes such as myxoid,

hyalinizationm, and calcification (Fig 6.95). About 20% of synovial sarcoma harbor calcification and foci of ossification ranging from inconspicuous to extensive masking of a large proportion of the tumor. Another peculiar feature

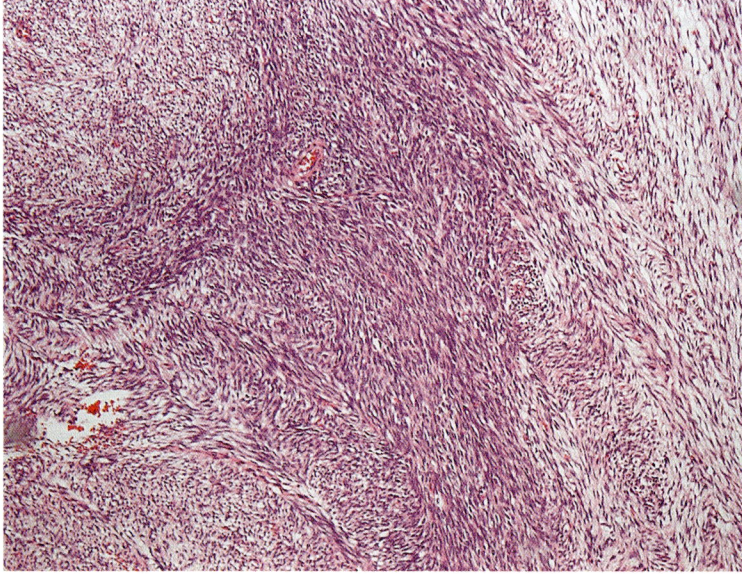

FIG 6.93 Synovial sarcoma, solid sheets of spindle cells indistinguishable from fibrosarcoma.

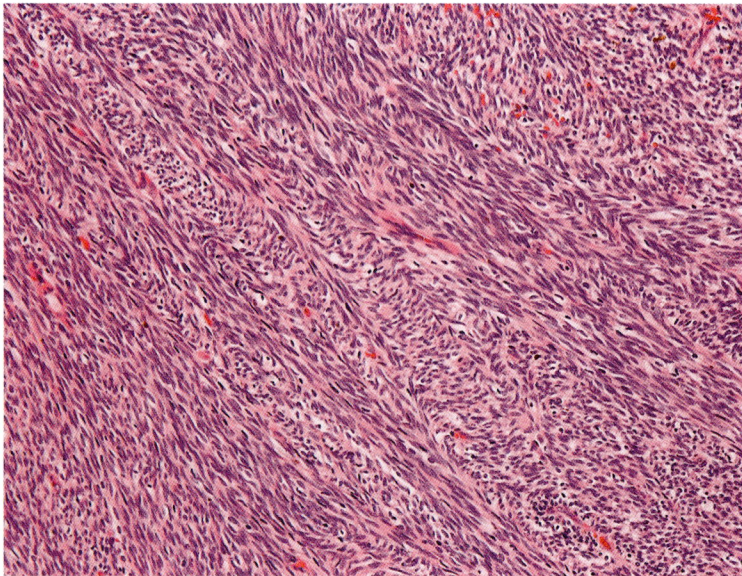

FIG 6.94 Herringbone pattern in fibrosarcoma.

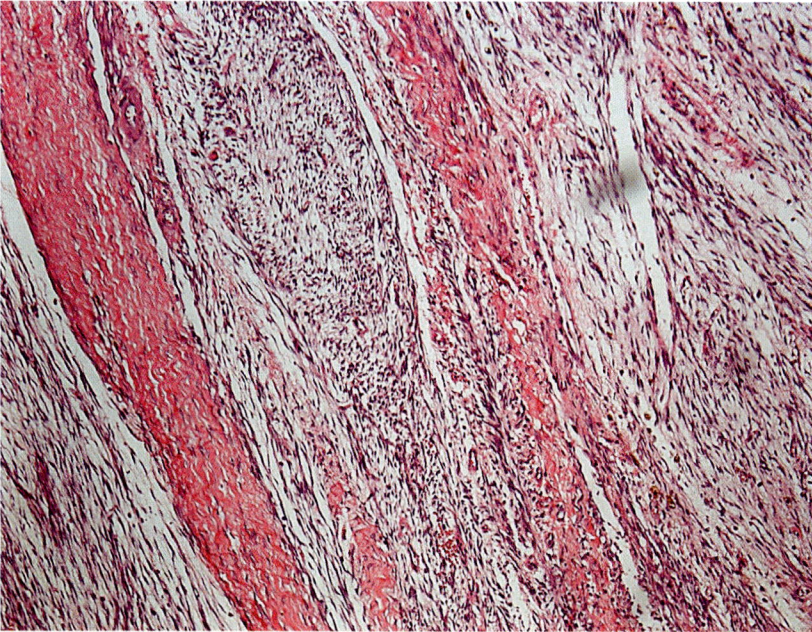

FIG 6.95 Synovial sarcoma, thick collagen bands with stromal hyalinization often present in monophasic subtype.

is the presence of well-developed vascular spaces resembling hemangiopericytoma, which is highly suggestive although not specific of the entity (Fig 6.96).

The immunohistochemical profile of synovial sarcoma, although not specific, is highly suggestive. Approximately 90% of synovial sarcomas are cytokeratin positive [112]. Only a few tumor cells express either cytokeratin or EMA in some cases hence the necessity to stain and examine sections from different portions of the tumors. Other antibodies of the selected panel for synovial sarcoma include protein S-100 (positive in 30%), CD99 (the product of the MIC2 gene showing cytoplasmic and membrane positivity), and bcl2 protein (positive in 75% of cases) that is strong and diffuse. CD34 is virtually always negative [113].

Cytogenetic and molecular genetics findings already have been emphasized. It is particularly useful for monophasic fibrous and poorly differentiated synovial sarcoma. Some disagreement has occurred in terms of correlation between histologic subtype and the gene breakpoint. Fusion transcript SSX-2 has been associated with monophasic fibrous synovial sarcoma and SSX-1 has been associated with the biphasic variety, criteria of importance to distinguish from solitary fibrous tumor. TLE1 is a nuclear protein that functions as a transcription repressor of Wnt/Beta catenin signaling. It is a potentially useful marker of synovial sarcoma as demonstrated by a multiple expression microarray study. It has been constantly identified as an excellent discriminator of synovial sarcoma [114].

6.3.2.2 Cytopathology. Synovial sarcoma usually displays highly cellular smears (Fig 6.97). Smears are characteristic and consistently consist of (classical pattern) a

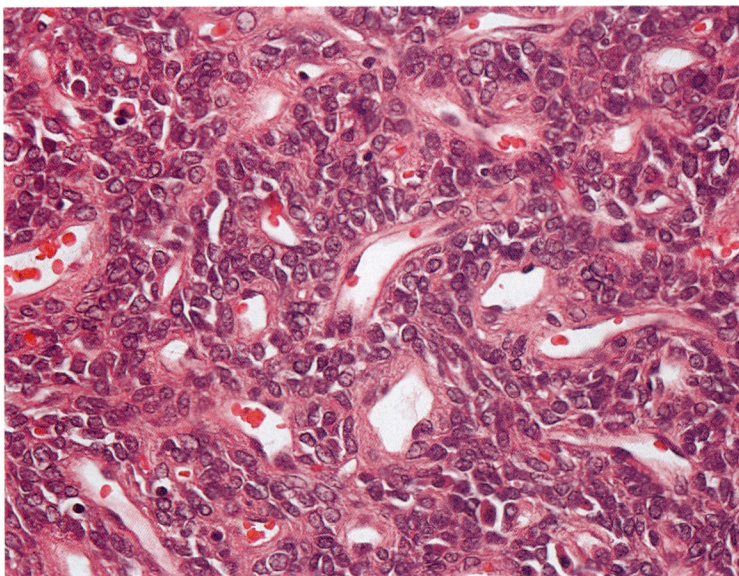

FIG 6.96   Synovial sarcoma, hemangiopericytoma-like vasculature frequently observed in monophasic subtype.

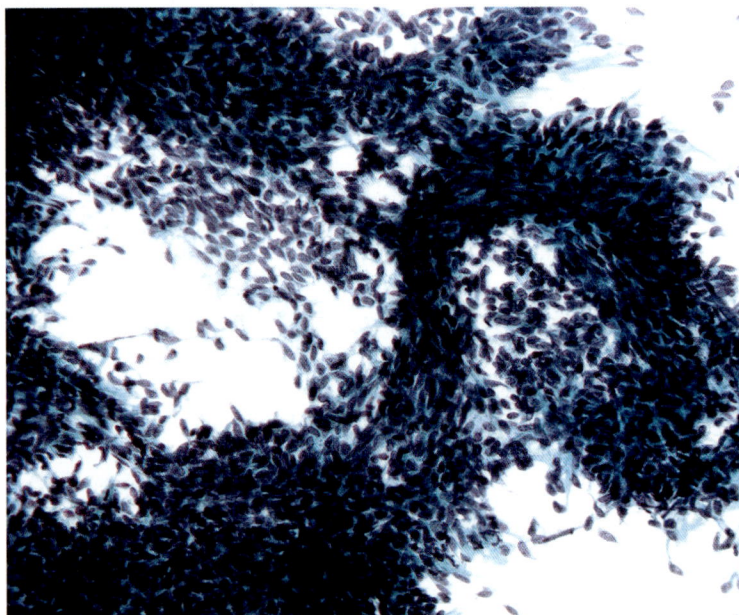

FIG 6.97   Synovial sarcoma, highly cellular smears.

mixture of dispersed or clusters of monomorphous cells (Figs 6.98 and 6.99) with bland chromatin, inconspicious nucleoli, oval-to-spindle-shaped cytoplasm, branching tumor tissue fragments (Figs 6.100 and 6.101), and vessel stalks. Cohesive

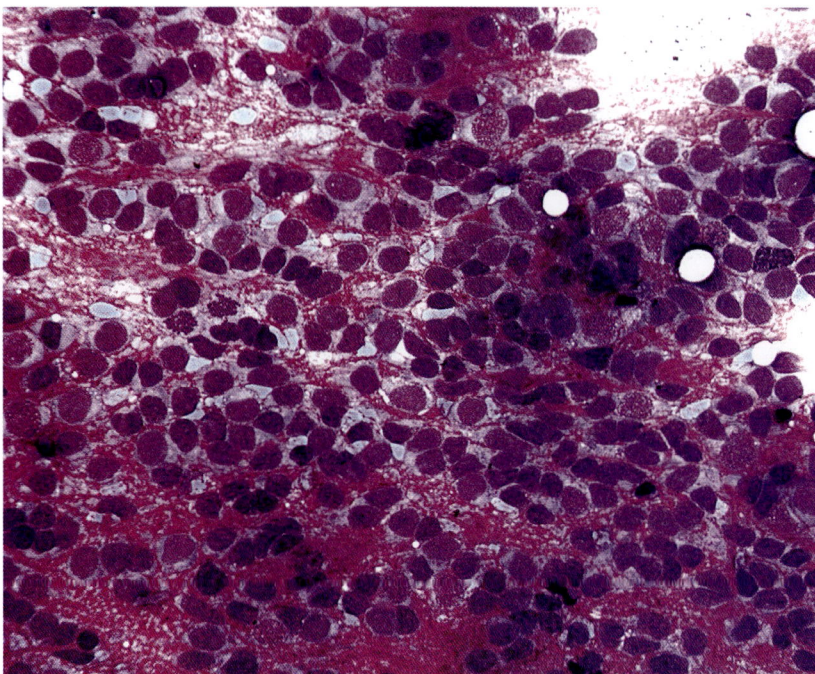

FIG 6.98 Synovial sarcoma, mixture of dispersed or clusters of monomorphous cells.

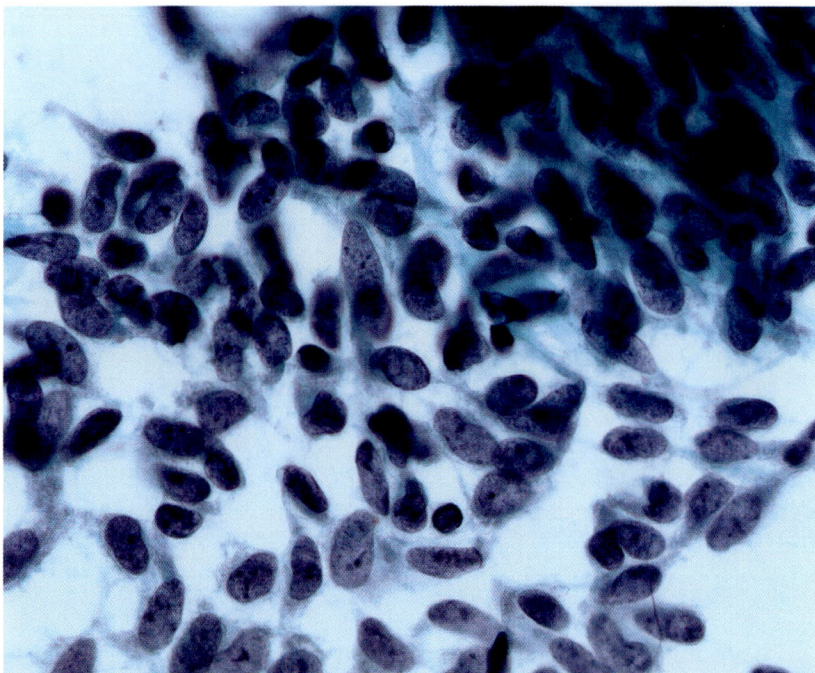

FIG 6.99 Synovial sarcoma, mixture of spindle cells, Papanicolaou stain.

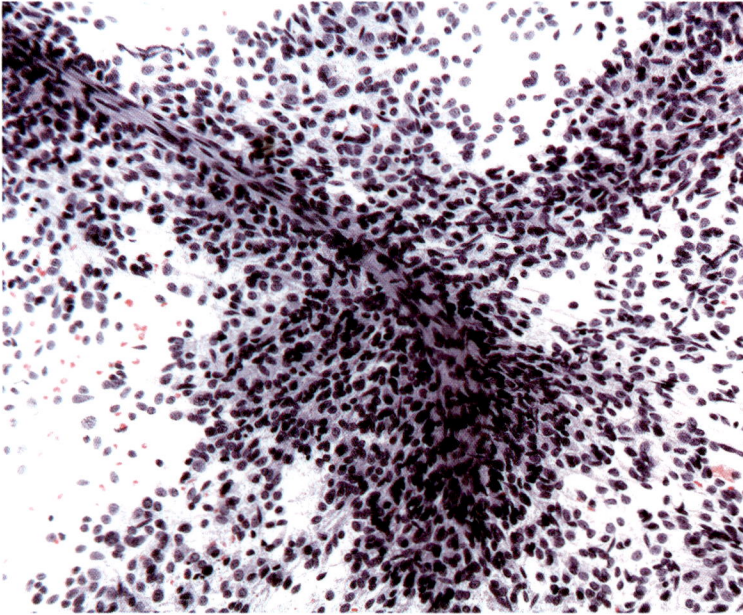

FIG 6.100   Synovial sarcoma, branching tumor tissue fragments. Connective, vascular cores are well evidenced using the Papanicolaou stain. This pattern is characteristic.

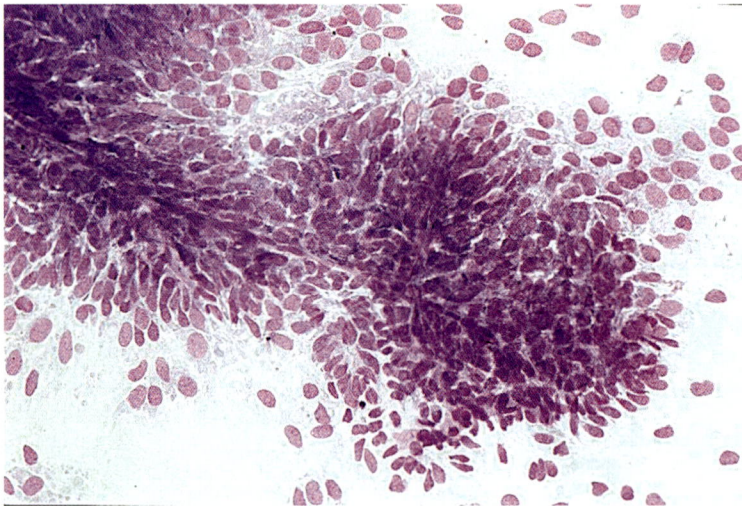

FIG 6.101   Synovial sarcoma, branching tumor tissue fragments. Same case as Fig 6.100. Higher magnification.

epithelial cells are observed in biphasic sybtypes (Figs 6.102 and 6.103). Mast cells, necrosis, comma-like nuclei, marked nuclear atypia, secretory mucin (Fig 6.104), rosette-like structures, mitotic figures, and connective stromal components are usually scarce.

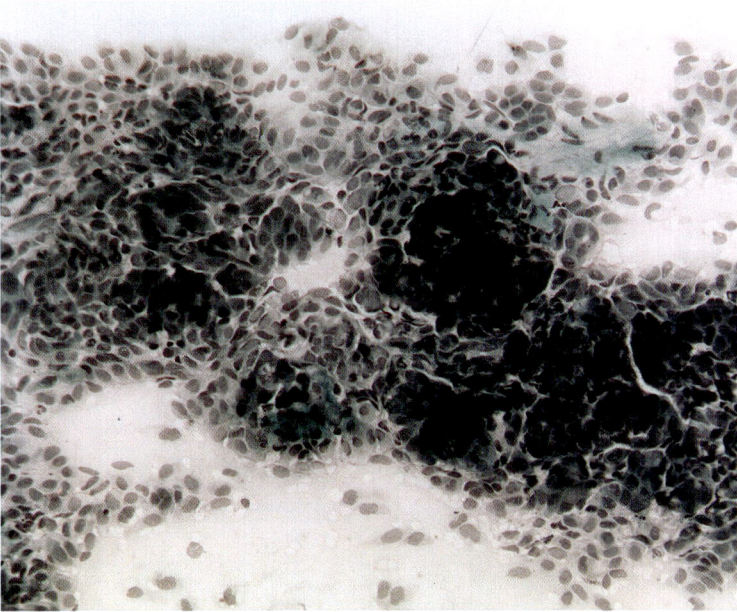

FIG 6.102 Synovial sarcoma, cohesive epithelial cells are well evidenced using the Papanicolaou stain.

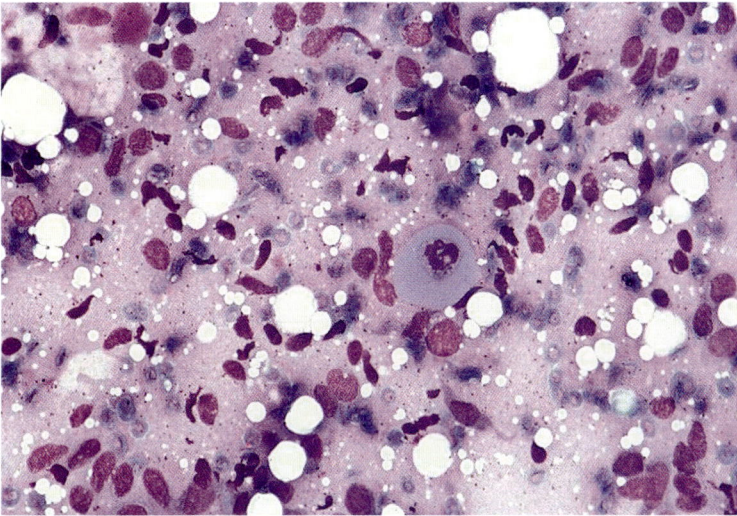

FIG 6.103 Synovial sarcoma, squamous cell suggesting a biphasic subtype.

6.3.2.3 Differential Diagnosis. The following entities should be differentiated from synovial sarcoma:

- Malignant peripheral nerve sheath tumor
- Leiomyosarcoma
- Solitary fibrous tumor
- Hemangiopericytoma

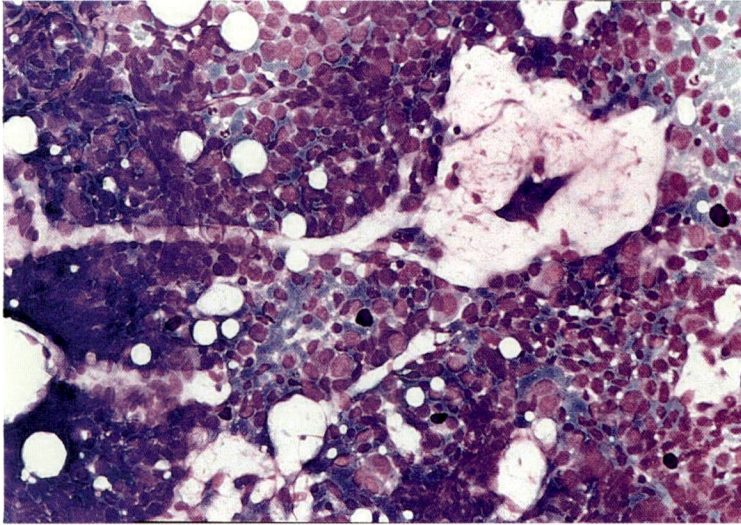

FIG 6.104 Synovial sarcoma, background of mucin in biphasic subtype.

TABLE 6.7 Cytological differential diagnosis in synovial sarcoma

	Synovial sarcoma	Hemangiopericytoma	Malignant peripheral nerve sheath tumor	Ewing sarcoma/ peripheral neuroectodermal tumor
Spindle cells	++	++	++	+/−
Round cells	+	+	−	++
Giant cells	+/−	−	+	−
Blunt-ends	−	−	−	−
Binucleated	−	−	+/−	−
Mitotic figures	+	−	+	++
Fibrous stroma	+/−	+	−	+/−
Myxoid stroma	+/−	+/−	+	−
Inflammation	+/−	−	−	++
Necrosis	+/−	−	+	++

++; Frequent, +; rare, +/− occasionally seen, −; absent.

Main entities to include in the differential diagnosis of synovial sarcoma are hemangiopericytoma, malignant peripheral nerve sheath tumor, and solitary fibrous tumor. Ewing sarcoma/peripheral neuroectodermal tumor and malignant melanoma also should be differentiated from poorly differentiated synovial sarcoma (Table 6.7).

Hemangiopericytoma and malignant peripheral nerve sheath tumor may have a similar morphology as synovial sarcoma [115]. In the absence of the classical pattern, or epithelial cells, the diagnosis of synovial sarcoma may be difficult and may require ancillary techniques such as immunocytochemistry, cell blocks, genetic studies, or electron microscopy. In the absence of a precise diagnosis, surgical biopsy is indicated. Differential diagnostic parameters like a vascular pattern in hemangiopericytoma, nuclear palisading in malignant peripheral nerve sheath tumor, and collagenosis or intersecting fascicles in fibrosarcoma may be present in synovial sarcoma but are more in the domain of histopathology than in cytopathology. Hemangiopericytoma remains a diagnosis of exclusion. There are tumors that show an overlapping morphology with synovial sarcoma, because of numerous spindle-shaped cells without nuclear pleomorphism [114]. In malignant peripheral nerve sheath tumor, a "wavy appearance," elongated and slender nuclei, focal prononced nuclear atypia, and fibrillary metachromic stroma are indicative of the diagnosis [116]. However, other features such as the location in the vicinity of a nerve, a history of neuroma or von Recklinghausen disease may help in the differential diagnosis.

Distinctive immunocytochemical analysis may be inconclusive because 30% of synovial sarcomas may show an unexpected S-100 protein positivity and only 50% of malignant peripheral nerve sheath tumor express S-100 protein [117]. Moreover, poorly differentiated synovial sarcoma may be keratin or epithelial membrane antigen negative, whereas several malignant peripheral nerve sheath tumors exhibit keratin positivity [118].

Solitary fibrous tumor, originally described as a pleural-based entity, has been well documented in numerous extrapleural sites including soft tissue. An architectural vascular pattern similar to hemangiopericytoma is often present, hence the necessity to distinguish from true hemangiopericytoma and synovial sarcoma with hemangiopericytoma-like features. The hemangiopericytoma-like vasculature of solitary fibrous tumor, however, is focal. Histologically malignant cases are very rare, and the spindle cell component express CD34, whereas synovial sarcoma never do.

Tumors in the spectrum Ewing sarcoma/peripheral neuroectodermal tumor are to be differentiated from poorly differentiated synovial sarcoma [105,119–122]. Ewing sarcoma/peripheral neuroectodermal tumor-like features are well known in synovial sarcoma [119–121]. Ewing sarcoma/peripheral neuroectodermal tumors usually consist of isolated or sparsely clustered round-to-oval cells with central nuclei. Pseudopapillary structures, usually observed in synovial sarcoma, are rare in Ewing sarcoma/peripheral neuroectodermal tumor. Periodic-acid-Schiff stain is strongly positive, and specific cytogenetic aberrations t(11;22) are common findings in these tumors. Achromic malignant melanoma may disclose cytologic findings similar to synovial sarcoma. The presence of epithelioid cells, spindle-shaped cells, macrophages with "dirty" cytoplasm, intranuclear inclusions, and binucleated cells are in favor of malignant melanoma.

6.3.2.4 Comments. Whatever monophasic, biphasic, or poorly-differentiated synovial sarcoma, cytologically a mixture of dispersed or clusters of monomorphous cells (classical pattern) is observed. Additionally, epithelial cells and/or secretory mucin are observed only in biphasic synovial sarcomas, whereas poorly differentiated round cells (Ewing sarcoma/peripheral neuroectodermal tumor-like pattern) are restricted to poorly differentiated synovial sarcomas. Comma-like nuclei are common and exclusive to monophasic fibrous variants. Highly versus poorly cellular smears do not differ significantly between morphological subtypes. Nuclear atypia, necrosis, and the presence of mast cells is not correlated with histological subtype. Finally, necrosis and mitotic figures are present more likely in grade II and grade III tumors. Secretory mucin is more likely observed in grade I tumors than in grades II and III tumors [105].

To improve the diagnostic criteria, ancillary studies of aspirated tumor cells are helpful [105, 122, 125]. It is now well established that cytogenetic analysis is a novel and objective tool for the diagnosis of soft tissue tumors and is more sensitive than conventional histologic and/or cytologic morphology, immunohistochemistry, or electron microscopic analysis. It has been demonstrated [124] that the analysis of karyotypes from cytology material in sarcomas is an accurate method of diagnosis. Cytogenetic studies also have revealed a specific chrosomal translocation t(X;18)(p11.2;q11.2), with a prevalence of 85% in synovial sarcoma [125]. In this context, it has been proposed that cytologic smears exhibiting a morphology suggestive of synovial sarcoma combined with a cytology-based cytogenetic analysis are sufficient for a definitive diagnosis of synovial sarcoma, rendering surgical biopsy unnecessary [126]. Similarly, cytology material also can be used for analysis of a specific translocation using the RT-PCR technique [127] or the SYT-SSX gene transcript [111].

The cytomorphology of 164 cases of synovial sarcoma were reported [105,115,122,126,128−134]. This entity is characterized by an important percentage of accurate/malignant rate. The false negative is negligible (0.2%).

6.3.2.5   *FNA Key Features.*   The following are in favor of the diagnosis:

- Highly cellular smears
- Dispersed or clusters of monomorphous cells
- Oval-to-spindle-shaped cytoplasm
- Branching tumor tissue fragments and vessel stalks
- Cohesive epithelial cells in biphasic subtype

The following are difficulties in the diagnosis:

- Mast cells
- Necrosis
- Comma-like nuclei
- Marked nuclear atypia
- Secretory mucin
- Rosette-like structures
- Mitotic figures and connective stromal components are usually scarce

The following are evidence against diagnosis:

- True rosettes
- Double population of roundish cells

6.3.3 Fibrosarcoma

Classical adult fibrosarcoma is now a rare tumor and, as already mentioned in this review, has become a diagnosis of exclusion. Despite a cellular component of compact sheets of spindle cells similar to other spindle cell sarcomas, it is defined by negative findings: the absence of a representative immunohistochemical profile (vimentin positive, occasional focal positivity for CD34) and, so far, neither recognizable cytogenetic nor molecular characterization. Most past adult fibrosarcomas fall into the group of monophasic synovial sarcomas, some others fall into solitary fibrous tumors of which they can closely resemble as well as low-grade malignant peripheral nerve sheath tumor and dermatofibrosarcoma protuberans.

Two recognized variants of adult fibrosarcoma deserve comments at this step of our review, (myxofibrosarcoma will be discussed later). Low-grade fibromyxoid sarcoma is now a well recognized nosologic entity [135] by virtue of its unique genetic and molecular characterization with the demonstration of the chimeric fusion transcript FUS/CREB3L2 resulting from the specific translocation t(7;16)(q33;p11) [136,137]. Identical molecular findings are found in hyalinizing spindle cell tumor with giant rosettes, which is now considered a variant of low-grade fibromyxoid sarcoma. The latter is a more cellular than myxoid tumor, hence, on cytohistological grounds it is to be included in the pattern of low-grade spindle cell lesions. These tumors also depict a network of curvilinear vessels also observed in other sarcomas such as myxofibrosarcoma.

So-called sclerosing epithelioid fibrosarcoma is an unusual variant of fibrosarcoma of which few cases were retrieved from our own material. Interestingly, one of us recently reported a small series of low-grade fibromyxoid sarcoma, and emphasis was focused on one recurrent case whose histology was characterized by a component of typical sclerosing fibrosarcoma admixed with pleomorphic areas indistinguishable from malignant fibrous histiocytoma [138]. Furthermore, immunohistochemical and molecular biology investigations tend to suggest that sclerosing epitheliod fibrosarcoma and low-grade fibromyxoid sarcoma are closely related entities sharing some morphological characteristics and depicting the same translocation [139].

6.3.3.1 *Histopathology.* Low-grade fibromyxoid sarcoma consists of an admixture of solid areas comprising of bland spindle cells lying in a collagenous stroma (Figs 6.105 and 6.106) and myxoid nodules containing spindle cells (Figs 6.107 and 6.108). The arrangement of spindle cells is characterized by a whorling growth pattern, better demonstrated at the interface between collagenous and myxoid areas. Arcades of small vessels and arterioles of medium size surrounded by sclerosis are focally present (Figs 6.109 and 6.110). Rare zones of increased cellularity and atypia can be observed.

Two morphological variants of low-grade fibromyxoid sarcoma have been identified: one is characterized by the presence of nodules whose central core consists of hyalinized collagen surrounded by epithelioid fibroblasts, hence the former appellation of "hyalinizing spindle cell tumor with giant rosettes" (Figs 6.111 and 6.112). Sclerosing epithelioid fibrosarcoma, a recently described variant of fibrosarcoma [140], is a deep-seated tumor usually well circumscribed, lobulated, or multinodular (Fig 6.113). At low magnification, the tumor is hypocellular with large

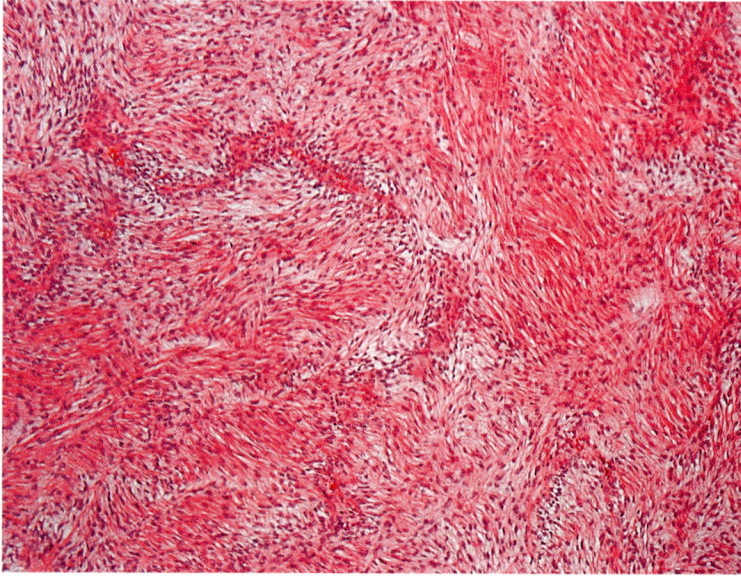

FIG 6.105 Low-grade fibromyxoid sarcoma, solid areas of bland spindle cells in a collagenous stroma.

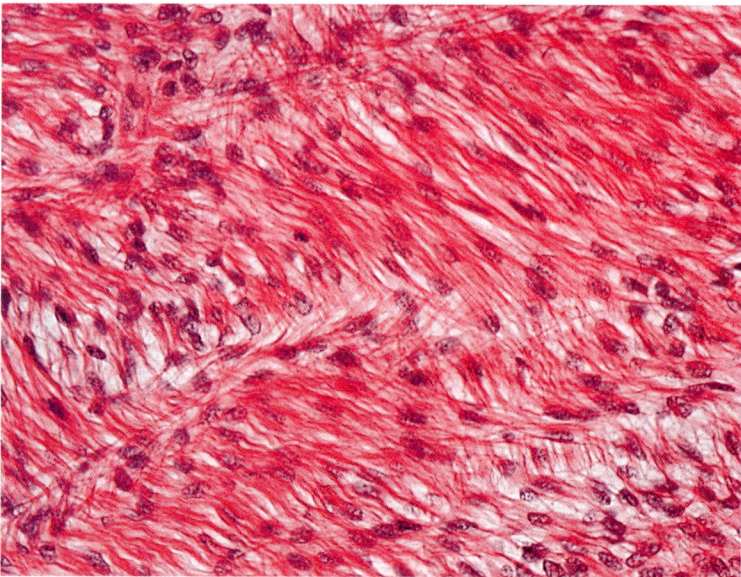

FIG 6.106 Low-grade fibromyxoid sarcoma, higher magnification.

areas of densely hyalinized stroma (Figs 6.114 and 6.115). Tumor cells are epithelioid and arranged in a variety of patterns, nests (Fig 6.116), cords (Fig 6.117), strands, and sometimes, alveolar and acinar. They are small-to-medium size with small basophilic nuclei, scant cytoplasm, and generally poor in mitosis, although some tumors depict a high mitotic rate. In contrast to typical fibrosarcoma, tumor cells express

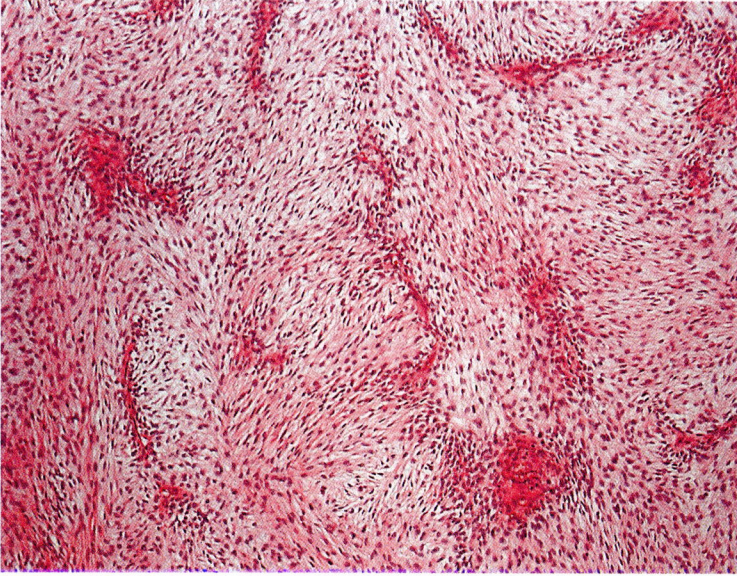

FIG 6.107   Low-grade fibromyxoid sarcoma, myxoid nodule with curvilinear blood vessels.

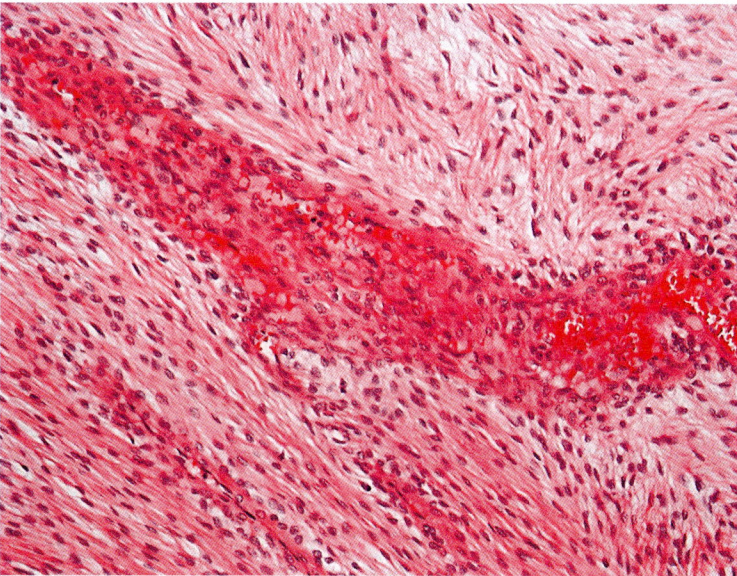

FIG 6.108   Low-grade fibromyxoid sarcoma, higher magnification.

a wide variety of antigens, vimentin, EMA (which could be confusing with malignant epithelial tumors, synovial sarcoma and epithelioid sarcoma), and neuron specific enolase (NSE, which can simulate a low-grade malignant peripheral sheath tumor.) Given the limited number of studies dealing with sclerosing epithelioid fibrosarcoma, their clinical behavior is difficult to precise. Recurrence

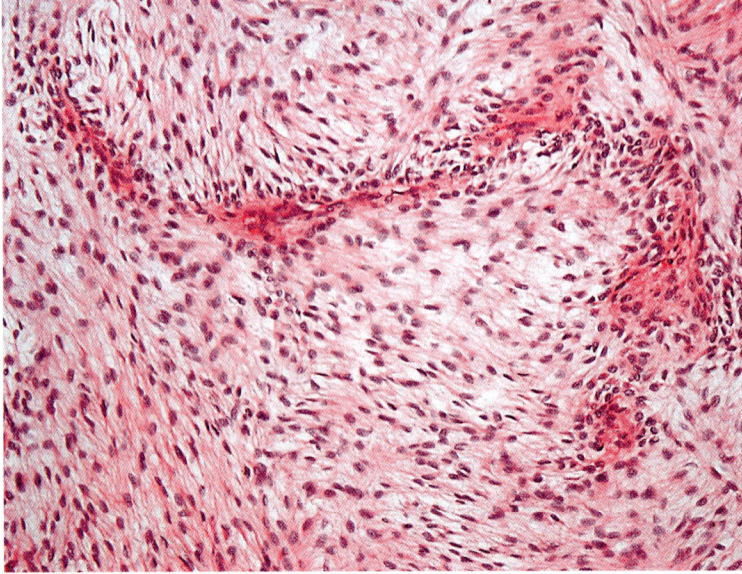

FIG 6.109   Low-grade fibromyxoid sarcoma, arcades of small vessels surrounded by sclerosis.

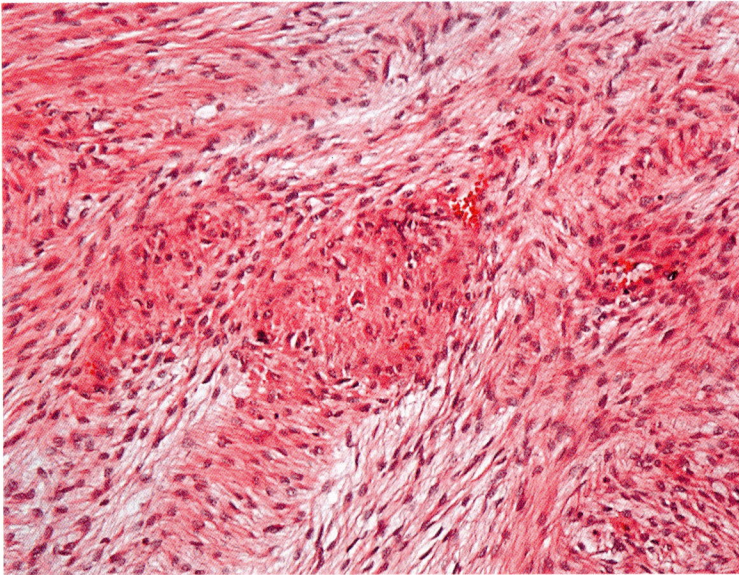

FIG 6.110   Low-grade fibromyxoid sarcoma, thick-walled vessels surrounded by epithelioid fibroblasts.

may be developed 4.8 years after the initial diagnosis and metastases developed in 43% of the patients [140].

6.3.3.2   *Cytopathology.* Smears in fibrosarcoma not otherwise specified (NOS) consist of isolated spindle-shaped cells showing moderate cytonuclear atypia. Occasionally, moderate cellular pleomorphism is observed. Cells may be in densely

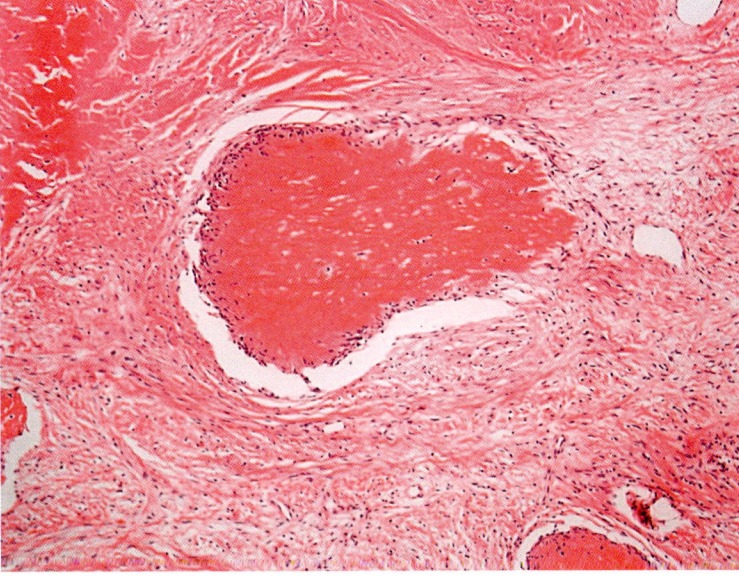

FIG 6.111 Low-grade fibromyxoid sarcoma, "giant hyalinized rosette" in a hyalinizing spindle cell tumor (courtesy of Dr. Gilles Théoret, Montréal, Canada.)

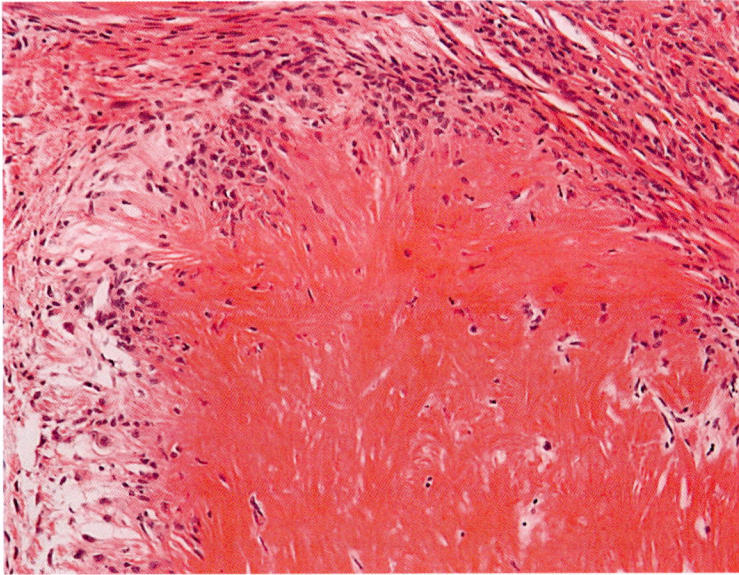

FIG 6.112 Low-grade fibromyxoid sarcoma. Higher magnification from Fig 6.111.

packed clusters in connective fragments. A storiform pattern and giant cells are not detected on cytology smears (Figs 6.118 and 6.119).

Cytologically low-grade fibromyxoid sarcomas are low-grade spindle cell malignancies with a scant and delicate myxoid component. The cellular component consists

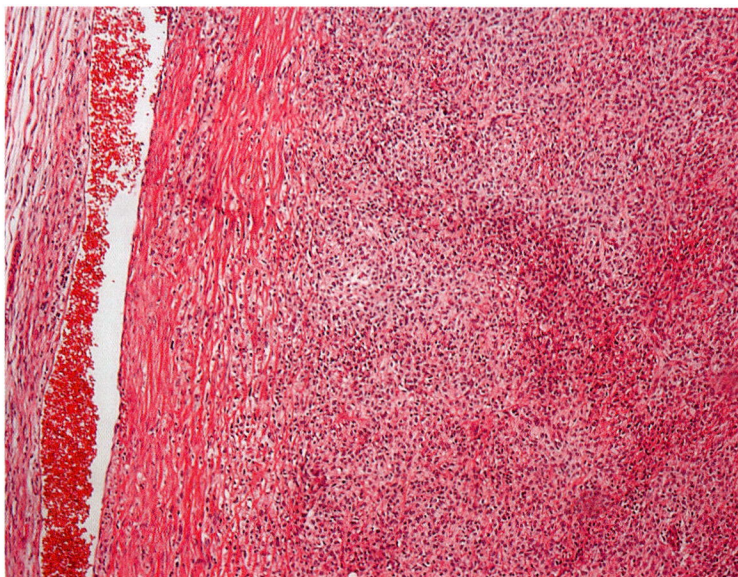

FIG 6.113 Epithelioid sclerosing fibrosarcoma, well-circumscribed tumor.

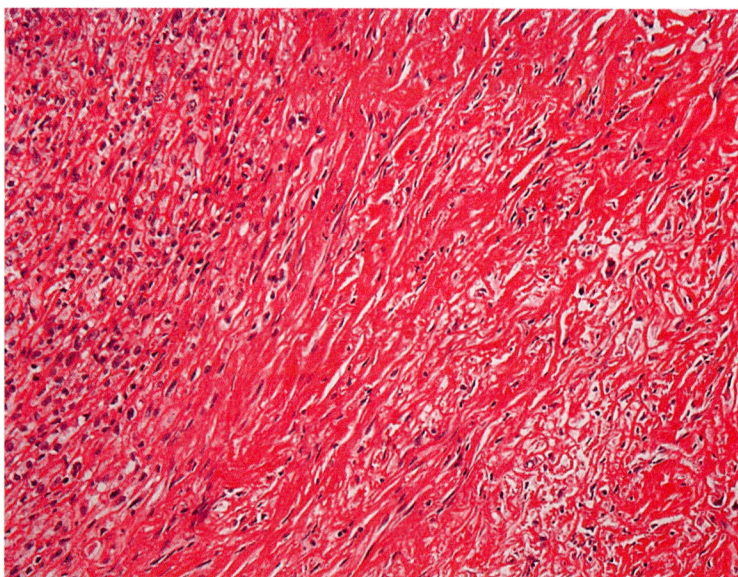

FIG 6.114 Epithelioid sclerosing fibrosarcoma, densely hyalinized area close to a more cellular one.

of uniform spindle and rounded cells embedded in a myxoid matrix (Fig 6.120). Cells may be in wavy fascicles or in three-dimensional clusters embedded in collagen. Cell borders are poorly defined. Nuclei are bare and occasionally slightly irregular. Some of them are spindle shaped. Nuclear grooves and pseudoinclusions may be observed. There is no mitotic activity. The matrix is scant and consists of myxoid and collagen

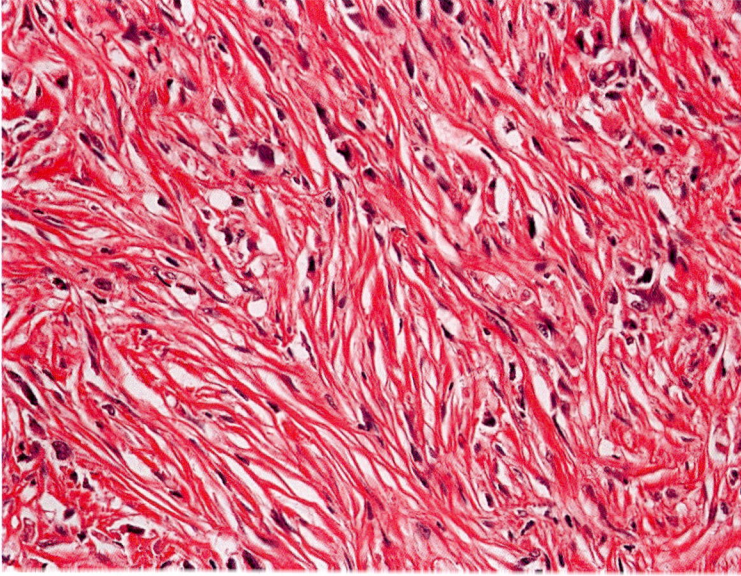

FIG 6.115   Epithelioid sclerosing fibrosarcoma, storiform pattern in a dense collagenous stroma.

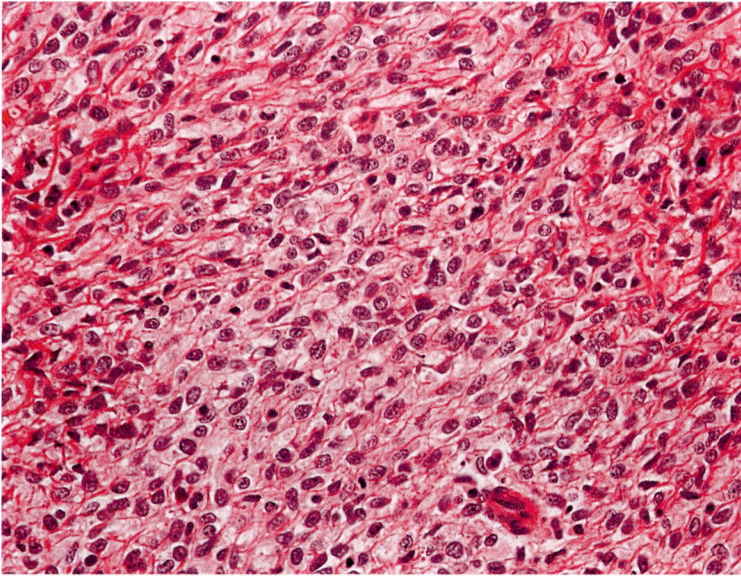

FIG 6.116   Epithelioid sclerosing fibrosarcoma, thightly packed epithelioid cells with minimal atypias.

fibers with rare vascular structures. Heterologous elements like striated muscle fragments and fat tissue also are found. In our material, tumors show scant myxoid background harboring dispersed oval and slightly irregular cells suggesting malignancy.

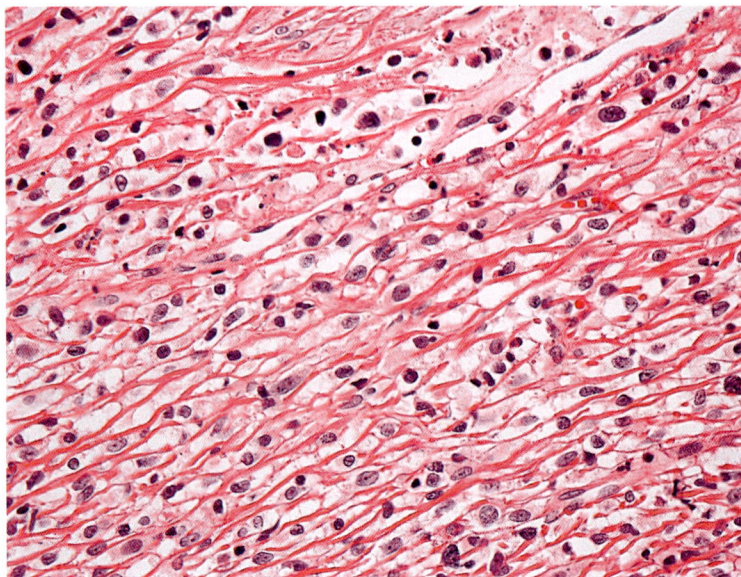

FIG 6.117 Epithelioid sclerosing fibrosarcoma, higher magnification with strands of epithelioid cells embedded in a "collagenous" network.

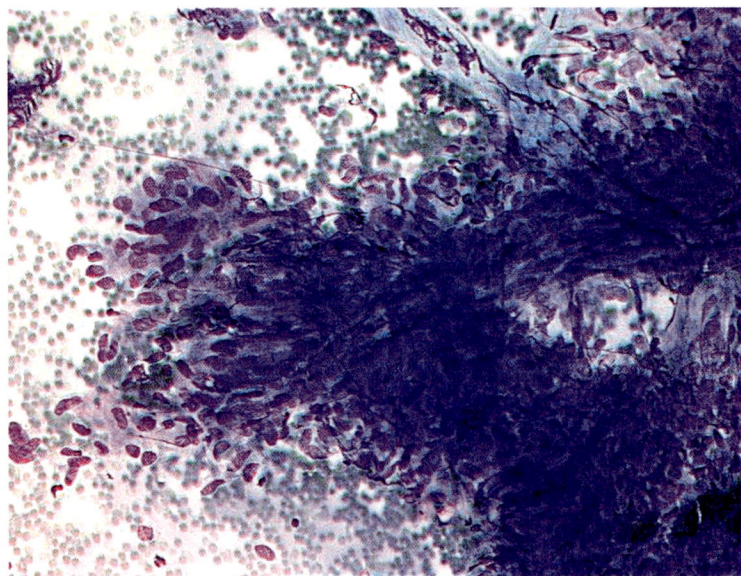

FIG 6.118 Fibrosarcoma, nonspecific and malignant spindle cells.

Primary sclerosing epithelioid fibrosarcoma has never been reported in cytology literature. Recently Tsuchido et al. [141] have described one case of metastatic sclerosing epithelioid fibrosarcoma in pleural effusion. It consisted of medium-sized clusters of epithelioid cells with dark-staining cytoplasm around the nuclei. Nuclei

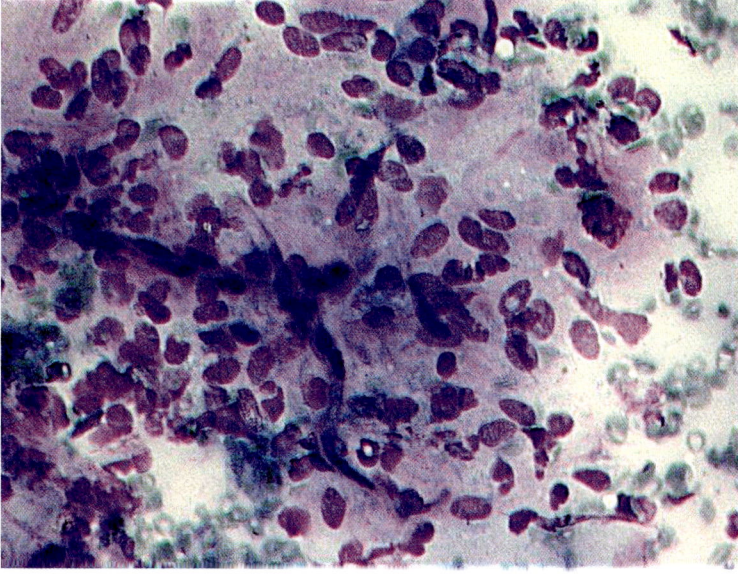

FIG 6.119 Fibrosarcoma, polymorphous cells within connective and collagen tissue.

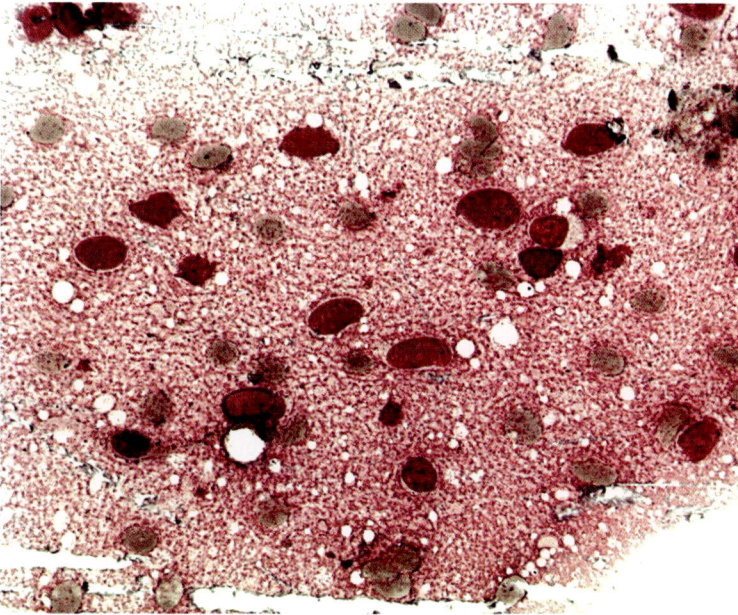

FIG 6.120 Low-grade fibromyxoid sarcoma. Isolated and regular spindle cells in delicate, scant myxoid matrix.

exhibited moderate pleomorphism and were oval, spindle, or cleaved with occasional multinucleation. In addition, some intranuclear inclusions were observed. We have observed three examples of sclerosing epithelioid fibrosarcoma, which consisted of two populations: small and regular spindle cells and roundish epithelioid cells. Nuclei

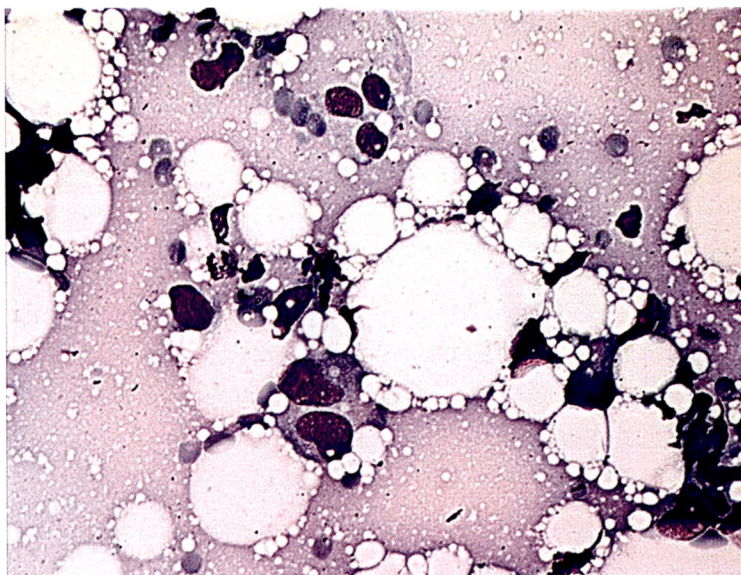

FIG 6.121 Sclerosing epithelioid fibrosarcoma, roundish malignant cells. Note the low cellularity of this smear.

exhibited slight pleomorphism and minute nucleoli. Cytoplasms were scant, spindle-shaped, homogenous, and densified around the nuclei (Fig 6.121).

6.3.3.3 Comments. Limited series of fibrosarcoma NOS have been published [142,143]. The diagnosis of malignancy was reached in all cases. Tumors consisted of spindle and roundish cells within collagen matrix. Only ten cases of low-grade fibromyxoid sarcoma were described cytologically [144–146]. Domanski et al. [146] have described eight tumors and compared their data with previously published cases. In their series, tumors consisted of spindled and polygonal cells in fascicles or isolated. A myxoid background was detected. We have observed 39 cases of fibrosarcoma NOS, 1 case of low-grade fibromyxoid sarcoma, and 3 cases of sclerosing epithelioid fibrosarcoma. All cases were diagnosed as malignant. In this group of malignancies, the cytologic features were not specific for an accurate diagnosis, but correlating the cytologic and clinical findings can narrow the range of diagnosis.

6.3.3.4 Differential Diagnosis. The following entities should be differentiated from fibrosarcoma:

- Dermatofibrosarcoma protuberans
- Myxofibrosarcoma
- Cellular myxoma

Fibrosarcoma, being a diagnosis of exclusion, should be differentiated from other low-grade spindle-shaped malignancies, especially from dermatofibrosarcoma protuberans and low-grade malignant peripheral nerve sheath tumor. Cytologically, low-grade fibromyxoid sarcoma should be differentiated from some other benign spindle-shaped cells tumors and from other myxoid low-grade tumors. High-grade malignant sarcomas may easily be excluded. Inversely, low-grade fibromyxoid sarcoma may be difficult to differentiate from myxofibrosarcoma, myxoid dermato-fibrosarcoma protuberans, and cellular myxoma. Myxofibrosarcoma shows an abundant myxoid matrix and spindle-shaped cells without cytonuclear atypia. It also shows the presence of arcade-type curvilinear vessels. However, clinical data are important: myxofibrosarcoma usually originates in the subcutaneous tissue of the extremities in elderly patients, whereas low-grade fibromyxoid sarcoma most often is observed as a deep soft tissue mass in young adults.

6.3.3.5 FNA Key Features of Fibrosarcoma. The following are in favor of the diagnosis:

— Spindle and polymorphous cells
— Aggregates of connective tissue
— Wavy fascicles
— No mitotic activity
— Deep soft tissue mass
— Exclusion of other spindle-shaped malignancy.

The following are difficulties in the diagnosis:

— Some smears may be paucicellular
— Roundish/epithelioid cells

The following are evidence against diagnosis:

— Giant cells
— Fibrillary stroma
— Epithelial cells
— High cellularity
— Lipoblast
— Mitotic figures

6.3.4 Malignant Fibrous Histiocytoma – Storiform Pattern

Does malignant fibrous histiocytoma exist? Numerous studies in the past 10–15 years have attempted to answer the question. Once considered as the most frequent sarcoma of adult life, its fate is similar to that of fibrosarcoma. It rather designates a spectrum of tumors, which share morphologic features that allow their inclusion in a distinct clinicopathologic setting, although they are not uniform in their histogenesis and pathogenesis. Over the recent years, better defined histologic criteria and comparative genomic analysis have resulted in the dismemberment of malignant fibrous histiocytoma, which is supported by findings showing, for example, similar genomic profiles such as, to name only a few, leiomyosarcoma and malignant fibrous histiocytoma [147, 148], liposarcoma, and malignant fibrous histiocytoma [149—151].

A previous study has attempted to define the cytological criteria in variants of malignant fibrous histiocytoma by comparing cytologic and histologic materials [152]. Indeed, because it was a retrospective study, some morphological criteria were identified that could fit in either variant of malignant fibrous histiocytoma or that correlate with cytological and histological findings. Retrospectively, and in overall agreement [153], the diagnosis of malignant fibrous histiocytoma should be avoided in fine needle aspiration material. Clinical and morphologic heterogeneity, even among the five different subtypes, account for the lack of representative accurate diagnostic criteria of tumoral phenotypes. The so-called storiform-pleomorphic variant could be included within the spindle cell pattern of soft tissue tumors by fine needle aspiration, although a pure form of spindle cell malignant fibrous histiocytoma is not frequent and probably corresponds to sarcomas of different phenotypes.

At the present time, the five variants of malignant fibrous histiocytoma have been reclassified based on morphological changes and molecular genetic profile. Storiform-pleomorphic malignant fibrous histiocytomas (Figs 6.122 and 6.123) usually are dedifferentiated liposarcomas or leimyosarcomas as well as inflammatory variant (Figs 6.124 and 6.125). Giant cell variant (Figs 6.126 and 6.127) belongs to the recently reclassified soft tissue malignant giant cell tumor. Myxoid (Figs 6.128 and 6.129) and angiomatous variants need to be revisited before they could move to another precise tumor phenotype. Cytomorphology corresponds to histological sybtype. Usually, tumors consist of spindle cells showing nuclear plomorphism (Figs 6.130—6.133). Some cases may show atypical, multinucleated cells (Fig 6.134), or roundish cells (Fig 6.135).

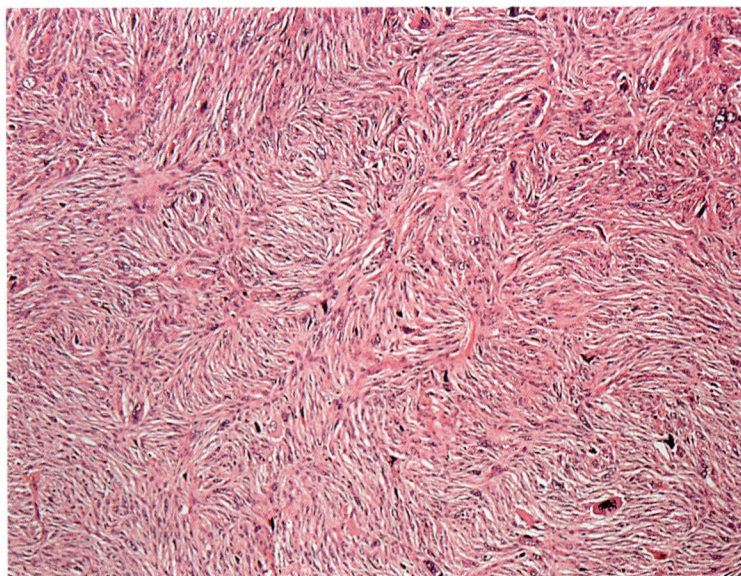

FIG 6.122 Malignant fibrous histiocytoma, storiform-pleomorphic variant.

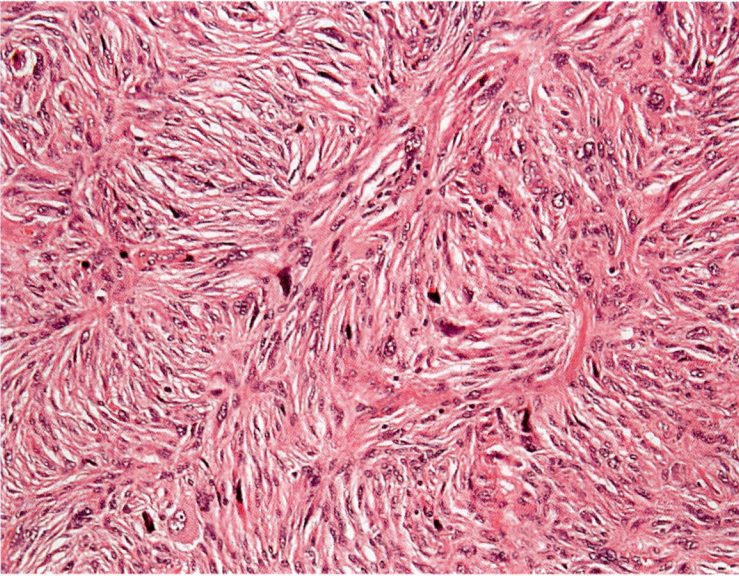

FIG 6.123   Malignant fibrous histiocytoma. Higher magnification from Fig 6.122.

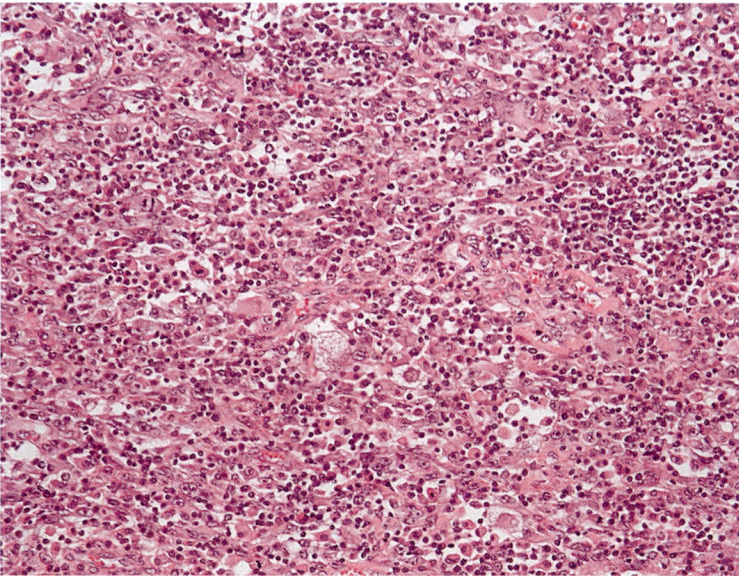

FIG 6.124   Malignant fibrous histiocytoma, inflammatory variant.

The angiomatoid malignant fibrous histiocytoma has been reclassified and renamed angiomatous fibrous histiocytoma. It is recognized as a well-defined nosologic entity by virtue of its morphologic, clinical, and molecular characteristics. This slow-growing neoplasm affects primarily children and young adults. It occurs in the extremities and rarely metastasises. Morphologically, it is characterized by an

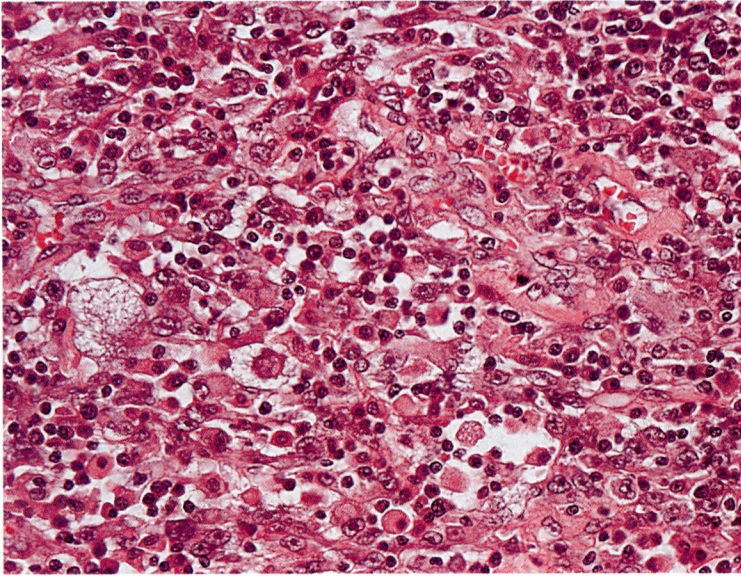

FIG 6.125 Malignant fibrous histiocytoma, inflammatory variant.

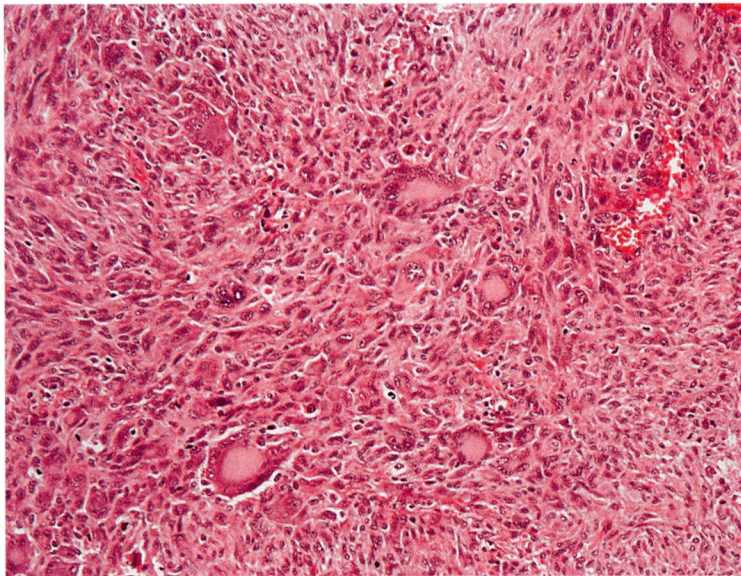

FIG 6.126 Malignant fibrous histiocytoma, giant cell variant.

irregular solid mass of histiocyte-like cells that are desmin positive (50% of cases) and by cystic areas of hemorrage and chronic inflammation. Molecular biology studies have shown that angiomatoid fibrous histiocytoma possesses a fusion gene that incorporates either EWRS1 or FUS gene and ATF1 [154]. Recently, another

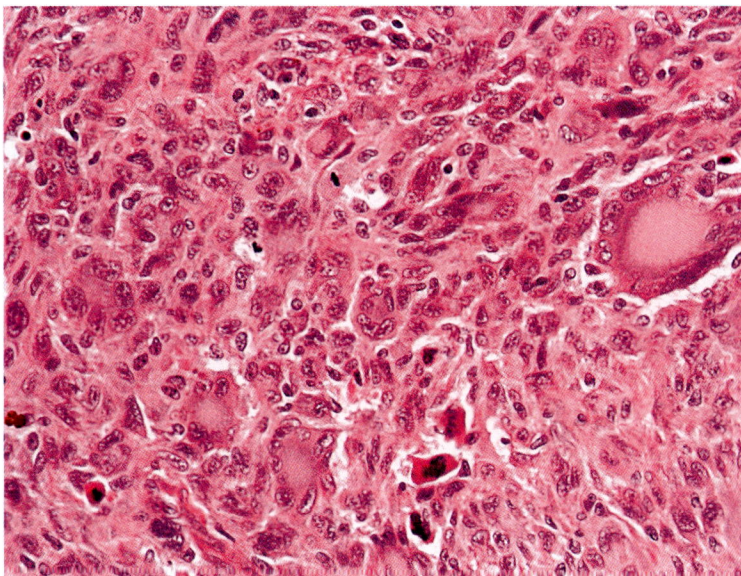

FIG 6.127 Malignant fibrous histiocytoma, giant cell variant.

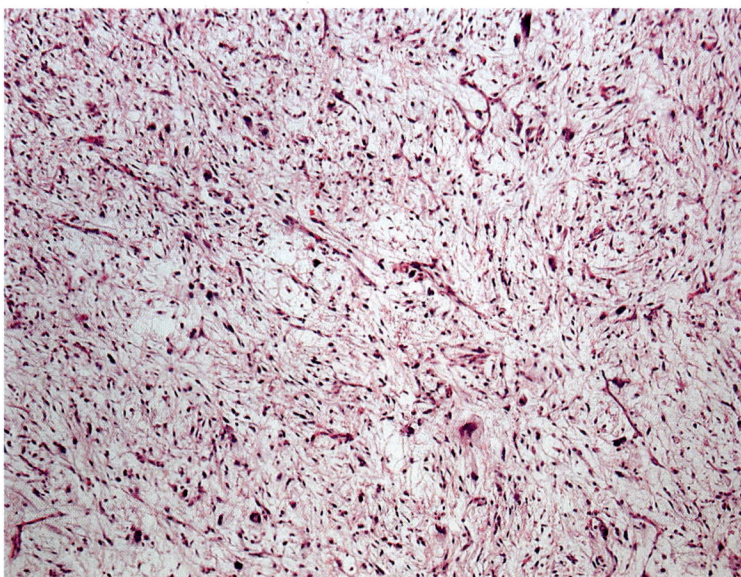

FIG 6.128 Malignant fibrous histiocytoma, myxoid variant.

study confirmed that the fusion gene EWRS1-CREBI is predominant in this entity [155].

It is out of the scope of that review to detail malignant fibrous histiocytoma and its recognized varieties because they better fit in previously discussed patterns, namely spindle cell, pleomorphic, and myxoid.

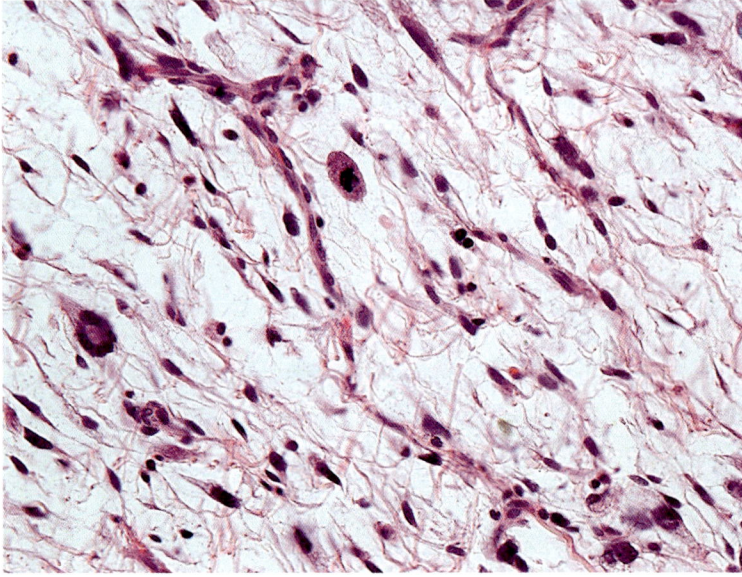

FIG 6.129 Malignant fibrous histiocytoma, myxoid variant.

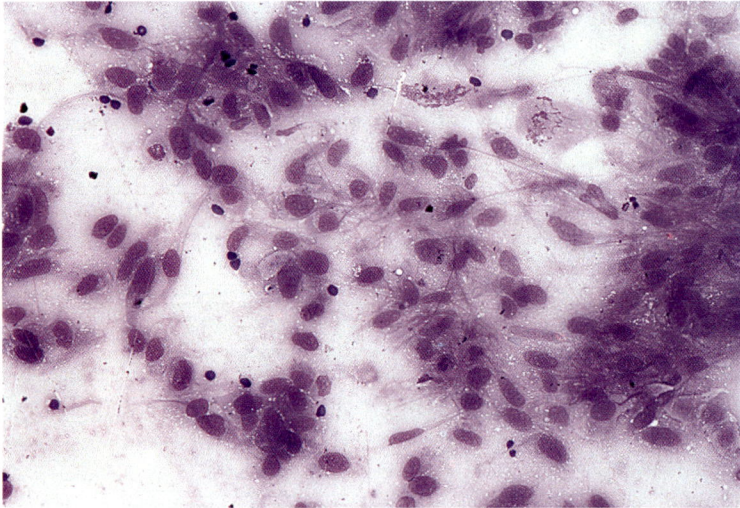

FIG 6.130 Malignant fibrous histiocytoma, storiform-pleomorphic variant. Spindle cells.

6.3.5 Malignant Peripheral Nerve Sheath Tumor

We have already drawn an overview of malignant peripheral nerve sheath tumor in the section devoted to low-grade spindle cell tumors (Figs 6.136–6.139). Similar general comments as well as morphologic cytological/histological findings could be applied to tumors of a higher degree provided they are not pleomorphic. Let us recall

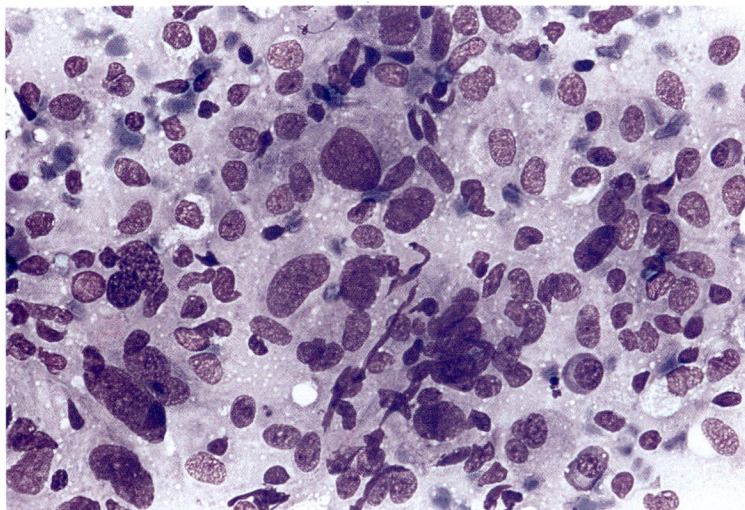

FIG 6.131 Malignant fibrous histiocytoma, storiform-pleomorphic variant. Large variety of spindle, roundish, and anaplastic cells. Malignant character is evident.

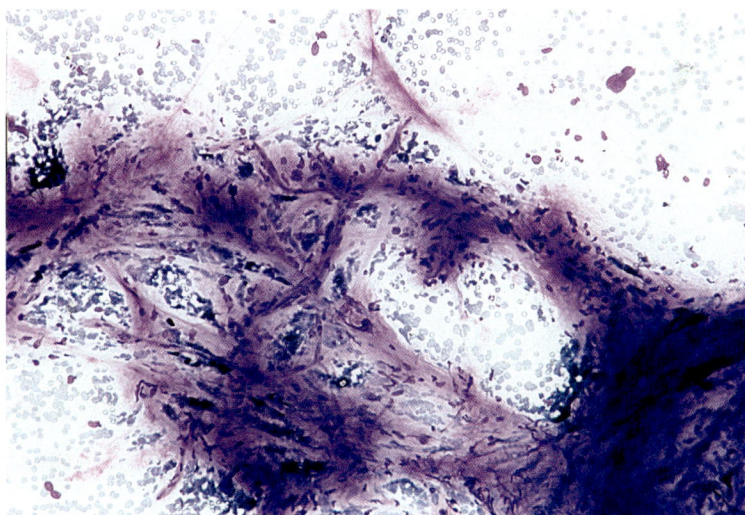

FIG 6.132 Malignant fibrous histiocytoma, storiform-pleomorphic variant. Spindle cells. Malignant character is evident.

that malignant peripheral nerve sheath tumor develops in three different settings: in the context of a documented neurofibromatosis, demonstration by electron microscopy of Schwann cell differentiation evidence, previous demonstration of a preexisting benign nerve sheath tumor [156].

We have previously completed a correlative cytologic and histologic study of 24 cases of malignant peripheral nerve sheath tumor [104]. Usually tumors consist of

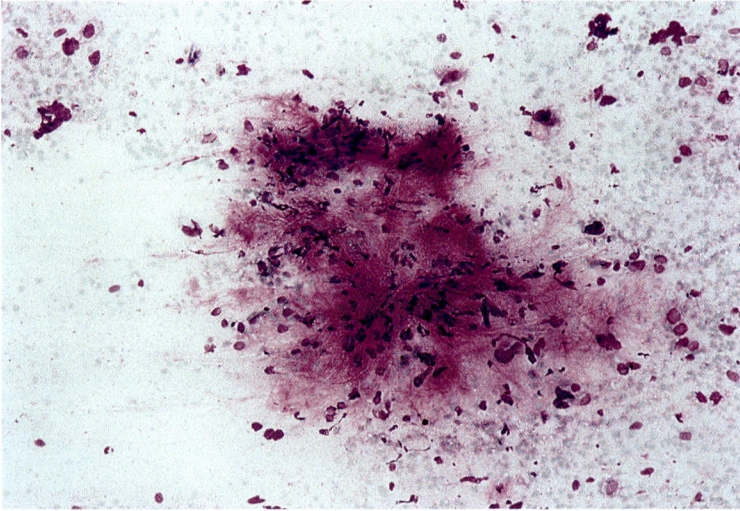

FIG 6.133 Malignant fibrous histiocytoma, storiform-pleomorphic variant. Variety of spindle cells and connective tissue fragments.

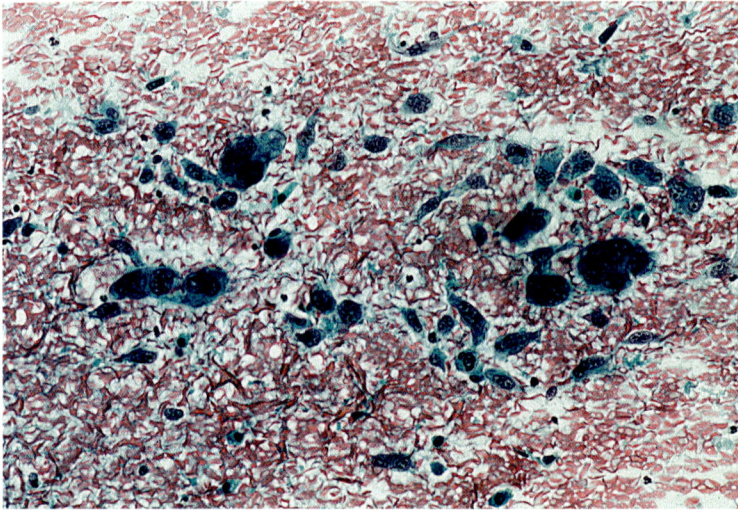

FIG 6.134 Malignant fibrous histiocytoma, storiform-pleomorphic variant, pleomorphic, and multinucleated cells.

spindle shaped cells (Figs 6.140–6.142), fishhook naked nuclei (Figs 6.143 and 6.144), and scant fibrillary stroma (Figs 6.145–6.147).

6.3.6 Spindle Cell Angiosarcoma

Angiosarcomas are rare malignant tumors that recapitulate functional and morphologic features of normal endothelium. Their morphologic aspect varies considerably

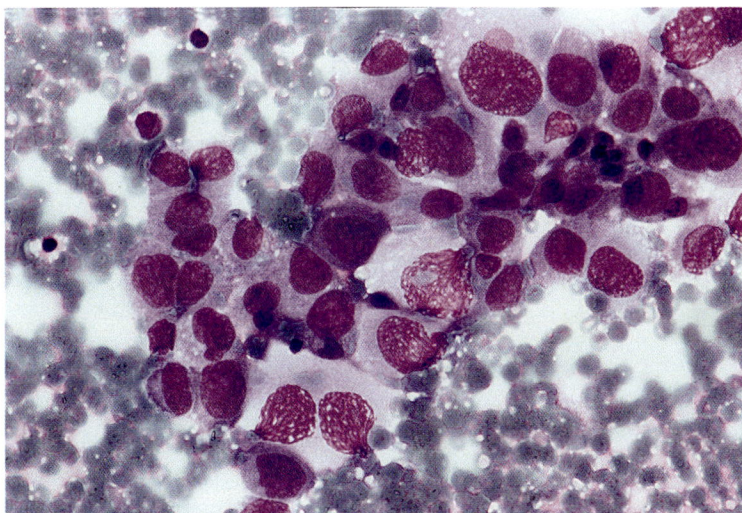

FIG 6.135   Malignant fibrous histiocytoma, storiform-pleomorphic variant comprising roundish cells.

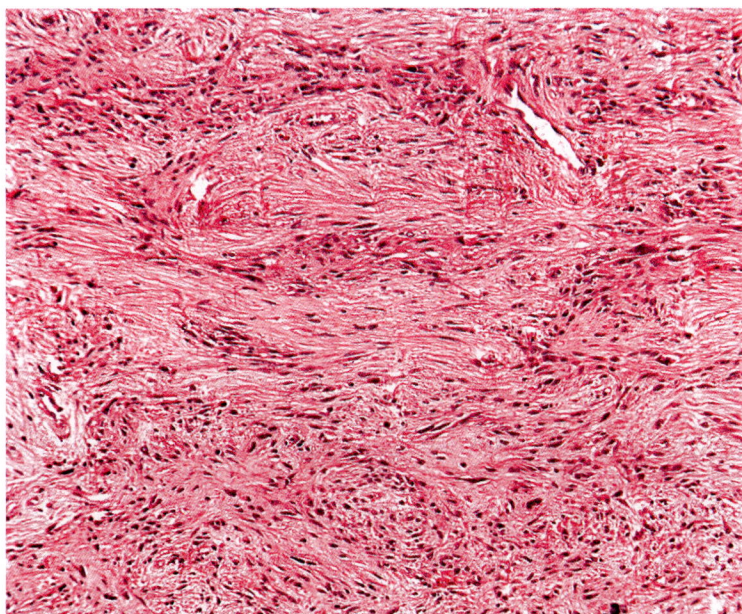

FIG 6.136   Malignant peripheral nerve sheath tumor, bland spindle cells in a myxoid stroma.

ranging from low-grade lesions resembling hemangioma to anaplastic tumors indistinguishable from carcinomas and melanomas by basic histopatholgy. This is one of the rarest soft tissue neoplasms. Although they occur at any site of location in the body, by contrast they rarely affect major vessels. They are typically skin tumors with rare cases in deep soft tissue. They predominate in elderly men and have a

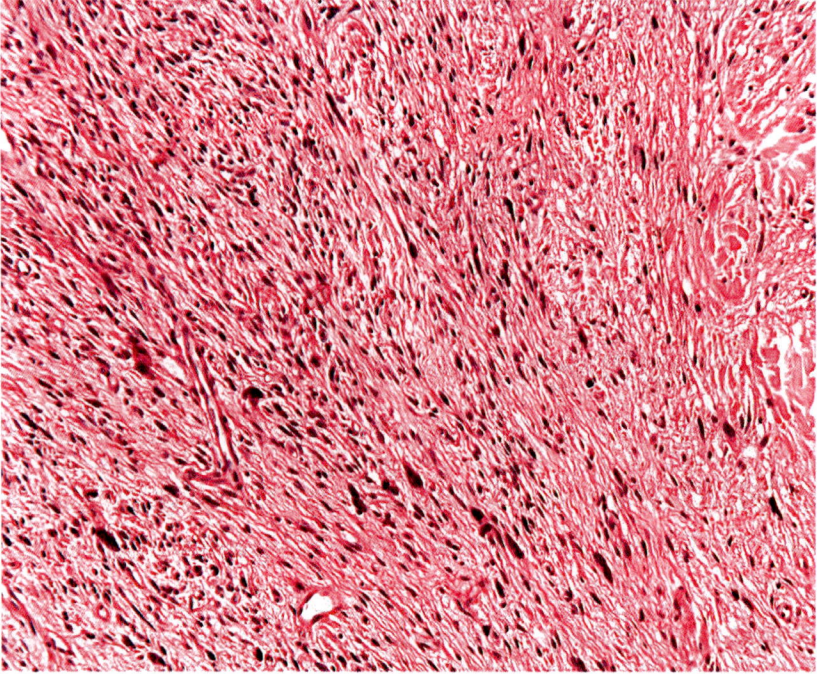

FIG 6.137 Malignant peripheral nerve sheath tumor, spindle cells separated by delicate collagen fibers.

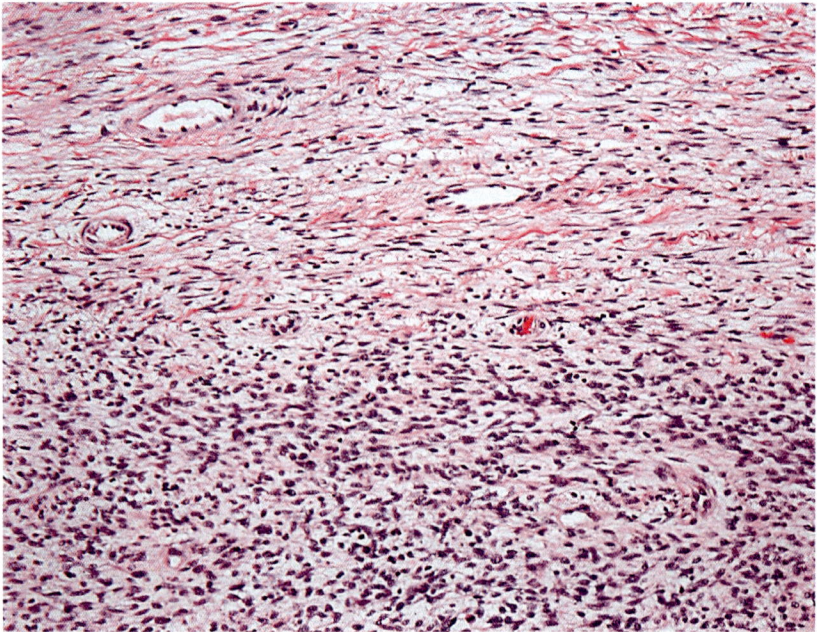

FIG 6.138 Malignant peripheral nerve sheath tumor, transition from low-grade to high-grade neoplasm.

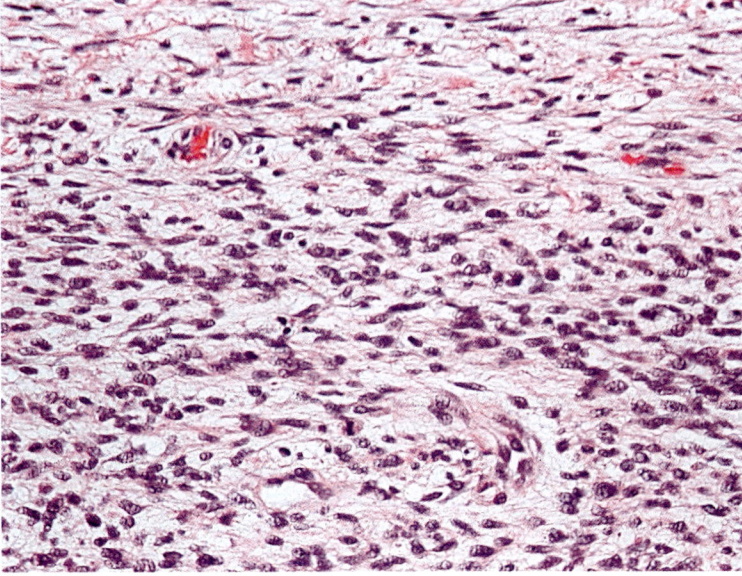

FIG 6.139 Malignant peripheral nerve sheath tumor, high-grade spindle cell sarcoma.

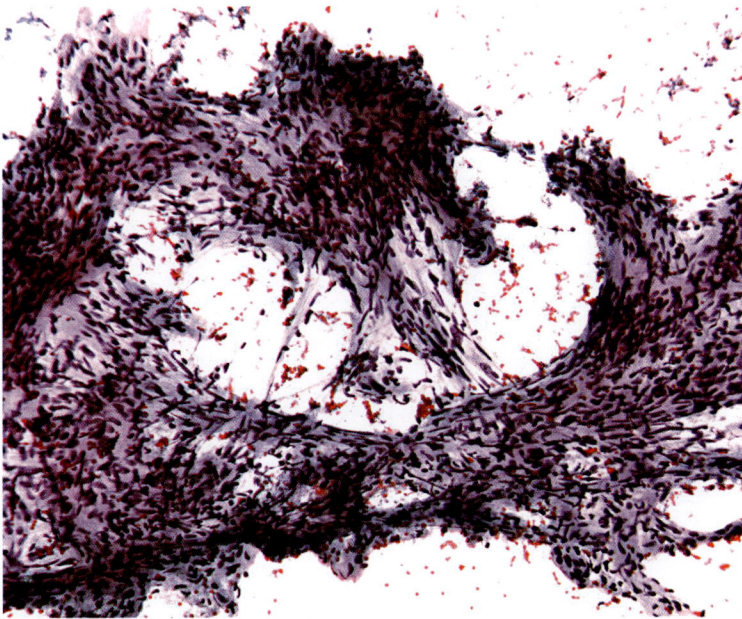

FIG 6.140 Malignant peripheral nerve sheath tumor, spindle cells in parallel aligment, suggesting neural origin.

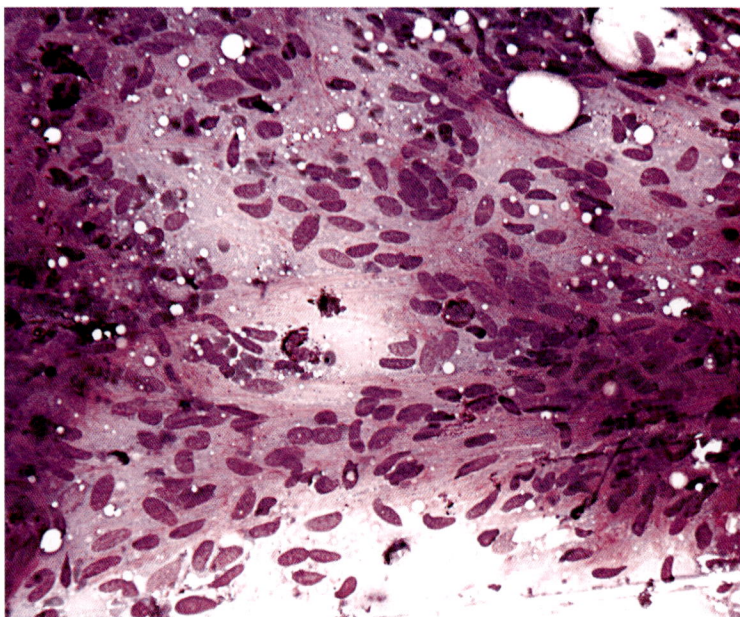

FIG 6.141   Malignant peripheral nerve sheath tumor, spindle cells.

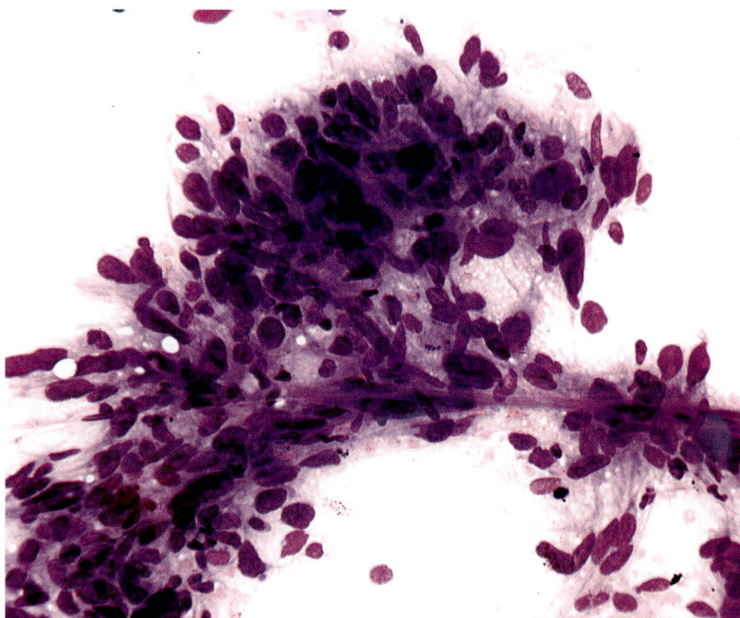

FIG 6.142   Malignant peripheral nerve sheath tumor, Pleomorphic cells.

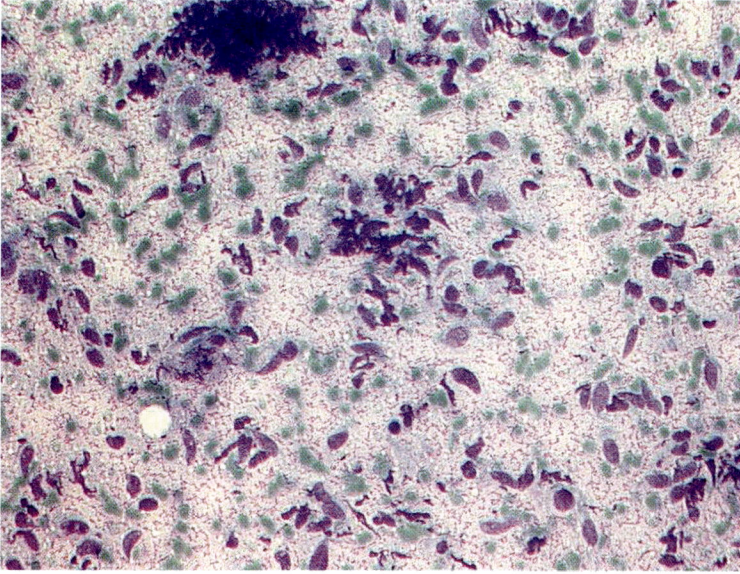

FIG 6.143 Malignant peripheral nerve sheath tumor, fishhook naked nuclei.

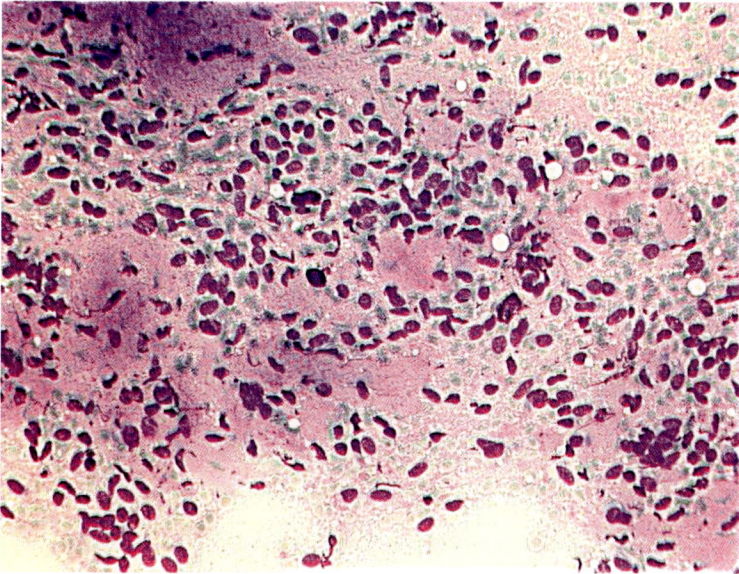

FIG 6.144 Malignant peripheral nerve sheath tumor. Fibrillary stroma.

predilection for the skin of the head and neck. Special varieties are angiosarcoma associated with lymphoedema after mastectomy and axillary dissection, and a few are late complications of radiation therapy. Based on their morphology, they must be differentiated from Kaposi sarcoma, other vascular or perivascular neoplasms, and from entities comprised in the whole spectrum of spindle cell pattern

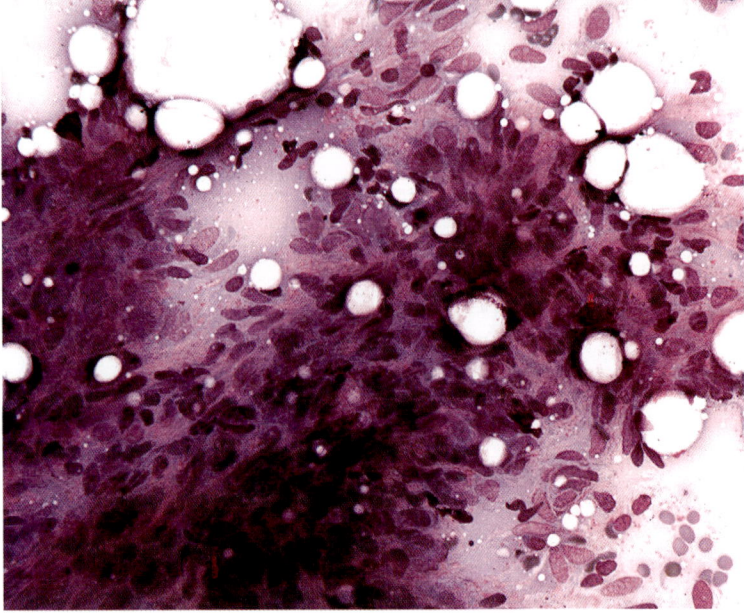

FIG 6.145 Malignant peripheral nerve sheath tumor, fibrillary stroma.

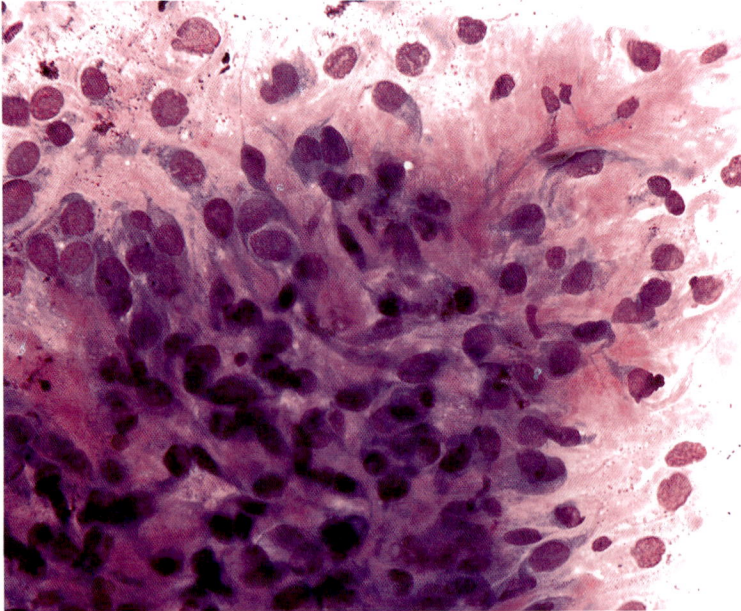

FIG 6.146 Malignant peripheral nerve sheath tumor, fibrillary stroma.

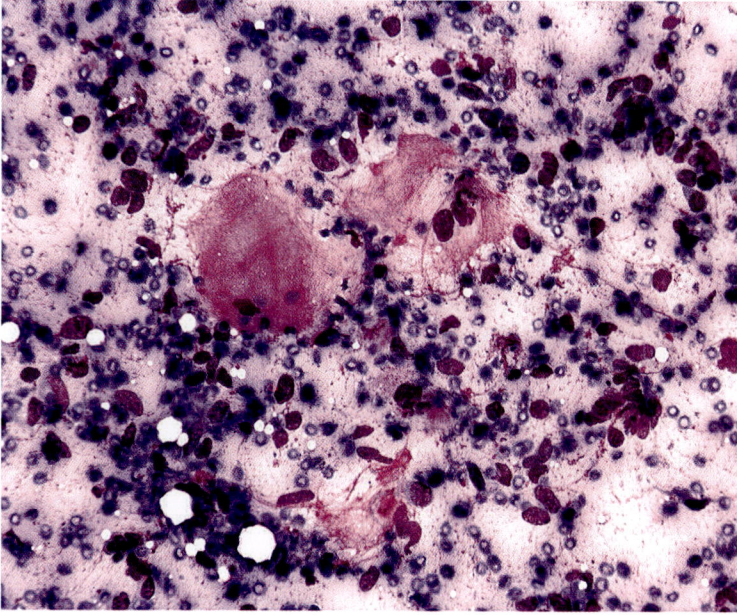

FIG 6.147 Malignant peripheral nerve sheath tumor, fibrillary stroma.

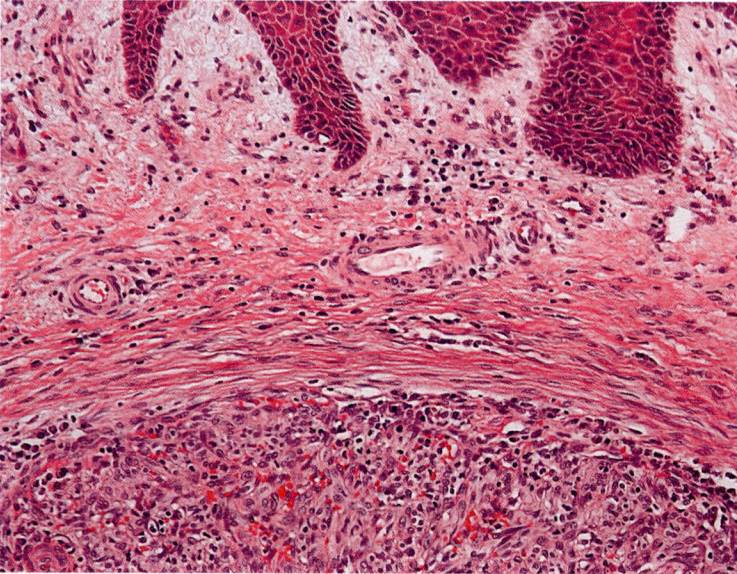

FIG 6.148 Spindle cell angiosarcoma, well-demarcated skin nodule in spindle cell variant.

The best-differentiated tumors (Fig 6.148) consist of irregularly anastomosing complex vascular channels (Fig 6.149) sometimes showing papillary projections. Higher grade tumors can easily be confused with fibrosarcoma (Fig 6.150), hence their inclusion in the group of spindle cell pattern. If occasional well-differentiated

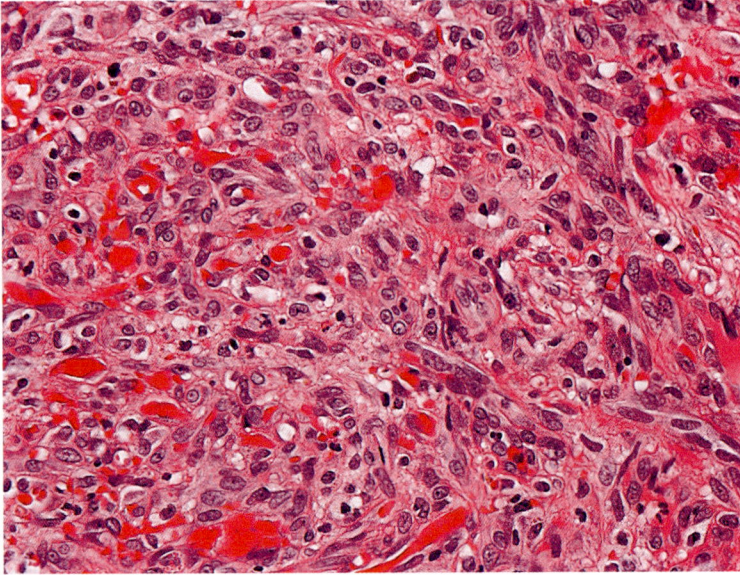

FIG 6.149   Spindle cell angiosarcoma, irregularly anatomizing complex vascular channels with virtual lumina.

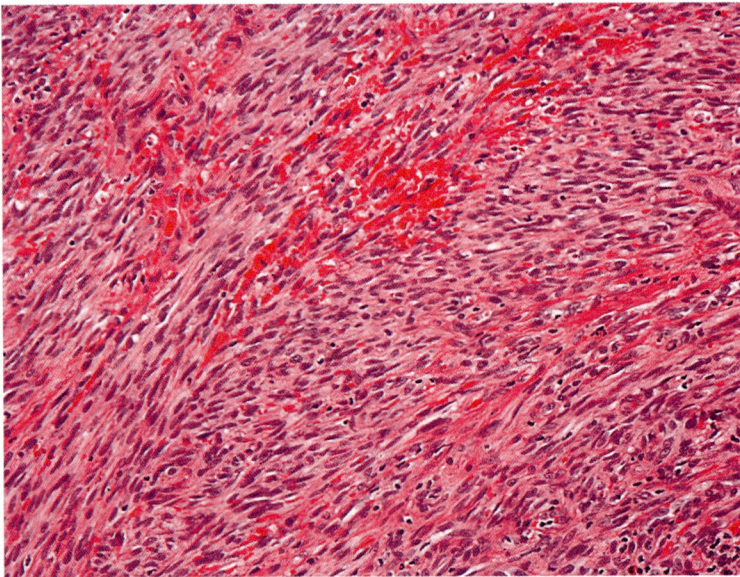

FIG 6.150   Spindle cell angiosarcoma, higher grade tumor resembling any of the spindle cell sarcoma group.

areas are present, then the diagnosis is facilitated. Depending on the degree of differentiation, atypia and mitosis (Fig 6.151) will vary in cell volume and shape as well as in atypia characterized by hyperchromasia and prominent nucleoli (Fig 6.152).

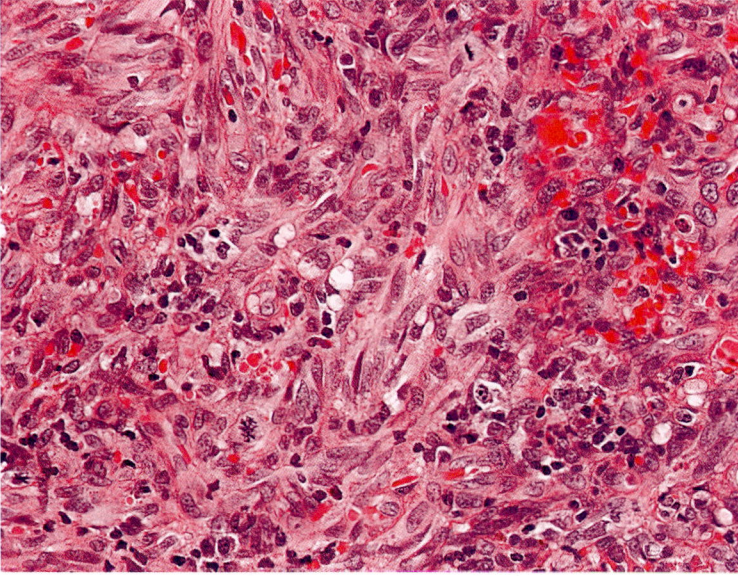

FIG 6.151 Spindle cell angiosarcoma, area showing atypical mitosis, paranuclear vacuoles, and extravasated red cells.

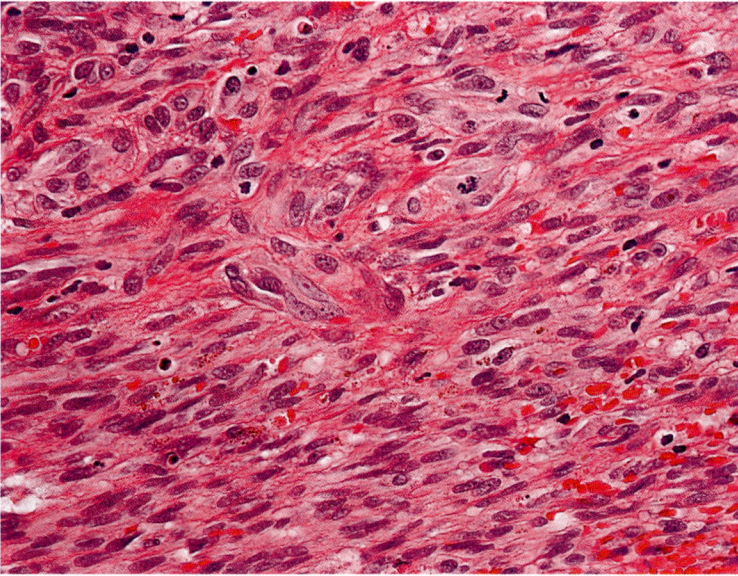

FIG 6.152 Spindle cell angiosarcoma, abortive vascular channels, predominance of a spindle cell component, and traces of iron pigment.

More solid tumors consisting of compact sheets of tumor cells are difficult to diagnose. In such cases, immunohistochemical profile is very helpful; most angiosarcomas stains for CD31, a lesser number stain for CD34, which is a nonspecific reaction, and FVIII-related antigen, which, although specific of endothelial cells, is less sensitive and, because of its presence in the plasma cells, can give false-positive results, particularly in areas of hemorrhage and necrosis. The results of a previous report of a series of 23 cases of angiosarcomas, 18 classic and 5 epithelioid, form the basis of the following review [157]. Cytologically, tumors present as a spindle cell sarcomas (Figs 6.153–6.155) within a hemorrhagic background. Prominent atypia is absent.

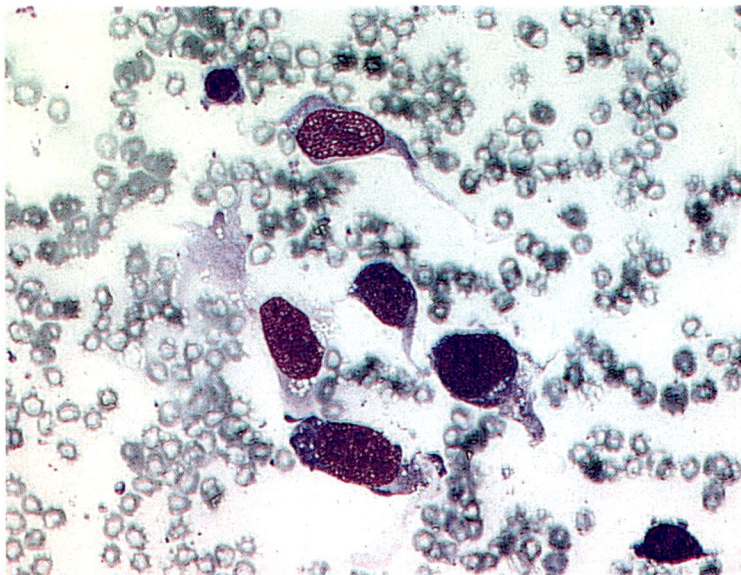

FIG 6.153 Spindle cell angiosarcoma. Malignant spindle cells.

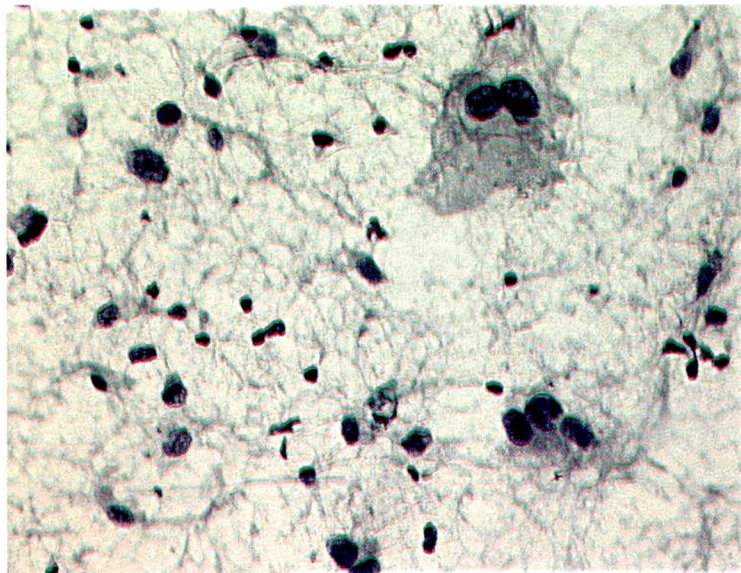

FIG 6.154 Spindle cell angiosarcoma. Polymorphous cells.

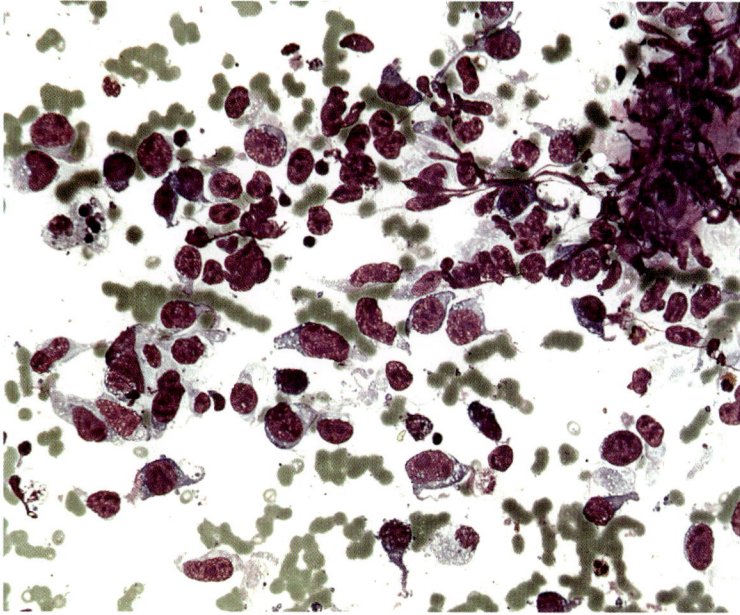

FIG 6.155 Spindle cell angiosarcoma, nonspecific malignant spindle shaped and polymorphous cells.

6.3.7 Kaposi Sarcoma

Kaposi sarcoma occurs in four different clinical settings: chronic, lymphadenopathic, transplantation-associated, and AIDS-related. The chronic form is observed in elderly men, generally of Mediterranean origin. The lymphadenopathic form occurs primarily in young African children whose presentation symptoms and physical signs are generalized lymphadenopathy with involvement of cervical, inguinal, and hilar lymph nodes. The two other forms are related to immunosuppression. The nodular cutaneous stage as well as later stages can be evaluated by fine needle aspiration.

6.3.7.1 Histopathology. The nodular phase of Kaposi sarcoma (Fig 6.156) is characterized by confluent and well-circumscribed proliferations of spindle cells. In the initial stages, they are bland and grouped around slit-like vascular channels. In more solid lesions, they tend to resemble fibrosarcoma or other sarcomas of spindle cell composition (Fig 6.157). Erythrocyte extravasation is frequent as are phenomenona of erythrophagocytosis (Fig 6.158). Periodic acid schiff-positive and diastase-resistant hyaline globules are engulfed within the cytoplasm of tumor cells and also lost in the extracellular stroma. These globules are also autofluorescent even in routine stains. Typical lesions of Kaposi sarcoma depict little pleomorphism and a low mitotic index (Fig 6.159), although more aggressive histologic cases can be observed.

The immunohistochemical profile has raised numerous controversies in reference to the nature of endothelial cells. Numerous antibodies have been tested and proved

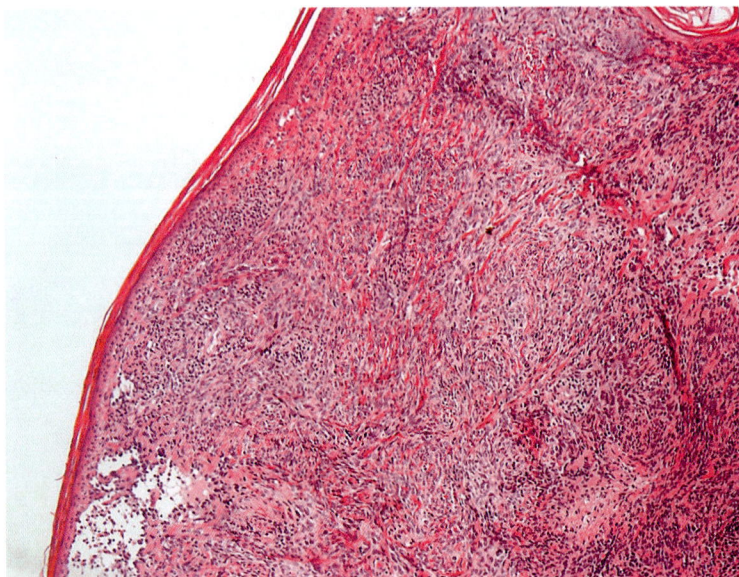

FIG 6.156   Kaposi sarcoma, nodular phase in a Kaposi sarcoma.

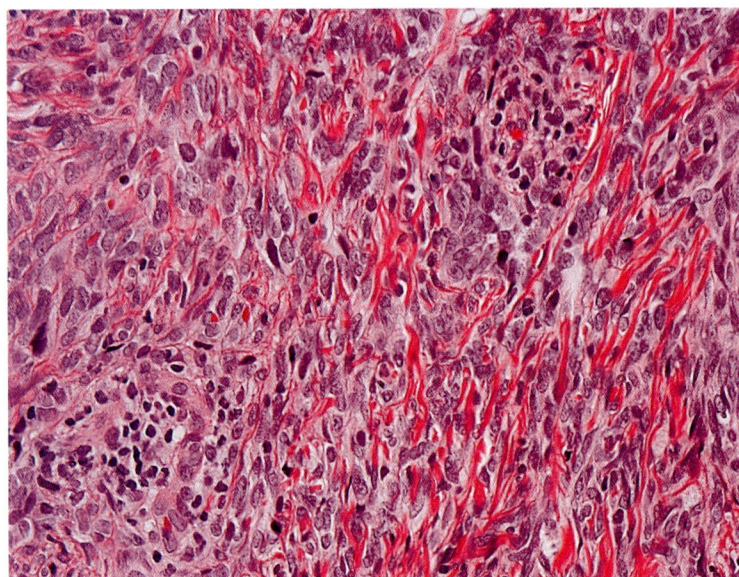

FIG 6.157   Kaposi sarcoma, solid area of spindle cells in the superficial dermis mimicking a spindle cell sarcoma.

nonconclusive; VEGFR-3 and HHV8 are recognized to give positive results, whatever the form of the disease.

6.3.7.2   Cytopathology. The smears are usually cell-rich and consist of spindle and plasmacytoid, sometimes epithelioid cells with a radial arrangement, and nuclear

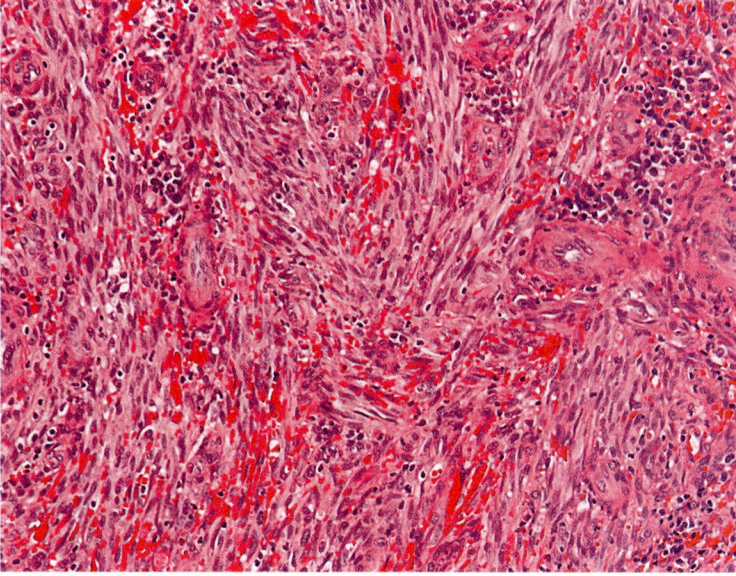

FIG 6.158 Kaposi sarcoma, erythocyte extravasation is frequent.

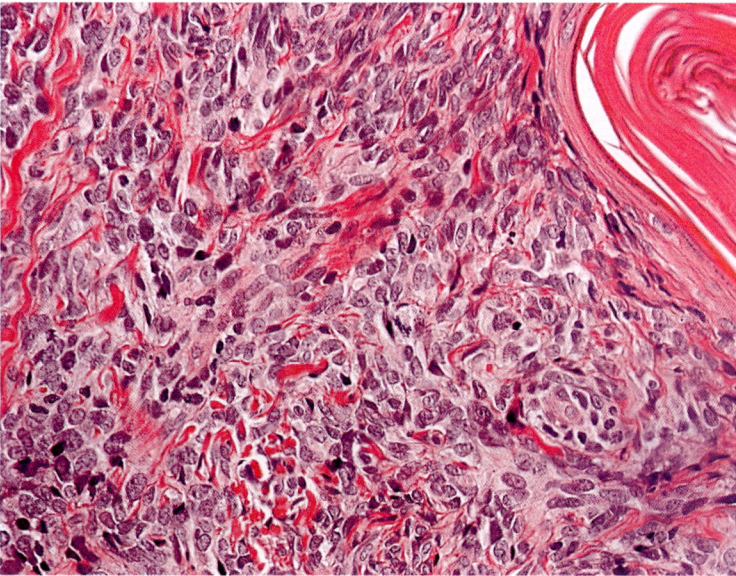

FIG 6.159 Kaposi sarcoma, higher magnification showing minimal pleomorphism and a low mitotic index.

crush artifacts (Fig 6.160). Chromatin is delicate. The most characteristic cytologic features are intact tissue fragments comprising of overlapping spindle cells with nuclear distortion and ill-defined cytoplasmic borders (Fig 6.161). The background may be hemorrhagic or necrotic.

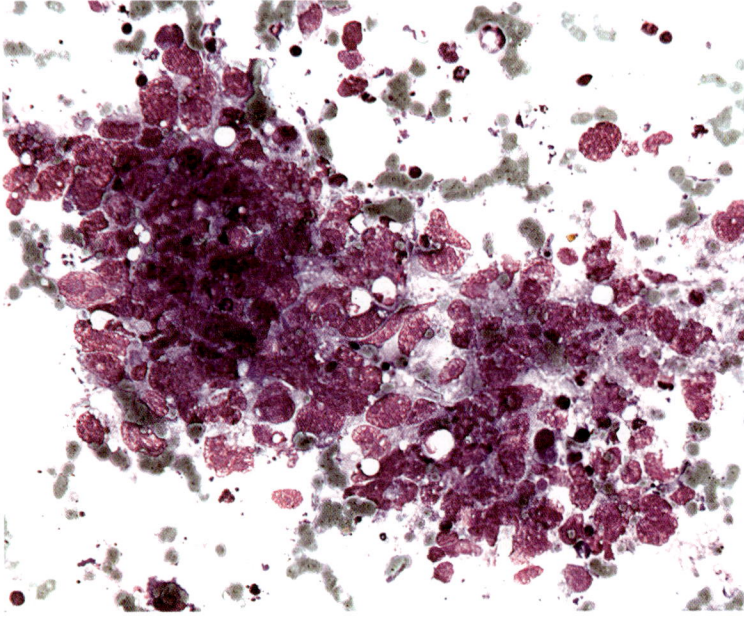

FIG 6.160 Kaposi sarcoma, epithelioid cells with nuclear crush artifacts. Necrotic background.

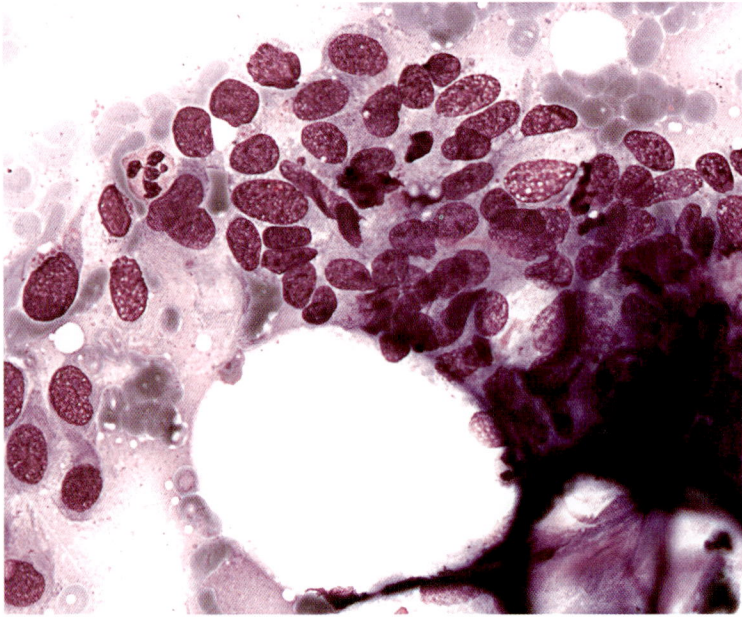

FIG 6.161 Kaposi sarcoma, overlapping spindle cells with nuclear distortion and ill-defined cytoplasmic borders.

6.3.7.3 Differential Diagnosis. Kaposi sarcoma should be differentiated from other spindle cell sarcomas, but in the appropriate clinical setting, cytologic features on fine needle aspiration are usually sufficient to be diagnostic of Kaposi sarcoma [158].

6.3.7.4 Comments. Thirty-six examples of fine needle aspiration of Kaposi sarcoma have been reported [159–163]. Epitrochlear lymph nodes are the most frequently aspirated site [161], and aspirated thyroid tumors in HIV negative patients also were described [160,162].

In the series of 15 cases described by Gamborino et al. [161], all aspirates allowed diagnoses of Kaposi sarcoma. Taking into consideration the high prevalence of AIDS and limited resources for diagnosis in Africa, FNA seems to be a useful method for the diagnosis of Kaposi sarcoma in developing countries, reducing the necessity for surgical lymph node excision. In an other large study of 15 cases [158] diagnosed by fine-needle aspiration biopsy, the diagnosis was confirmed by tissue biopsy in 8 cases. All patients were homosexual males, and 13 had a previous diagnosis of AIDS. In our series, we have observed four cases, in which two were diagnosed accurately, one was diagnosed as fibrosarcoma, and finally, one was not satisfactory for diagnosis.

6.4 MYXOID TUMORS

Several soft tissue tumors could be included in this pattern category. Survey of the literature shows that myxoid lesions exhibit variable biological behavior, from harmless entities (like intramuscular myxoma) to malignant sarcoma (like extraskeletal myxoid chondrosarcoma). In this part of the review, the focus is on predominantly benign and malignant myxoid tumors. The main candidates are myxoid liposarcoma, myxoid malignant fibrous histiocytoma, myxoma, and extraskeletal myxoid chondrosarcoma.

The value of fine needle aspiration in the differential diagnosis of adult myxoid sarcoma has been already investigated largely [164] and proved to represent a valuable diagnostic tool. Myxoid sarcomas present probably the greatest challenge when attempting to make an accurate diagnosis with cytologic methods, but the recognition of myxoid soft tissue tumor is not complicated because of the presence of a characteristic myxoid substance. Comparative cytological studies of myxoid tumors were analyzed in a large series [164,165] in a logistic regression study of sarcomas with a myxoid background. As an example, Layfield et al. [165] found that the presence of pleomorphic giant cells and fibroblast-like cells are most predictive of myxoid malignant fibrous histiocytoma. Compared with other myxoid soft tissue tumors, physaliphorous cells were more representative of chordoma, chondroid fragments of chondrosarcoma, and lipoblasts of liposarcoma. Other comparative cytological studies of myxoid tumors were reported [166–168] and disclosed similar results.

6.4.1 Myxoid Liposarcoma (With or Without Round or Spindle Cells)

Liposarcoma is the most frequent soft tissue sarcoma of adult life since the reclassification of malignant fibrous histiocytomas. Myxoid variant of liposarcoma is the most frequent subtype acconting for approximately 50% of all liposarcomas. Although given separated designation in the literature, its round cell variant represents the less well-differentiated end of the same nosologic spectrum. This has been substantiated by the demonstration of the typical t(12;16)(q13;p11) and t(12;22) (q13;q12) chromosomal translocations in both morphological variants [169]. They are also similar in terms of age and location. In comparison with well-differentiated and dedifferentiated liposarcomas, they occur in a younger age group. They originate principally in the lower extremities, thigh and popliteal area, and rarely in the abdominal cavity and retroperitoneum. A typical well-differentiated myxoid liposarcoma is a low-grade sarcoma characterized by recurrences, whereas the round cell tumors are prone to result in metastasis. Howewer, it is still debated and unclear which proportion of round cells is indicative of a metastatic potential. One study has suggested the following scheme: 0 to 5% of round cells = 23% of risk, 5 to 10% round cells = 35%, and >25% round cells = 58% [170]. According to Weiss and Goldblum [171], the following labels have been attributed to round cell myxoid liposarcoma grade I with less than 10% of round cells, grade II for 10−25% round cells, and the remainder is grade III. Of interest, if myxoid/round cell liposarcoma metastasizes to usual sites like lung and bone, then they tend also to extend to other soft tissue sites. The immunohistochemical profile of myxoid liposarcoma does not contribute significantly to the precision of diagnosis. For more difficult cases, the molecular genetic profile is very helpful.

6.4.1.1 Histopathology. Typically, the predominantly myxoid liposarcomas are multinodular, gelatinous masses, whereas the round cell type depicts some white opaque nodules with a fleshy appearance when totally composed of round cells. The overall morphology of myxoid liposarcoma has been compared with developing fat, hence the former designation "embryonal lipoma" and the suggestion that they could originate from the brown fat. They consist of varying numbers of small round-to-stellated cells dispersed in an abundant myxoid stroma within a delicate plexiform capillary network designated as a "chicken-wire" pattern (Fig 6.162). Mitosis,

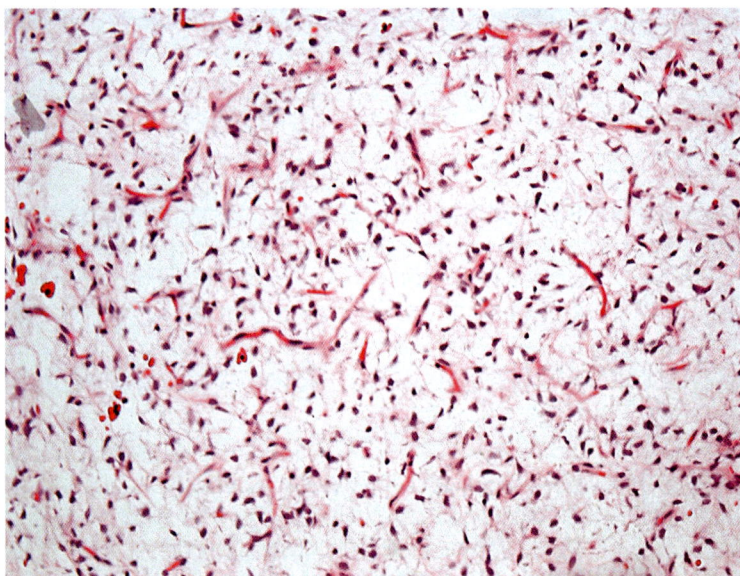

FIG 6.162 Myxoid liposarcoma, varying numbers of small round-to-stellated cells interspersed within a delicate plexiform capillary network of "chicken-wire pattern".

pleomorphism, and tumoral necrosis are absent. Variable numbers of lipoblats are observed (Fig 6.163). Small-to-large anastomosing "pools" of mucin are observed readily and, when extreme, can simulate a lymphangioma (Fig 6.164). The round cell

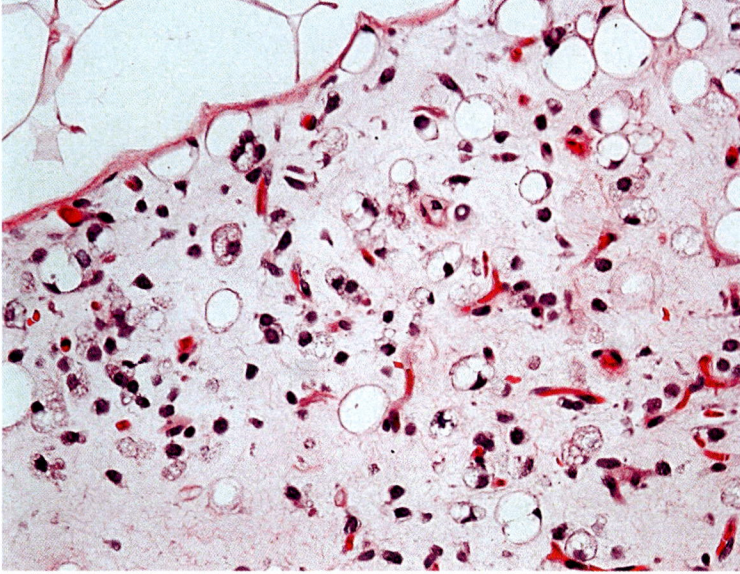

FIG 6.163   Myxoid liposarcoma, lipoblasts at different stages of maturation.

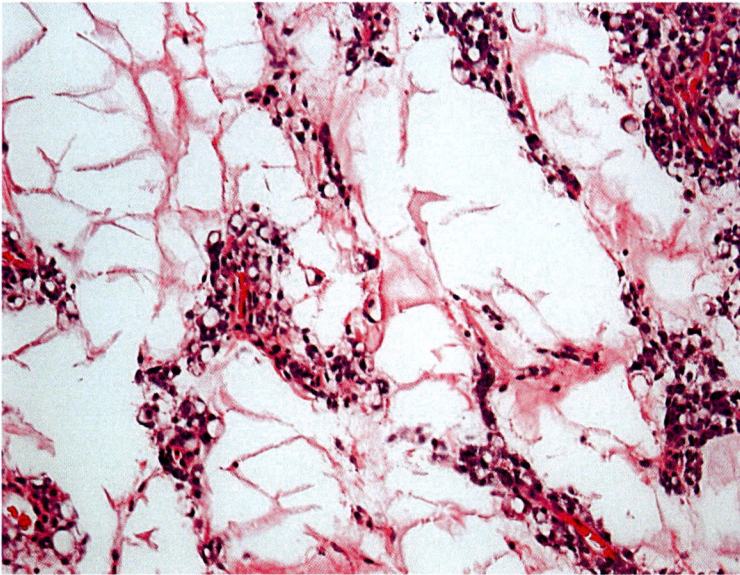

FIG 6.164   Myxoid liposarcoma, cords of rounds cells interspersed between mucin pools in the round cell variant.

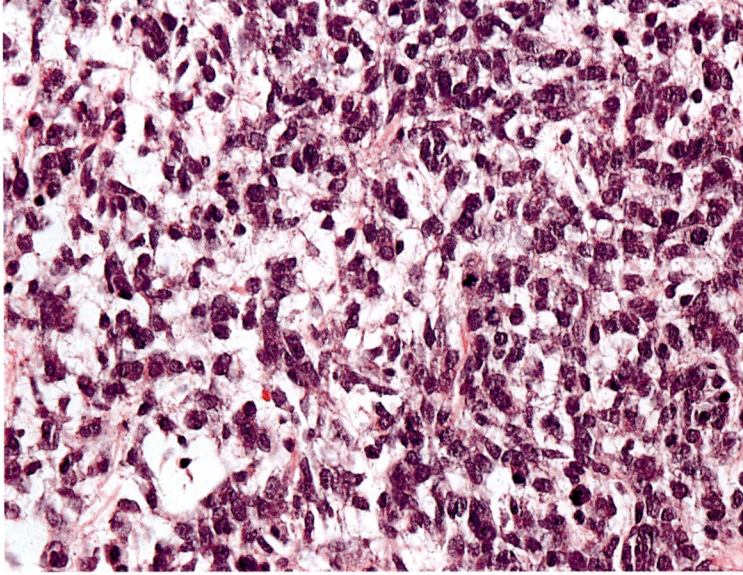

FIG 6.165 Myxoid liposarcoma, solid sheaths or cord-like of round cells without intervening myxoid stroma.

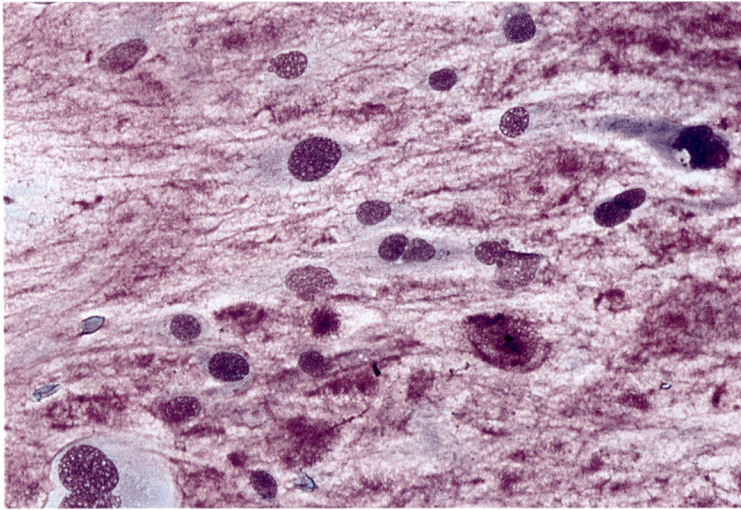

FIG 6.166 Myxoid liposarcoma, myxoid background.

variant is characterized by solid sheaths or cord-like primitive round cells showing a high cytonuclear ratio with small nuclei, without intervening stroma (Fig 6.165). Some unusual morphological features may be present (e.g., predominance of a spindle cell component or rhabdomyoblastic differentiation).

6.4.1.2 Cytopathology. Most pure myxoid liposarcomas are stroma-rich and cell-poor. Some parts of smears show an abundant myxoid background (Figs 6.166 and 6.167) and typical vascular arborizing structures (Fig 6.168). Tumor cells, if present,

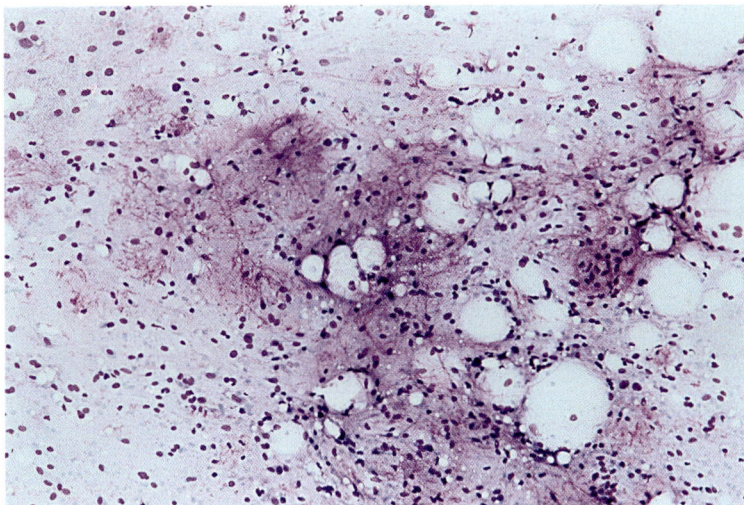

FIG 6.167 Myxoid liposarcoma, spindle malignant cells.

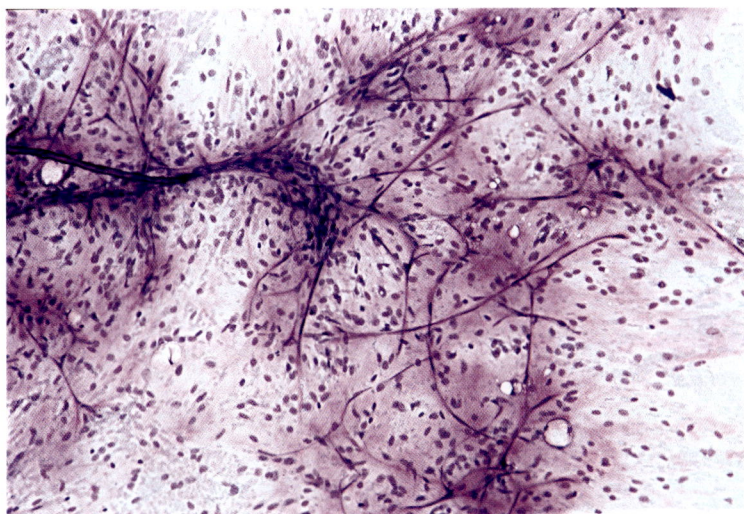

FIG 6.168 Myxoid liposarcoma, vascular arborizing structures.

are round or spindle. Lipoblasts are observed in half of cases (Figs 6.169–6.171). The combination of lipoblasts and a myxoid background is characteristic and allows an accurate tumor typing. Round cell myxoid liposarcoma is also stroma-rich and mainly consists of a myxoid background, vascular arborizing structures, round cells (Fig 6.172), and less frequently, lipoblasts. They also can be entirely round cell, although they are less well developed than typical liposarcomas. Spindle cell myxoid liposarcoma show, similar to round cells counterparts, a myxoid background and vascular arborizing structures. Spindle cells usually are found (Figs 6.173–6.175), and round cells are found in half of cases. Both round cell and spindle cell tumors show relatively frequent cytonuclear atypia and mitotic figures.

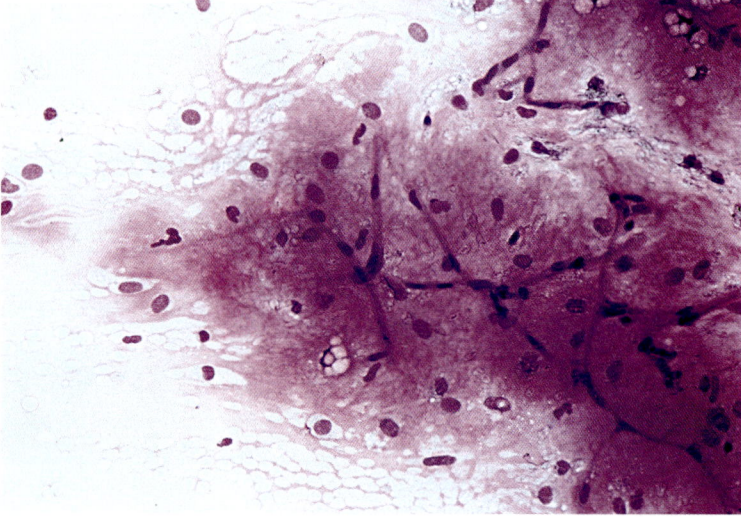

FIG 6.169 Myxoid liposarcoma, dispersed and single lipoblasts, myxoid matrix and vessels.

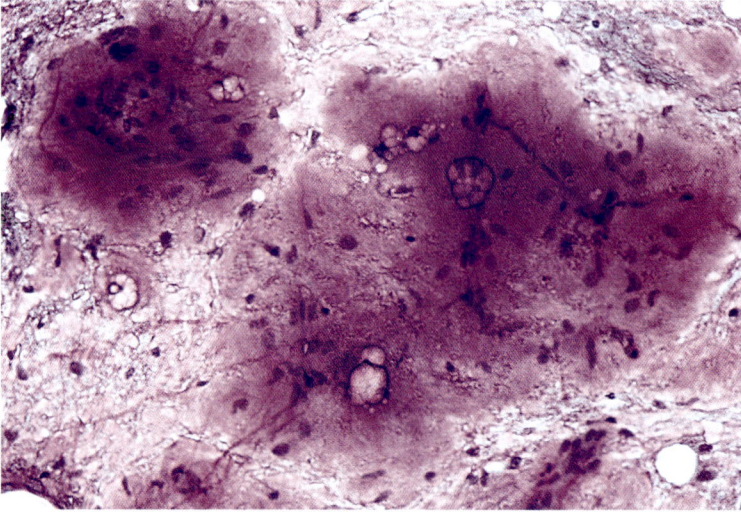

FIG 6.170 Myxoid liposarcoma, dispersed and single lipoblasts within myxoid matrix.

6.4.1.3 Differential Diagnosis. The following entities should be differentiated from myoxid liposarcoma:

- Myxoid malignant fibrous histiocytoma
- Extraskeletal myxoid chondrosarcoma
- Myxoma
- Myxofibrosarcoma
- Lymphangioma

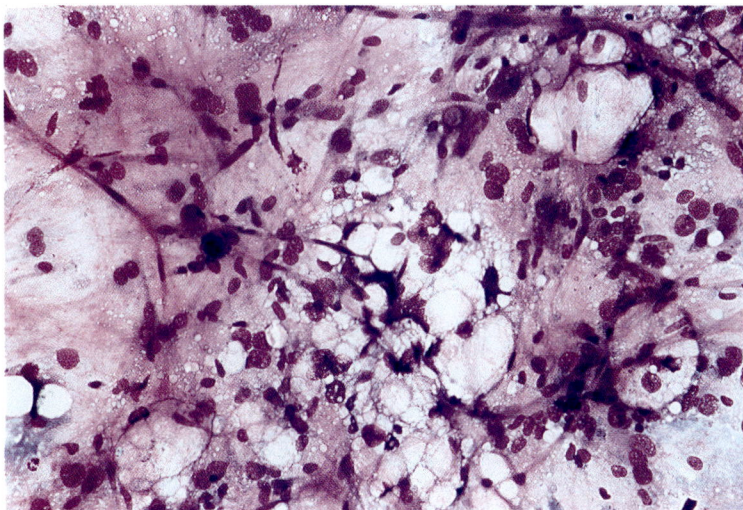

FIG 6.171 Myxoid liposarcoma, spindle cells. Note the presence of myxoid and lipoblasts.

The main entities to consider in the differential diagnosis (Table 6.8) are benign myxoma; howewer, they are devoid of lipoblasts and of the typical vasculature of myxoid liposarcoma and myxoid malignant fibrous histiocytoma. They are different by some degree of cellular pleomorphism and polymorphism as well as extraskeletal myxoid chondrosarcoma by the quality of the mucin stroma consisting of acid mucopolysaccharides with sulfated radicals and also by a different genetic profile.

The distinction between myxoid liposarcoma and myxoid malignant fibrous histiocytoma could be impossible in many cases, especially on smears without lipoblasts. Moreover, numerous "pseudolipoblasts" are present in the myxoid portion of myxoid malignant fibrous histiocytoma. The typical curvilinear vasculature of myxoid malignant fibrous histiocytoma is not differentiated easily from the chicken-wire arborizing vasculature of myxoid liposarcoma. Layfield et al. [165] performed a logistic regression analysis of myxoid sarcoma and found that the presence of lipoblasts is a significant clue for the diagnosis of myxoid liposarcoma. The finding of arborizing vascular structures was not sufficiently distinctive to establish a diagnosis of myxoid liposarcoma because similar structures are also observed in 15% of myxoid malignant fibrous histiocytoma and 6% of chondrosarcomas.

If fine needle aspiration plays a role in the orientation of the treatment of various types of sarcomas, then one has to keep in mind that, given the morphological heterogeneity of mesenchymal sarcomes, many pitfalls are inherent to this method of diagnosis. Clinicopathological correlations are strongly indicated to avoid risks of under/overdiagnosis of these neoplams. When lipoblasts are not detected, myxoid liposarcoma should also be differentiated from myxoid leiomyosarcoma. The main differential diagnostic tool is the immunocytochemical detection of muscular markers [168].

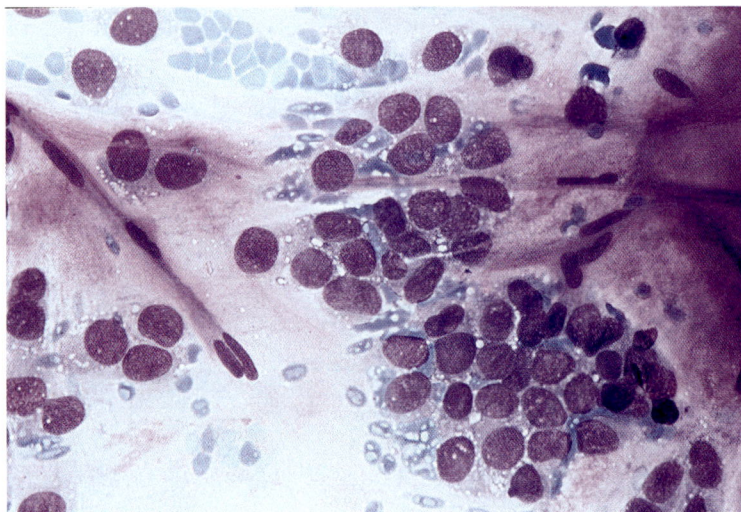

FIG 6.172   Myxoid liposarcoma, round cells.

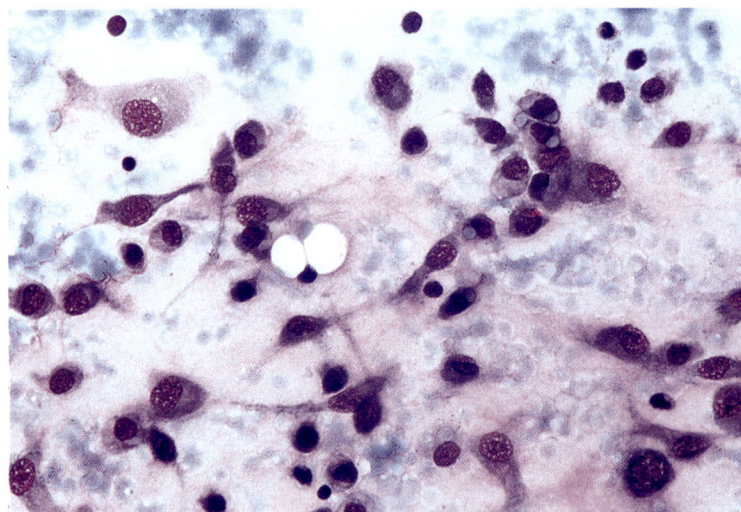

FIG 6.173   Myxoid liposarcoma, spindle cells. Note the presence of lipoblasts.

6.4.1.4 *Comments.* Pure myxoid liposarcomas were well characterized in previous cytologic studies [164,165,167,172–179]. The cytological features are fairly
typical in most cases: "a myxoid background matrix, tissue fragments with arborizing capillary network, and small to medium-sized rounded to ovoid, slightly atypical
tumors cells and typical uni- or multivacuolated lipoblasts with scalloped nuclei"
[180]. The univacuolated lipoblasts display various shapes, with the more immature
cells being elongated with a small vacuole, whereas the more mature lipoblasts show
a large vacuole displacing the nucleus at the periphery. The multivacuolated
lipoblasts are somewhat round to polygonal, and the nuclei could be deformed

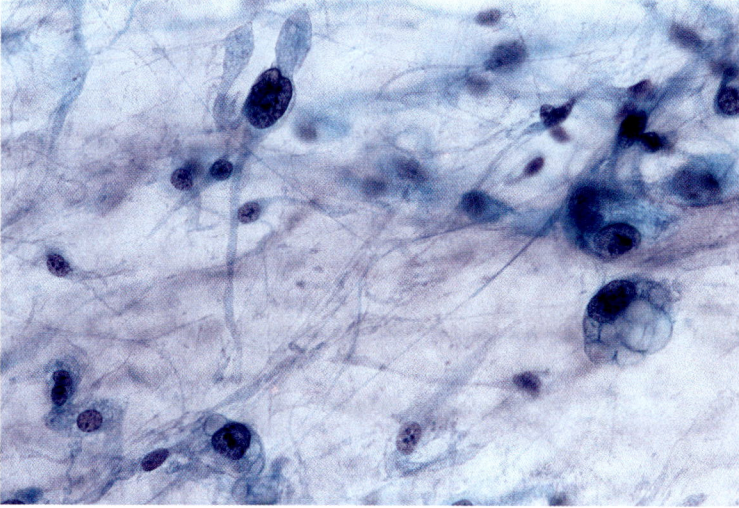

FIG 6.174 Myxoid liposarcoma, Same case as in Fig 6.173, Papanicolaou.

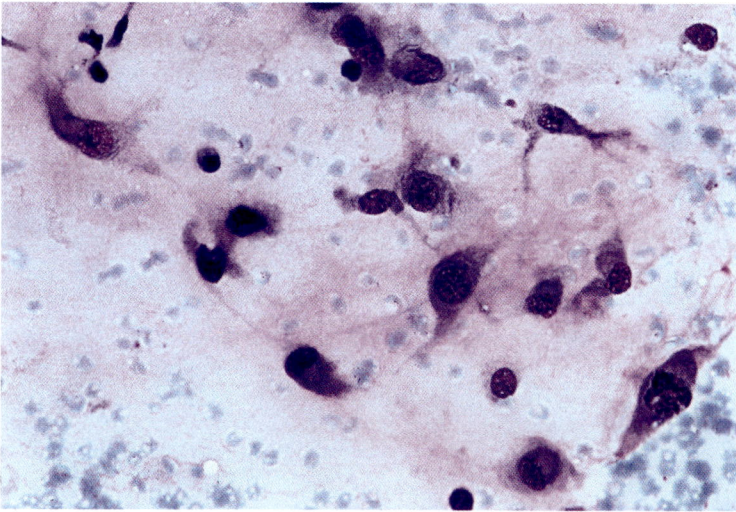

FIG 6.175 Myxoid liposarcoma, spindle cells.

strongly by compression of vacuoles on their cell membrane [172]. Our findings [167] are in agreement with the following observations: myxoid liposarcomas comprised a myxoid background in 94% of cases, arborizing vascular structures in 61%, and moderate quantities of round or spindle cells (present in 67% and 61%, respectively). Lipoblasts were observed in 42% of cases.

Reported features of round cell myxoid liposarcoma consist of a predominantly single-cell population of round-to-monomorphic slightly oval cells without cellular cohesion. Mitotic figures usually are present. Inversely, myxoid background, lipoblasts, and vascular arborizing structures are hardly observed [180,181]. In our

TABLE 6.8 Cytological differential diagnosis of myxoid liposarcoma and related myxoid tumors

	Myxoid liposarcoma			Myxoid MFH and myxofibrosarcoma	Myxoid leiomyosarcoma	Extraskeletal myxoid chondrosarcoma
	Pure	Round cells	Spindle cells			
Myxoid	++	++	++	++	++	++
Lipoblasts	+	+	+	−	−	−
Round cells	+	++	−	++	++	++
Spindle cells	+	+/−	++	++	++	+/−
Chondroid	−	−	−	−	−	+/−

++; Frequent, +; rare, +/− occasionally seen, −; absent.

study [167], a myxoid background was observed in 76% of cases and round cells in 76% of cases. Lipoblasts and vascular arborizing structures were noted in 53% and 35% of cases, respectively. To our knowledge, cytological characteristics of spindle cell myxoid liposarcoma hitherto have been reported once in the literature [167] and showed constant presence of spindle malignant cells with an admixture of round cells in approximately half of the cases. A myxoid background was present in 62% of cases and arborizing vascular structures were present in 38% of cases. Some tumors may show cytonuclear atypia, but mitotic figures are absent. More than 110 cases of myxoid liposarcoma were reported [164,167,172,174,176,182,183]. The typical translocation t(12;16)(q13;p11) detected by cytogenetical analysis as well as the fusion transcript CHOP-TLS also detected by molecular analysis strongly confirm the accurate diagnosis.

6.4.1.5 *FNA Key Features.* The following are in favor of the diagnosis:

— Aboundant myxoid background
— Lipoblasts
— Round cells and/or spindle-shaped cells
— Vessels

The following is a difficulty in diagnosis:

— Lack of lipoblasts

The following is evidence against a diagnosis:

— Physalipherous cells

6.4.2 Myxofibrosarcoma

Once considered a specific type of malignant fibrous histiocytoma, the myxoid variant has been reclassified as a low-grade myxoid fibrosarcoma and as a myxoid malignant fibrous histiocytoma grade II. Such designation is applied to malignant spindle cell tumors depicting a morphological component of more than 50% of myxoid matrix. For the purpose of this review, we will consider both entities under the same roof. They do differ by their cellular characteristics, with myxofibrosarcoma depicting spindle cells with minimal atypia, hence some overlap with entities included in the "low-grade spindle cell pattern," and myxoid malignant fibrous histiocytoma consist of spindle/round cells with moderate-to-marked atypia. Whatever their designation, they are members of the same nosologic entity at different stages of maturation.

Myxofibrosarcoma, a term coined by Scandinavian investigators [184], originally designated a mesenchymal tumor characterized by a myxoid matrix and a spindle cell component of fibroblastic differentiation. Nearly at the same time, similar tumors were included in the group of "myxoid variant of malignant fibrous histiocytoma" [185]. The concept of malignant fibrous histiocytoma has been revisited extensively, and myxofibrosarcoma has become a well-accepted term and studies particularly have focused on the low-gade variant of myxofibrosarcoma [186,187]. Myxofibrosarcoma, as a whole group, is a common sarcoma in the extremities and affects elderly patients. Trunk, head and neck, and retroperitoneum are also sites of predilection. In one large series of cases [186], nearly 70% were located in the dermal and subcutaneous tissues. Local recurrence was independent of histologic grade, but metastasis was related to intermediate- and high-grade neoplasms. As expected, the deeper the tumors, the higher the incidence of metastasis. It also is well recognized that tumors tend to become high grade in recurrences. The low-grade fibromyxosarcoma deserves particular attention given its better prognosis, provided that its morphological criteria are well identified (i.e., superficial location and cellular composition) and that proper treatment is instituted to avoid local recurrence and progression to a higher neoplastic process.

Cytomorphological analysis of myxofibrosarcoma is limited particularly in its low-grade variant [188,189] with more emphasis having been demonstrated extensively for the higher grade neoplasms. In their morphological composition, they resemble more myxoid areas of fasciitis, myxoid dermatofibrosarcoma protuberans, and cellular myxoma from which they are to be differentiated.

6.4.2.1 *Histopathology.*

A wide spectrum of morphologic features characterize myxofibrosarcoma. The low-grade variant depicts more than 50% of the myxoid component. As already stated, they tend to be smaller tumors, frequently developing in the dermal and subcutaneous tissues. They are sometimes multinodular, limited by a pseudocapsule. The degree of cellularity is inversely proportional to the amount of myxoid stroma. The cellular component with spindle, polygonal, or stellated cells show minimal atypia (Fig 6.176). The matrix contains a network of curvilinear-shaped blood vessels, often depicting a virtual lumen more or less reminiscent of myxoid liposarcoma (Figs 6.177 and 6.178. Vacuolated cells are different from true lipoblasts because they stain for mucins and not neutral fat and constitute matrix pseudoinclusions within the cytoplasm, such it has been demonstrated by electron microscopy [190].

Their immunohistochemical profile does not contribute to the precision of the diagnosis, nor to their molecular genetic profile showing complex karyotypes, some

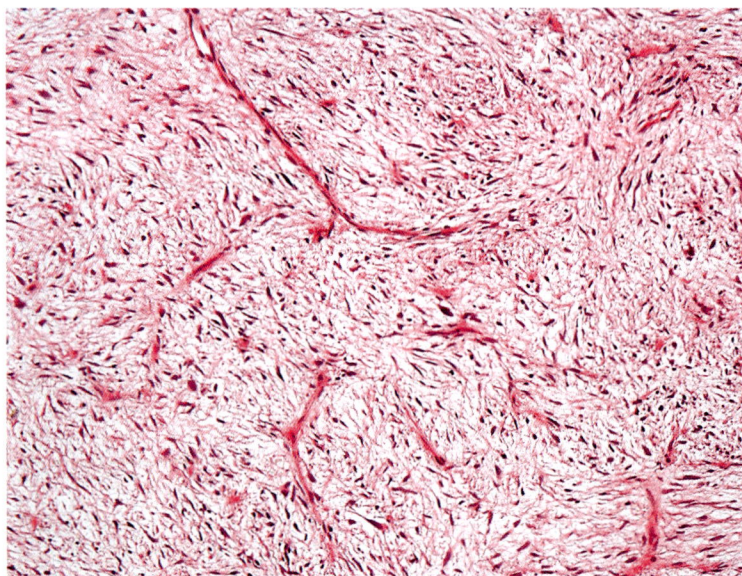

FIG 6.176 Myxofibrosarcoma, low-grade myxofibrosarcoma depicting spindle polygonal, or stellated cells in an abundant myxoid stroma.

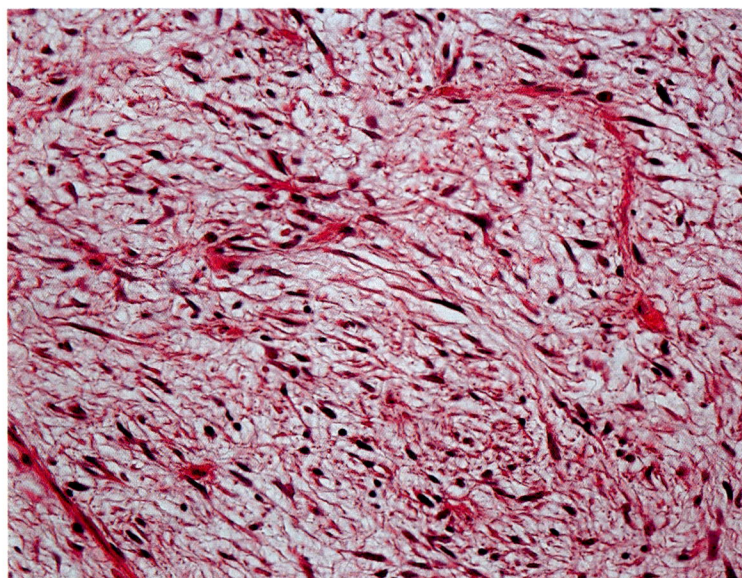

FIG 6.177 Myxofibrosarcoma, curvilinear-shaped vasculature sorrounded by atypical spindle and stellated cells with minimal atypias.

of which are shared with other high-grade sarcomas. Rare examples of low-grade myxofibrosarcoma harbor a supernumerary ring chromosome like in other low-grade sarcomas (e.g., dermatofibrosarcoma protuberans and juxtacortical osteosarcoma [191,192]).

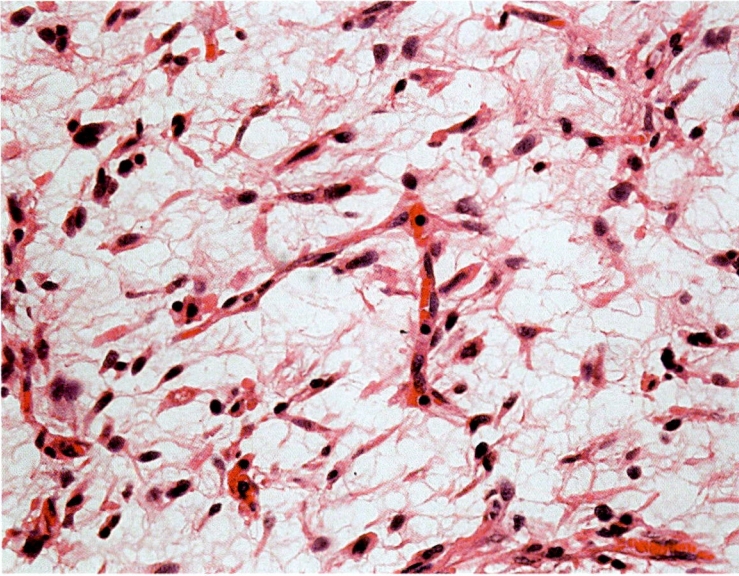

FIG 6.178 Myxofibrosarcoma, same case as in Fig 6.177. Higher magnification.

6.4.2.2 Cytopathology. Smears are cell-rich and stroma-rich. They are consistently composed of isolated and regular small spindle-shaped and stellated cells with elongated nuclei containing small inconspicuous nucleoli (Figs 6.179 and 6.180). Cytoplasm is pale with elongated processes. Roundish cells without a specific pattern are also observed in most cases. Moderate cytonuclear atypia (Figs 6.181 and 6.182) and occasional multinucleated giant cells may be present. A background of an abundant myxoid stroma (Fig 6.183), as well as curvilinear vascular structures, are always observed (Figs 6.184 and 6.185). Few ramifications of capillaries are observed (Fig 6.186). Those are isolated or intermingled with clusters of spindle-shaped cells. There are no eosinophilic fragments of connective tissue.

6.4.2.3 Differential Diagnosis. The following entities should be differentiated from myxofibrosarcoma:

— Myxoid liposarcoma
— Myxoma
— Myxoid malignant fibrous histiocytoma

Myxofibrosarcoma should be differentiated from other myxoid tumors like myxoid malignant fibrous histiocytoma, myxoid liposarcoma, and myxoma, but this differentiation is difficult because of overlapping features with many other low-grade myxoid lesions.

Myxoid malignant fibrous histiocytomas consist of fibroblast-like cells and histiocyte-like elongated cells with slight-to-moderate nuclear atypia predominant in low-grade tumors, whereas polygonal or round cells with one or more nuclei and marked nuclear atypia predominate in high-grade tumors [188]. Malignant fibrous

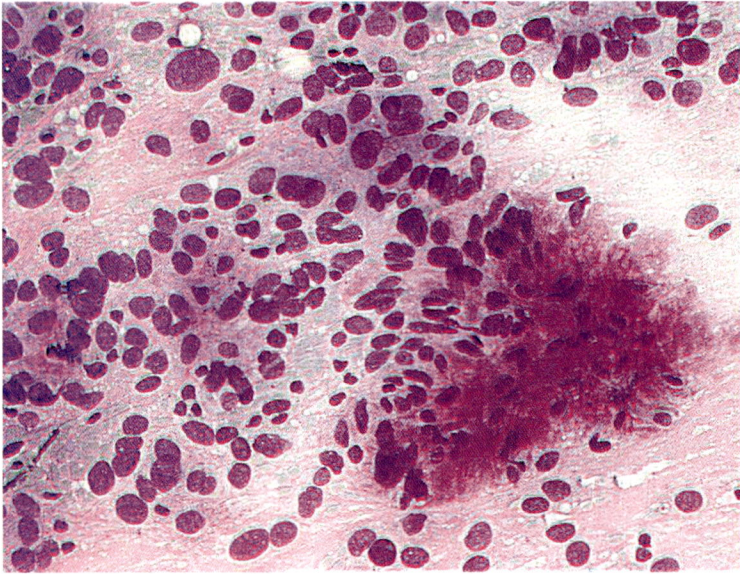

FIG 6.179   Myxofibrosarcoma, isolated and regular small spindle-shaped and stellated cells. Myxoid background.

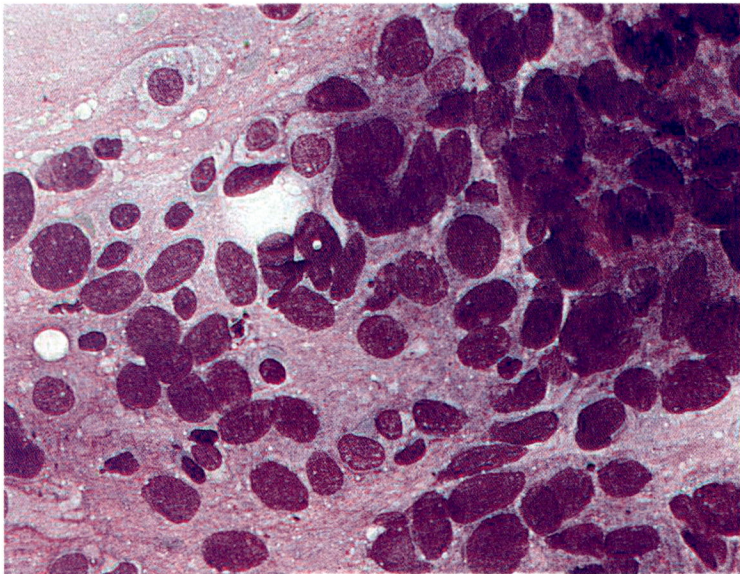

FIG 6.180   Myxofibrosarcoma, isolated and regular small spindle-shaped and stellated cells. Malignant character is evident.

histiocytomas are morphologically similar, but cytonuclear atypia usually is present. Cytologically, low-grade myxofibrosarcoma is different from myxoid malignant fibrous histiocytoma, because the former shows an abundant myxoid background as well as oval-to-spindle cells with minimal plemorphism. Inversely, high-grade

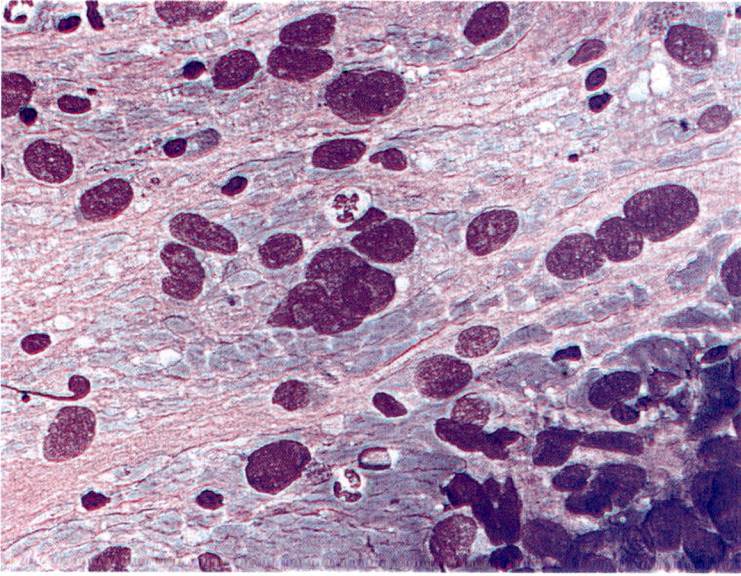

FIG 6.181   Myxofibrosarcoma, moderate cytonuclear atypia.

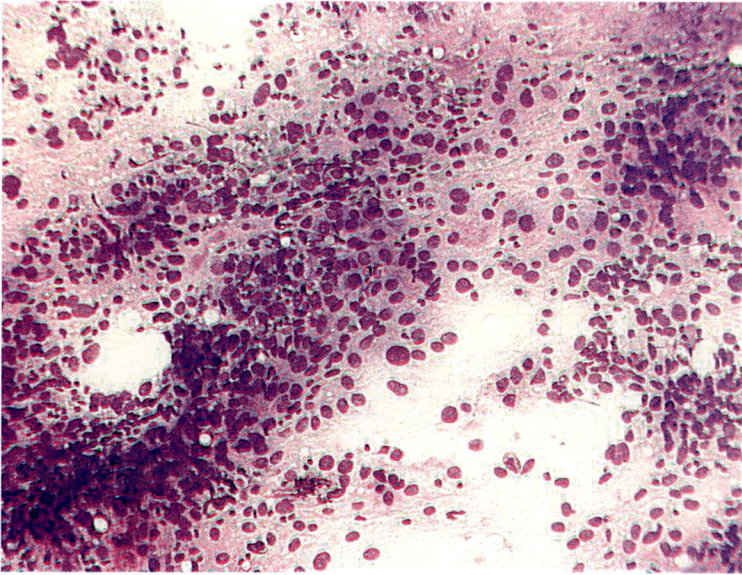

FIG 6.182   Myxofibrosarcoma, moderate cytonuclear atypia. Myxoid background.

myxofibrosarcoma is similar to myxoid malignant fibrous histiocytoma because cytonuclear atypia and giant cells may be observed.

Myxoid liposarcoma also could resemble myxofibrosarcoma, but usually, smears show the presence of lipoblasts. When absent, differential diagnosis is not possible.

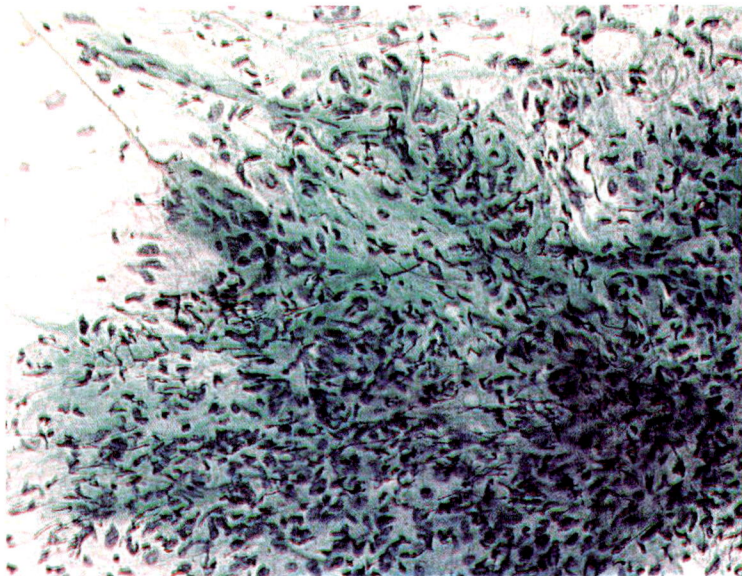

FIG 6.183 Myxofibrosarcoma, abundant myxoid stroma.

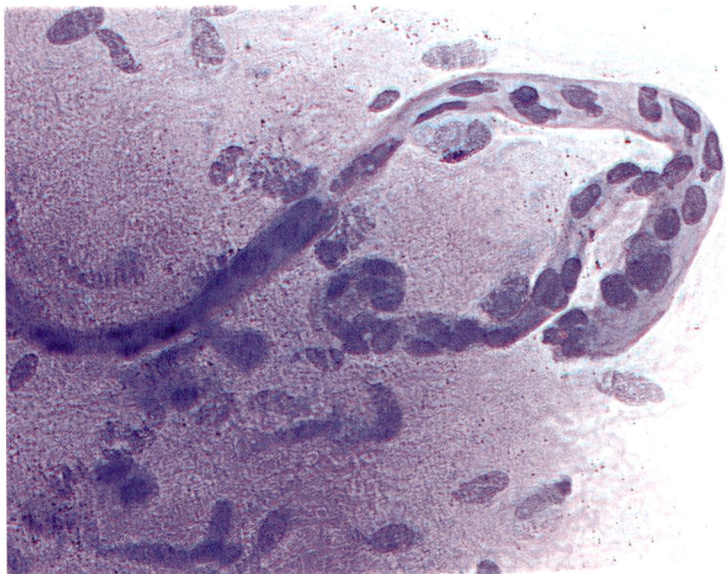

FIG 6.184 Myxofibrosarcoma, curvilinear vascular structures.

In round or spindle-shaped cells variants of myxoid liposarcoma, the tumors are more cellular and atypical; this is helpful to differentiate from myxofibrosarcoma. The vascular network observed in both myxofibrosarcoma and myxoid liposarcoma could be responsible for the difficulty in separating both tumors [167].

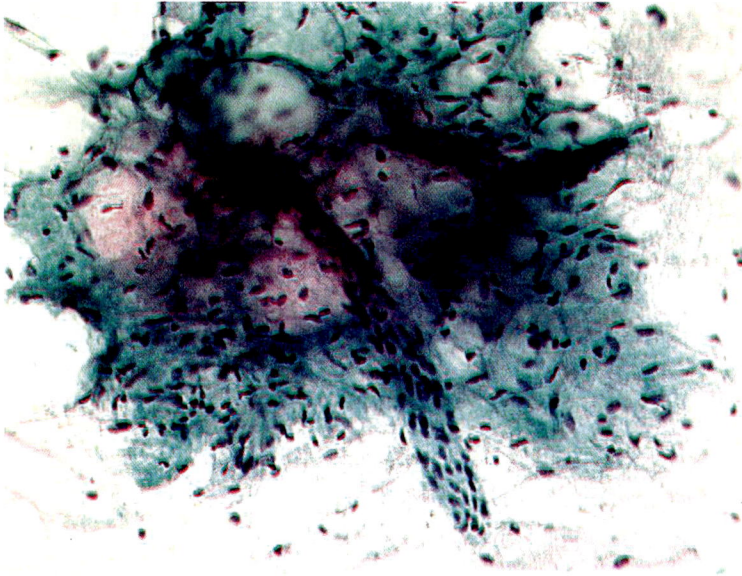

FIG 6.185 Myxofibrosarcoma, curvilinear vascular structures.

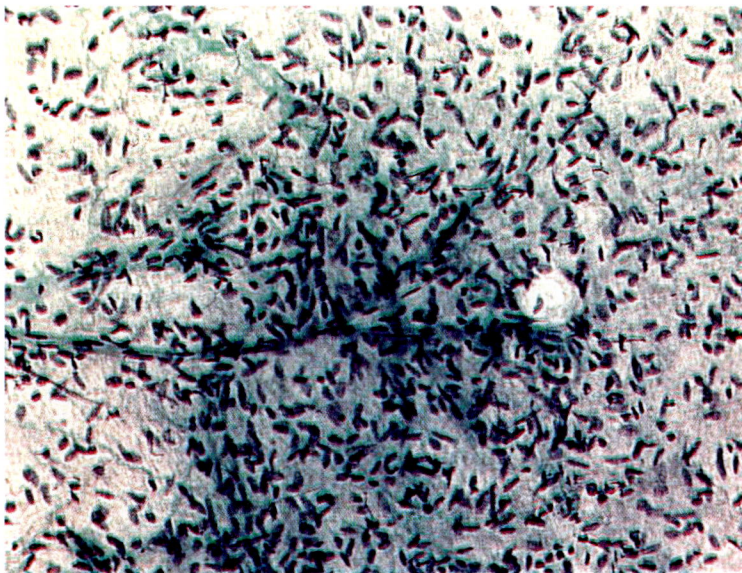

FIG 6.186 Myxofibrosarcoma, ramifications of capillaries.

Cellular myxoma is an intermediate lesion between intramuscular myxoma and low-grade myxoid fibrosarcoma. This entity may be difficult to differentiate because the smears show the presence of atypical cells with some elongated nuclei in a myxoid background. However, typical myxofibrosarcoma is a tumor of the superficial soft tissues of the extremities and is considered as a low-grade sarcoma.

6.4.2.4 Comments. The volume of the myxoid material is inversely proportional to the cellularity and grade. High-grade myxofibrosarcoma is more difficult to diagnose and is not distinguished easily from other adult pleomorphic sarcomas. In our series of 14 cases, 3 were rendered false-negative. There is a limited number of studies dealing with the cytology description of myxofibrosarcoma, particularly its low-grade variant, with more emphasis focused on higher grade neoplasms [188,193–195]. Only 21 cases have been reported in the English literature [170]. A series [194] of 13 cases showed that tumors consisted of spindle-shaped and roundish cells arranged in clusters. Other cases have shown an abundant myxoid background, spindle-shaped cells, and curvilinear vessels. In six additional cases [188,193] similar features were found, including spindle, stellated, and polymorphous cells within a myxoid granular to filamentous background. Capillary curvilinear vessels were also found but inconstantly. In our series, similar pitfalls to previous studies were noted [189]. All cases consisted of small regular, isolated, or clustered spindle-shaped cells, curvilinear vessels, and a myxoid background. Mild atypia was unusual and rather occurred in recurrent tumors. Two of 5 primary tumors were misdiagnosed as benign conditions, given the lack of cytonuclear atypia, mitotic figures, and necrosis. These results can be explained by the benign morphologic appearance of some myxoid neoplasms and by the limited number of such cases observed by the pathologists.

6.4.2.5 Clinical and FNA Key Features. The following are in favor of the diagnosis:

— Abundant myxoid background
— Isolated and regular small spindle-shaped and stellated cells
— Curvilinear-shaped blood vessels
— Extremities dermal and subcutaneous localization

The following are difficulties in the diagnosis:

— Round cells
— Giant multinucleated cells
— Lack of cytonuclear atypia

The following are evidence against a diagnosis:

— Lipoblasts
— High-grade atypical cells and mitotic figures
— Deep localization

6.4.3 Myxoid Leiomyosarcoma

Leiomyosarcoma has been discussed in the present review in the section of malignant spindle cell pattern. There is a limited number of studies in the literature deal with the so-called myxoid variant [196]. As a group, they do not differ significantly from their classical counterpart save for the presence of a myxoid stroma occupying more than 50% of the tissue examined. As expected, their occurrence in female patients is largely outnumbered by 14 to 4 in male patients. They have been described under three major histological architectures: fascicular, reticular/microcystic, and "myxofibrosarcoma-like," hence their inclusion in the differential diagnosis of the lesions of myxoid pattern.

In our previous study [168], myxoid leiomyosarcomas consisted of large amounts of myxoid matrix containing large spindle-shaped and giant tumor cells. Granular cytoplasm, blunt-ended nuclei, and intranuclear inclusions were consistently absent. Cases of myxoid leiomyosarcoma studied by cytology and retrieved from the literature showed the presence of an abundant myxoid matrix intermixed with randomly distributed isolated tumor cells or arranged in large cohesive clusters. The neoplastic cells vary from ovoid to spindle. Nuclei are round to ovoid, moderately pleomorphic, and contain small nucleoli.

The differentiation of myxoid leiomyosarcoma from other myxoid sarcomas (myxoid fibrosarcoma, myxoid liposarcoma, myxoid chondrosarcoma, and myxoid malignant fibrous histiocytoma) may be difficult. The presence of large numbers of tumor cell clusters and aggregates on cytologic smears is more representative of leiomyosarcoma and would be unusual in other myxoid malignancies (Figs 6.187–6.190).

6.4.4   Myxoma and Cellular Myxoma

Myxoma of soft tissue occurs in different body sites and is designated according to the following respective clinical settings: intramuscular myxoma, nerve sheath myxoma, and cutaneous myxoma. The present review only focuses on the intramuscular

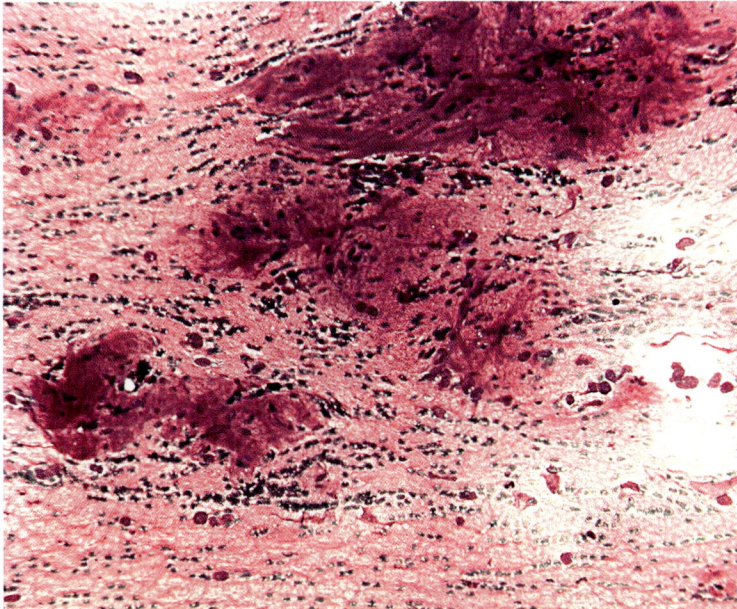

FIG 6.187   Myxoid leiomyosarcoma, myxoid background.

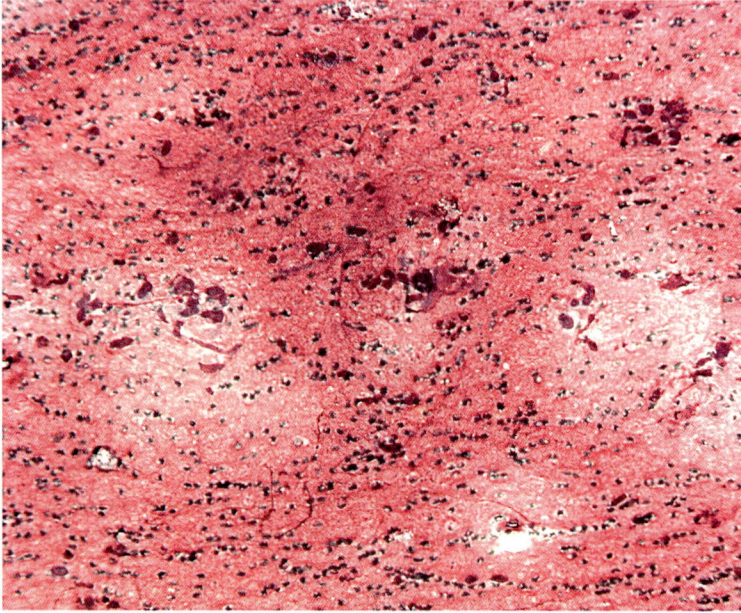

FIG 6.188 Myxoid leiomyosarcoma, myxoid background and scant cellularity.

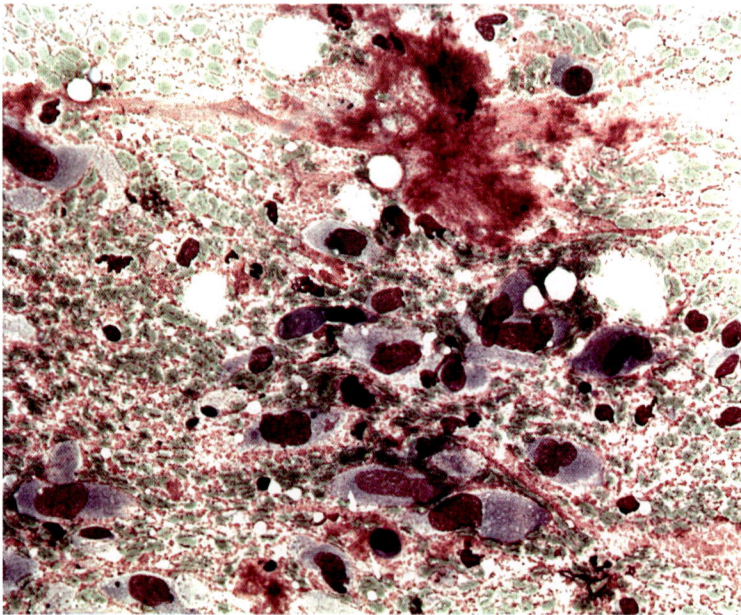

FIG 6.189 Myxoid leiomyosarcoma, spindle shaped, clearly malignant cells.

myxoma. The cellular variant of the latter also deserves some comment because its histologic composition, greater cellularity, and hypervascularization could raise concern of a myxoid sarcoma, although a large series has confirmed its indolent clinical behavior [147].

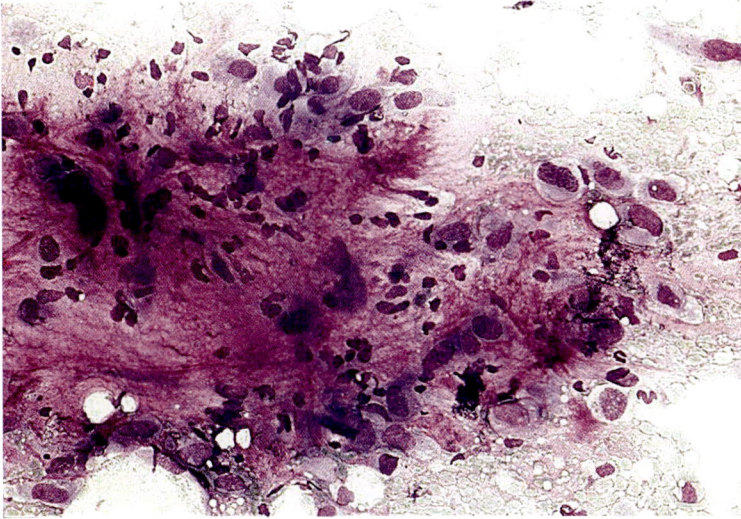

FIG 6.190 Myxoid leiomyosarcoma, roundish cells. This pattern may be present in other varieties of myxoid sarcomas.

Intramuscular myxoma is a benign soft tissue lesion of adult life with a female predominance (66%) and occurs predominantly in the limbs and is solitary. Multiple lesions are associated with fibrous dysplasia of the bone. Complete excision is curative. Their inclusion in the category of myxoid sarcoma is pertinent and justified. Because of their frequent deep location and their infiltrative character, they can easily simulate malignant myxoid sarcoma.

6.4.4.1 Histopathology. The following main features characterize benign myxoma: abundant myxoid matrix, small number of bland inconspicuous spindle-shaped or stellate-shaped cells, and a poorly developed vasculature (Fig 6.191). Despite their gross appearance of well-circumscribed lesions, they may infiltrate the adjacent musculature deeply (Fig 6.192). The immunohistochemical profile does not contribute to their differential diagnosis, save for the absence of expression of S-100 protein, in comparison with a positive expression of lipoblasts of myxoid liposarcoma. The matrix stains for mucins, which are digested completely by hyaluronidase. Apart from myxoid liposarcomas and other myxoid sarcomas, the following benign entities should be differentiated in the diagnosis, but they will not be discussed here: fasciitis, neurothekoma, myxoid neurofibroma, juxtaarticular myxoma, and "ganglion," entities in the group of angiomyxoid lesions of the genital tract such as aggressive angiomyxoma (Fig 6.193).

6.4.4.2 Cytopathology. In both myxoma and cellular myxoma, the smears are of low cellularity. Droplets of a highly viscous fluid typically characterize an aspirate (Fig 6.194). The cells have elongated cytoplasm (Fig 6.195). The nuclei are fusiform to oval with a bland chromatin pattern (Fig 6.196). Stellate cells and delicately branching capillaries also are present (Fig 6.197).

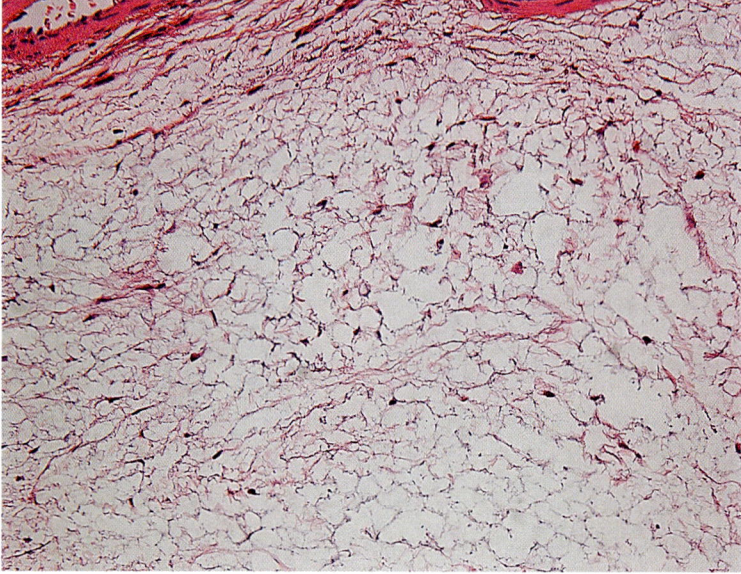

FIG 6.191 Myxoma, abundant myxoid stroma, paucity of cellular component, poorly developed vasculature are typical.

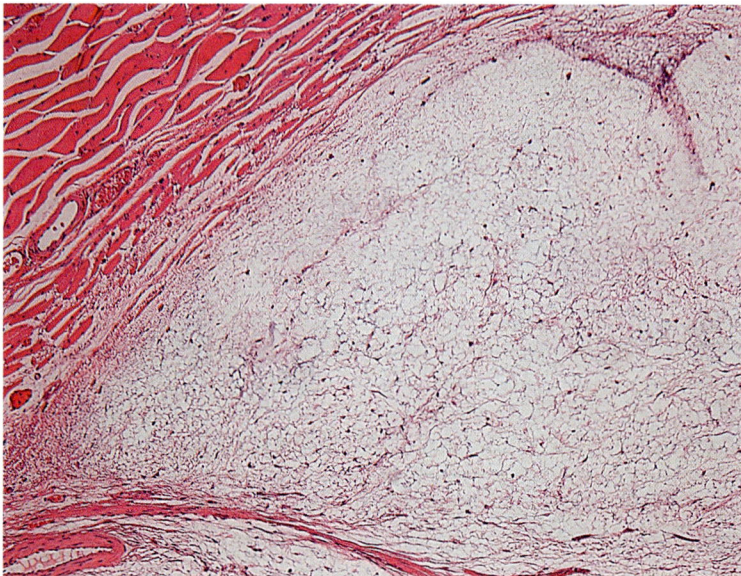

FIG 6.192 Myxoma, infiltration of adjacent muscle fibers.

6.4.4.3 *Differential Diagnosis.* The following entities should be differentiated from myxoma and cellular myxoma:

- Myxoid liposarcoma
- Low-grade myxofibrosarcoma
- Schwannoma, Antoni type B
- Neurofibroma
- "Ganglion" cyst

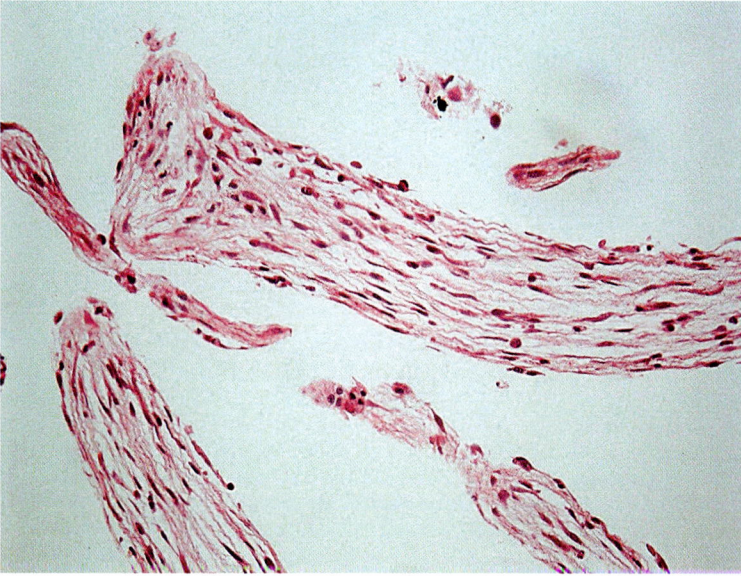

FIG 6.193 Cellular myxoma, biopsy specimen showing areas of relatively denser cellularity.

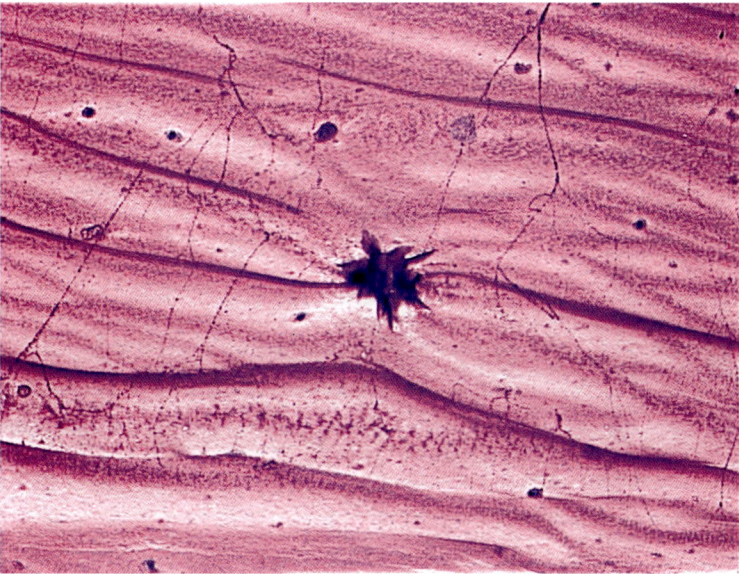

FIG 6.194 Myxoma, typical viscous and acellular fluid.

Myxomas should be differentiated from malignant myxoid sarcomas like low-grade myxofibrosarcoma and myxoid liposarcoma [198] as well as from benign myxoid lesions of the extremities, including myxoid schwannoma and neurofibroma, mesenchymal repair, and ganglion cyst [199] (Table 6.9). Once the myxoid stromal nature of the proliferation is recognized, a differential diagnosis of myxoid lesions can be considered along with a recommendation for open biopsy to establish the definitive diagnosis [200].

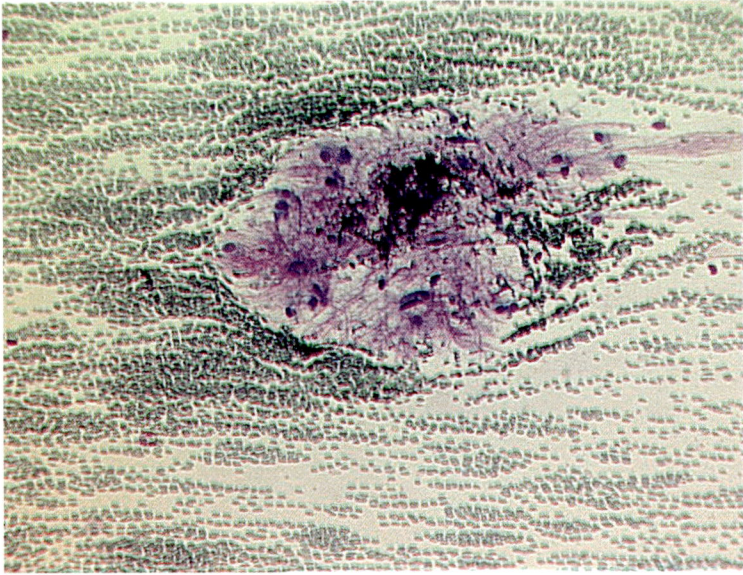

FIG 6.195 Myxoma, scant cells with elongated cytoplasm. Delicate myxoid background.

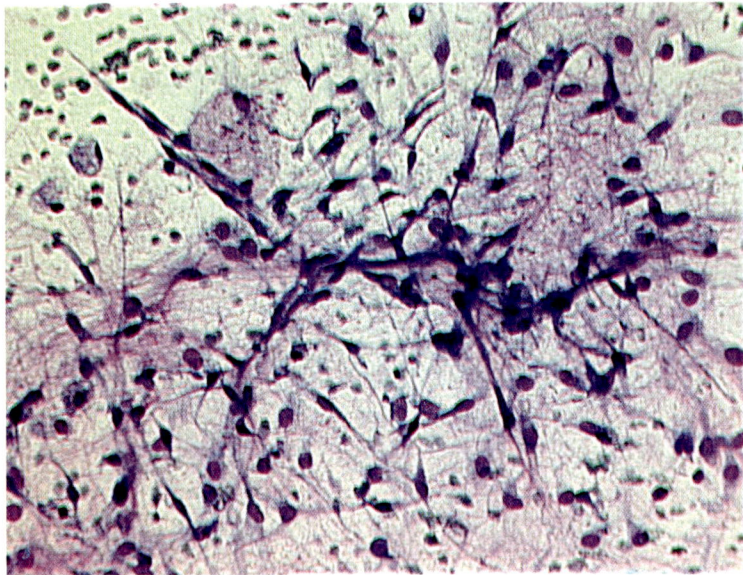

FIG 6.196 Cellular myxoma, fusiform-to-oval cells with a bland chromatin pattern.

6.4.4.4 Comments. Twenty-seven examples of myxoma have been published [198–201]). We have seen 13 examples of such a tumor. One case was misdiagnosed as myxoid sarcoma. Although the cytologic features are suggestive of myxoma, a definitive diagnosis is often difficult, owing to scant cellularity and to a lack of distinctive cytologic features. The radiology imaging findings may be used as an adjunct to the cytologic features to suggest a more confident diagnosis of

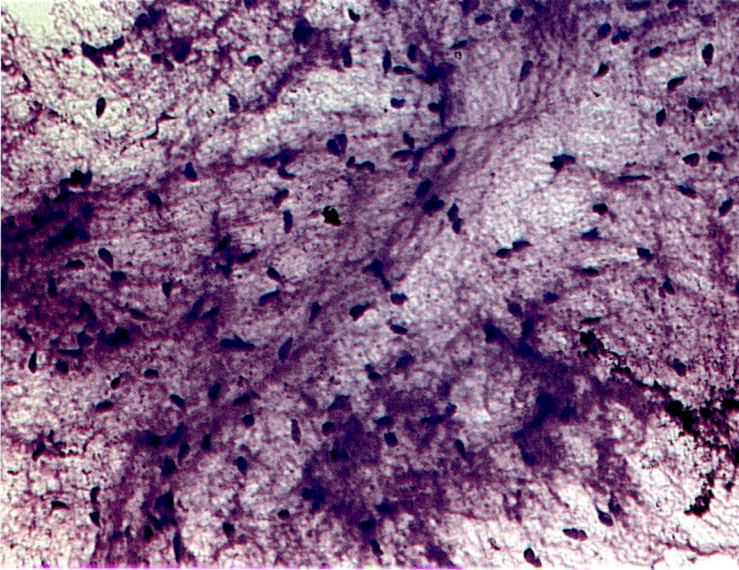

FIG 6.197   Cellular myxoma, stellate cells and delicately branching capillaries.

TABLE 6.9   Cytological differential diagnosis of myxoma

	Myxoma	Myxofibrosarcoma	Myxoid liposarcoma
Myxoid	++	+	++
Lipoblasts	−	−	+
Round	+/−	+	+
Spindle	++	++	+
Stellate	+	−	−

++; Frequent, +; rare, +/− occasionally seen, −; absent.

intramuscular myxoma [199]. Wakely et al. [201] studied the practicality of issuing a cytologic diagnosis of myxoma/juxta-articular myxoid lesion/ganglion. All cases except one (fat necrosis) were diagnosed correctly as benign myxoid lesions.

Aggressive angiomyxomas are uncommon but distinct soft-tissue neoplasms occurring predominantly in the pelvis and peritoneum of females, but they have been reported occasionally in association with inguinal hernias in males [200].

6.4.4.5   *FNA Key Features.*   The following are in favor of the diagnosis:

- Aboundant myxoid background with scant cellular component
- Stellate cells.

The following are difficulties in a diagnosis:

- Acellular myxoid material
- Occasionnal atypical cells

The following is evidence against a diagnosis:

- Lipoblasts
- High grade atypical cells
- Mitotic figures
- Vessels

6.4.5 Chordoma

Chordoma is a malignant tumor originating in the notochordal tissue and belongs to the group of bone tumors. Because of their rather indolent course characterized by a slowly growing tumor and an extension to adjacent soft tissues, they are discussed briefly in the present section of myxoid tumors. Chordomas are easily accessible for investigation by fine needle aspiration. Most chordomas do not present major problems of differential diagnosis because of their clinical features—location, and destruction of osseous structures—and their unique cellular composition. Extra-skeletal myxoid chondrosarcoma, myxopapillary ependymoma, and metastatic mucinous carcinoma of the colon can be confused with chordoma.

6.4.5.1 Histopathology. Histological composition is characterized by nests and cords of large, polygonal vacuolated cells embedded in a myxoid matrix (Fig 6.198). The cellularity is variable from tumor to tumor in terms of density and pleomorphism (Fig 6.199). There are two cell types: large uni- or multivacuolated cells sharply demarcated by delicate strands of cytoplasm (Fig 6.200)—the typical physalipherous cells—and smaller less numerous polygonal cells with moderate amounts of cytoplasm. The immunohistochemical profile is an adjuvant to

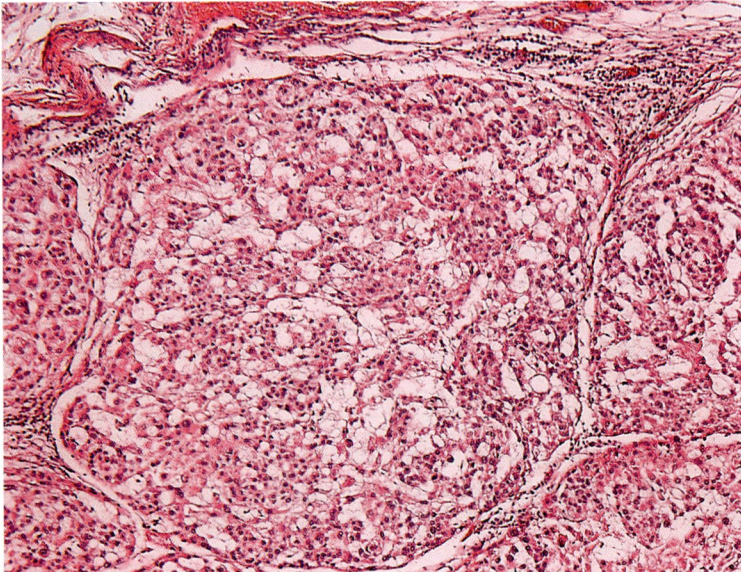

FIG 6.198 Chordoma, nests and cords of large, polygonal vacuolated cells.

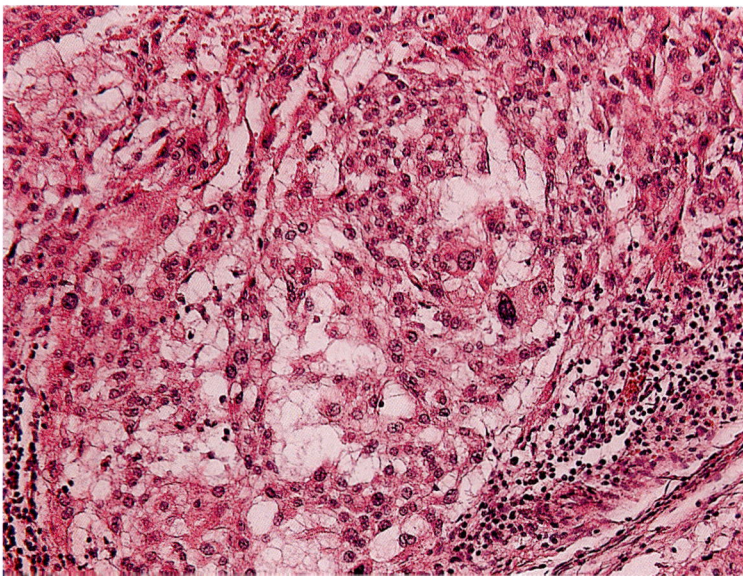

FIG 6.199 Chordoma, cellular density and pleomorphism are variable in the same tumor.

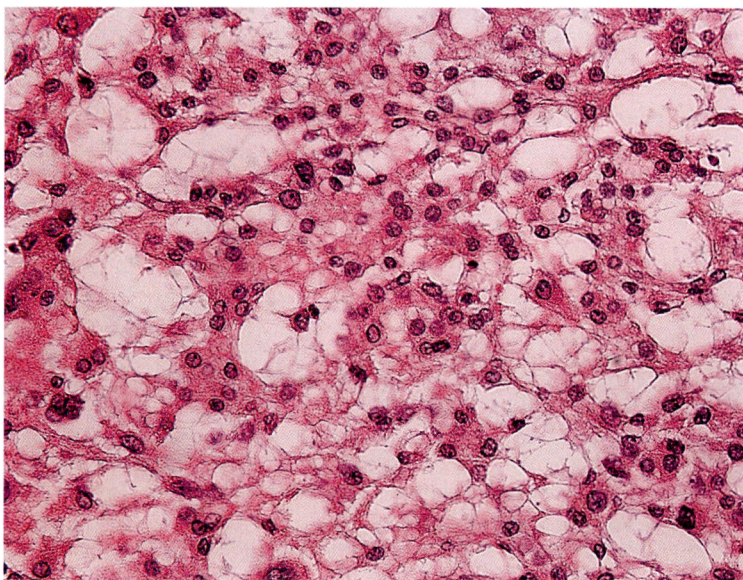

FIG 6.200 Chordoma, large physaliferous, multivacuolated, and smaller polygonal cells.

diagnosis. Chordoma express cytokeratin 19 and S-100 protein, whereas metastatic colon carcinoma express CK20 and is negative for S-100 protein, and myxoid chondrosarcoma is positive for S-100 protein (50% of cases) and rarely positive for CK20, but if it is, it is very focal.

6.4.5.2 *Cytopathology.* Smears are cell-rich and stroma-rich and are character-istic and unique in their morphology. Cells show two distinct populations; one consists of small, epithelial-like cells, and the other is characterized by physalipher-ous cells with clarified cytoplasm (Figs 6.201 and 6.202). Mitotic figures, multi-nucleated cells, and anaplastic cells also may be observed.

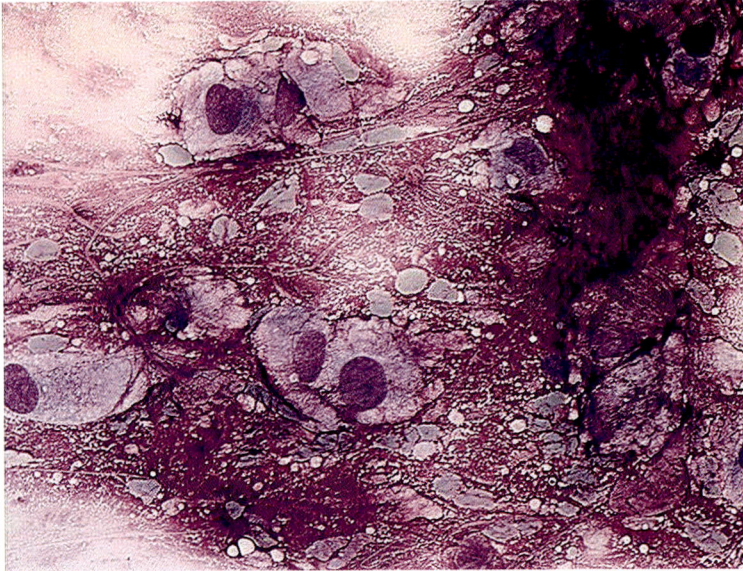

FIG 6.201 Chordoma, physaliphorous cells and specific magenta matrix.

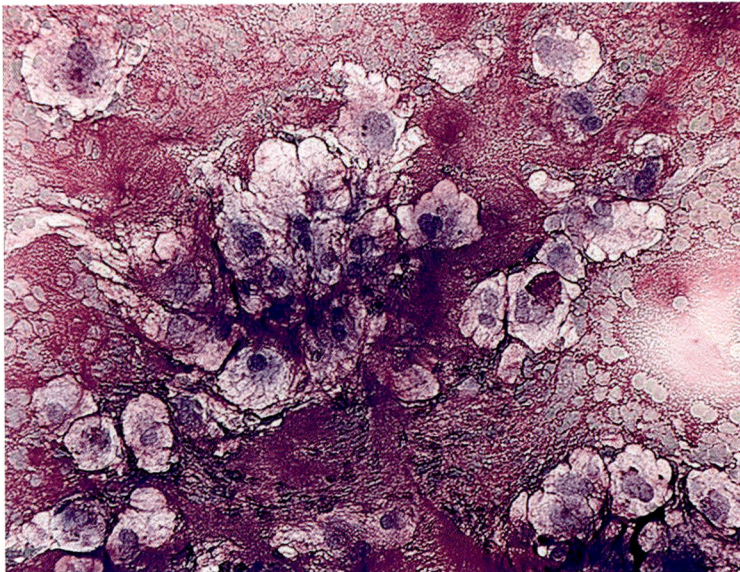

FIG 6.202 Chordoma, physaliphorous cells and specific magenta matrix. This pattern is characteristic.

The tinctorial reddish characteristic of chondroid matrix (in May–Grunwald-Giemsa [MGG] stain) is different than pink myxoid and greatly helps in the differential and accurate diagnosis.

Immunohistochemical demonstration of epithelial markers is useful to distinguish from chondrosarcoma.

6.4.5.3 Differential diagnosis. Because of various cytologic presentations and overlapping, chordoma should be differentiated from chondrosarcoma and metastatic clear cell carcinoma (Table 6.10). In chondroid chordomas, the smears are similar to those of well-differentiated chondrosarcomas, but they show a positive reaction for epithelial markers [202].

6.4.5.4 Comments. The cytologic features of chordoma are characteristic, especially on MGG-stained slides. Most smears are diagnosed accurately because of the cellular material and fibrillary background. Chordomas, however may show a large spectrum of differentiation. Chondroid chordomas may demonstrate polymorphous cells and stain positively for epithelial markers [202]. Dedifferentiated chordomas show sarcomatous components and need to be differentiated from malignant fibrous histiocytoma, fibrosarcoma, or osteosarcoma. Slides in such cases reveal a tumor of a high-grade malignancy comprising short atypical spindle cells containing modest amounts of granular cytoplasm. Physalipherous cells are absent, and myxoid material is scant [203]. Numerous examples of chordoma have been described in the cytology literature in the series and case reports [202–207]. We have studied 15 examples of chordoma. Eleven cases were diagnosed accurately, three cases were misdiagnosed as chondrosarcoma and one case was unsatisfactory for diagnosis.

6.4.5.5 Clinical and FNA Key Features. The following are in favor of the diagnosis:

- Clinical presentation
- Cellular material and fibrillary background
- Physalipherous cells

The following are difficulties in the diagnosis:

- Dedifferentiation resembling polymorphous sarcoma with myxoid
- Lack of physalipherous cells

The following is evidence against diagnosis:

- Chondroblasts, osteoblasts, spindle shaped cells

6.4.6 Extraskeletal Myxoid Chondrosarcoma

Although extraskeletal myxoid chondrosarcoma is a rare soft tissue sarcoma, much has been reported on all aspects of this neoplasm in the 30 last years. Once named "chordoid sarcoma," the designation of extraskeletal myxoid chondrosarcoma has come to be recognized despite a morphological spectrum varying from predominantly myxoid tumors to more solid ones [208]. The demonstration of a recurrent

TABLE 6.10 Cytological differential diagnosis between chordoma and chondrosarcoma

	Chordoma	Myxoid chondrosarcoma	Myxopapillary ependymoma
Myxoid	++	++	++
Chondroid	+/−	+	−
Round cells	++	++	++
Spindle cells	−	+/−	++
Physaliphorous cells	++	−	−

++; Frequent, +; rare, +/− occasionally seen, −; absent.

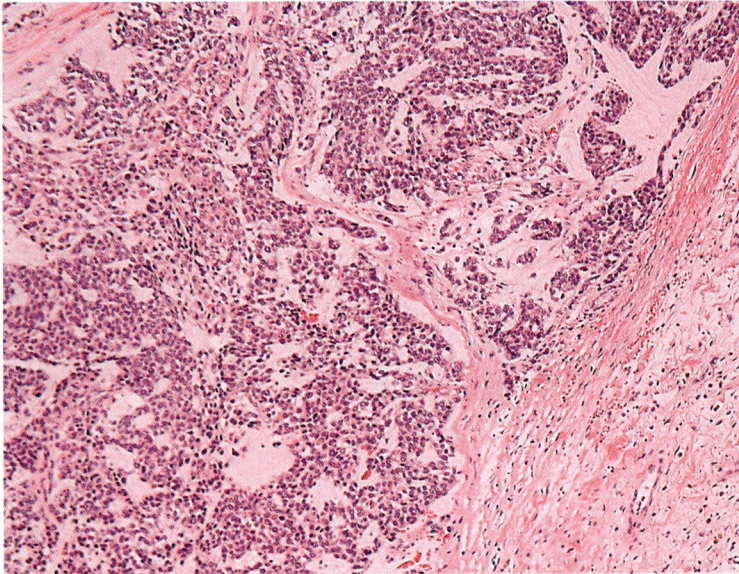

FIG 6.203 Extraskeletal myxoid chondrosarcoma, well-circumscribed tumor with lobular architecture.

t(9;22)(q22;q12) chromosome translocation resulting in the EWS/TEC protein has been well demonstrated with a prevalence of about 75% [209]. Less often, a second translocation t(9;17)(q22;q11) also is present.

Extraskeletal myxoid chondrosarcoma occurs principally in the deep soft tissues of the extremities. Similar tumors are found in the bones but does not harbor the afore-mentioned molecular genetics findings. Biologic behavior of extraskeletal myxoid chondrosarcoma is characterized by recurrence and metastasis, sometimes several years after the initial excision. Controversies surround its histoprognosis, with some reports suggesting that tumor cellularity could be predictive of its outcome [208,210−212]. Principal entities to consider in the differential diagnosis are myxoid liposarcoma, myxoid malignant fibrous histiocytoma, and for more solid tumors, mixed tumors of epithelial origin like chondroid syringoma.

6.4.6.1 *Histopathology.* Grossly, extraskeletal myxoid chondrosarcoma is a lobular-to-nodular mass, generally well circumscribed with a fibrous capsule, which is well demonstrated at low-power microscopic examination (Fig 6.203). Tumor cells

are grouped in short anastomosing cords, strands, or pseudoacini creating a lace-like pattern (Fig 6.204). Decreasing cellularity from the periphery of the lobules to their central parts creates a so-called "cobweb pattern." Pleomorphism is rare and the mitotic figures in typical cases are few in number (Fig 6.205). The extracellular

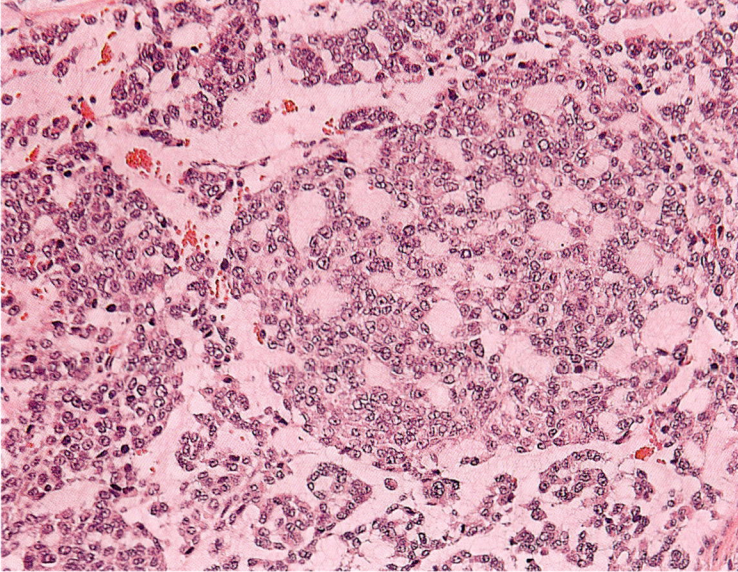

FIG 6.204   Extraskeletal myxoid chondrosarcoma, tumor cells are grouped in short anastomotic cords or strands.

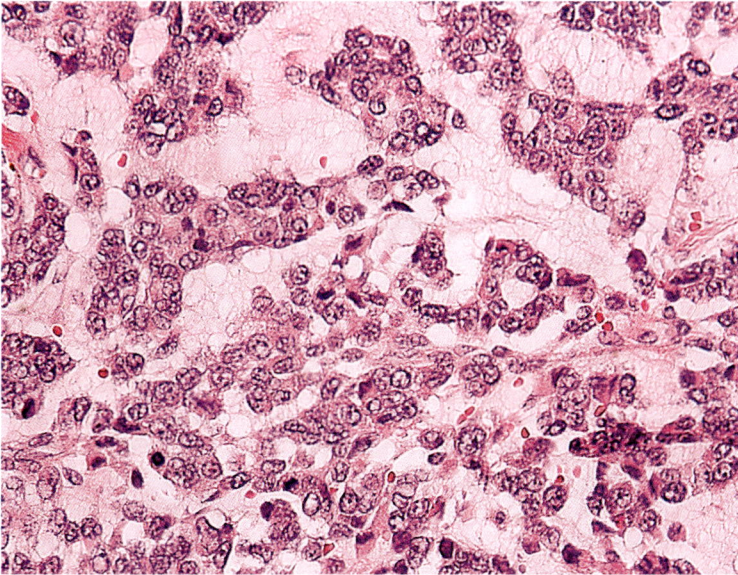

FIG 6.205   Extraskeletal myxoid chondrosarcoma, monotonous cell component with occasionnal mitosis and pseudoacini entrapping the myxoid stroma.

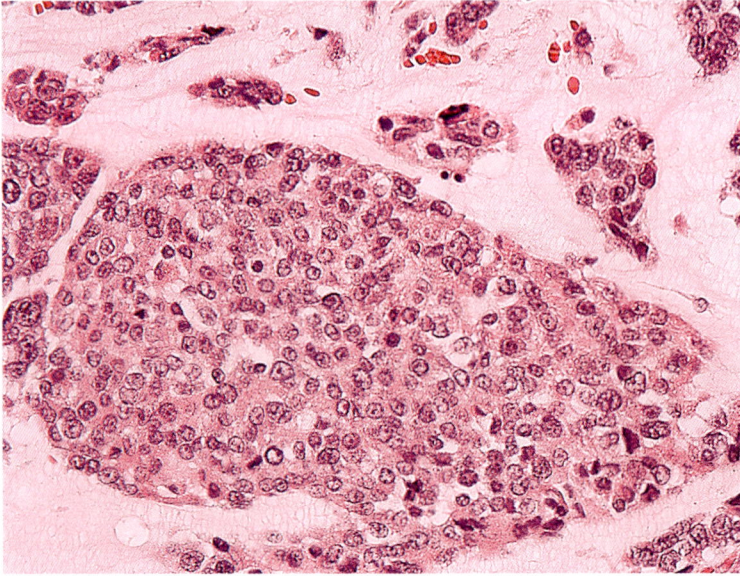

FIG 6.206 Extraskeletal myxoid chondrosarcoma, solid area of tumor cells surrounded by a rich myxoid stroma.

mucinous component is abundant (Fig 6.206) and stains with alcian blue that resists hyaluronidase digestion, which is indicative of acid mucopolysaccharides of sulfated radicals like chondroitin sulfates 4 and 6 and keratin-sulfates. The immunohisto-chemical profile is characterized by the expression of vimentin, S-100 protein in about 50% of the cases, and rarely, focal keratin positivity. As already stated, problems of differential diagnosis can be resolved by molecular genetic investigations. More solid areas of greater cellularity without any recognizable pattern resemble poorly differentiated carcinoma. The presence of islands of well-differentiated cartilagineous matrix containing chondrocytes grouped in rosettes is a feature occasionally observed.

6.4.6.2 Cytopathology. Cytological features in extraskeletal myxoid chondrosarcoma are distinct. Usually, smears are cell-poor and matrix-rich, but their presentation may vary depending on tumor histology. Cytology samples taken from chondroid areas contain a thin chondroid and metachromatic background that stains red using the MGG method. When matrix is abundant, chondroid lacunae with cells may be observed (Fig 6.207). Cytology samples taken from cellular areas contain either monotonous uniform, middle-sized, and roundish cells with frequently vacuolated cytoplasms or atypical polymorphous cells (Fig 6.208) with bland nuclei and grooves or pseudoinclusions. Occasionally, larger cells with pseudoepithelial morphology (Fig 6.209) and cells depicting a perinuclear halo are present. However, smears may show a cordlike pattern mimicking plates of hepatocytes. Mitotic activity is almost absent.

Ancillary techniques (FISH) show a positive 22q12 translocation, which confirms a diagnosis.

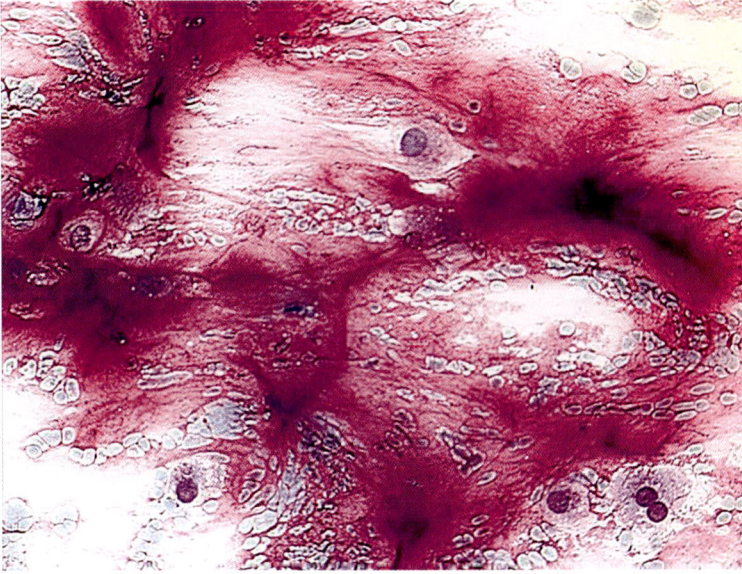

FIG 6.207 Extraskeletal myxoid chondrosarcoma, smears are cell-poor and matrix-rich.

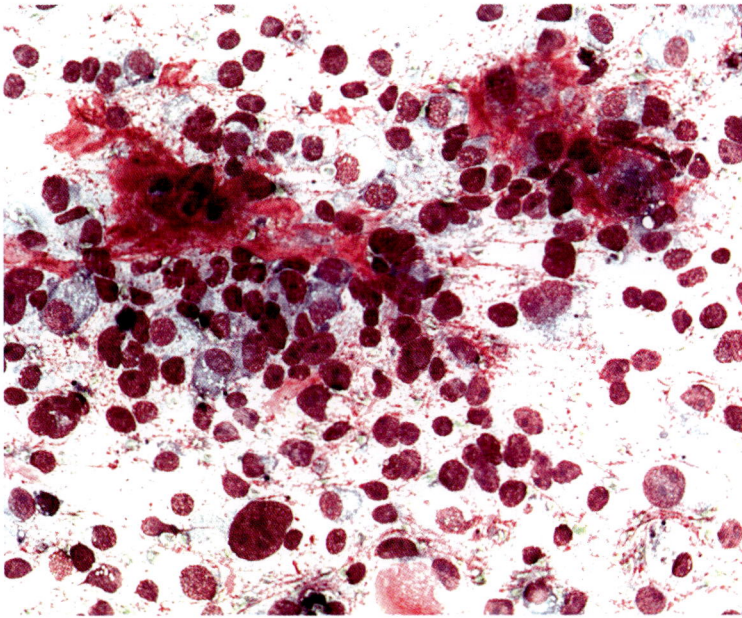

FIG 6.208 Extraskeletal myxoid chondrosarcoma, middle-sized, polymorphous roundish cells with frequently vacuolated cytoplasms. Scant myxoid.

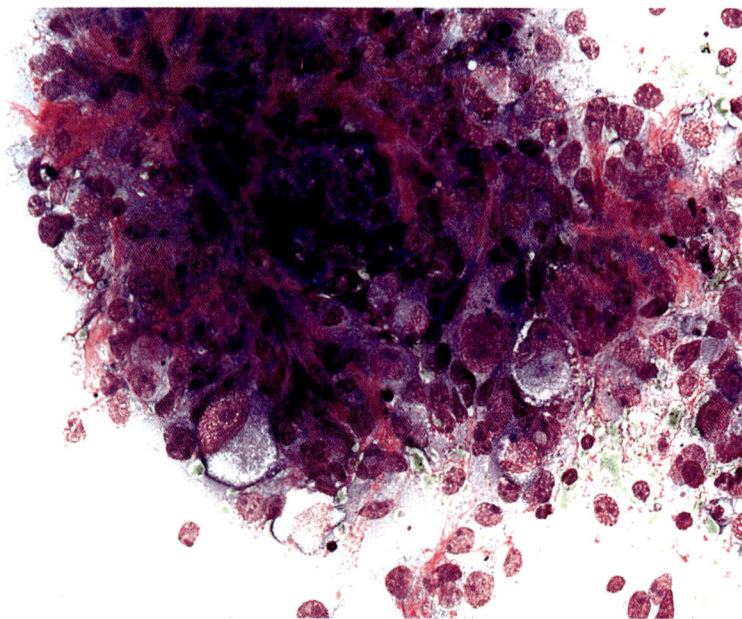

FIG 6.209 Extraskeletal myxoid chondrosarcoma, larger cells with pseudoepithelial morphology.

6.4.6.3 *Differential Diagnosis.* The following entities should be differentiated from extra sekeltal myxoid chondrosarcoma:

- Myxoid liposarcoma
- Chondroid syringioma
- Metastatic mucinous carcinoma
- Myxoid malignant fibrous histiocytoma
- Myxofibrosarcoma
- Myxoma

Extraskeletal myxoid chondrosarcoma should be differentiated from other tumors showing myxoid/chondroid stroma. Extraskeletal myxoid chondrosarcomas are different from myxoid liposarcomas in the lack of typical vasculature and lipoblasts. Myxofibrosarcoma show more nuclear atypia and pleomorphism. Myxomas usually consist of a myxoid background with rare stellate cells. Low-grade fibromyxoid sarcoma usually exhibits the spindle cell population and is a tumor predominantly cellular-rich and stroma-poor in mucin. Moreover, the cordlike arrangement is usually observed in extraskeletal myxoid chondrosarcoma, although it is observed rarely in other entities like the round cell variant of myxoid liposarcoma [213]. Chordoma, myxopapillary ependymoma, and metastatic mucinous adenocarcinoma are candidates in the differential diagnosis spectrum. Physaliperous cells and binucleation are specific for chordoma. "Goblet" or "signet ring" cells with a single distinct vacuole are in favor of mucinous adenocarcinoma [214].

6.4.6.4   Comments. FNA of extraskeletal myxoid chondrosarcoma can be accurate even in the absence of obvious chondroid differentiation but, in general, depends on the presence of uniform, round-to-oval chondroblasts often arranged in cords and set in an abundant myxoid/chondromyxoid background. Ancillary techniques are confirmatory when coupled with characteristic morphology [211,215]. Approximately 40 cases of extraskeletal myxoid chondrosarcoma have been reported [213,215,216]. We have noted three other examples; one was misdiagnosed as Ewing sarcoma because of numerous roundish cells.

6.4.6.5   FNA Key Features. The following are in favor of the diagnosis:

- Aboundant metachromatic myxoid background with lacunar spaces containing single cells
- Monotonous roundish cells with cordlike pattern or pseudoepithelial morphology

The following is a difficulty in making a diagnosis:

- Mitotic figures, hypercellularity

The following is evidence against a diagnosis:

- Vessels, lipoblasts, spindle-shaped cells

6.5   ATYPICAL LIPOMATOUS TUMORS

"The unpredictable fatty tumors" a paper written by Dr. A.P. Stout in the early 1950s in Annals of Surgery could be applied today for some atypical fatty tumors. However, better defined clinical and pathological features of those tumors in conjunction with cytogenetic and molecular analysis gained importance and help in characterizing those atypical lesions. Nevertheless, one has to recognize that in day-to-day practice the pathologist/cytologist still is faced with the difficult task of accurately diagnosing some fatty tumors. Entities such as spindle cell lipoma and its morphological variant, pleomorphic lipoma, and well-differentiated liposarcoma/atypical lipoma are included in this category. The wide variety of benign lipomas are excluded from the present review (e.g., angiolipoma, myolipoma, chondroid lipoma, etc).

6.5.1   Well-Differentiated liposarcoma / Atypical Lipoma

In the World Health Organization (WHO) classification of liposarcomas, well-differentiated liposarcoma is subclassified in lipoma-like, inflammatory, and sclerosing types. Dedifferentiated tumors belong also to this subgroup given their cytogenetic and molecular characteristics. It is now accepted that well-differentiated liposarcoma, atypical lipoma, and atypical lipomatous tumor are different terms of the same entity (i.e. well-differentiated liposarcoma). Tumors originating in the subcutaneous tissues of limbs and trunk preferably are termed "atypical lipoma" given their biological behavior, devoid of metastatic potential and serious consequences, whereas similar morphologic tumors in deep locations of the limbs (e.g., intramuscular) and the retroperitoneum are called well-differentiated liposarcoma. Well-differentiated liposarcoma is the most common form observed during late adult life. Peak incidence is reached during the sixth and seventh decades of life. Armed Forces Institute of Pathology (AFIP) and Mayo clinic files [217,218] show that 75% developed in deep muscles of the extremities and 20% in the retroperitoneum, with the remainder affecting the groin and other various sites. They are usually large and multilobular masses often mistaken for lipomas at gross examination. As already mentioned, they are nonmetastasizing tumors. However, their rate of recurrence and disease-related mortality are influenced strongly by their location. The recurrence rate for the retroperitoneal tumors approaches nearly 100%. A second harmful outcome is dedifferentiation, and in such cases, sarcomas of intermediate and high grades are found.

6.5.1.1 Histopathology. Lipoma-like liposarcoma, as its name indicates, resembles lipoma. Subtle differences such as variation in volume and configuration of adipocytes could be the only feature found (Fig 6.210). The number of lipoblasts is variable, and it is recognized that they are not a "sine qua non" for the diagnosis of well-differentiated liposarcoma, hence the limitation of fine needle aspirates in the diagnostic approach. The occurrence of variable numbers of spindle cells with hyperchromatic nuclei could be suggestive of malignancy, although it is not specific (Fig 6.211). Hypercellular tumors, which often require extensive sampling of the tumor, could be present. Sclerosing forms have a predilection for the groin and the retroperitoneum (Fig 6.212). In large tumors, it is not rare for the three subtypes of liposarcoma to merge and overlap. Obviously, the entities to consider in the

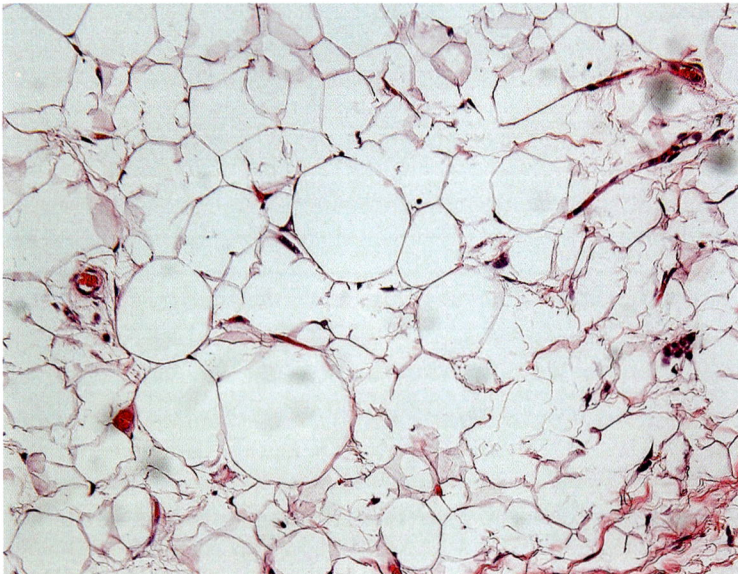

FIG 6.210 Well-differentiated liposarcoma/atypical lipoma, variation in volume and configuration of adipocytes

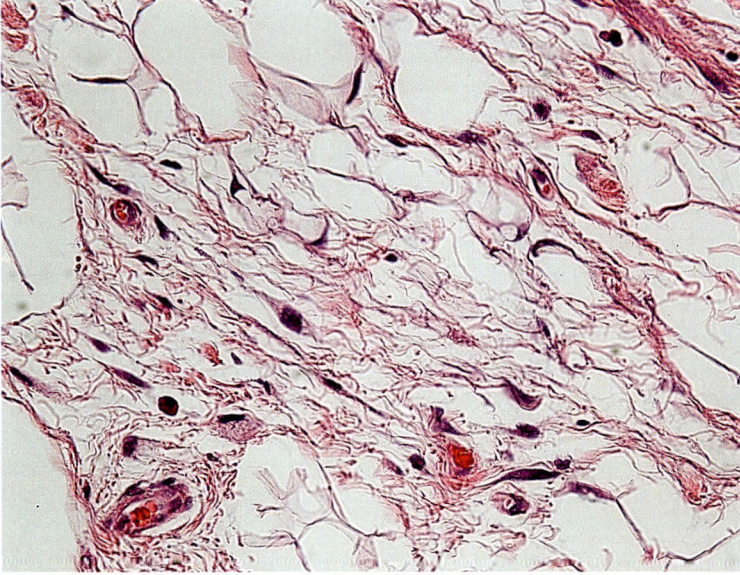

FIG 6.211 Well-differentiated liposarcoma/atypical lipoma, spindle cells with hyperchromatic nuclei admixed with adipocytes of variable configuration.

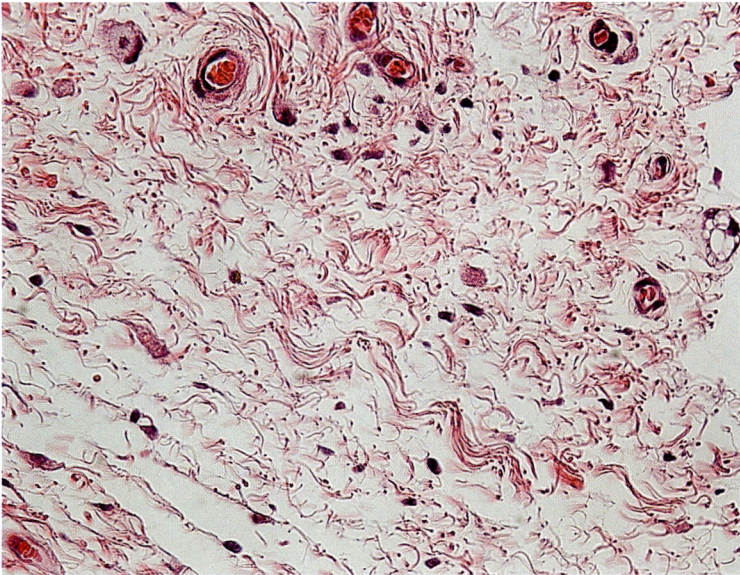

FIG 6.212 Well-differentiated liposarcoma/atypical lipoma, area of a lipoma-like liposarcoma depicting multivacuolated lipoblast and small round atypical cells.

differential diagnosis are lipomas and their morphological variants including spindle cell and pleomorphic lipoma.

The immunohistochemical profile does not contribute to the precision of the diagnosis. However, well-differentiated liposarcoma have unique and specific genetic and molecular features. They consistently show amplified sequences of 12q13-q15 [219,220]. *MDM2* and CDK4 genes harbor the mutations that can be demonstrated readily by immunohistochemical methods. They are specific and constitute an example of a sarcoma with a simple genetic profile, similar to recognized translocations. This is a powerful tool to differentiate well-differentiated liposarcoma from some forms of large infiltrating lipomas.

6.5.1.2 *Cytopathology.* Smears are cell-poor and stroma-poor. Interestingly, well-differentiated liposarcoma constantly consist of adult lipocytes, occasional lipoblasts (Fig 6.213), and an admixture of round or spindle cells (Figs 6.214 and 6.215). Usually, the characteristic adipocytic cells with intracytoplasmic vacuoles of variable size are observed (Figs 6.216–6.218). Nuclei are usually small and regular. Low-grade dedifferentiated and sclerosing liposarcomas mainly consist of spindle or round cells (Fig 6.219), but lipoblasts also may be present. Cytonuclear atypia or mitotic figures are rare. Myxoid or vascular arborizing structures are extremely scant or absent.

6.5.1.3 *Differential Diagnosis.* The following entities should be differentiated from well-differentiated liposarcoma:

– Lipoma
– Spindle cell lipoma
– Pleomorphic lipoma

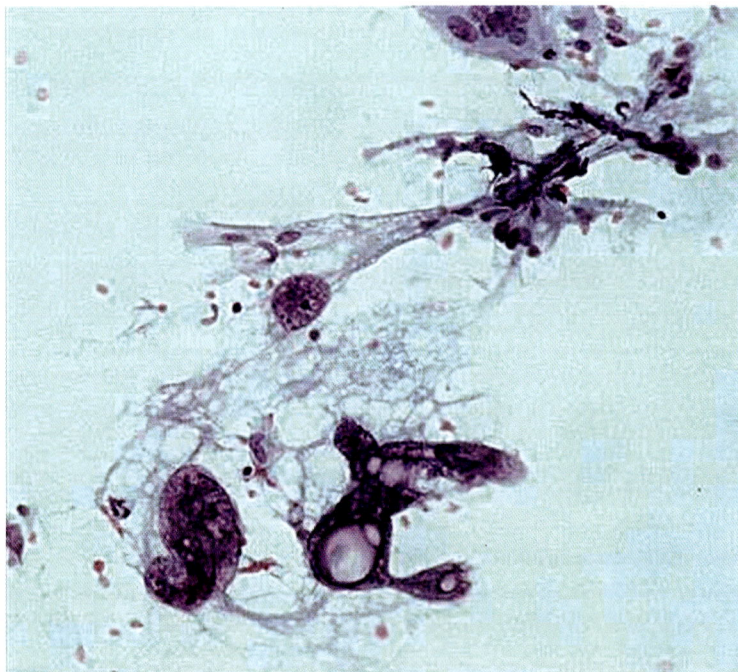

FIG 6.213 Well-differentiated liposarcoma, atypical adipocytic cells.

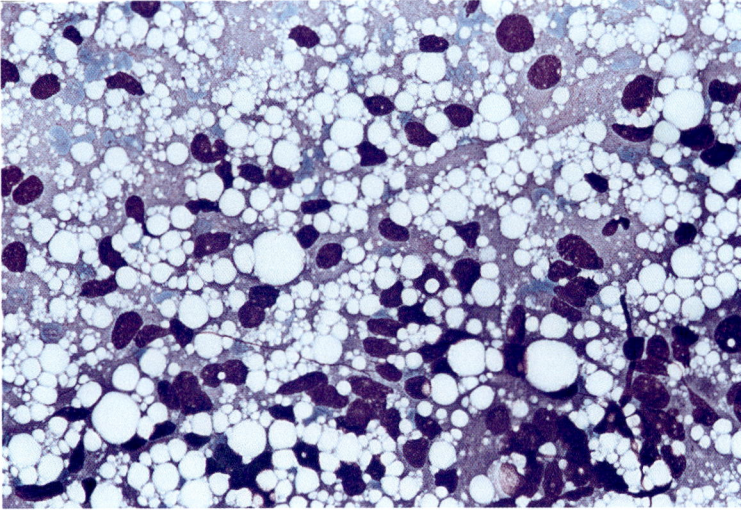

FIG 6.214 Well-differentiated pleomorphic liposarcoma. Microvacuolated lipoblasts.

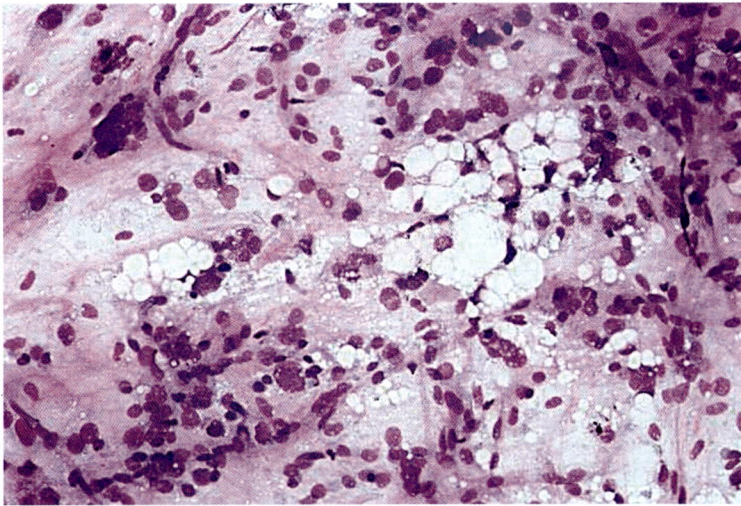

FIG 6.215 Well-differentiated liposarcoma, area of cells with scant myxoid. Numerous lipoblasts.

Well-differentiated liposarcoma should be differentiated from atypical lipoma and hibernoma, spindle cell lipoma, and pleomorphic lipoma (Table 6.11). Well-differentiated liposarcoma and atypical lipoma are cytologically similar. They are better categorized based on their anatomical location, with the term of atypical lipoma being privileged for tumors of superficial location in the trunk and the extremities, whereas tumors of deep soft tissues of extremities and retroperitoneum are classified as well-differentiated liposarcoma. Moreover, the extreme rarity of typical lipoblasts in superficial well-differentiated liposarcoma/atypical lipomas does not allow differentiating the entities from classical lipomas. Spindle cell lipoma presents the following distinctive cytological

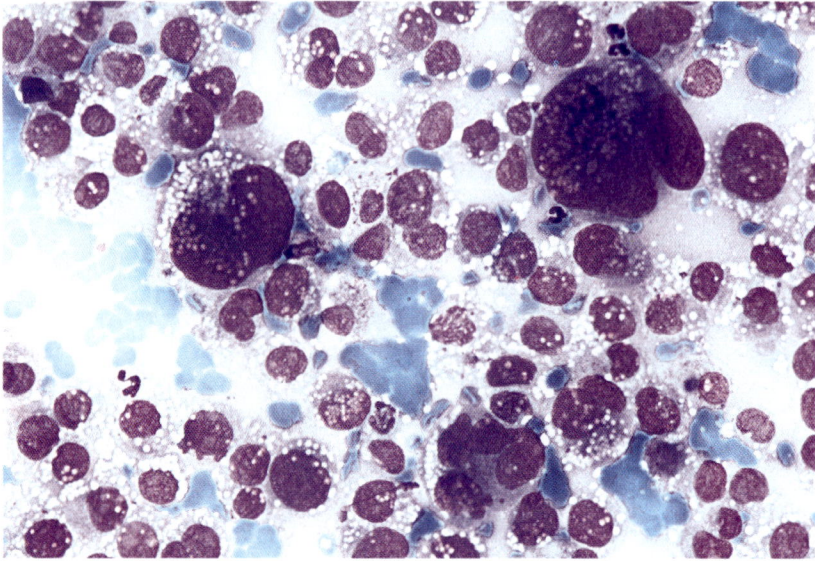

FIG 6.216   Well-differentiated liposarcoma, adipocytic cells with intracytoplasmic vacuoles of variable size and shape.

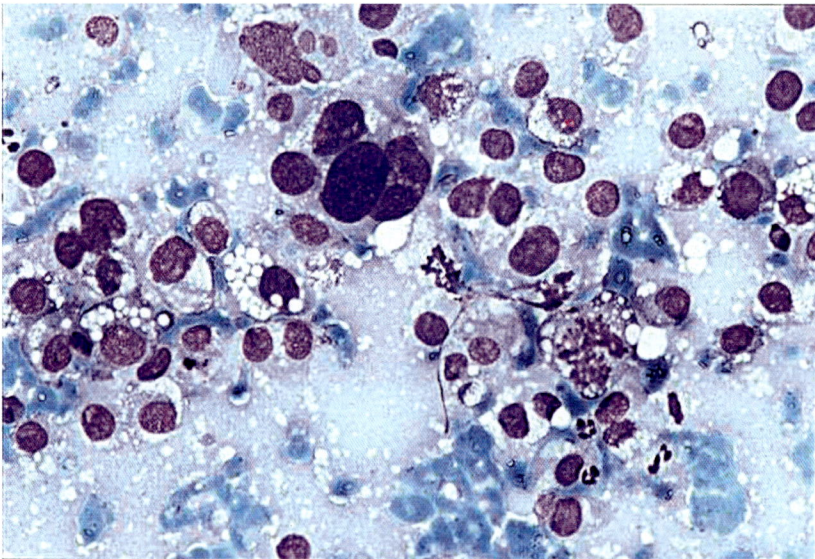

FIG 6.217   Well-differentiated liposarcoma, lipoblasts and atypical cells.

features: mature adipocytes, uniform spindle cells, and bundles of collagen [221]. Uniformity of spindle cells also may be present in well-differentiated liposarcoma. Hibernoma may have cytological characteristics overlapping with well-differentiated liposarcoma. Cytologically, hibernoma consists of small, round, and brown fat-like cells

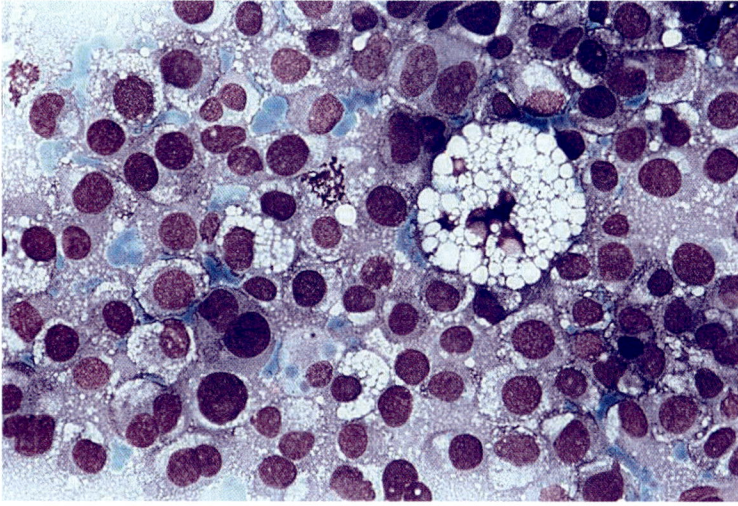

FIG 6.218 Well-differentiated liposarcoma, polymorphous cells and lipoblasts. This pattern is characteristic.

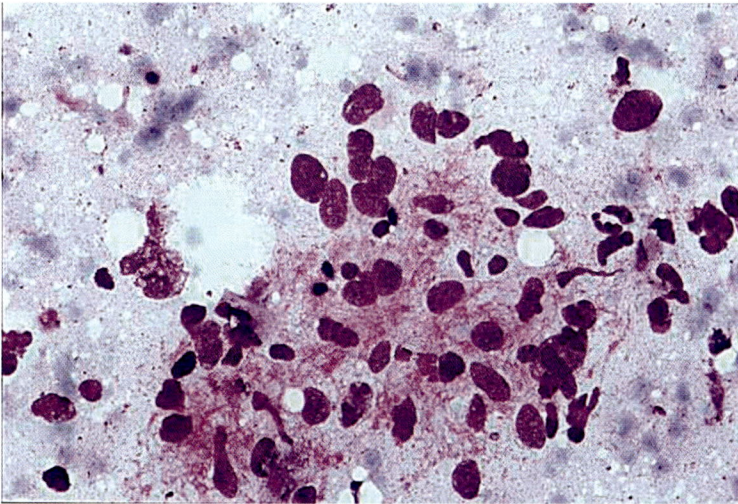

FIG 6.219 Slerosing liposarcoma, spindle or round cells with nonspecific connective fragments.

with uniform cytoplasmic vacuoles and regular round nuclei. Arborizing vascular structures and mature adipocytes also are noted [222]. Pleomorphic lipoma may simulate cytologically well-differentiated liposarcoma.

6.5.1.4 Comments. Cytologic features of well-differentiated liposarcoma have been well delineated in previous studies. Pure well-differentiated liposarcoma are characterized by mature-appearing adipose tissue admixed with rare lipoblasts, round or spindle cells [223–226]. Sclerosing variants of well-differentiated

TABLE 6.11 Cytological differential diagnosis of atypical lipomateous tumors

	Well differentiated liposarcoma/ atypical lipoma	Sclerosing liposarcoma	Pleomorphic lipoma
Adipocytes	++	+	+
Lipoblasts	++	+	−
Connective tissue fragments	+	++	+/−
Cytonuclear atypia	+	+/−	++

++; Frequent, +; rare, +/− occasionally seen, −; absent.

liposarcoma are very rare in the cytologic literature. Tumors are characterized by the presence of fibrous, partially edematous tissue and lipoblasts [226]. Gonzalez-Campora et al [227] have described such a case occurring in the retroperitoneum whose correct cytological diagnosis was supported by the presence of lipoblasts, giant cells, fibrous and adipose tissue. Palmer et al [228] have reported two cases, but in both instances, samples were not satisfactory for diagnosis. In our series [226] the 3 such cases were all misdiagnosed as fibrosarcoma in two instances and as sarcoma not otherwise specified in one case. All tumors were composed of fibrous tissue and atypical isolated spindle cells. Lipoblasts were seen in only one smear. Numerous studies have attempted to characterize the cytologic morphology of different variants of liposarcoma [223,224,226,228–232] totalizing 82 cases.

6.5.1.5 *FNA Key Features.* The following are in favor of the diagnosis:

— True lipoblasts
— Mature cells with irregular nuclei

The following is a difficulty in the diagnosis:

— Well differentiated lipoblasts may resemble mature cells

The following is evidence against a diagnosis:

— Myxoid background

6.5.2 Spindle Cell and Pleomorphic Lipoma

Spindle cell and pleomorphic lipoma are two distinctive pathologic variants of the same nosologic entity. Clinically, they show identical settings; most of patients are men between 45 and 65 years of age (91% in AFIP series), and they originate in the subcutaneous tissue in the posterior neck or shoulder. They are also described, although rarely, in unusual sites. Howewer, much caution is indicated when dealing with a presumed spindle cell and pleomorphic lipoma outside the classic body sites of occurrence, as are such lesions presumed in children and females. Classical tumors are well circumscribed or encapsulated nodules in the subcutaneous tissue. Local excision is curative, but rare recurrences have been reported.

6.5.2.1 *Histopathology.* The histological picture may vary from predominantly adipocytic tumors with restricted areas of dispersed spindle cells (Fig 6.220) to hypercellular lesions (Fig 6.221) resembling dermatofibrosarcoma protuberans and the solitary fibrous tumor, with which they share the same immunohistochemical profile with a diffuse expression of CD34. Tumor cells are elongated with a single narrow nucleus and bipolar cytoplasmic processes (Fig 6.222). Mitotic figures and necrosis are extremely rare. Tumor cells are deposited in a myxoid matrix and, if abundant, can be confused with myxoma. The vasculature is variable ranging from small-to-medium-sized vessels to a well-developed plexiform pattern similar to myxoid liposarcoma or a prominent hemangiopericytoma-like pattern (Fig 6.223).

Pleomorphic lipoma differs from spindle cell lipoma by the presence of large cells, often multinucleated with significant degrees of nuclear atypia and pleomorphism. The large bizarre cells frequently show a concentric floret-like arrangement of multiple hyperchromatic nuclei (Figs 6.224 and 6.225). Like classical spindle cell lipoma, the quality of the stroma is variable in terms of collagen fibers, myxoid changes, and the presence of mast cells. Pleomorphic lipoma has been already grouped under the term of atypical lipoma, which presently is not justified given their distinct clinical, morphologic, and genetic features.

6.5.2.2 *Cytopathology.* Spindle cell lipoma consists of a dispersed or clustered admixture of mature adipocytes and of spindle-shaped and bland-looking cells. Occasionally, a myxoid background with mast cells may be observed. Collagen-hyaline fibers are common. No prominent cytonuclear atypia or atypical lipoblasts

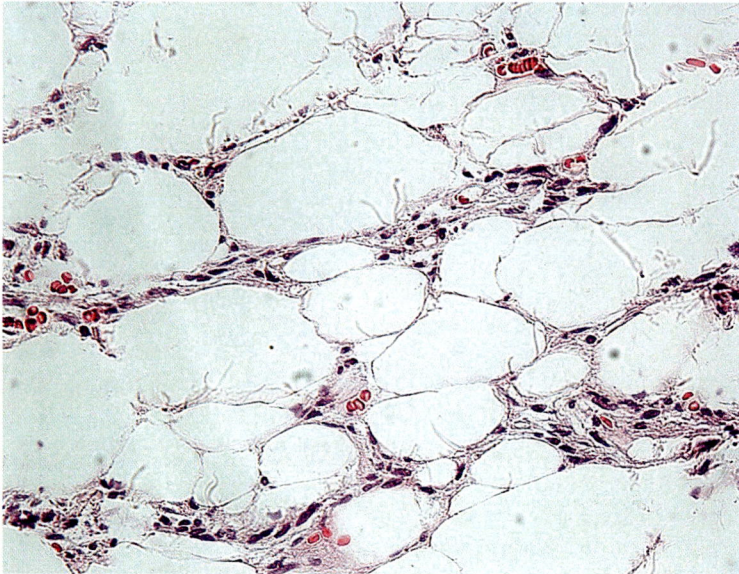

FIG 6.220 Spindle cell lipoma, predominantly adipocytic tumor with rare clusters of spindle cells.

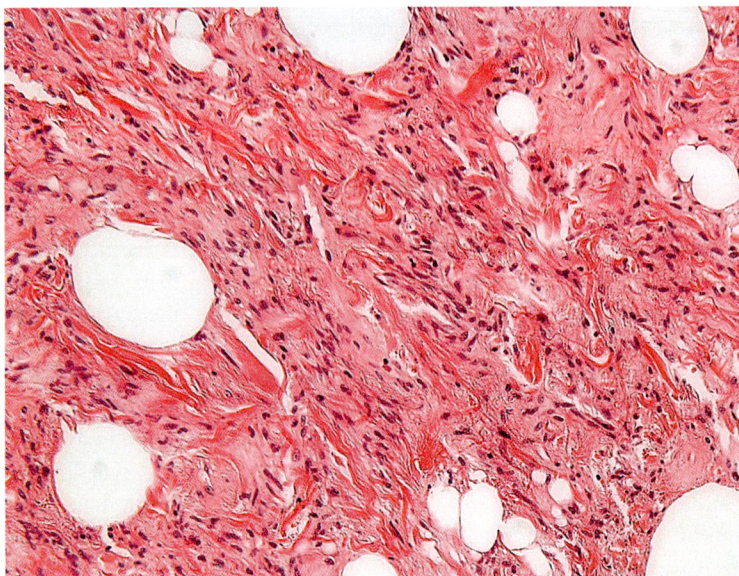

FIG 6.221 Spindle cell lipoma, hypercellular and stroma-rich area with adipocytes resembling solitary fibrous tumor.

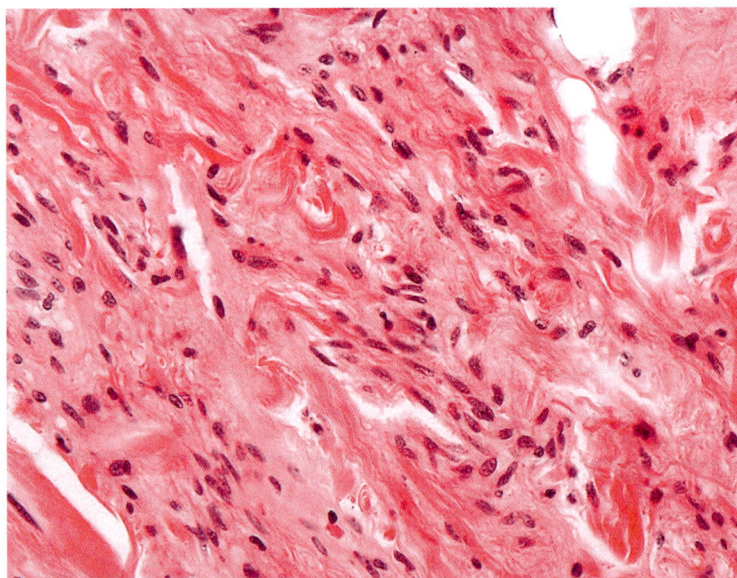

FIG 6.222 Spindle cell lipoma, elongated spindle cells with a single narrow nucleus devoid of mitosis.

are present [221]. In pleomorphic variants of lipoma, smears may present different-sized mature adipocytes mixed with rounded cells with nuclei in rings (floret cells), giant multinucleated cells, fibroblasts, collagen fragments, and even a myxoid background (Figs 6.226 and 6.227). Vasculature is scant.

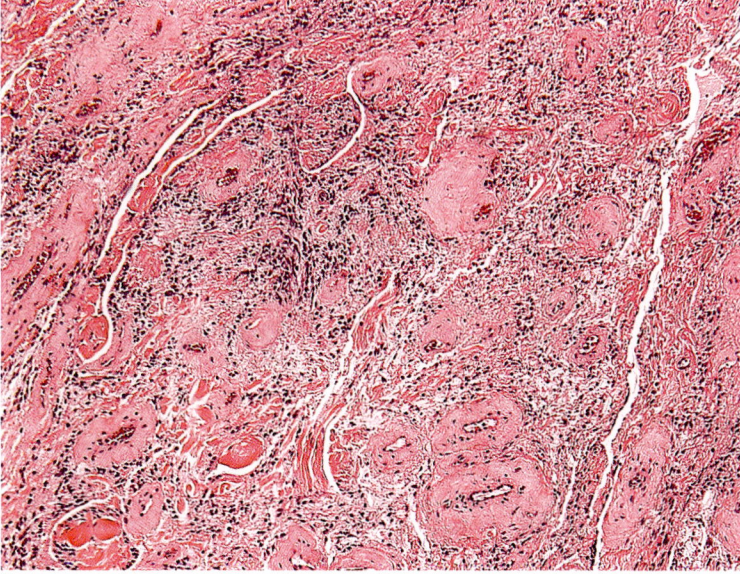

FIG 6.223 Spindle cell lipoma, thick-walled hyalinized blood vessels with clusters of spindle cells and absence of adipocytes.

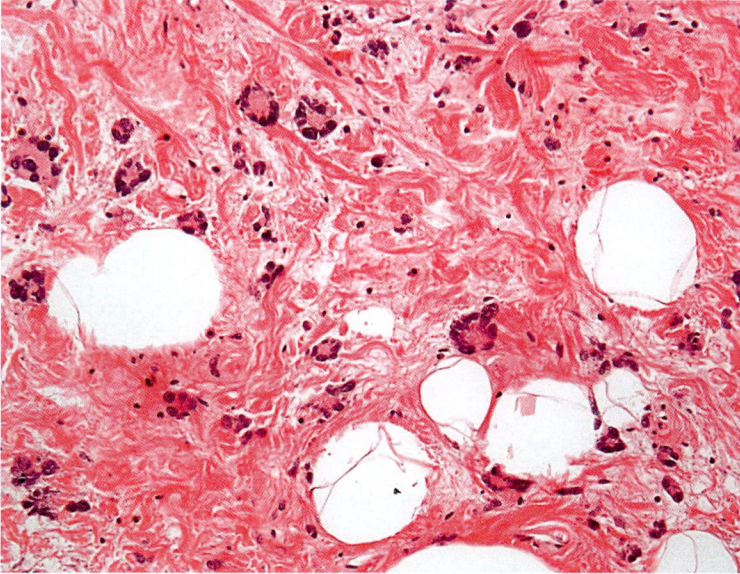

FIG 6.224 Pleomorphic lipoma, "floret-like" bizarre cells in a pleomorphic lipoma.

6.5.2.3 Differential Diagnosis and Comments. The following entities should be differentiated from spindle cell and pleomorphic lipoma:

— Well-differentiated liposarcoma/Atypical lipoma
— Solitary fibrous tumor

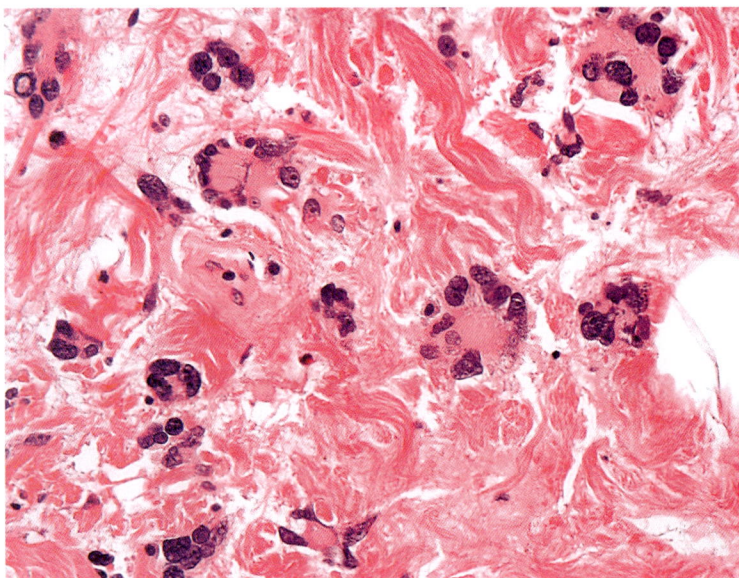

FIG 6.225 Pleomorphic lipoma, "floret-like" bizarre cells. Higher magnification.

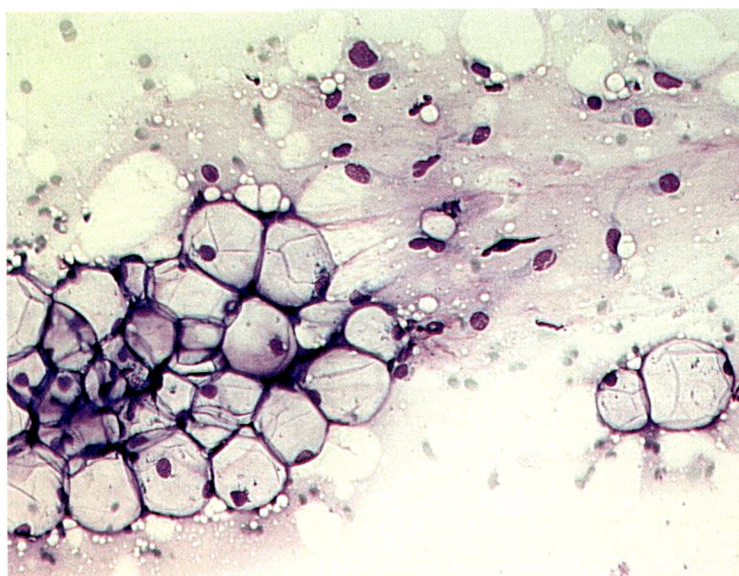

FIG 6.226 Spindle cell lipoma. Mature adipocytes, spindle and roundish cells.

Variants of benign lipomatous tumors include angiolipoma, myolipoma, spindle cell lipoma, pleomorphic lipoma, and chondroid lipoma. Spindle cell lipoma and pleomorphic lipoma are morphologically similar [233–237] on smears and should be differentiated from well-differentiated liposarcoma/atypical lipoma, well-differentiated sclerosing liposarcoma, and solitary fibrous tumor. One of the most important points in

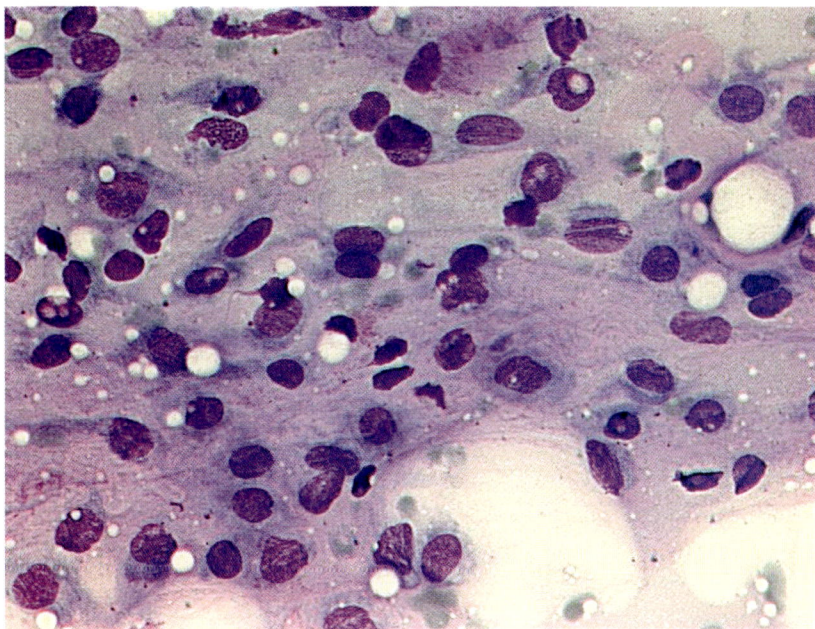

FIG 6.227 Spindle cell/and pleomorphic lipoma. Mature adipocytes and spindle or roundish cells, higher magnification.

the differential diagnosis is the clinical presentation and the presence of atypical lipoblasts in well-differentiated liposarcoma/atypical lipoma. However, pleomorphic lipoma develops characteristically in the head and neck area as well as the shoulder and back regions in aged men [238]. The immunohistochemical profile with an expression of CD34 is representative of spindle cell lipoma, dermatofibrosarcoma protuberans, and solitary fibrous tumor. Knowledge of the clinical presentation of lesions is helpful. In more difficult tumors to classify, a cytogenetical profile could be indicative of the following: spindle cell lipoma and pleomorphic lipoma, which depict characteristic abnormalities exhibiting an loss of 16q material and less frequently 13q material. The presence of a supernumerary ring12 chromosome and the typical t(17;22) tranlocation is diagnostic of dermatofibrosarcoma protuberans. Well-differentiated liposarcoma shows a different profile already discussed. The immunohistochemical profile of solitary fibrous tumor is different from spindle cell lipoma; if it shows positivity for CD34, then it expresses variably bcl-2 and rarely desmin.

6.6   EPITHELIOID TUMORS

The epithelioid pattern is less frequent in the fine needle aspiration in soft tissue tumor. It includes benign lesions such as granular cell tumor and granular rhabdomyoma and sarcomas of epithelioid-like appearance. The latter comprises epithelioid angiosarcoma, epithelioid leiomyoma/leiomyosarcoma (GIST), epithelioid sarcoma, rhabdoid tumor, metastatic from carcinomas and malignant melanoma. A few of those are well-characterized entities (e.g., epithelioid sarcoma), whereas others are not. Their general morphologic pattern has already been described (see section 5.1.6). Entities within this group have been redefined partially by their immunohistechemical profile, cytogenetics and molecular features.

6.6.1 Epithelioid Sarcoma

Epithelioid sarcoma is a relatively rare soft tissue tumor, whose classical variant occurs in the distal portions of extremities, hand, and wrist. It easily could be confused with benign and malignant conditions, especially inflammatory granulomatous process, synovial sarcoma, and ulcerated squamous cell carcinoma. Typically, the neoplasm principally affects adolescents and young adults with a proportion of 2:1 male/female. With progression, multiple small nodules may develop and progress along the fascias and neurovascular structures. The proximal type of epithelioid sarcoma has been described [239,240]. It is deeply situated, and pursues a more aggressive clinical course than the classical epithelioid sarcoma. Most proximal types of epithelioid sarcoma originate in the pelvis, peritoneum, and genital tract. They consist of multinodular masses of large epithelioid and rhabdoid-like cells with marked cellular atypia, vesicular nuclei and prominent nucleoli. Classical epithelioid sarcoma is often confused with benign processes because of its harmless histologic picture, featuring necrotizing granuloma particularly in the early stages of the disease. Frequently, superficial tumors are multinodular, although multinodular deep-seated tumors has already been observed.

6.6.1.1 Histopathology. The principal microscopic characteristics are a distinct nodular arrangement of tumor cells, tending to undergo central degeneration and necrosis simulating necrotizing granuloma (Figs 6.228 and 6.229), the epithelial appearance with eosinophilic cytoplasm (Fig 6.230) indicate of the presence

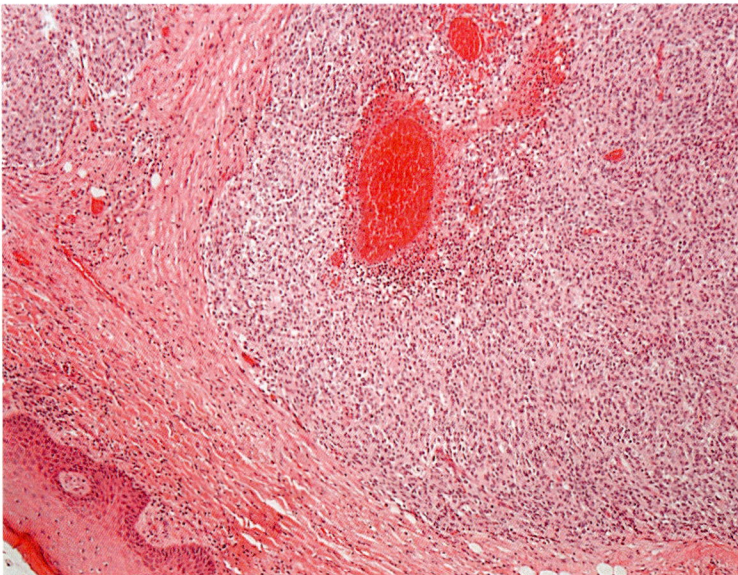

FIG 6.228 Epithelioid sarcoma, distinct nodular arrangement of tumor cells.

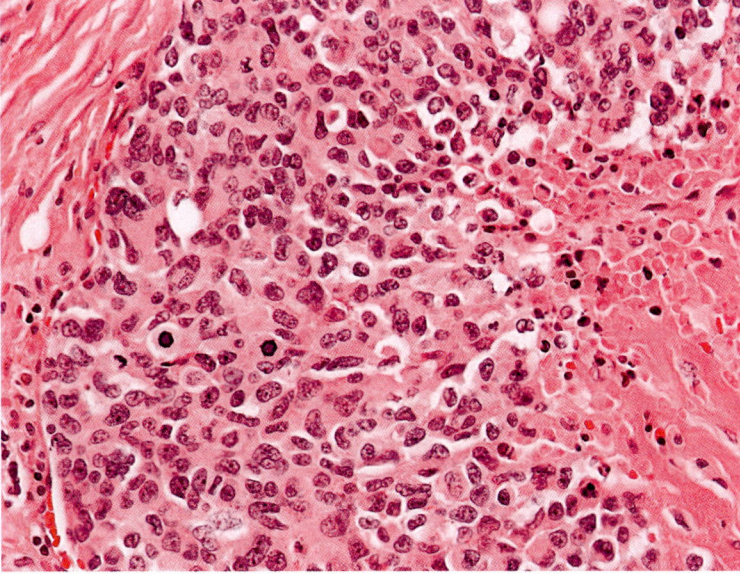

FIG 6.229   Epithelioid sarcoma, central necrosis in a nodule simulating necrotizing granuloma.

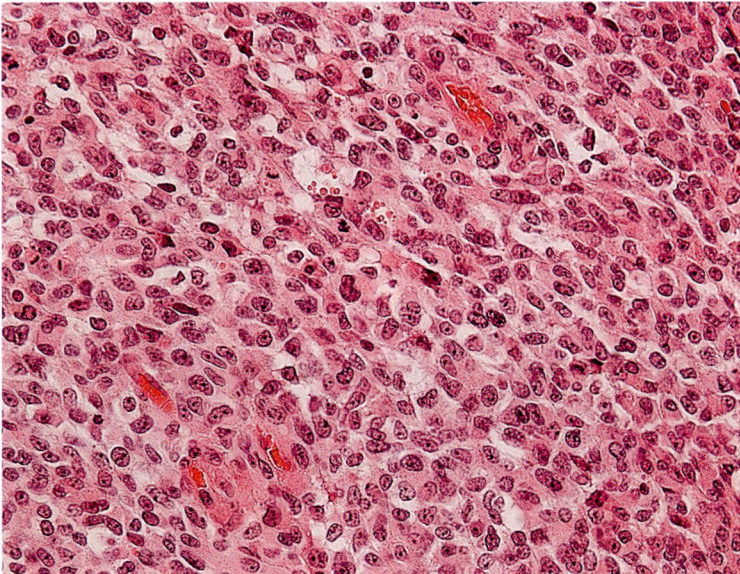

FIG 6.230   Epithelioid sarcoma, epithelial appearance with eosinophilic cytoplasm.

of cytoplasmic filaments. The fusion of nodules creates a geographic lesion with scalloped margins. Extension of the lesion into the dermis often ulcerates, mimicking an ulcerated squamous cell carcinoma. Large polygonal and eosino-philic cytoplasm cells could be mistaken for rhabdomyoblasts (Fig 6.231). Recently, a mutation/deletion similar to rhabdoid tumors, involving the gene *INI1*, a member

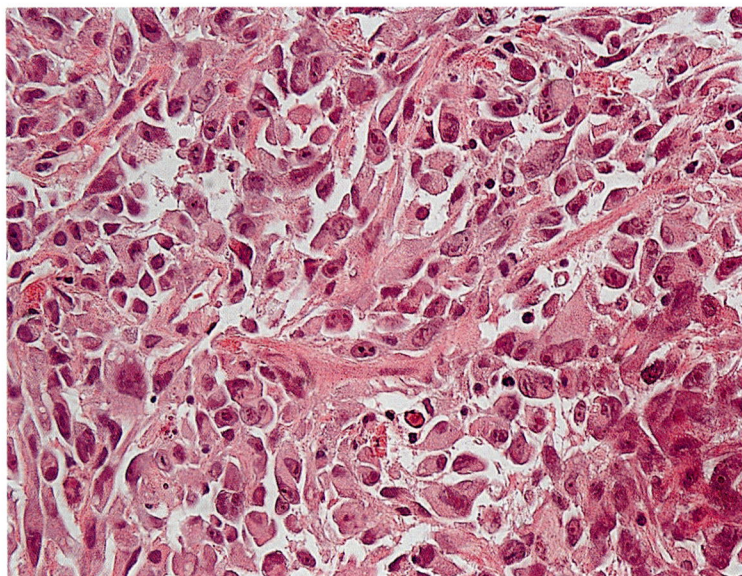

FIG 6.231   Epithelioid sarcoma, area of large polygonal cells resembling rhabdomyoblasts.

of the SW1/SNF chromosome and remodeling complex on chromosome 22q11.2, has been reported the in conventional type of epithelioid sarcoma [240]. The immuno-histochemical profile shows a dual expression of epithelial and mesenchymal markers (i.e., EMA, cytokeratin, and vimentin).

6.6.1.2 Cytopathology. Smears in epithelioid sarcoma are usually hypercellular and stroma-poor. They consist of aggregated and isolated epithelioid tumor cells that are round to polygonal (Figs 6.232 and 6.233), with eccentrically located nuclei. The tumor cells show severe-to-moderate atypia (Figs 6.234 and 6.235), irregularity in size, and many mitoses. Binucleation is common. Occasionally, spindle cells also are present and show important cellular pleomorphism. A matrix mimicking osteoid also may be observed. The background is usually necrotic and inflammatory. Certain "proximal-type" tumors show predominant rhabdoid or plasmacytoid features with globular intracytoplasmic inclusions positive for cytokeratin, vimentin, and CD34. Moreover, the immunocytochemical stains show diffuse cytoplasmic positivity for cytokeratins (CAM 5.2) and both cytoplasmic and cell membrane positivity for vimentin, whereas S-100 protein and HMB 45 immunostaining were negative, thus supporting the cytological diagnosis of epithelioid sarcoma, which was subsequently proven on the surgical samples.

6.6.1.3 Differential Diagnosis. The following entities should be differentiated from epithelioid sarcoma:

- Necrotizing granuloma
- Epithelioid malignant peripheral nerve sheath tumor
- Epithelioid angiosarcoma
- Rhabdoid tumor

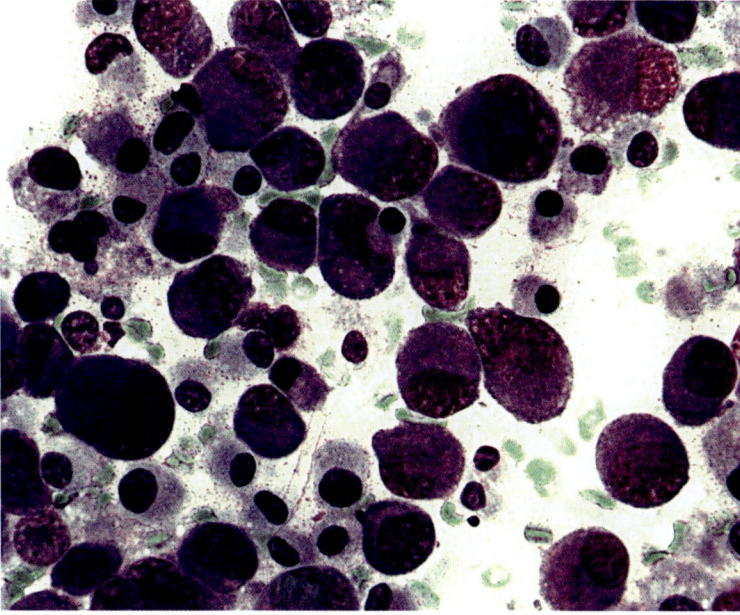

FIG 6.232 Epithelioid sarcoma, aggregated and isolated epithelioid tumor cells that are round to polygonal.

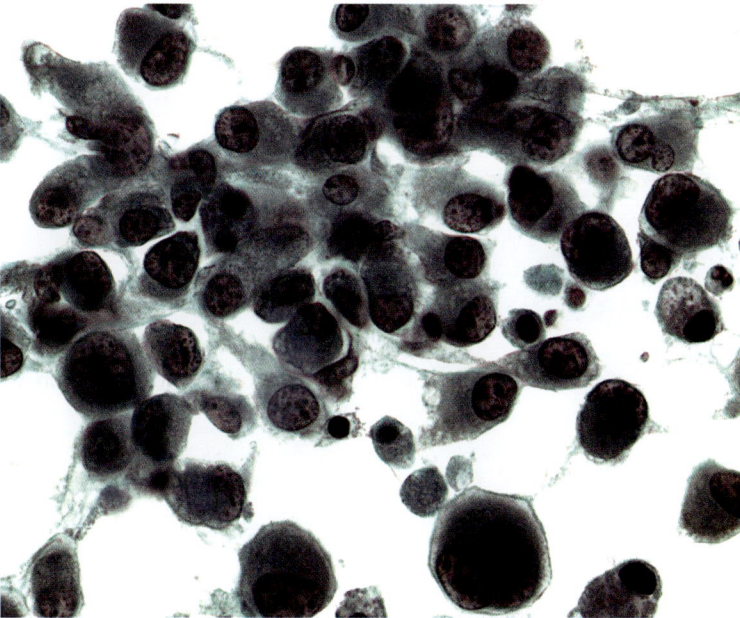

FIG 6.233 Epithelioid sarcoma, same case as Fig 6.232. Papanicolaou.

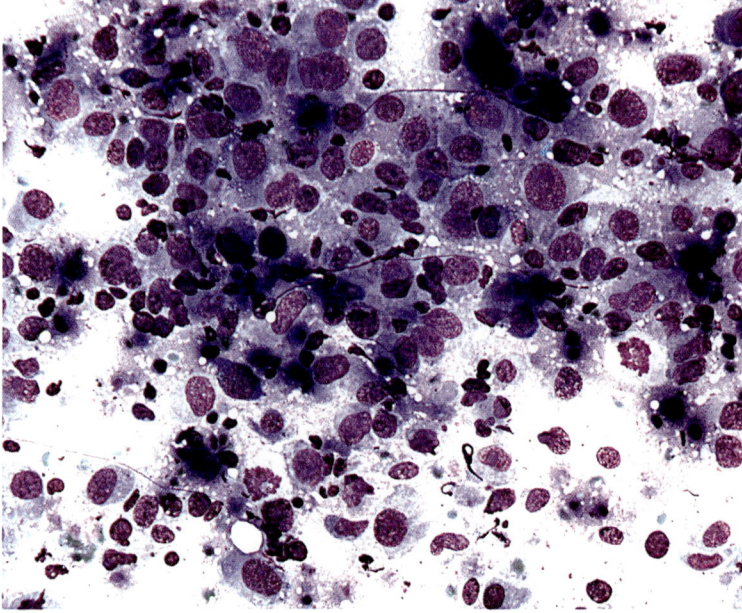

FIG 6.234 Epithelioid sarcoma, severe-to-moderate atypia, irregularity in size and mitoses.

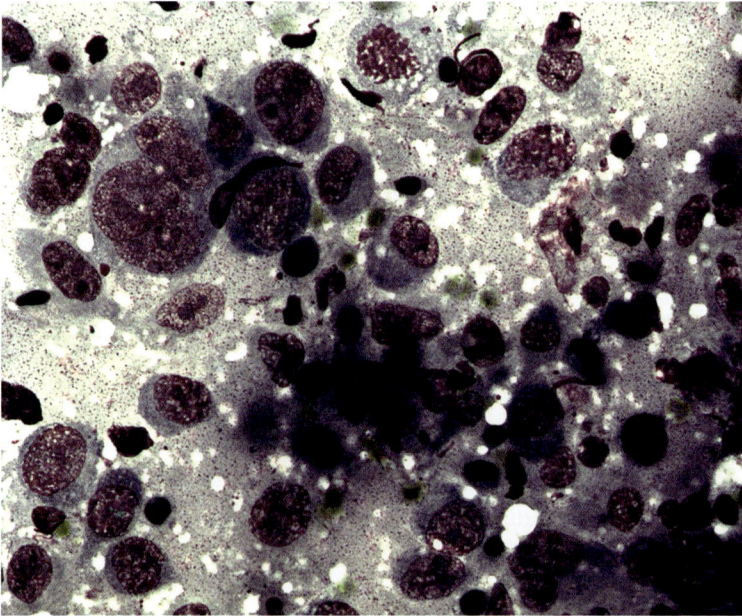

FIG 6.235 Epithelioid sarcoma, higher magnificaiton.

Differential diagnosis includes entities like necrotizing granuloma, epithelioid malignant peripheral nerve sheath tumor, epithelioid angiosarcoma, rhabdoid tumor, and melanoma. A well selected panel of antibodies can help to precise the diagnosis

TABLE 6.12   Cytologic differential diagnosis of epithelioid sarcoma

	Epithelioid sarcoma	Epithelioid angiosarcoma	Malignant melanoma
Epithelioid clusters	++	++	+/−
Spindle-shaped cells	+	++	++
Round cells	++	+	++
Erythrophagocytosis	−	+	−
Hemorrhagic background	−	++	−

++; Frequent, +; rare, +/− occasionally seen, −; absent.

Epithelioid malignant peripheral nerve sheath tumor and other mesenchymal epithelioid tumors can easily be confused. However, they are differentiated by their immunohistochemical profile; typically, most epithelioid sarcomas express low- and high-molecular weight cytokeratins, EMA, and vimentin. They also express CD34 in a proportion of about 70% of epithelioid sarcoma. Endothelial and neurogenic markers are typically negative. In the past, cytogenetic data were limited. Recently, a mutation of the gene *hSNF5/INI1* similar to rhabdoid tumor has been reported [240]. Nevertheless, there is still no consensus about the definite phenotype of epithelioid sarcoma. The recent description of that gene mutation raises concern.

Epithelioid angiosarcoma consists of isolated or clustered polymorphous cells. Clusters in angiosarcoma may exhibit epithelial morphology, whereas epitheliod sarcoma rather consists of isolated epithelioid and rounded cells. Erythrophagocytosis is absent. Both tumors may show necrosis and mitotic figures. Differentiation from rhabdoid tumor may be challenging and necessitates immunohistochemical (cytokeratin perinuclear positivity) and genomic analyses because both entities are morphologically similar. Amelanotic malignant melanoma is a serious candidate to consider in the differential diagnosis. Intranuclear inclusions and spindle-shaped cells are more in favor of malignant melanoma.

Table 6.12 summarizes the cytologic differential diagnosis of epithelioid sarcoma.

6.6.1.4   Comments. Epithelioid sarcoma is an uncommon tumor with a wide range of differential diagnosis, especially in cytology specimens. In the presence of classic cytologic findings, the diagnosis of epithelioid sarcoma can be suggested. Subsequent histologic examination and immunohistochemistry can confirm the diagnosis [241].

Thirty cases of epithelioid sarcoma were investigated in the cytology literature [241–250]. All tumors were diagnosed accurately as sarcoma. We have collected five other examples of epithelioid sarcoma. One case was rendered false negative, three cases were diagnosed as pleomorphic high-grade sarcoma, and only one case was diagnosed accurately.

6.6.1.5   Clinical and FNA Key Features. The following are in favor of the diagnosis:

— Hypercellular smear
— Epithelioid cells

- Prominent cytonuclear atypia
- Huge nucleoli, aboundant cytoplasm
- Binucleated cells
- Necrosis or poorly preserved cells

The following are difficulties in the diagnosis:

- Cells may resemble rhabdoid tumor, rhabdomyosarcoma, or melanoma
- Prominent inflammatory background

The following are evidence against a diagnosis:

- Melanin, Squamous cells
- Intrarenal tumor
- Pediatric age

6.6.2 Gastrointestinal Stromal Tumor (GIST)/Epithelioid Leiomyosarcoma

The term GIST is recognized as the right designation for a group of mesenchymal spindle cell and/or epitheliod neoplasms originating in the abdominal cavity and gastrointestinal tract. Throughout the previous 40–50 years, several appellations were coined such as leiomyoblastoma (benign/malignant), epitheliod leiomyoma/ leiomyosarcoma, stromal tumor, and for a limited number of identical morphological neoplasms, gastrointestinal autonomic nervous tumor (GANN). Previous immunohistochemical investigations tend to identify different subgroups of entities according to profiles of antibody expression, smooth muscle, nervous, or neither, of which 60–70% were positive for CD34.

A consensus approach defined the key elements to address the role of Kit immunopositivity in the diagnosis of GIST [251]. Most GISTs express Kit (gene Kit mutation at 4q11) and have a constitutional activation of tyrosine kinase receptor Kit and *PDGFRA*. However, some uncertainties are to be precised in terms of histogenesis and biological behavior. Of the GIST resected, approximately 50% will recur or metastasize. If large size and high mitotic activity are associated strongly with malignant behavior, then smaller tumor size, and an absence of mitotic activity do not preclude malignant behavior. Tumors of similar morphology but developing at different locations along the gastrointestinal tract differ widely in their biologic behavior. Also, increased activity of the Kit protein in an absence of the gene Kit mutation has been demonstrated. There is a wide variety of anatomical localization along the whole gastrointestinal tract including the esophagus and gallbladder, mesentery, omentum, retroperitoneum, and even urinary bladder. Within the gastrointestinal tract, 50–60% originate in the stomach and 20–30% originate in the small intestine. The former pursues a relative good prognosis, whereas tumors of the small intestine do not.

6.6.2.1 Histopathology. The following different histologic patterns of GIST have been recognized: spindle cell (70%), epithelioid (20%) (Fig 6.236), mixed (Fig 6.237), myxoid, and nested (paraganglioma-like) (Fig 6.238). The expression of CD117 reveals

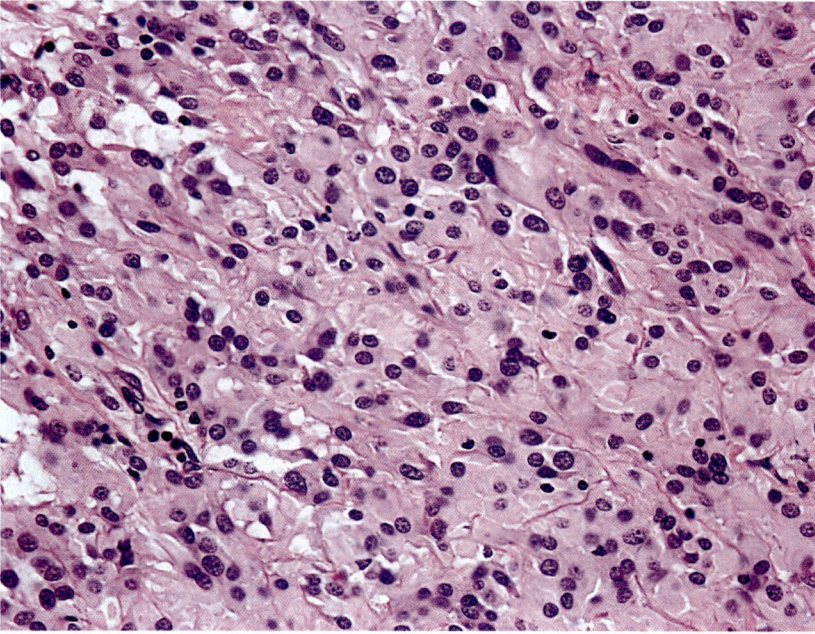

FIG 6.236 Gastrointestinal stromal tumor, cohesive epithelioid cells with eosinophilic cytoplasm without significant atypias.

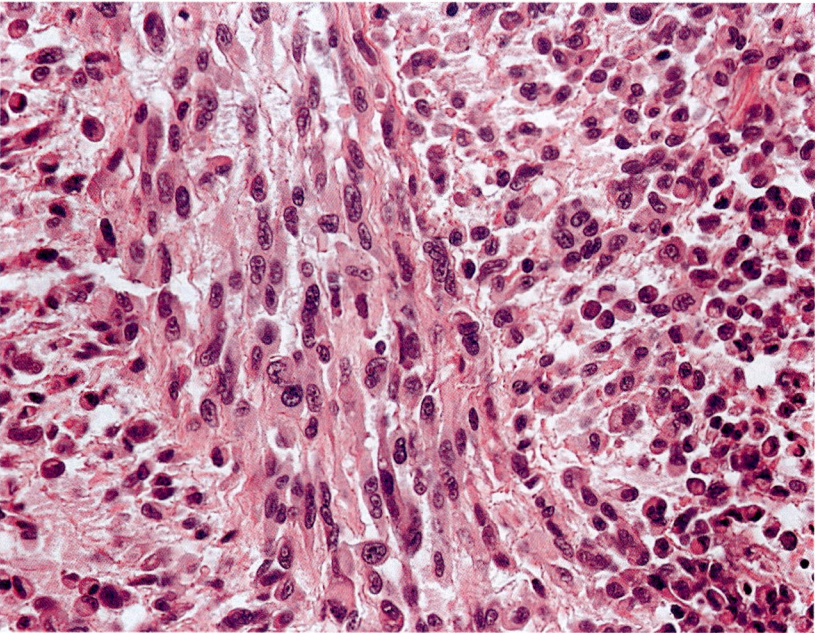

FIG 6.237 Gastrointestinal stromal tumor, irregular fascicles of epithelioid cells and spindle cells with eosinophilic cytoplasm.

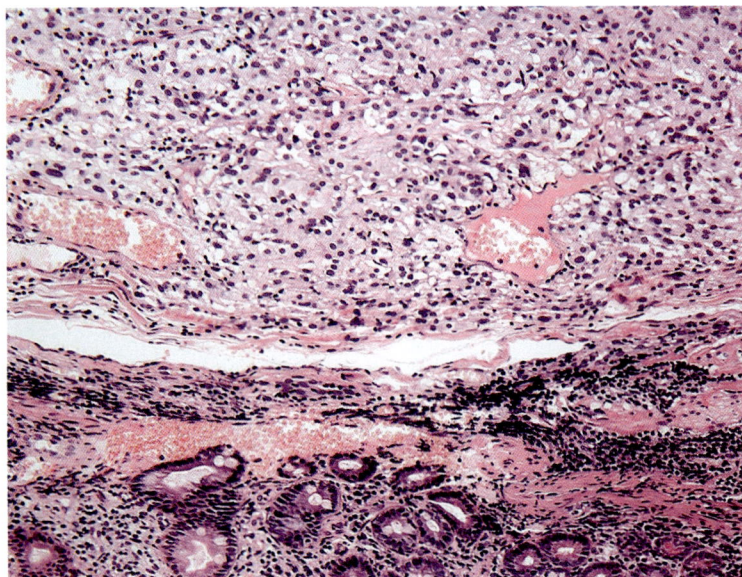

FIG 6.238   Gastrointestinal stromal tumor, submucosal tumor comprising nests of epithelioid cells, some with clear cytoplasm.

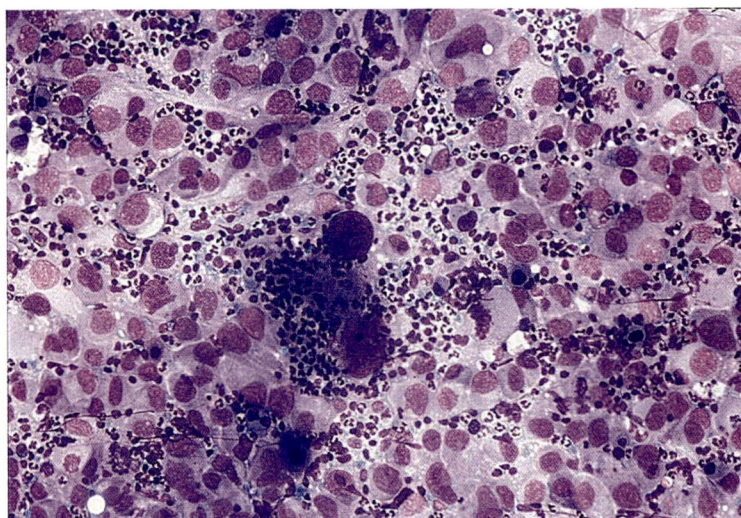

FIG 6.239   Gastrointestinal stromal tumor, isolated epithelioid cells with inflammatory background.

different patterns of marking including strong cytoplasmic (most of them), a cytoplasmic dot, a cellular membrane with a high percentage of tumor cell positivity, and more rarely, show focal positivity.

6.6.2.2 Cytopathology. The aspirates reveal mainly single or small clusters of isolated epithelioid cells (Fig 6.239) or arranged in fascicles that exhibit focal,

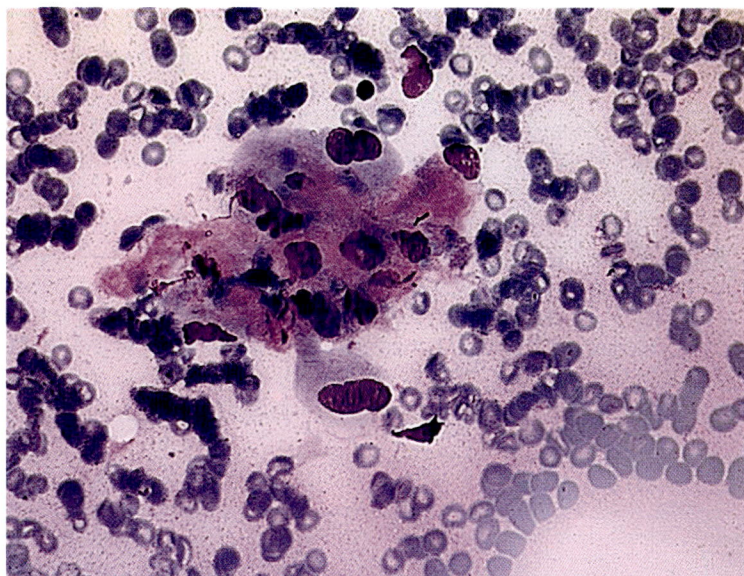

FIG 6.240 Gastrointestinal stromal tumor, collagenous stroma with single spindle cells.

nuclear palisading. Cytoplasms depicting a basophilic appearance, are of moderate amount, and are granular to clear with indistinct cytoplasmic borders. Frequently, tumor cells have long, delicate, filamentous extensions. Nuclei are small and uniform with mild-to-marked nuclear envelope irregularities, and no significant atypia or mitosis is detected. Binucleation and intranuclear inclusions are frequent findings. Collagenous stroma is present in most cases (Fig 6.240), often in the hemorrhagic background.

6.6.2.3 *Differential Diagnosis.* The following entities should be differentiated from GIST/epitheloid leiomyosarcoma.

- "True" leiomyosarcoma
- Malignant peripheral nerve sheath tumor
- Malignant melanoma
- Neuroendocrine carcinoma

GISTs may cause significant diagnostic confusion on fine needle aspiration with carcinomas, neuroendocrine tumors, and melanoma, particularly with metastatic neoplasms [252,253]. However, GIST should be differentiated from true epithelioid leiomyosarcomas [254–256]. Differentiation between carcinomas and melanomas is made using classic cytologic analysis. Adenocarcinomas and neuroendocrine carcinomas consist of epithelial cells, mostly clustered or isolated. Neuroendocrine carcinomas frequently show characteristic immature chromatin and nuclear molding. Amelanotic melanomas consist of epithelioid or spindle-shaped cells with frequent binucleation and intranuclear inclusions. Differentiation from epithelioid leiomyosarcoma may be more problematic. The epithelioid leiomyosarcomas show three-dimensional, tightly cohesive, sharply marginated syncytia of spindle cells, often with a nuclear crush artifact. The cytoplasm and stroma have a distinct wiry, refractile appearance [254]. However, true epithelioid leiomyosarcoma have a relatively poor intercellular cohesion and occur singly and rarely in cohesive groups, whereas tumor cells in GIST often manifest in cohesive groupings with a syncytial appearance and delicate cytoplasmic processes. Furthermore, tumor cells from epithelioid leiomyosarcoma exhibit apparent variation in nuclear size and have scanty or no recognizable cytoplasm [257]. Tumor cells in GIST appear more uniform and regular and have abundant cytoplasm with ill-defined cell borders [254,255]. Ancillary studies such as immunohistochemical stains are usually helpful in making a definitive diagnosis. Epithelioid cells without prominent cytonuclear atypia c-kit positive are characteristic features of GIST and can help to distinguish these tumors from leiomyosarcoma in cytologic specimens [254].

6.6.2.4 Comments. For practical purposes and in term of histoprognosis, GIST has been subgrouped into four categories according to size and mitotic activity: very low risk (<2 cm, <5/50), low risk (2−5 cm, <5/50), intermediate (<5 cm, 6−10/50) (5−10 cm, <5/50), high risk (>5 cm, > 5/50); (>10 cm, any rate of mitosis), (any size, >10/50) [251].

The most important in sampling submucosal tumors of the gastrointestinal tract is to make an accurate diagnosis and to predict a tumor of malignant potential. GIST is a distinct group of mesenchymal neoplasms shown to exhibit differentiation toward interstitial Cajal cells. C-kit (CD117), an immunocytochemical marker consistently expressed in normal interstitial Cajal cells, is demonstrable in 81−100% of GISTs [258]. Schmitt et al. [259] analyzed c-Kit mutations in GIST, and it was found in 61% of tumors. Nearly 95% of c-Kit-mutant tumors carried exon 11 mutations. Mutation analysis was possible in fine needle aspiration cell blocks and can assist in the diagnosis and therapeutic decisions in GIST cases. More recently, Stelow et al. [260] studied material obtained by fine needle aspiration for the diagnosis of subepithelial intramural gastrointestinal mesenchymal neoplasms. Using immunocytochemistry in 95 cases, they could differentiate GISTs from leiomyomas, peripheral nerve sheath tumors, and other neoplasms by cytologic examination. Immunoreactivity with antibodies to CD117, not previously diagnosed accurately, confirms a GIST at follow-up; 15 of 16 cases immunoreactive with antibodies to CD34 were GISTs at follow-up. Similarly, Yoshida et al. [261] reviewed a correlative cytologic and histologic study of 49 cases of gastrointestinal submucosal tumors. Both cytological and histological findings were examined for c-Kit. With cytology, cellular clusters were classified into type A (piled clusters with high cellularity showing a fascicular pattern), type B (thin layered clusters with high cellularity showing a fascicular pattern), and type C (monolayered clusters or scattered cells). Types A and B were associated strongly with a histological diagnosis of GIST. Type C clusters needed confirmation of c-Kit positivity and histology. Thus, the cell cluster pattern was informative in routine diagnosis for GIST.

Fine needle aspiration material also was considered a predictive factor of malignant potential. Analyses were either purely morphologic or combined with immunocytochemistry. The assessment of the degree of maligncy is difficult based on cytology alone. In a previous study [262], parameters like the presence of spindle or epithelioid cells with minimal nuclear atypia or pleomorphism and a moderate amount of cytoplasm could not distinguish benign and malignant tumors with reliability. Inversely, the presence of necrosis or mitoses in cytologic specimens correlated with a diagnosis of malignancy [262]. Thus, in appropriate clinical and radiological settings, a confident diagnosis of primary or metastatic GIST can be established by fine needle aspiration and cell blocks with combined immunohisto-chemistry [253]. Positive immunostaining of p53 has been evaluated as a predictive factor of the outcome of GIST and proved reliability, whereas Ki-67 and bcl-2 were not [263].

Numerous correlative cytological and histological studies of GIST, totalizing more than 300 cases, have been reported [253,254,256,258,259,262–268]. A high level of diagnostic accuracy was reached, provided that ancillary immunohistochemistry was combined with routine cytology. In most of these reported cases, deep-seated tumors were sampled either by endoscopic ultrasound-guided fine needle aspiration (EUS-FNA) or by transcutaneous aspirations.

6.6.2.5 FNA Key Features. The following are in favor of the diagnosis:

- Single or small clusters of epithelioid cells
- Fascicles and nuclear palisading
- Granular to clear cytoplasms
- Uniform nuclei, binucleation
- Clinicoradiological evidence of gastrointestinal tumor

The following is a difficulty in the diagnosis:

- Mitotic figures and moderate cytonuclear atypia

The following are evidence against a diagnosis:

- Melanin
- Nuclear molding
- Carcinomatous morphology

6.6.3 Epithelioid Angiosarcoma

Epithelioid angiosarcomas account for a limited number of malignant soft tissue neoplasms, which encompass a spectrum of entities rather than a single one. Whatever the clinical setting in which they originate, epithelioid angiosarcoma, unlike angiosarcoma of the skin, are more commonly deep tumors and seem to be more aggressive neoplasms [269], which result in local recurrences and distant metastasis, most often to the lung, lymph node, bone, and soft tissue. Features that are statistically associated with a bad prognosis are older age, retroperitoneal location, large size, and index of cell proliferation (ki-67).

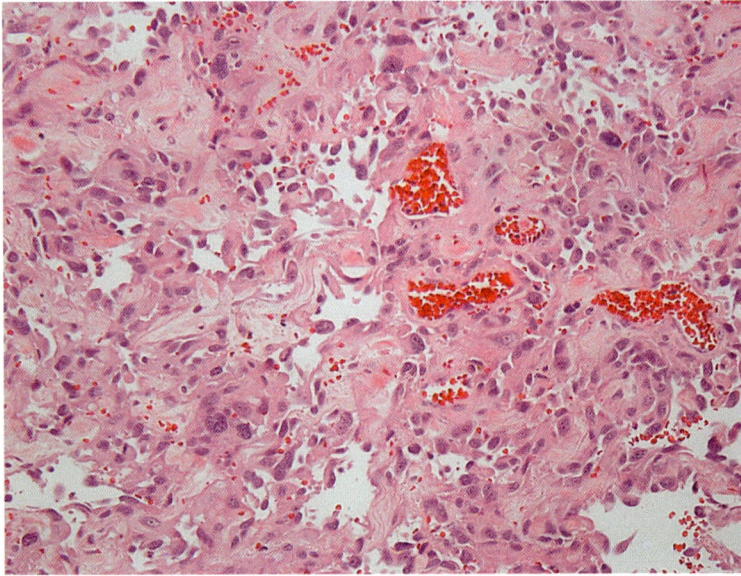

FIG 6.241 Epithelioid angiosarcoma, irregular vascular channels lined by atypical epithelioid cells.

6.6.3.1 *Histopathology.* From a morphological point of view, the angiosarcomas are divided into classical (well, moderately, and poorly differentiated) and epithelioid subtypes [270].

Epithelioid angiosarcomas consist of sheets of highly atypical round cells with prominent nuclei, sometimes depicting intracytoplasmic lumens (Fig 6.241). They are associated with erythrophagocytosis (Figs 6.242 and 6.243). Most of epithelioid angiosarcoma stain for endothelial markers CD31, occasionally FVIII-related antigen, and in nearly 50% of cases, cytokeratin of low-molecular weight, and cam 5.2, hence the difficulty in separating epithelioid angiosarcoma from epithelioid sarcoma and metastatic carcinoma.

6.6.3.2 *Cytopathology.* Cell composition varies depending on tumor differentiation. In general, epithelioid angiosarcomas show predominant pseudoepithelial morphology, making a differential diagnosis from carcinoma but atypical spindle cells also are present. The reported findings in well- and moderatety differentiated epithelioid angiosarcomas do not allow drawing an overall uniform cytopathologic picture. Half of the smears are cell-rich and half are cell-poor with a hemorrhagic background. In well-differentiated epithelioid angiosarcomas, the population of tumor cells is polymorphous and consists of predominant spindle-shaped cells (Figs 6.244 and 6.245), some round to oval cells, polygonal epithelioid cells (Figs 6.246 and 6.247), and giant cells in various proportions. In moderately differentiated epithelioid angiosarcomas, spindle-shaped cells of inter-mediate size (Fig 6.248) are less frequent, and round to oval cells as well as polygonal epithelial-like cells (Fig 6.249) predominate. The cytoplasm in epitheli-oid cells may show vacuolizations/lumina. Frequently, these cells are grouped in clusters. In poorly differentiated epithelioid sarcomas, numerous roundish

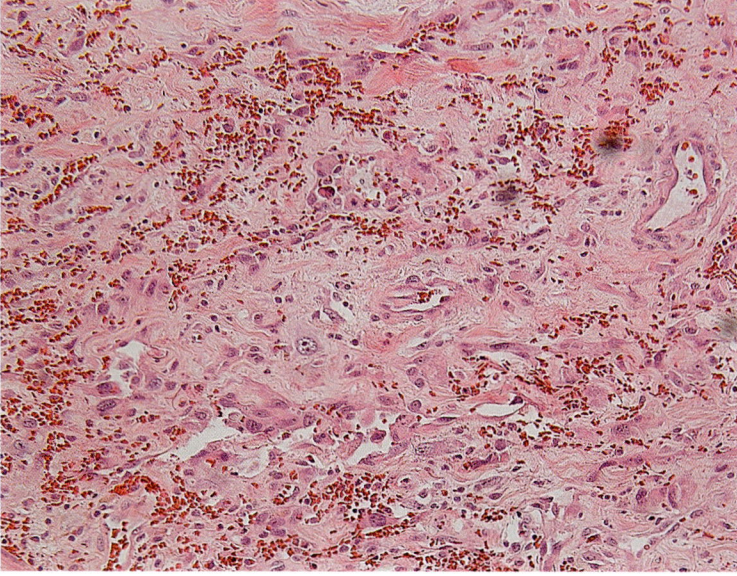

FIG 6.242 Epithelioid angiosarcoma, slit-like and opened-lumen vascular channels as well as erythrocytes extravasation.

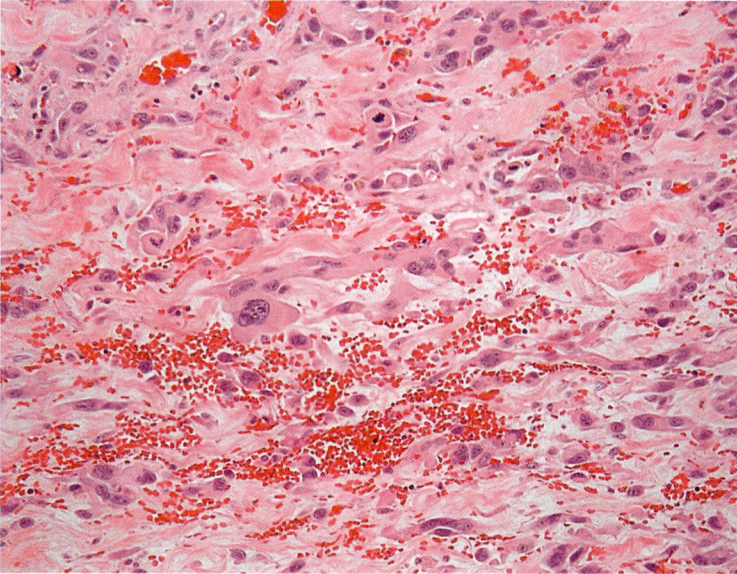

FIG 6.243 Epithelioid angiosarcoma, pleomorphic epithelioid cells mixed with erythrocytes.

and cohesive epithelioid cells are present. Their nuclei are irregular, strongly nucleolated, and their cytoplasms stain dark blue with MGG. Giant cells, anaplastic spindle cells, erythrophagocytosis, and mitotic figures are frequent. Stromal fragments are always scant.

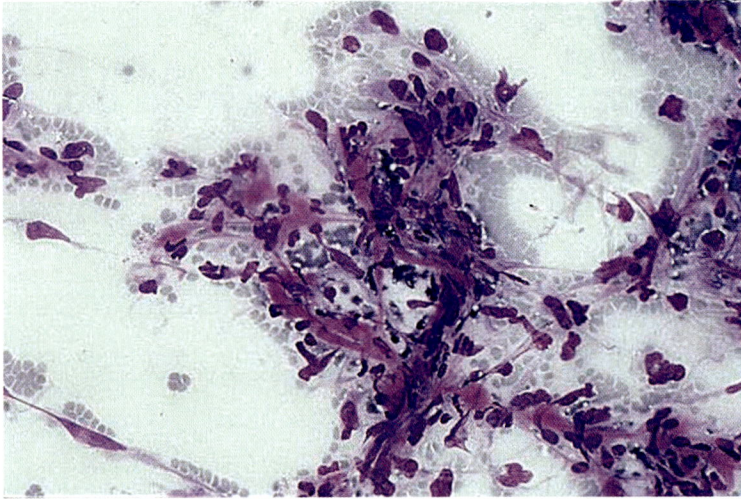

FIG 6.244 Epithelioid angiosarcoma, vascular structures are well seen.

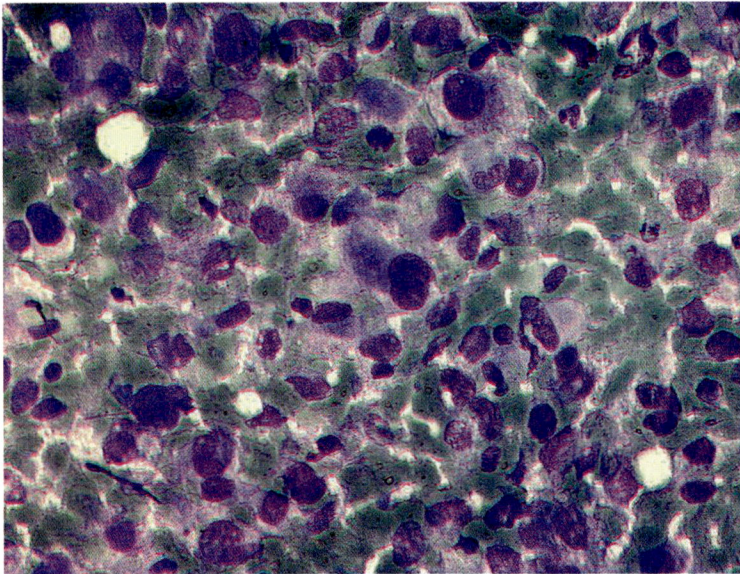

FIG 6.245 Epithelioid angiosarcoma, polymorphous and spindle-shaped cells.

6.6.3.3 *Differential Diagnosis.* The following entities should be differentiated from epithelioid angiosarcoma:

— Epithelioid sarcoma
— Rhabdomyosarcoma
— Malignant melanoma
— Metastatic/recurrent carcinoma

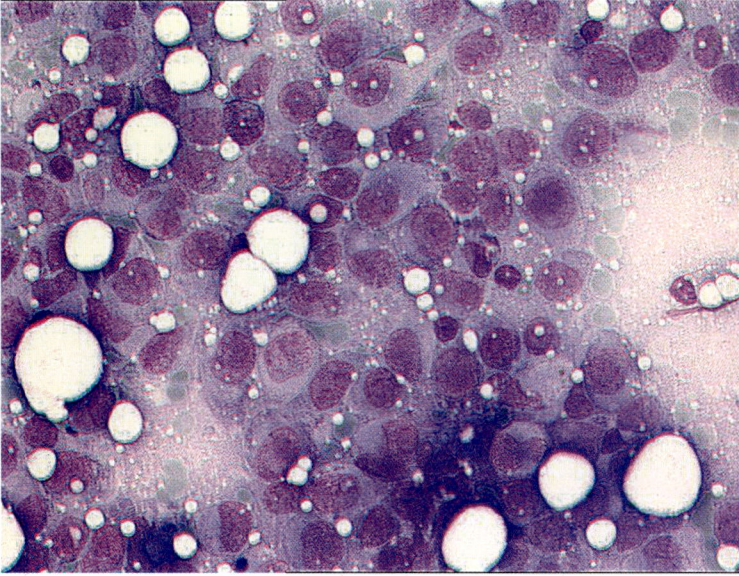

FIG 6.246   Epithelioid angiosarcoma, epithelioid cells similar to carcinoma.

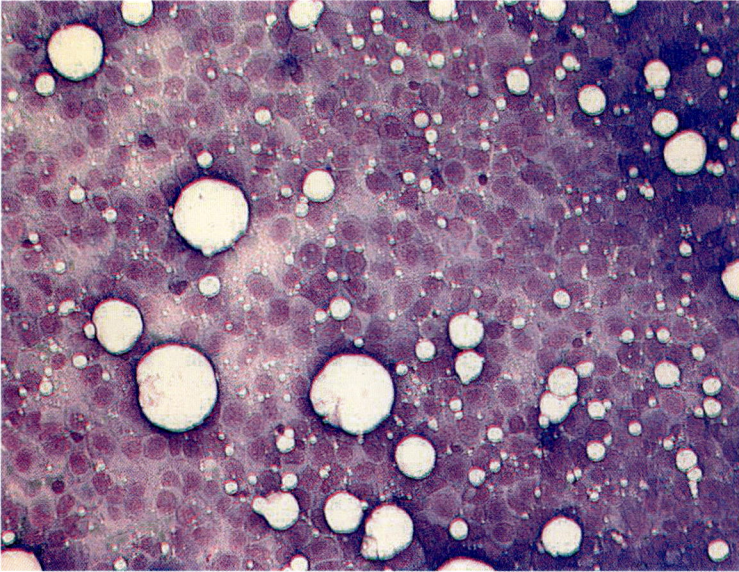

FIG 6.247   Epithelioid angiosarcoma, round-to-oval cells.

Classic and epithelioid angiosarcomas should be differentiated from adenocarcinoma, epithelioid sarcoma, rhabdomyosarcoma, and malignant melanoma (Table 6.12). The presence of spindle-shaped, giant, and round-to-oval cells are rather in favor of sarcoma and are against carcinoma. This distinction is particularly important in

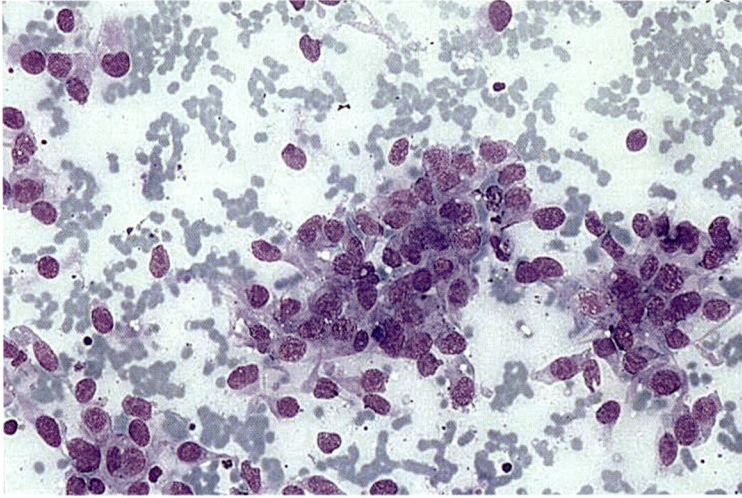

FIG 6.248 Epithelioid angiosarcoma, spindle-shaped and roundish cells of intermediate size.

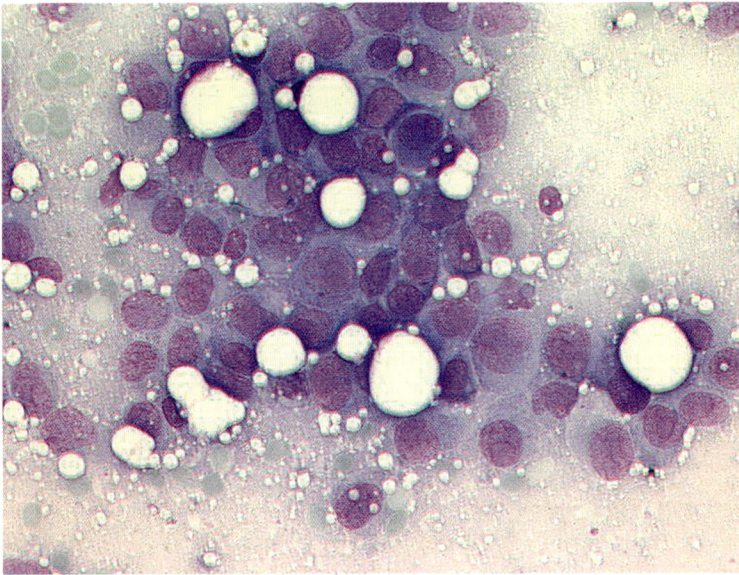

FIG 6.249 Epithelioid angiosarcoma, polygonal epithelial-like cells in loose clusters.

patients treated previously for breast carcinoma to differentiate between radio-induced angiosarcoma from recurrent carcinomas. Epithelioid sarcoma may share similar cytological features with epithelioid angiosarcoma [271,272]. Smears of epithelioid sarcoma show a single cell pattern of oval cells containing eccentric nuclei, abundant cytoplasm, and occasional cytoplasmic vacuoles. However, dense perinuclear zone and less opaque cell margins are observed. Rhabdomyosarcomas consist of isolated or clustered round-to-oval or spindle-shaped cells with eccentric nuclei and characteristic plasmacytoid cytoplasms. Binucleated cells with finely vacuolated cytoplasms are frequently observed [273,274]. Periodic acid-Shiff and muscular markers are strongly positive. In addition, rhabdomyosarcomas have a uniform morphology, and the admixture of different types of cells is usually not present.

Several malignant melanomas consist of oval cells with single or two nuclei. Intranuclear inclusions, admixed with macrophages containing melanin desposits, help to precise the diagnosis. Intracytoplasmic hemosiderin deposits (brown in MGG stain) in angiosarcomas may be distinguished easily from the melanin (grey in MGG stain) in melanotic malignant melanoma.

6.6.3.4 *Comments.*

Rare cytologic studies of epithelioid angiosarcomas are reported [275–279]. Cytological smears are similar in all cases but may be relatively hypocellular because of the dilutional effects of abundant red cells [277]. Smears of epithelioid angiosarcoma are always cell-rich, whereas the smears in classic angiosarcomas are cell-rich in only half of tumors [279]. Epithelioid angiosarcomas constantly consist of round-to-oval cells and polygonal, epithelial-like cells with frequent clusterization. Erythrophagocytosis is present. In contrast, classic angiosarcomas show morphological diversity and consist of an admixture of spindle, round-to-oval, epithelial-like, and giant cells in various proportions. Erythrophagocytosis also may be observed. When correlating the histological grade with the cytological findings, the smears in high-grade (grade III) angiosarcomas are always cell-rich and frequently consist of round-to-oval and epithelial-like cells with clusterization. Erythrophagocytosis is also more frequent in high-grade than in low-grade (grades I and II) tumors. Epithelioid angiosarcoma is diagnosed more accurately than classic angiosarcoma, particularly if epithelioid cells are associated with erythrophagocytosis. Moreover, classic angiosarcoma shares some cytological features with epithelioid angiosarcoma [279].

Angiosarcomas are one of the rarest variants of malignant soft tissue neoplasms. So far, the limited number of cytomorphological studies does not allow their characterization. Several cytological studies of angiosarcomas totaling approximately 79 cases have been reported [275–282] of which only 3 [276,279,282] dealt with more than 10 cases. Cases of angiosarcomas in sites such as the liver, lung, breast, subcutaneous tissue, bone, kidney, thyroid, and parotid glands have been reported.

6.6.3.5 *FNA Key Features.*

The following are in favor of the diagnosis:

- Deep tumor
- Pleomorphic epithelial-like cells with a tendency to be clustered
- Erythrophagocytosis
- Important cytonuclear atypia.

The following are difficulties in the diagnosis:

- Numerous clusters
- Hemorrhagic background

The following is evidence against a diagnosis:

- Melanin

6.6.4   Granular Cell Tumor

The granular cell tumor is a fairly common lesion of controversial origin. Originally considered a muscle tumor, immunohistochemical studies have allowed documenting its neural nature. Its morphological appearance is sufficiently distinctive to separate it from other neural tumors, namely neurofibroma and schwannoma. It occurs at any body site including the orofacial region, of which numerous observations have been reported including the tongue, with the latter accounting for 75% of granular cell tumors at this site. The latter may pose a problem of differential diagnosis because it frequently is associated with a pseudoepitheliomatous hyperplasia of the overlying epithelium, which is a pitfall to avoid when dealing with a superficial biopsy specimen. As a rule the lesion is characterized by a solitary nodule located in the dermis and the subcutis and less frequently in the submucosa or in the smooth or striated muscle. Not infrequently, it is organ-associated (e.g., the larynx, the bile duct, etc). This is a benign lesion, and recurrence is rare save for the malignant tumors, which are less than 2% of all granular cell tumors.

6.6.4.1   Histopathology. There is a considerable pattern of growth. The histological picture is characterized by a poorly circumscribed tumor, accompanying acanthosis and pseudoepitheliomatous hyperplasia of overlying epithelium as well as a close association of granular cells with peripheral nerves. Tumor cells are rounded to polygonal with moderate nuclear atypia (Fig 6.250). The main feature is the observation of eosinophilic cytoplasm (Fig 6.251) containing coarse granules that stained positive for PAS and are resistant to digestion. Immunohistochemical investigations have attested to its neural nature; S-100 protein, myelin protein, and myelin-associated glycoprotein frequently are demonstrated. Apart from the aforementioned immunohistochemical profile, CD68 can be expressed, which indicates numerous cytoplasmic phagolysosomes

6.6.4.2   Cytopathology. Smears in granular cell tumor are cell-rich and stroma-poor. Tumor material is characteristic and consists of both large cohesive groups of cells with a syncytial appearance and single cells. These cells are of large size and have ill-defined abundant granular cytoplasm and bland regular small nuclei (Figs 6.252 and 6.253). Nucleoli are inconspicuous. Neither mitoses nor necrosis are noted.

6.6.4.3   Differential Diagnosis. The most important differential diagnosis in our experience is breast cancer because of the frequent occurrence in this setting. Recognition of granular cell tumor is important because the clinical, radiological, and gross appearance of granular cell tumors of the breast often simulate carcinoma.

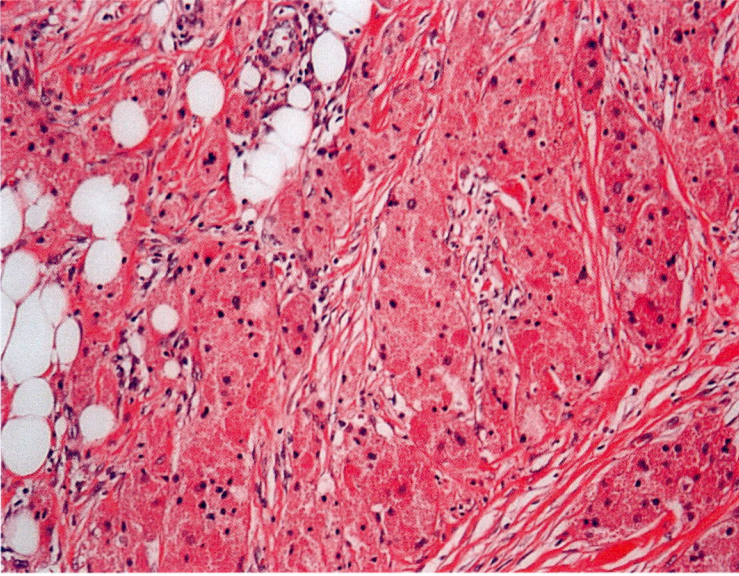

FIG 6.250   Granular cell tumor, sheets and cords of eosinophilic epithelioid cells containing coarse granules.

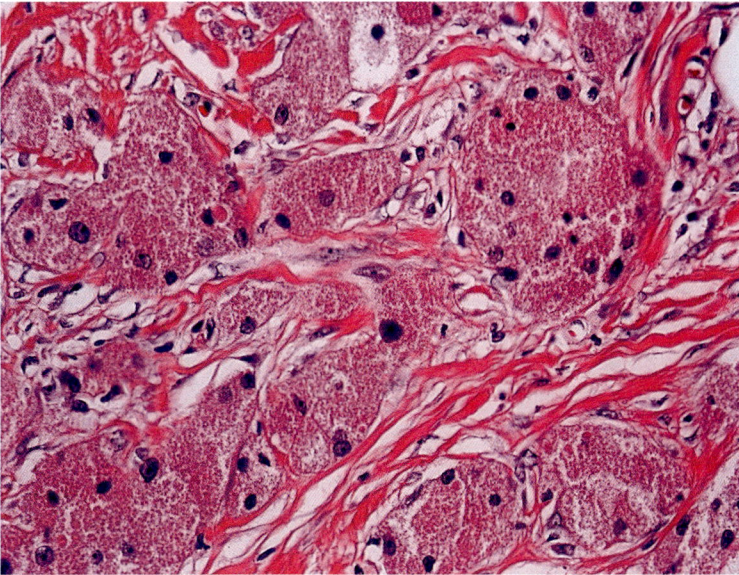

FIG 6.251   Granular cell tumor, higher magnification of granular cells.

Cytologically, the tumors consist of cohesive groups of cells with a syncytial appearance, with abundant, finely eosinophilic cytoplasmic granules and small round-to-slightly-oval nuclei, whereas breast cancer consists of clearly epithelial cells with well-defined cytoplasmic borders [283, 284].

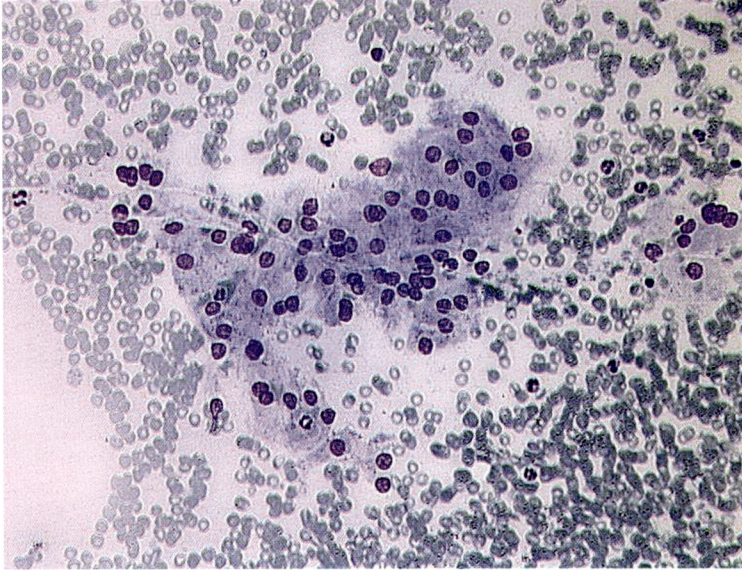

FIG 6.252   Granular cell tumor, typical cells with ill-defined cytoplasmic borders.

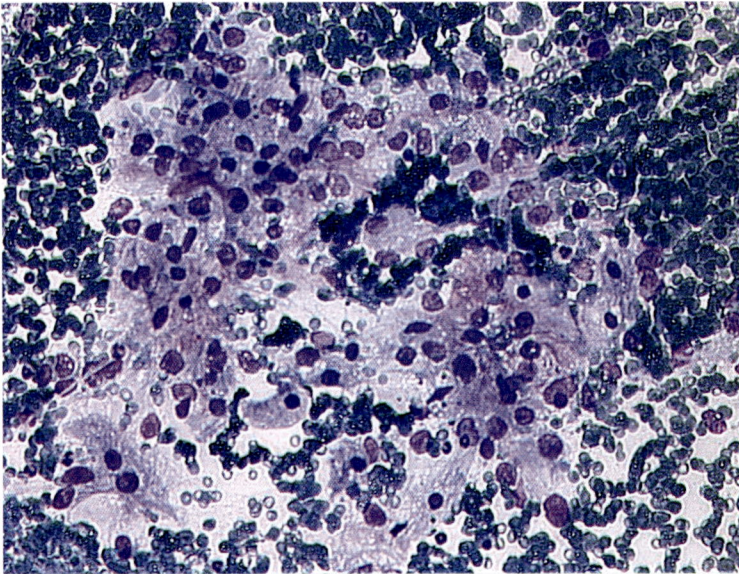

FIG 6.253   Granular cell tumor, typical cells with small, dark nuclei.

6.6.4.4 Comments. There is a limited number of cytological large series of granular cell tumor [284–286], whereas many publications are case reports. A consensus has been reached concerning the morphology of the granular cell tumor, which is highly characteristic. Some reports describe malignant evolution [285,287,288]. For some authors [287], malignant transformation may be extremely difficult or impossible to diagnose unless metastatic disease is demonstrated.

For others [285], malignant granular cell tumors demonstrated characteristic cytologic features that differ from those of benign granular cell tumors. Evidence of mild-to-moderate cytologic atypia, increased mitotic activity, and DNA ploidy analysis may be helpful in predicting malignant behavior [287]. A previous study of 3 malignant and 17 benign granular cell tumors was reported [285]. It was concluded that hyperchromasia, coarse chromatin, an increased cytonuclear ratio, nuclear pleomorphism, and vesicular nuclei with enlarged nucleoli and spindle cell morphology mostly were associated with malignancy.

Numerous examples of granular cell tumor were reported in the literature, of which many cases were breast lesions. Granular cell tumors of the breast are rare and may mimic an invasive carcinoma [286]. However, the accurate diagnosis is rather straightforward. In our series of 15 cases, only one case was misdiagnosed as metastasis of head and neck squamous cell carcinoma.

6.6.4.5 Clinical and FNA Key Features. The following are in favor of the diagnosis:

- Cohesive groups of cells with a syncytial appearance
- Abundant, finely eosinophilic cytoplasmic granules and small round-to-slightly-oval nuclei
- Ill defined cytoplasmic borders

The following are difficulties in the diagnosis:

- Malignant behaviour in rare cases, unusual localizations
- Nuclear pleomorphism

The following is evidence against the diagnosis:

- Well-delimitated cytoplasmic borders

6.6.5 Rhabdoid Tumor

Originally described in the kidney and reported as a "rhabdomyosarcomatous variant of Wilms' tumor," the rhabdoid tumor is a distinct clinicopathologic entity. Subsequent descriptions of similar tumors developing in every extrarenal anatomic site have been well documented. Indeed, most rhabdoid tumors originate in the kidney in children less than 1 year of age and pursue an aggressive clinical course. It is important to better define extrarenal rhabdoid tumor because a wide variety of carcinomas with rhabdoid features have been described, including urothelial carcinoma, renal cell carcinoma, and colorectal carcinoma. Similar features are also part of melanoma, mesothelioma, lymphoma, and sarcomas of various types. Besides its clinical course, the rhadboid tumor has unique immunohistochemical and cytogenetic profiles. Aberrations of chromosomes 11 and 22 have been reported, suggesting the presence of a muted suppressor gene at this locus. The gene *hSNF5/INI* has been reported to be mutated and is presently a serious candidate for the development of the tumor [240].

6.6.5.1 Histopathology. As indicated by its name, the rhabdoid tumor consists of a population of large polygonal cells, with eccentric nuclei, prominent nucleoli, and abundant cytoplasm (Figs 6.254 to 6.256) containing hyaline PAS+ globoid inclusions (Fig 6.257) that correspond by electron microscopy to accumulations of

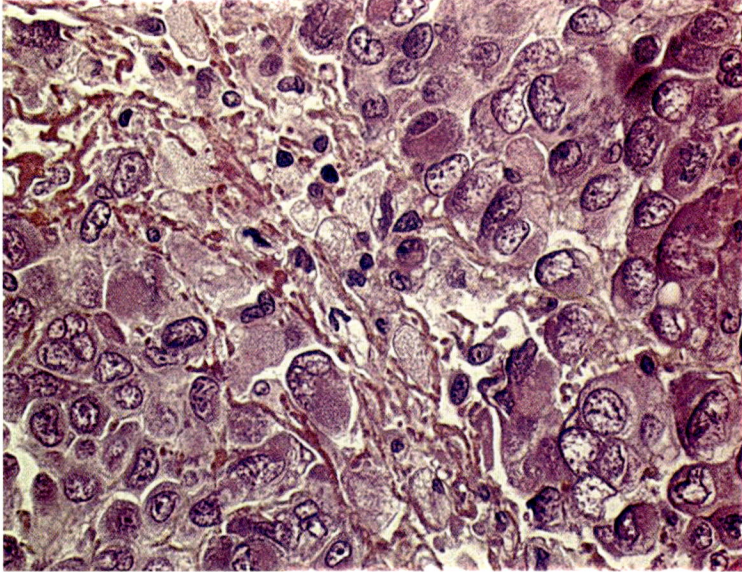

FIG 6.254 Rhabdoid tumor, large polygonal and ovoid cells, with abundant cytoplasm.

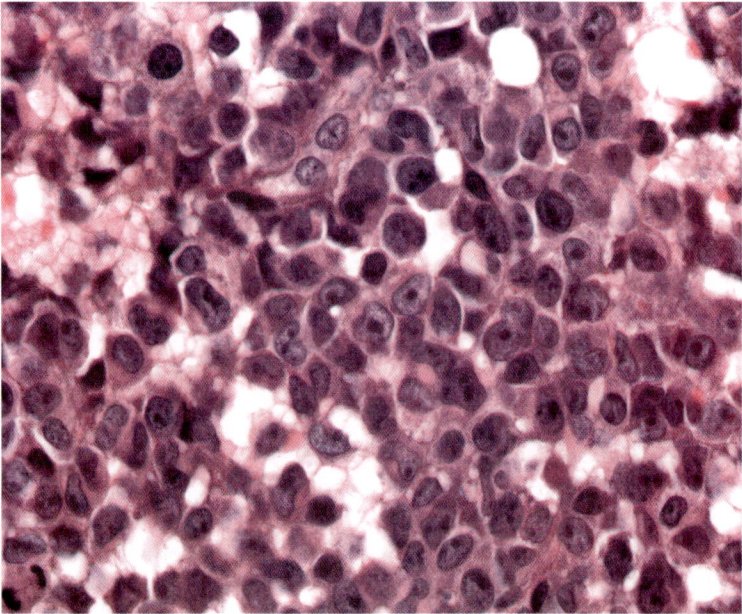

FIG 6.255 Rhabdoid tumor, large polygonal and ovoid cells, with eccentric nuclei, and prominent nucleoli.

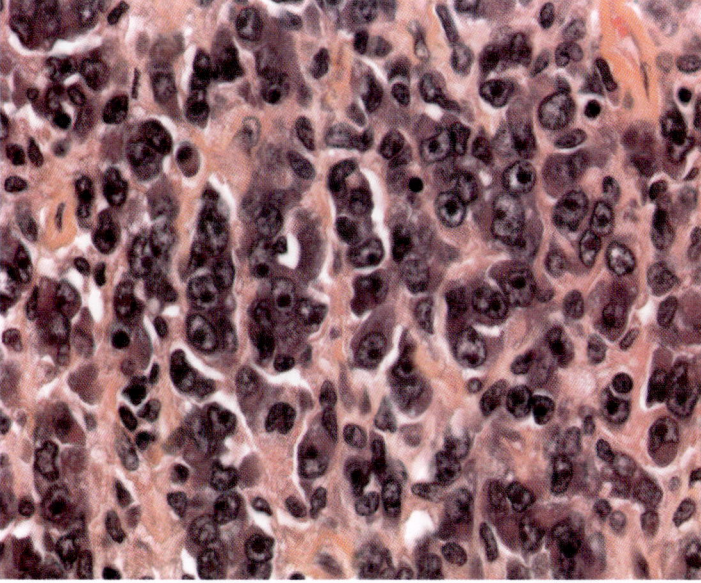

FIG 6.256 Rhabdoid tumor, large polygonal and ovoid cells.

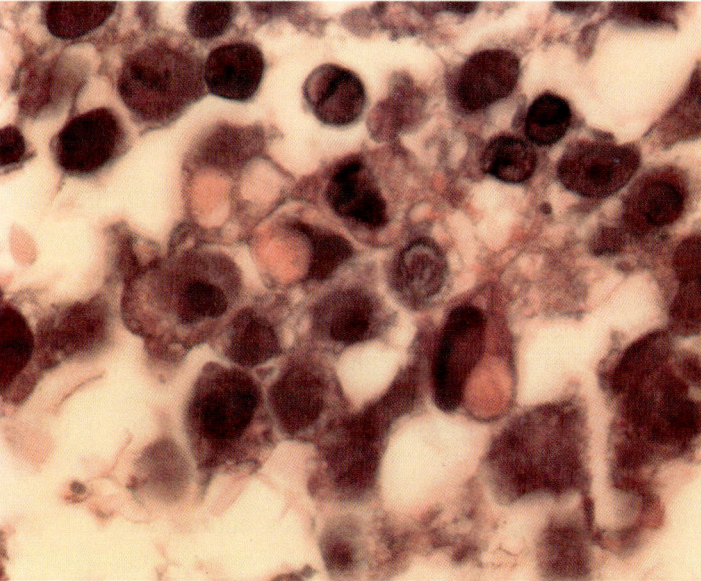

FIG 6.257 Rhabdoid tumor, hyaline globoid paranuclear inclusions.

paranuclear intermediate filaments. They express vimentin, cytokeratin of low-molecular weight, and neural antigens.

6.6.5.2 *Cytopathology.* Smears in the rhabdoid tumor are hypercellular and stroma-poor. They are relatively similar from case to case and invariably consist of atypical, anaplasic, and pleomorphic cells showing a rhabdomyoblast-like

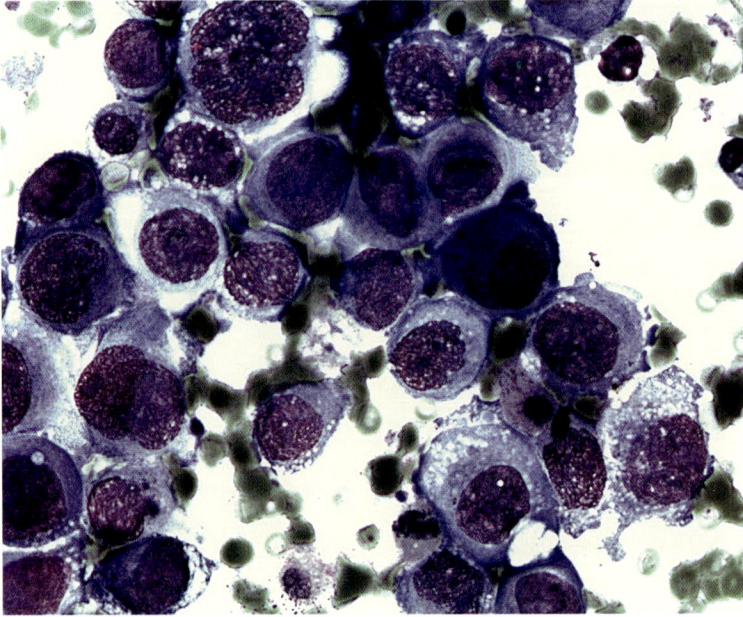

FIG 6.258 Rhabdoid tumor, atypical, anaplastic cells.

morphology (Figs 6.258 and 6.259) and an important variability in size. Cells usually are isolated but also clustered. Binucleation also is observed occasionally. In large cells, nuclei are irregular, with coarse chromatin with one or numerous nucleoli (Fig 6.260). Some nuclei are kidney-shaped. In smaller cells, nuclei are roundish with dark, homogenous chromatin. Numerous mitotic figures usually are present. Cytoplasms are large, grayish, and usually microvacuolated. In some cells, cytoplasms are reduced to a thin perinuclear rim; in others they are large and ill-delimitated. Some cytoplasms show peripheral densifications being clarified in perinuclear space. In some cases, tumor cells show homogenous, globoid inclusions adapting a plasma-like morphology (Fig 6.261). Inclusions are positive for epithelial markers (Fig 6.262). Spindle-shaped cells also are observed (Figs 6.263 and 6.264). Some cases show an abundant necrotic background. Connective tissue fragments, calcifications, rosettes, or papillary clusters are not present.

6.6.5.3 Differential Diagnosis. The following entities should be differentiated from rhabdoid tumor:

— Rhabdomyosarcoma
— Alveolar soft tissue sarcoma
— Epithelioid sarcoma

In renal localizations, rhabdoid tumors should be differentiated from nephroblastomas with rhabdoid features [289] (Table 6.13). This distinction is essential for therapeutic purposes. The presence of blastematous cells and epithelial structures are pathognomic for nephroblastoma. In extrarenal localisations,

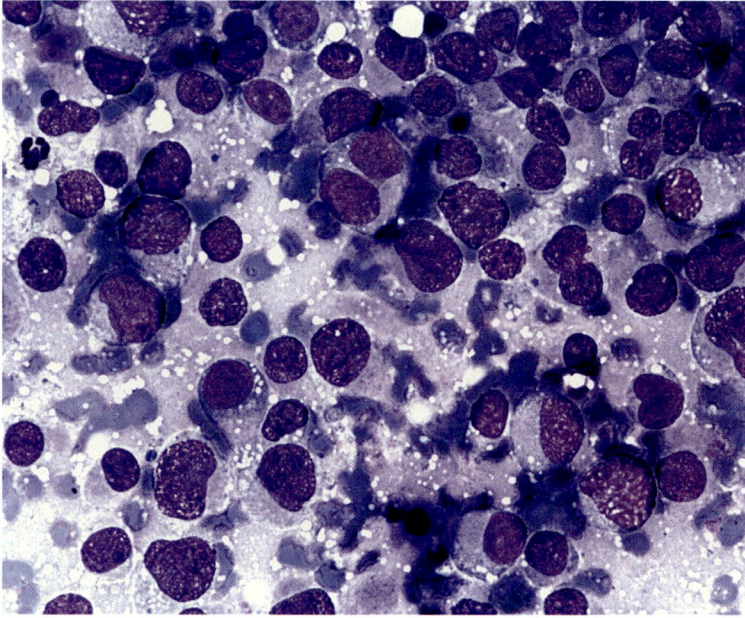

FIG 6.259   Rhabdoid tumor, atypical cells showing rhabdomyoblast-like morphology.

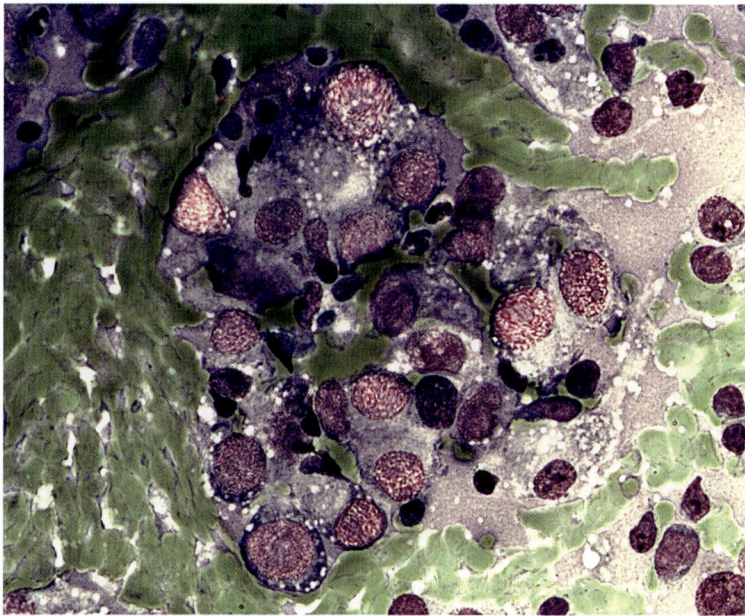

FIG 6.260   Rhabdoid tumor, epithelioid pattern and coarse chromatin with prominet nucleoli.

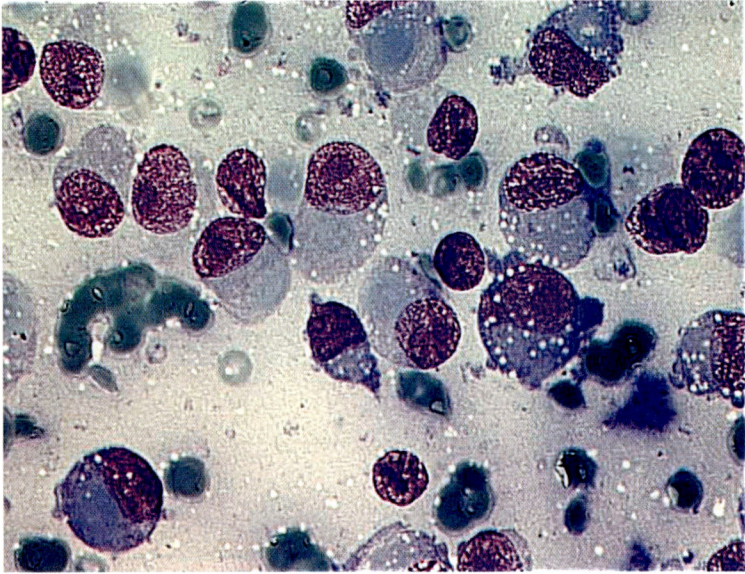

FIG 6.261 Rhabdoid tumor, homogenous, globoid Intracytoplasmic inclusions, adapting a plasma-like morphology.

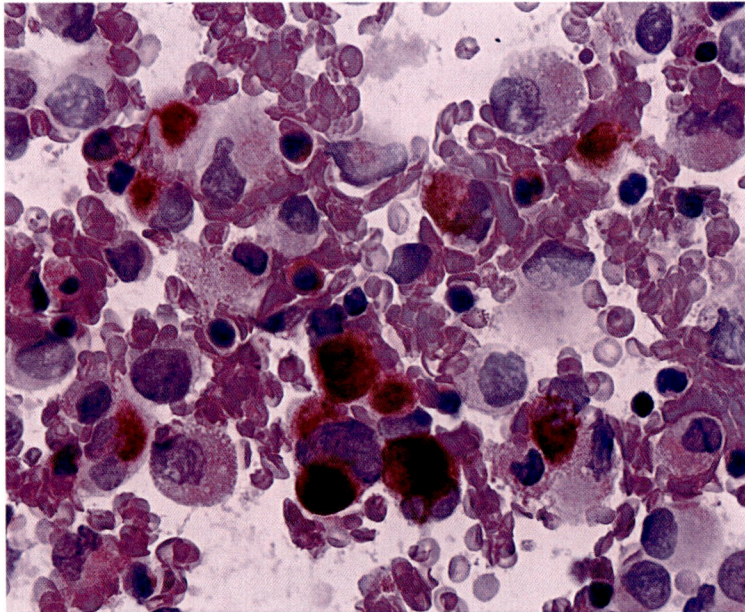

FIG 6.262 Rhabdoid tumor, inclusions are positive for epithelial markers (KL1).

rhabdoid tumors should be differentiated from rhabdomyosarcoma and alveolar soft part sarcoma using immunocytochemical, molecular, and eventually, ultra-structural methods [274]. Rhabdomyosarcomas, however, show a more mono-morphous morpholody. Similarly, rhadboid tumors should be differentiated from

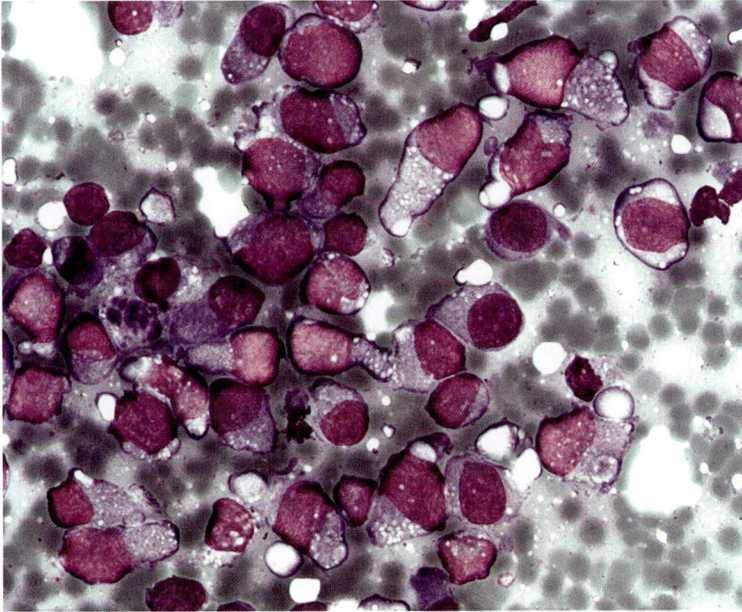

FIG 6.263   Rhabdoid tumor, elongated and epithelioid cells.

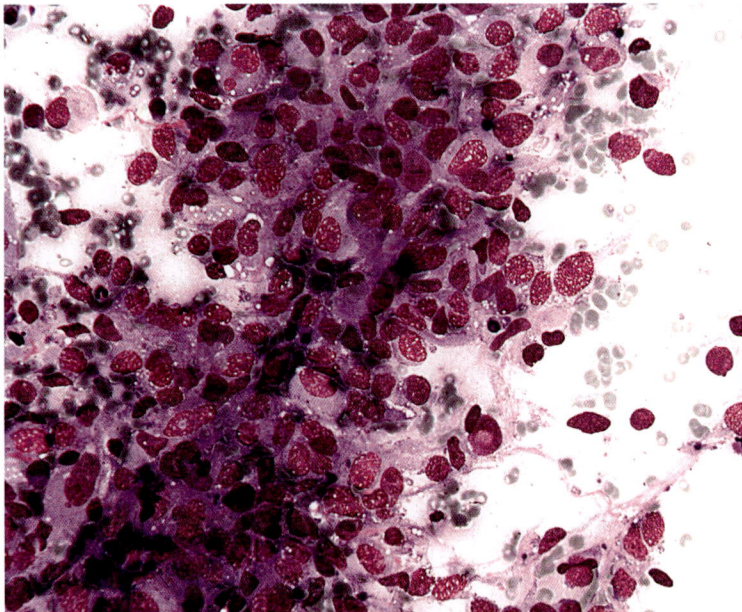

FIG 6.264   Rhabdoid tumor, spindle-shaped and polymorphous cells.

TABLE 6.13   Cytologic differential diagnosis of extrarenal rhabdoid tumor

	Rhabdoid tumor	Rhabdomyosarcoma	Alveolar soft part sarcoma	Epithelioid sarcoma
Epithelioid Clusters	+/−	−	+	++
Rhabdomyoblastic- like cells	++	++	+/−	+/−
Round Cells	++	++	++	++
Spindle shaped Cells	+	+	+/−	+
Cytoplasm	Perinuclear inclusions	Vacuolated	Crystalloids	Vacuolated

++; Frequent, +; rare, +/− occasionally seen, −; absent.

epithelioid sarcoma. Once again, both entities show immunohistochemical and genomic specificities that allow an accurate diagnosis. Immunocytochemical study shows muscular markers negativity (HHF and desmin) as well as cytokeratin and/ or EMA positivity.

6.6.5.4 *Comments.* Cytoplasmic eosinophilic densities correspond to cytoplasmic eosinophilic globules observed in the histologic sections and cytoplasmic filamentous inclusions observed ultrastructurally [290]. Diagnosis of malignant rhabdoid tumor of the kidney may be suggested from fine needle aspiration smears; however, additional confirmation of the diagnosis by histologic or ultrastructural examination is desirable [291].

More than 40 rhabdoid tumors were reported in the cytology literature [291–298]. In reported series, smears are hypercellular and stroma-poor. Cells are predominantly round to oval, singly, or arranged in irregularly shaped clusters. Tumor cells do not differ much in shape and exhibit clear, empty nuclei with prominent nucleoli; the cytoplasm is abundant and sometimes eosinophilic [296, 298]. Occasionally, smears show characteristic rhabdoid cells (i.e., cells with a large, vesicular nucleus with a prominent nucleolus and cytoplasm exhibiting a large, dense, and paranuclear inclusion) [295, 298]. Consequently, a consensus has been reached that rhabdoid tumors are pleomorphic neoplasms showing rhabdomyoblastic and polygonal features. The presence of rhabdoid-like cells may pose diagnostic problems because of its broad morphologic spectrum, but immunohistochemistry shows cytokeratin or EMA positivity [294]. Ultrastructural examination shows the presence of intermediate cytoplasmic filaments. Similar features have been observed in our series. Nineteen cases were characterized constantly by an anaplastic morphology with rhabdomyoblastic features and atypical, strongly nucleolated nuclei. Only a few tumors showed perinuclear cytoplasmic inclusions. The high level of accurate diagnosis was related to the use of immunocytochemistry (EMA and/or cytokeratin).

6.6.5.5 *Clinical and FNA Key Features.* The following are in favor of the diagnosis:

- Young age, kidney localization
- Round-to-oval rhabdomyoblastic cells

- Perinuclear inclusions that are keratin positive.

The following is a difficulty in the diagnosis:

- Lack of perinuclear densities.
- Epithelioid pattern with clusters

The following is against the diagnosis:

- True rhabdomyoblasts, alveolar structures

6.6.6   Alveolar Soft Part Sarcoma

Alveolar soft part sarcoma is a rare malignant tumor of unusual clinical behavior originally described in 1952 [299]. Despite several immunohistochemical and electron microscopic studies, its exact nature and its nosologic classification are uncertain, although it recently was characterized better by the documentation of a recurrent, nonreciprocal translation, der (17)t(x;17)(p11.2;q25) [300,301]. Despite a controversial histogenesis and cryptic behavior, its histopathological picture is characteristic. Most alveolar soft part sarcomas occur in adolescents and young adults with a predilection for females during the first 2 years of life [299]. Muscles and soft tissue of the extremities are the most common sites of involvement followed by the trunk, head and neck, and the retroperitoneum. At the time of diagnosis, several patients have metastatic disease [302]. A 5-year survival rate could reach up to 80% [303] even if the ultimate prognosis is nevertheless poor. The most important parameters of clinical outcome are age at diagnosis, tumor size, and presence of metastases at initial diagnosis.

6.6.6.1   Histopathology. In most cases, the histopathological diagnosis is straightforward, with rare cases showing atypical features simulating, for example, metastatic renal cell carcinoma, paraganglioma, or granular cell tumor. Typically, tumor cells are large, polygonal/epithelioid, and grouped in well-defined nests or pseudoalveoles separated by thin-twilled vascular channels lined by a simple layer of endothelial cells (Fig 6.265). Cytoplasm is abundant eosinophilic, rarely vacuolated, and often countains glycogen as well as PAS+ and diastase-resistant rhomboid or rod-shaped crystals (Fig 6.266), which could be confirmed by electron microscopic examination. Mitotic figures are rare. The nests or pseudoalveoles are delimited by fine reticulin fibers, which do not penetrate between individual tumor cells in contrast to paraganglioma.

A plethora of immunohistochemical studies have attempted to determine the phenotype of alveolar soft part sarcoma. As a rule, constituent cells are immunoreactive for vimentin, muscle-specific actin, and desmin. There are inconsistent reports on the detection of nuclear-MyoD1. As already mentioned, alveolar soft part sarcoma depicts a well-characterized cytogenetic translocation [304]. It has been suggested that the female predominance could be influenced by the possession of an extra X chromosome, which doubles the likehood of developing alveolar soft part sarcoma [305].

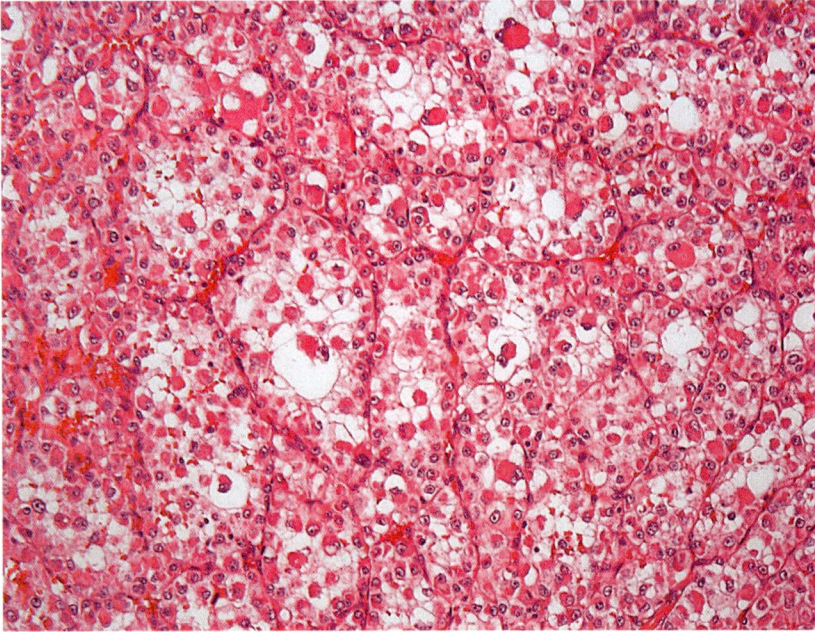

FIG 6.265 Alveolar soft part sarcoma, well-defined nests of pseudoalveoles separated by thin-walled vessels.

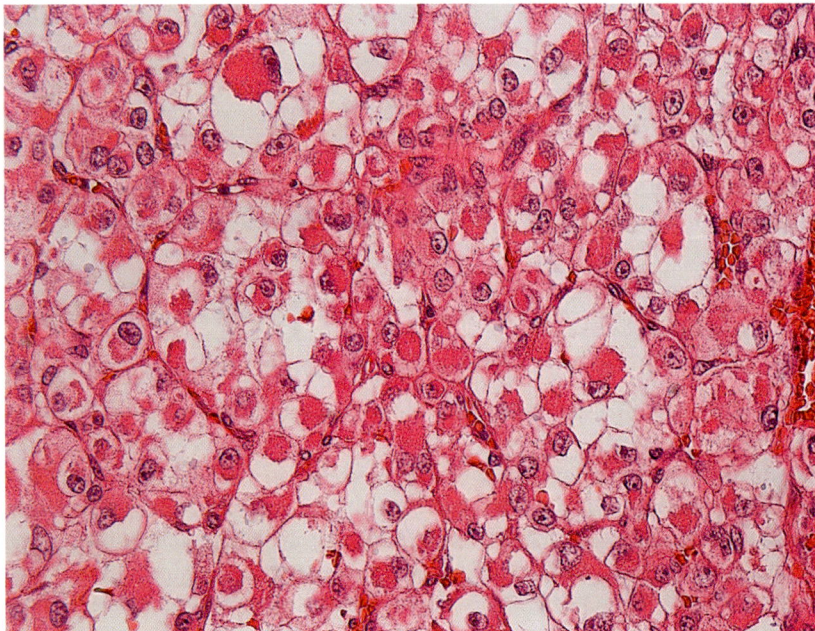

FIG 6.266 Alveolar soft part sarcoma, cohesive tumor cells countaining rod-shaped or rhomboid crystals.

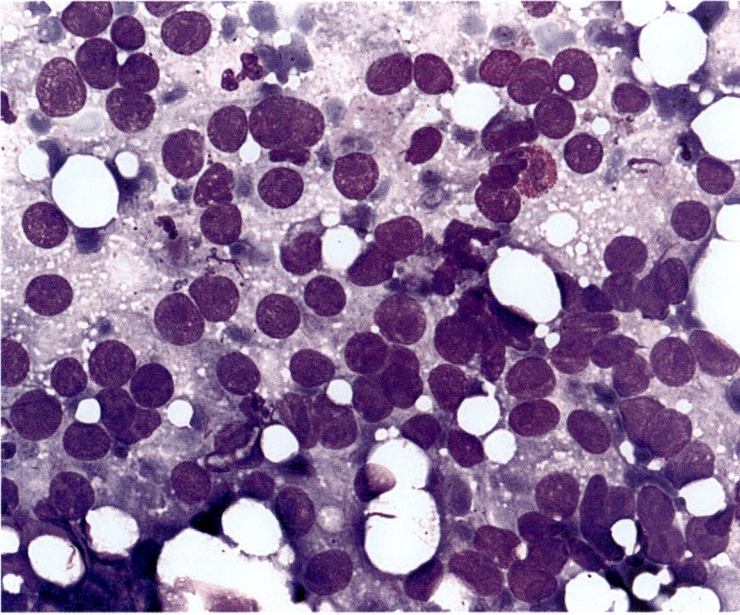

FIG 6.267   Alveolar soft part sarcoma, roundish, strongly nucleolated cells.

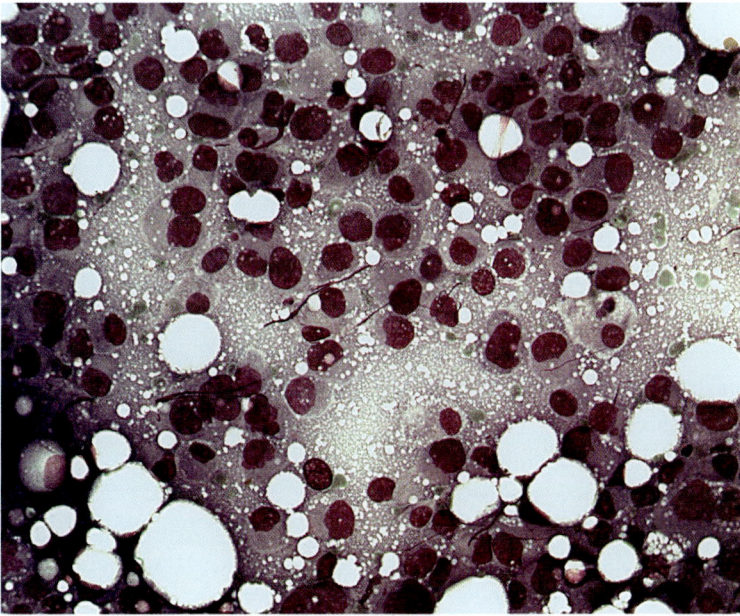

FIG 6.268   Alveolar soft part sarcoma, monotonous cells.

6.6.6.2   *Cytopathology.* Smears in alveolar soft part sarcomas are hypercellular, stroma poor, and similar in all cases when observed randomly. Cells may be roundish (Figs 6.267 and 6.268), rhabdomyoblastic-like (Fig 6.269), or spindle-shaped (Fig 6.270). They are isolated or arranged in syncytial groups with occasional

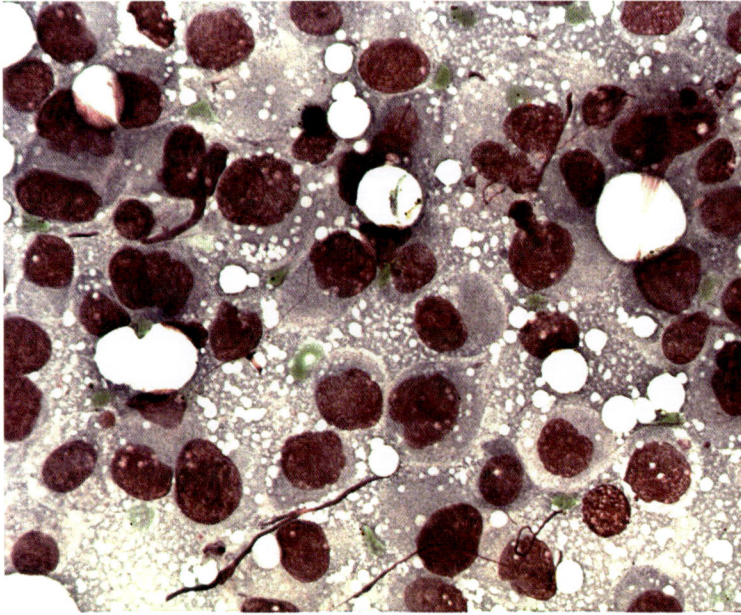

FIG 6.269 Alveolar soft part sarcoma, rhabdomyoblastic pattern.

acinar-type architecture. Cytoplasms are large, granular, and variably vacuolated or microvacuolated. Cytoplasmic fragility and granularity with abundant, atypical, and naked nuclei are present. Mitotic activity is clearly present. The characteristic perinuclear crystals are observed in some cells and are especially well detected with Papanicolaou-stained smears within the cytoplasm and in the background near the tumor cells.

6.6.6.3 *Differential Diagnosis.* The following entities should be differentiated from alveolar soft part sarcoma:

— Metastatic renal cell carcinoma
— Paraganglioma
— Granular cell tumor (malignant)
— Alveolar rhabdomyosarcoma
— Rhabdoid tumor
— Epithelioid sarcoma

The differential diagnosis should include rhabdomyosarcoma, epithelioid sarcoma rhabdoid tumor, and eventually, granular cell tumor [306]. In general, the differential diagnosis may be difficult in this group of epithelioid/roundish cells sarcomas and is assisted by immunohistochemistry and genomic results. Rhabdomyosarcoma usually consists of the following varieties of cells: roundish, spindle-shaped, rhabdomyo-blastic, and plasmacytoid, sometimes binucleated with excentric nuclei. Numerous

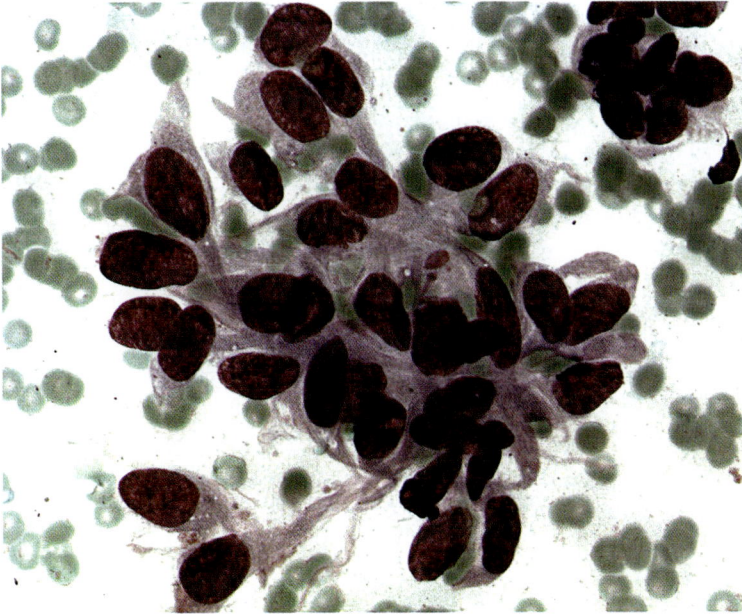

FIG 6.270 Alveolar soft part sarcoma, spindle-shaped cells.

mitotic figures, prominent cytonuclear atypia, and sometimes an important necrotic background, are observed. Moreover, multinucleated cells are frequent in well-differentiated (embryonal) rhadbomyosarcoma, whereas this feature is exceptionnal in alveolar soft part sarcoma [274]. Epithelioid sarcoma consists of aggregated and isolated epithelioid cells that are round to polygonal, with eccentrically located nuclei. The tumor cells show severe-to-moderate atypia and pleomorphism. This pattern may simulate alveolar soft part sarcoma. Rhabdoid tumor consists of atypical, anaplasic, and pleomorphic cells showing rhabdomyoblast-like morphology and an important variability in size. Cells usually are isolated as well as clustered. Binucleation also is observed occasionally. Detailed analysis allows finding peri-nuclear inclusions. A malignant granular cell tumor also should be differentiated. Cells in alveolar soft part sarcoma are more epithelioid with well-deliminated cells borders than those in malignant granular cell tumor. Ultrastructurally, peculiar, needle-like intracytoplasmic crystalline rhomboid cytoplasmic inclusions typical of alveolar soft part sarcoma are identified [307,308]. TFE3 staining is an extremely helpful antibody in confirming the diagnosis of alveolar soft part sarcoma.

Table 6.13 summarizes the differential diagnosis of alveolar soft part sarcoma.

6.6.6.4 Comments. Alveolar soft part sarcoma is a rare neoplastic entity that shows an uncharacteristic cytologic image of epithelioid/roundish cell sarcoma. Distinctive histopathological patterns may be absent in smears. A pseudoalveolar pattern, observed in tissue specimens, is absent or inconspicious in aspirates. Similarly, crystalloids also typical for alveolar soft part sarcoma may be identified occasionally with success using MGG stain. Wakely et al. [309] reported the largest series of alveolar soft part sarcoma. They compared their results with literature data. Needle-shaped crystals were reported only in one-third of cases. They concluded that although they are helpful when present, the crystals are an uncommon finding in aspirates or imprint smears of alveolar soft part sarcoma, and their absence should not be negative of diagnosis. When correlated with an adequate clinical context, it allows specific preoperative recognition. Although while immunocytologic studies are helpful to exclude other neoplasms, ultrastructure and core biopsy may result in a precise diagnosis [310].

Twenty-four examples of alveolar soft part sarcoma were reported in the cytology literature [306–311]. The diagnosis of malignancy was reached in all cases. In nine other examples of our series, only one tumor was diagnosed, accurately and eight others were misdiagnosed as another type of sarcoma, rhabdomyosarcoma, or synovial sarcoma.

6.6.6.5 Clinical and FNA Key Features. The following are in favor of the diagnosis:

- Hypercellular smear
- Roundish cells with frequently vaculoated cytoplasms
- Regular nuclei with well visible nucleoli
- Mitotic figures
- Acinar structures
- Needle-like crystalloids

The following is a difficulty in the diagnosis:

- Lack of cytonuclear atypia, monomorphous character

The following are evidence of the diagnosis:

- Clinical evidence of renal cell carcinoma or paraganglioma
- Perinuclear inclusions

6.6.7 Clear Cell Sarcoma

Clear cell sarcoma of tendons and aponeuroses, formerly referred to as malignant melanoma of soft parts, is a rare malignant neoplasm derived from neural crest cells. Both females and males are affected, although women are affected more frequently. The median age of occurrence is 36 years. Most tumors occur in the extremities, with the trunk and head and neck being involved more rarely. They are medium-sized neoplasms averaging 4–5 cm in largest diameter and are well circumscribed, lobulated, or multinodular. The prognosis is poor. Large series of cases have shown a 5-year survival rate of around 55% (AFIP and the Netherland's tumor registry). A more recent study from the Japanese Oncology Group reports an overall survival rate of 45% at 5 years and 36% at 10 years [312].

In the past, many studies attempted to verify the nosologic classification of clear cell sarcoma and its distinction from other similar morphologic entities, particularly malignant melanoma to which it has been closely associated. Electron microscopic and immunohistochemical investigations had shown a melanocytic differentiation for clear cell sarcoma. However, a cytogenetic hallmark of clear cell sarcoma has been demonstrated: a translocation t (12;22)(q13;q12) resulting in the chimeric *EWS-ATF1* gene. Although preliminary reports tended to show that this genetic abnormality was isolated, additional studies confirmed that detection of *EWS-ATF1* was highly prevalent and therefore could be used as a sensitive diagnostic tool [313,314]. Now convincing evidence has been found that clear cell sarcoma could be separated from malignant melanoma based on the molecular findings [315].

6.6.7.1 Histopathology. Clear cell sarcoma is characterized by a histological pattern of uniform, epitelioid/polygonal to spindle cells (Figs 6.271 and 6.272) with clear eosinophilic cytoplasm, grouped in variable size clusters (Fig 6.273), and separated by fibrous septa. The clear cell appearance (Fig 6.274) is a result of the presence of cytoplasmic glycogen. Pleomorphism is absent or minimal, and mitotic figures are rare. Scattered multinucleated giant cells are observed frequently. The demonstration of melanin pigment by histochemical methods is inconsistent and, of particular interest, could be abundant in metastasis, whereas the primary tumor was completely devoid of.

The immunohistochemical profile is characterized by positive reactions for S-100 protein, HMB-45, Melan-A, and microphtalmia transferring factor (MCTF), all of which reflect a melanin synthesis. Demonstration by electron microscopy of melanosomes at different stages of maturation could complete the morphological phenotype of clear cell sarcoma.

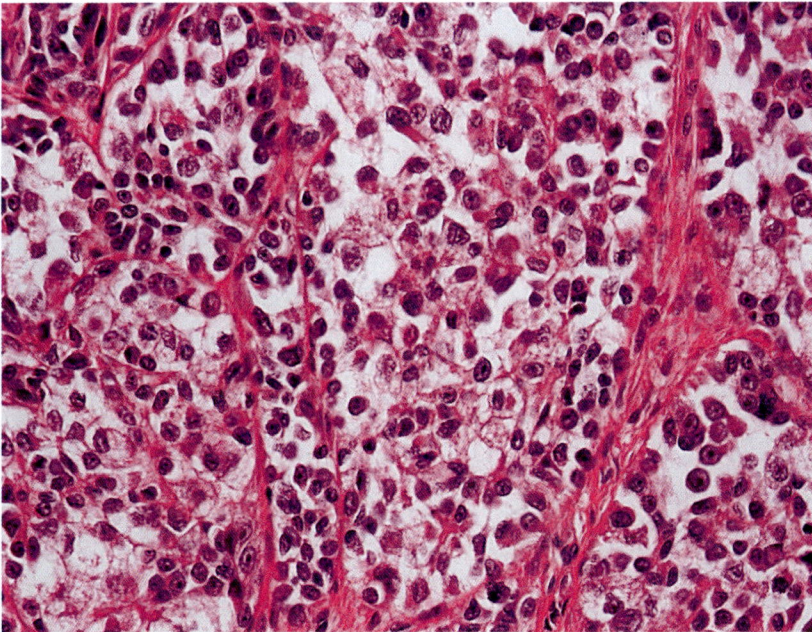

FIG 6.271 Clear cell sarcoma, nests of epithelioid clear cells.

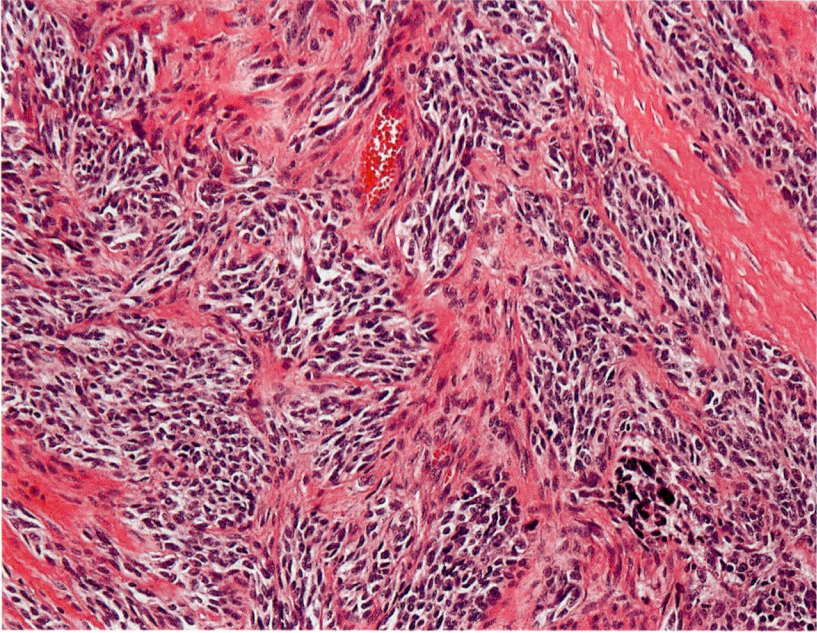

FIG 6.272   Clear cell sarcoma, area comprising neoplastic cells dissecting tendon sheaths.

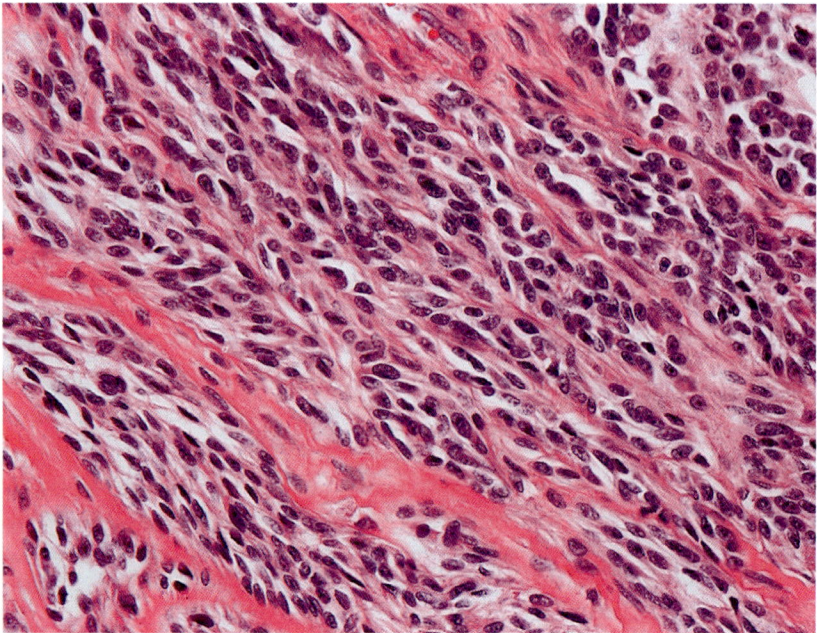

FIG 6.273   Clear cell sarcoma, higher magnification of spindle cell bundles.

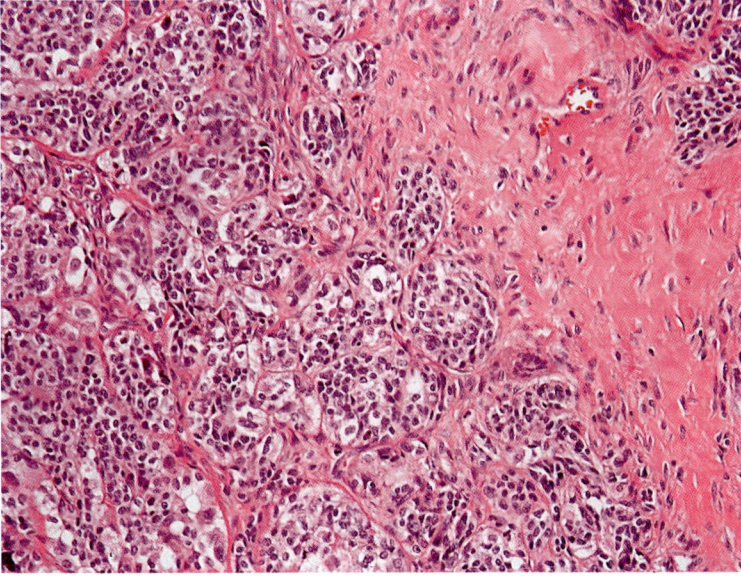

FIG 6.274 Clear cell sarcoma, nests of uniform epithelioid clear cells separated by fibrous septa.

6.6.7.2 Cytopathology. Aspirates in clear cell sarcomas are hypercellular and stroma-poor (Fig 6.275). Cellular material consists of dispersed and noncohesive epithelioid cells with large cytoplasm showing cytonuclear atypia. Cells may be polymorphous, rounded (Fig 6.276), polygonal (Figs 6.277 and 6.278), or spindly shaped (Fig 6.279). Occasional multinucleated cells also are noted (Fig 6.280). Nulei are hyperchromatic, and nucleoli are central and prominent. Cytoplasms are clarified, and are shown especially well using Papanicolaou stain. Microacinar structures are observed. Moreover, the so-called "tigroid background" also was described in clear cell sarcoma. Some cases may show abundant melanin, making diagnosis easier.

6.6.7.3 Differential Diagnosis. The following entities should be differentiated from clear cell sarcoma:

- Alveolar soft part sarcoma
- Malignant melanoma
- Metastatic carcinoma

The main differential diagnoses are melanoma and metastatic clear cell carcinoma. Multinucleation may be a feature of clear cell sarcoma and is exceptional in alveolar soft part sarcoma.

6.6.7.4 Comments. The cytology pattern is similar to the histological findings. Cells are monomorphic and characteristic. Ther are large-sized and vary in shape going from epithelioid to spindle-shaped. In general, the cytology is comparable with the cytology of classical cutaneous malignant melanoma. In rare cases, tumors show

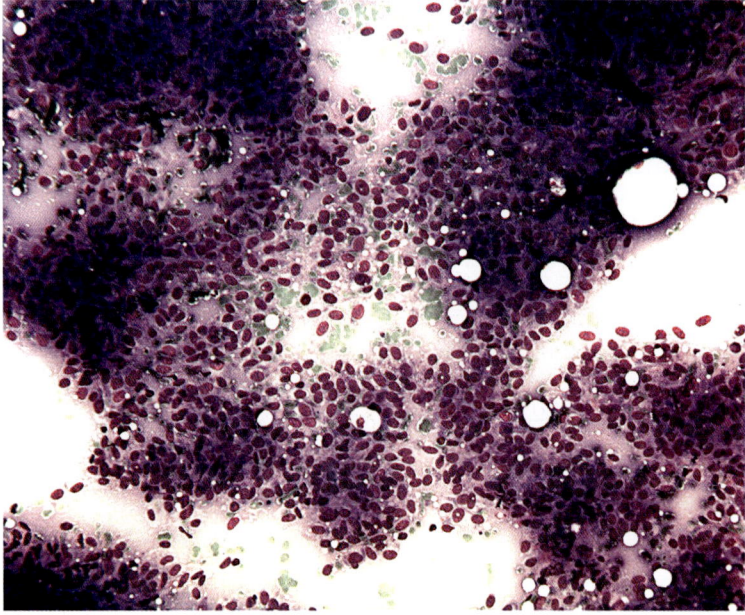

FIG 6.275   Clear cell sarcoma, hypercellular and stroma-poor smear.

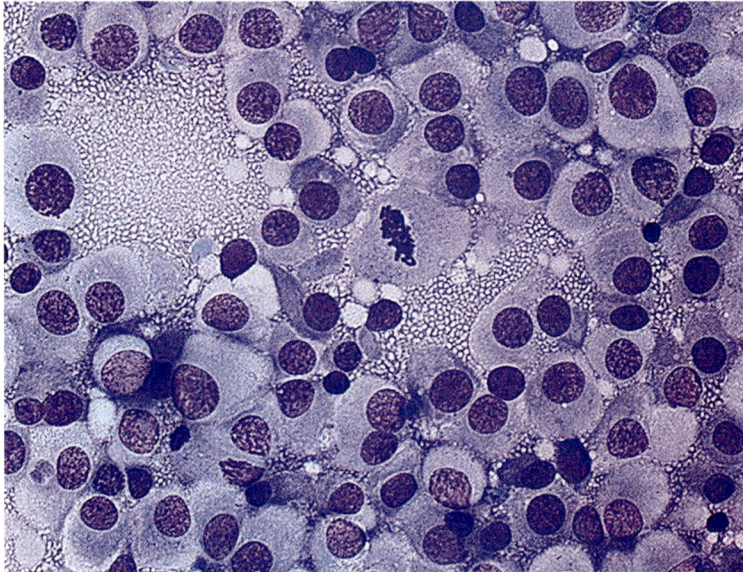

FIG 6.276   Clear cell sarcoma, rounded cells and epithelioid.

a pure population of spindle-shaped cells. Cytoplasmic clarification is not always well detected.

Only small series were reported, totalizing 22 cases [316–318]. All cases were diagnosed as malignancies. In 10 other personal examples of clear cell sarcomas, all

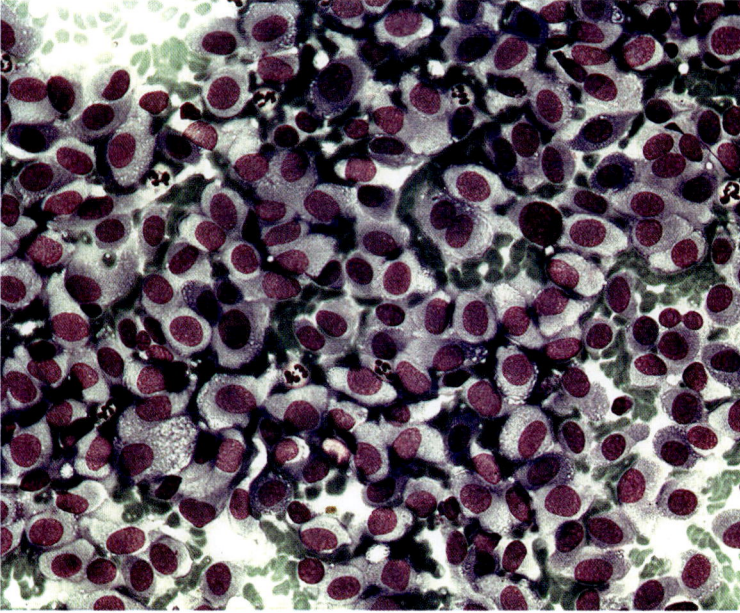

FIG 6.277 Clear cell sarcoma, polygonal cells.

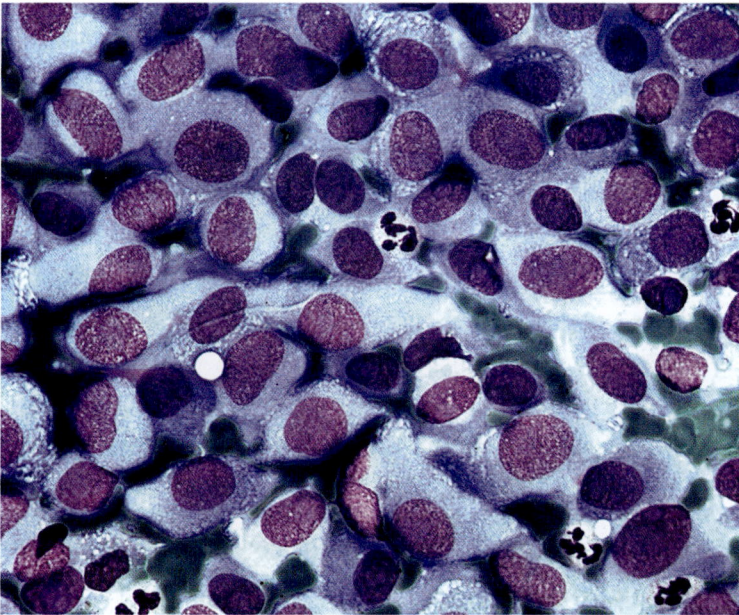

FIG 6.278 Clear cell sarcoma, roundish cells resembling melanoma. Compare to Fig 6.282.

cases were diagnosed as malignant, but only 3 were diagnosed accurately. Other tumors were misdiagnosed as synovial sarcoma, malignant hemangiopericytoma, or Ewing sarcoma.

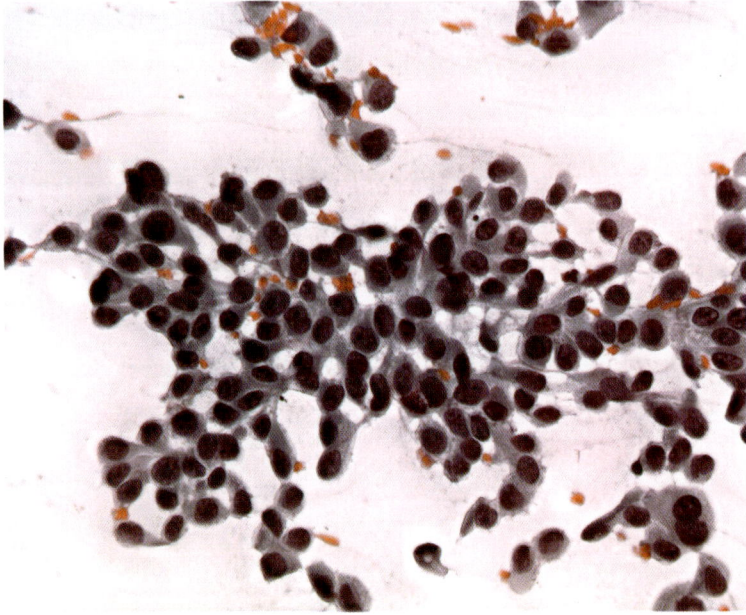

FIG 6.279 Clear cell sarcoma, spindly shaped cells, Papanicolaou. Compare to Fig 6.283.

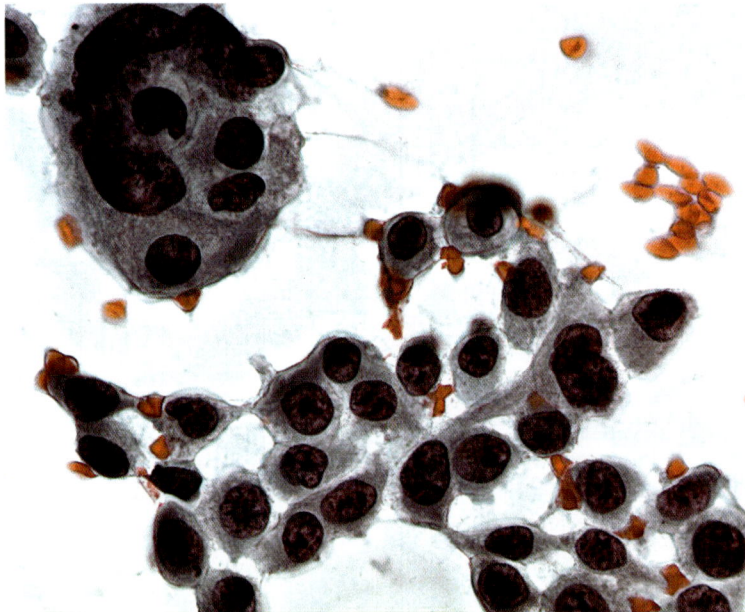

FIG 6.280 Clear cell sarcoma, multinucleated cells, Papanicolaou.

6.6.7.5 *FNA Key Features.* The following are in favor of diagnosis:

- Monomorphous roundish/epithelioid cells
- Cytoplasmic clarification

  – Melanin
  – Central nuclei with prominent nucleoli, multinucleation, and tigroid background

The following are difficulties in the diagnosis:

  – Spindle-shaped cells
  – Lack of mitotic figures

The following are evidence against the diagnosis:

  – Perinuclear inclusions
  – Needle-like crystals
  – Cohesive epithelial clusters

6.6.8   Malignant Melanoma and Metastases

Malignant melanoma, metastatic renal cell, and lung carcinomas are great imitators of sarcomas as they are coined frequently by pathologists. Such entities are emphasized often in the differential diagnosis of tumors occurring in the soft tissues. Presently, it is not necessary to develop the general clinical features and histopathology of those tumors because it is a "per se nota" when evaluating a soft tissue lesion. A typical example is the differentiation among renal cell carcinoma, rhabdoid tumor, and alveolar soft part sarcoma or between malignant melanoma and soft part clear cell sarcoma (Figs 6.281–6.283).

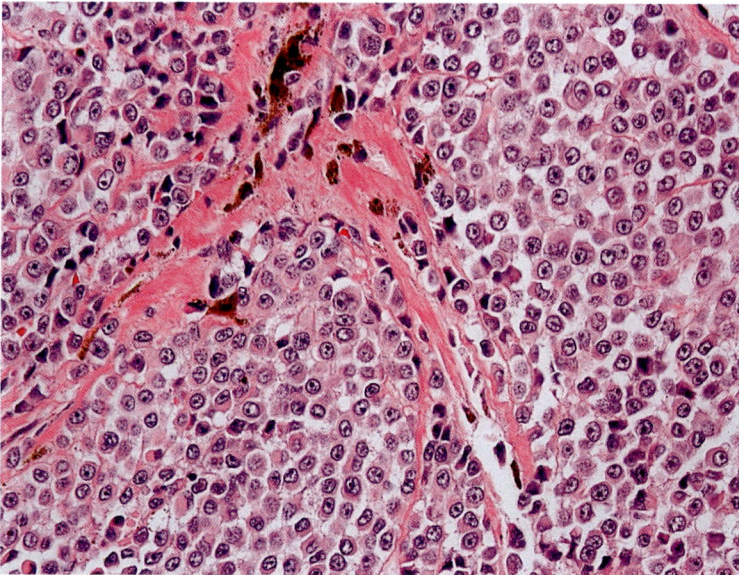

FIG 6.281 Metastatic epithelioid melanoma.

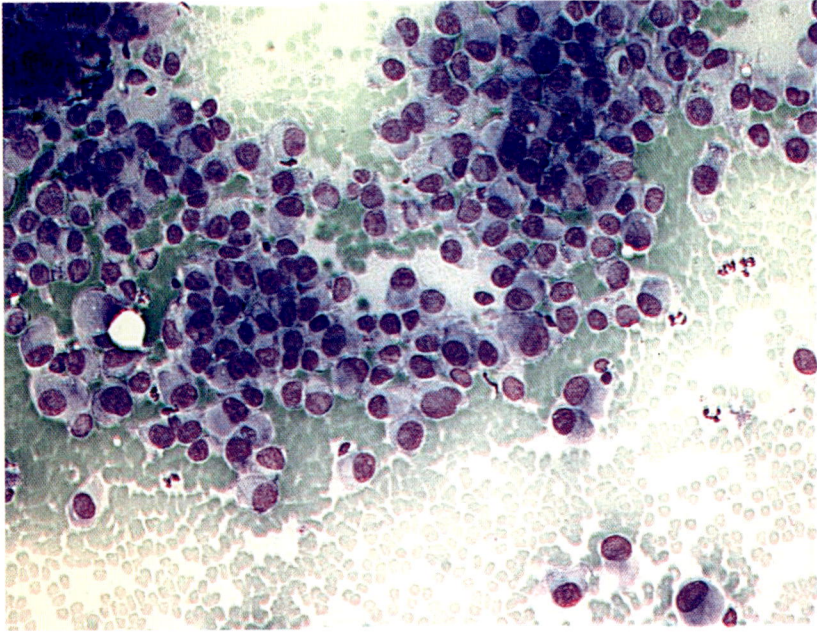

FIG 6.282   Metastatic epithelioid melanoma.

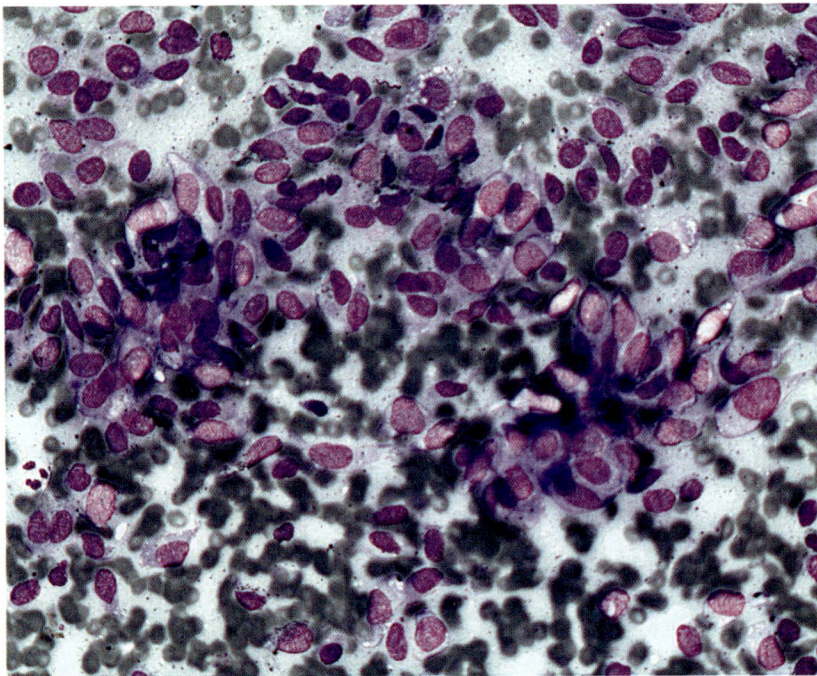

FIG 6.283   Metastatic epithelioid and spindle cell melanoma.

6.7 PLEOMORPHIC SARCOMAS

Plemorphic sarcoma for a long time has been considered a wastebasket of sarcomas whose phenotype could not be determined with accuracy. Not long ago, pathologists suscribed to the assertion that "attempts to precise the diagnosis of pleomorphic sarcoma is a frustrating, time-consuming and futile exercise" in terms of treatment approach and histoprognosis. The adjuncture of more recent ancillary techniques such as cytogenetics and molecular biology added to newer immunohistochemical panels of antibodies, allowed separating distinct entities within the group of plemorphic sarcoma. Some of these studies also have shown that these distinctions were important in view of the poor prognosis associated with particular groups of pleomorphic sarcomas, and therefore, the histopathological reclassificatuion of pleomorphic sarcomas of soft tissue had clinical relevance. Candidates to include in that category are malignant fibrous histiocytoma (pleomorphic variant), liposarcoma, leiomyosarcoma, malignant peripheral nerve sheath tumor, rhabdomyosarcoma, as well as the rare cases of soft tissue osteosarcoma and chondrosarcoma. Previous correlative histological/cytological studies have attempted to delineate some cytological features that, in conjunction with ancillary techniques, could be helpful in the precision of diagnosis of pleomorphic sarcoma.

6.7.1 Pleomorphic Malignant Fibrous Histiocytoma

Presently, most entities included in the subgroups of malignant fibrous histiocytoma have been reclassified, either by immunohictochemical studies or by molecular genetics investigations. Approximately 15 years ago, it was postulated that, with sufficient effort, a specific line of differentiation could be identified in most pleomorphic malignat soft tissue sarcomas including malignant fibrous histiocytoma [319]. Later on, studies from the CHAMP GROUP demonstrated that because of the karyotype complexity of pleomorphic sarcoma, it seems unlikely that cytogenetic analysis could assist in the diagnosis and subclassification of pleomorphic sarcoma, including malignant fibrous histiocytoma [320]. Additional investigations nevertheless have shown that despite karyotypic complexities, some pleomorphic sarcomas, particularly malignant fibrous histiocytoma and liposarcoma, malignant fibrous histiocytoma, and leiomyosarcoma, could share similar genomic imbalances [321–323]. Tissue microarray studies now tend to identify genetic profiles among some pleomorphic sarcomas of which pleomorphic malignant fibrous histiocytomas are candidates.

6.7.1.1 Histopathology. Much has been said and written on the five subgroups of malignant fibrous histiocytoma. Turning to the pleomorphic variant, the overall histologic picture could be similar to other pleomorphic sarcomas except for those that show restricted foci of better differentiation, such as those that could be observed at the periphery of some tumors. As a rule, the tumors of the storiform/pleomorphic type depict a highly variable morphologic pattern with frequent transitions from storiform to pleomorphic areas. Although only one pattern is seldom observed within a given tumor, emphasis is directed toward the pleomorphic

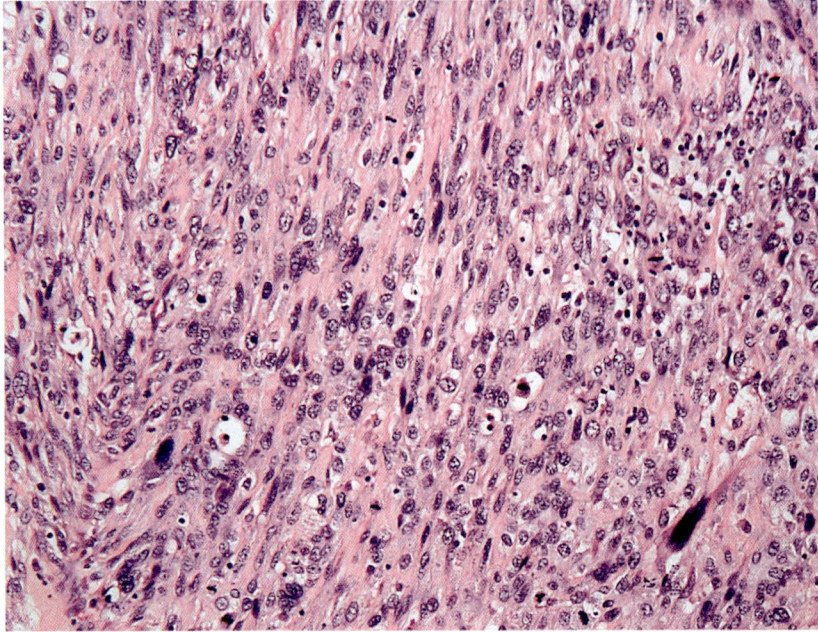

FIG 6.284 Pleomorphic malignant fibrous histiocytoma, atypical spindle, round, and polygonal cells without any recognizable pattern of growth.

variety. It consists of plumper spindle cells of fibroblast type and, round or polygonal "histiocytic cells" with large numbers of giant cells with multiple hyperchromatic nuclei (Fig 6.284). Extreme degrees of pleomorphism and bizarre giant cells also are present (Fig 6.285). Stromal and secondary alterations vary from tumor to tumor in terms of components of collagen fibers, inflammatory cells, myxoid changes, and vascular architecture.

Numerous studies have attempted to characterize the immunohistochemical profile of malignant fibrous histiocytoma and have given negative results in view of precising its phenotype. Howewer, they allow revealing distinction from non-mesenchymal anaplastic tumors (e.g., anaplastic carcinoma, melanoma, and ana-plastic large cell lymphoma). In some cases, specific reactions have demonstrated foci of better differentiation, which confirms the concept of tumor progession morpho-logically corresponding to a malignant fibrous histiocytoma pattern.

6.7.1.2 Cytopathology. Cytologically pleomorphic malignant fibrous histiocy-toma presents as polymorphous high-grade sarcoma (Figs 6.286 and 6.287). Samples are usually hypercellular and the material consists of various proportions of spindle-shaped (Fig 6.288), round, and pleomorphic giant cells (Figs 6.289 and 6.290). Occasionally, osteoclastic-like cells and cells with granular cytoplasm also are observed (Fig 6.291). Blunt-ended nuclei, erytrophagocytosis, and cohesive pseudo-papillary clusters around a fibrovascular core may be observed occasionally (Fig 6.292). All smears are stroma poor. However, other features like eosinophic-magenta myxoid background, inflammatory cells (Fig 6.293), and extensive necrosis are described.

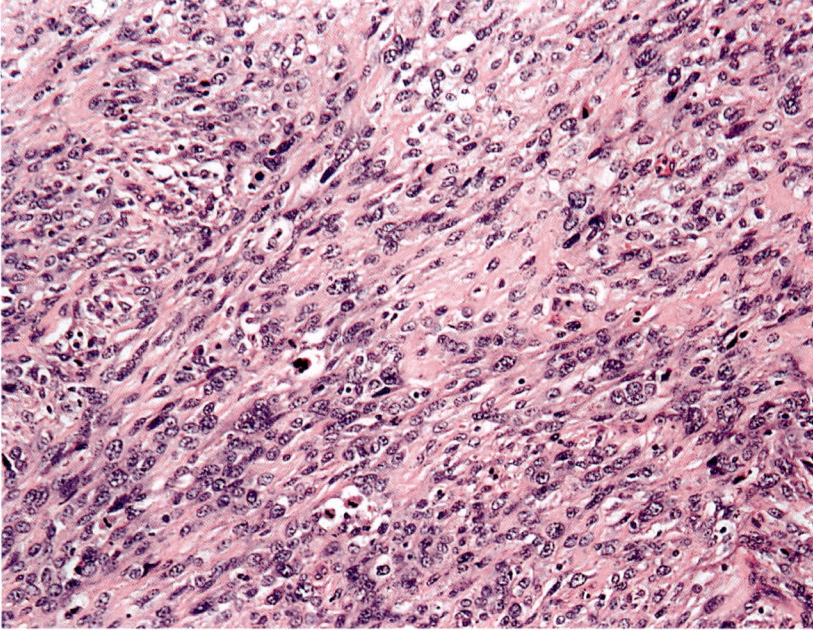

FIG 6.285 Pleomorphic malignant fibrous histiocytoma, numerorus cellular atypias and atypical mitosis.

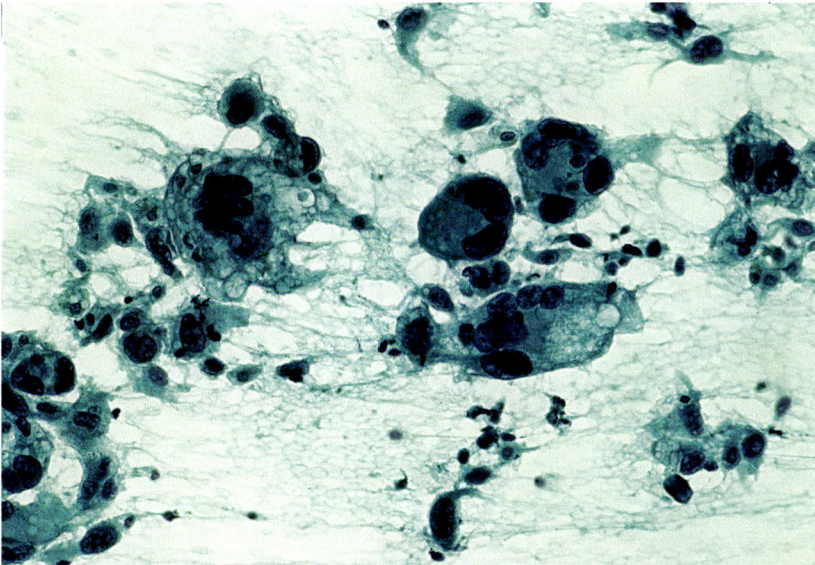

FIG 6.286 Pleomorphic malignant fibrous histiocytoma, typical pleomorphic pattern consisting in anaplastic and multinucleated cells, Papanicolaou.

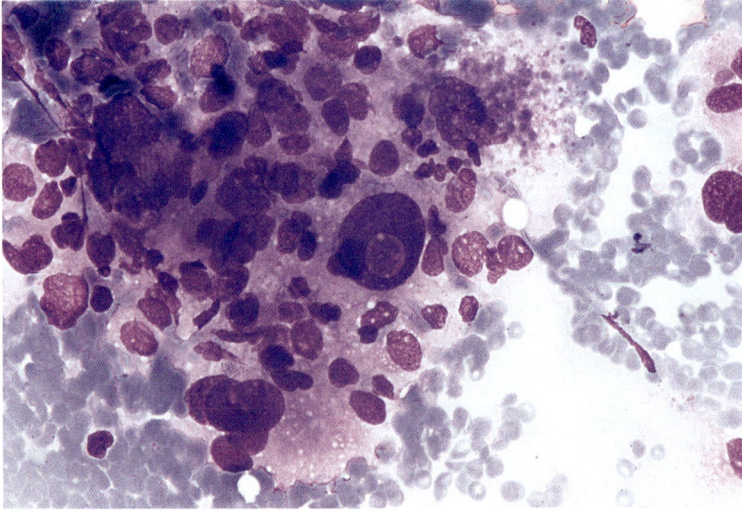

FIG 6.287 Pleomorphic malignant fibrous histiocytoma, typical pleomorphic pattern.

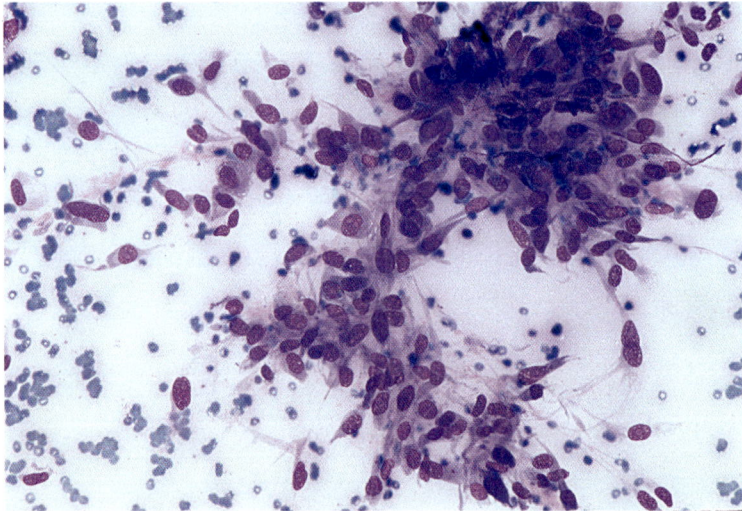

FIG 6.288 Pleomorphic malignant fibrous histiocytoma, spindle-shaped cells.

6.7.1.3 *Differential Diagnosis.* One of the main differential diagnoses of pleomorphic malignant fibrous histiocytoma is classical (high-grade) leiomyosarcoma, because the cellular pleomorphism is a common feature of both leiomyosarcoma and malignant fibrous histiocytoma [324,325]. Immunocytochemistry, using muscular markers, helps to differentiate between these tumors. Other variants of malignant fibrous histiocytoma (giant cell and inflammatory) may be differentiated from pleomorphic malignant fibrous histiocytoma. The smears of giant cell malignant fibrous histiocytoma are hypercellular and similar to the storiform variant. However, the presence of osteoclast-like giant cells with multiple bland nuclei has been

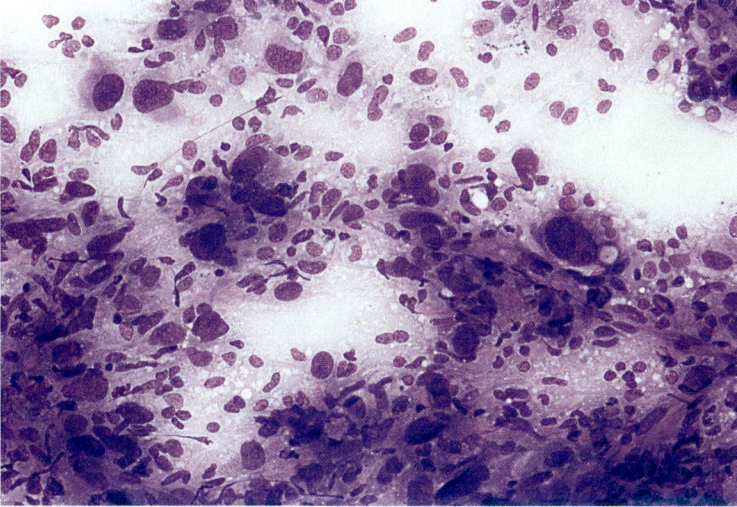

FIG 6.289 Pleomorphic malignant fibrous histiocytoma, pleomorphic cells.

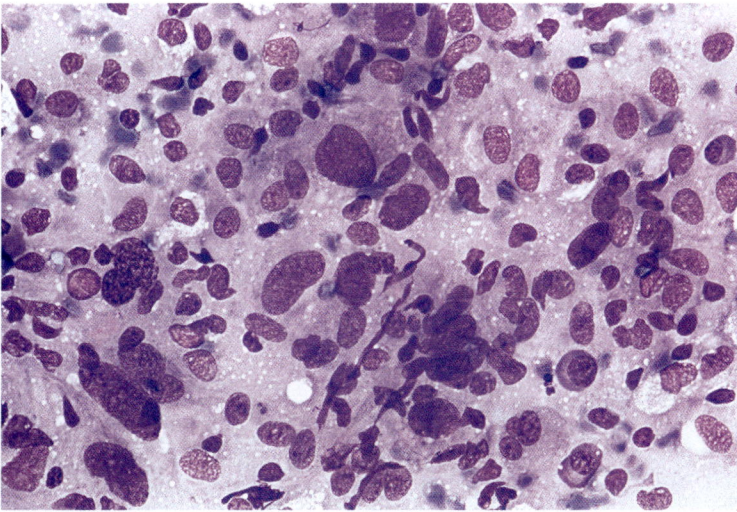

FIG 6.290 Pleomorphic malignant fibrous histiocytoma, pleomorphic cells. Higher magnification.

suggested as a feature of these tumors [326–329]. Few examples of inflammatory malignant fibrous histiocytoma have been described [325,330]. Similar to our observations, this entity consists of pleomorphic sarcomatous cells within an abundant inflammatory background.

Table 6.14 illustrates the differential diagnosis of pleomorphic malignant fibrous histiocytoma.

6.7.1.4 *Comments.* Storiform/pleomorphic malignant fibrous histiocytoma smears are always cell-rich and stroma-poor and suggestive of diagnosis. Any morphological parameter is indicative or exclusive for this tumor type. However, the

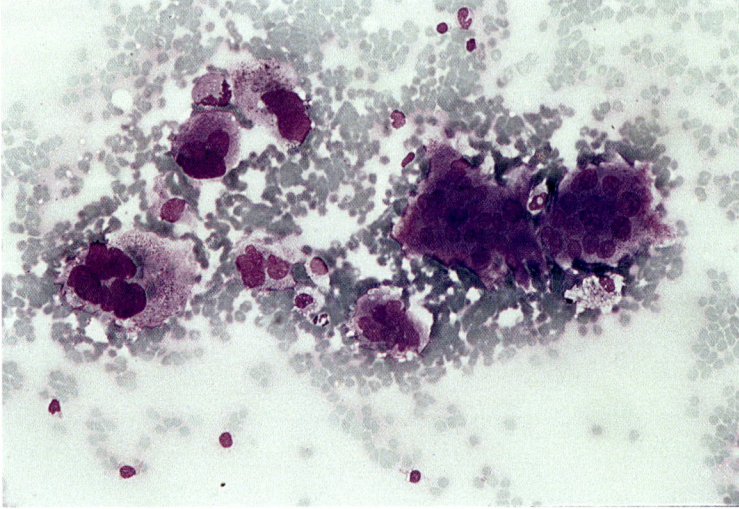

FIG 6.291 Pleomorphic malignant fibrous histiocytoma, osteoclastic-like cells.

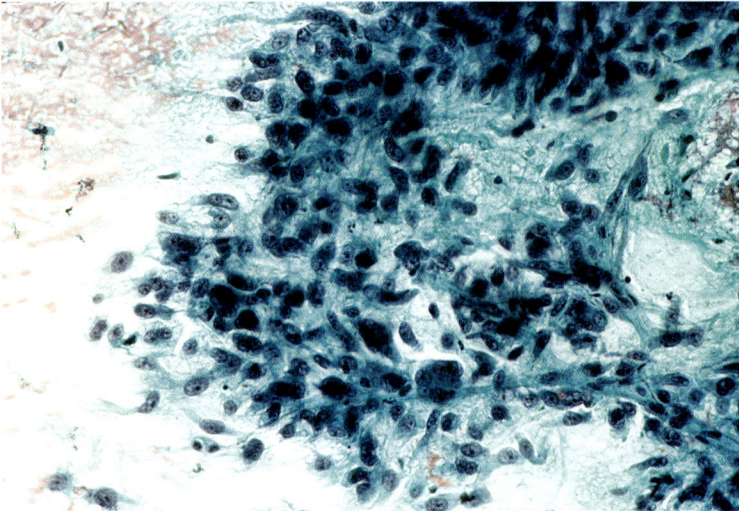

FIG 6.292 Pleomorphic malignant fibrous histiocytoma, pseudopapillary clusters around fibro-vascular core, Papanicolaou.

combination of spindle-shaped, round, and giant cells is a frequent feature. Giant cell and inflammatory variants of malignant fibrous histiocytoma are high-grade sarcomas. Rare morphologic details such as blunt-ended nuclei and erytrophago-cytosis are present exclusively in a storiform variant of malignant fibrous histiocytoma. Other morphological parameters such as pseudopapillary structures and mitotic figures also are distributed equally in all variants of malignant fibrous

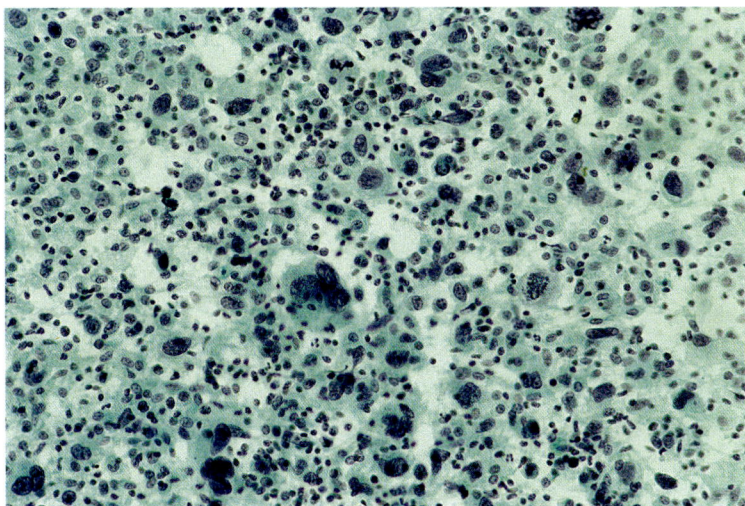

FIG 6.293 Pleomorphic malignant fibrous histiocytoma, inflammatory variant, Papanicolaou.

TABLE 6.14 Quantitative cytological differential diagnosis of pleomorphic sarcomas

	Pleomorphic malignant fibrous histiocytoma	Pleomorphic leiomyosarcoma	Pleomorphic liposarcoma
Cells			
Spindle	++	++	++
Round	++	++	++
Giant	++	++	+
Granular	+/−	+/−	−
Blunt-ends	+/−	+	−
Binucleated	+/−	−	−
Mitoses	+	+	+
Stroma			
Fibrous	+/−	+/−	+/−
Myxoid	+/−	−	−
Inflammatory	−	+/−	−
Necrosis	+	+	+/−

++; frequent, +; common, +/−; occasionally seen, −; usually not seen.

histiocytoma. High-grade tumors are more cell-rich and show more round and more malignant giant cells [325].

Numerous studies have attempted to characterize the cytologic morphology of malignant fibrous histiocytoma [325,326,330–334]. More than 380 cases of such tumors were investigated. A comprehensive assessment of the cytological findings representative of malignant fibrous histiocytoma is therefore difficult given the variability of the criteria used for classification. The subclassification of spindle cell and pleomorphic sarcomas may be largely academic because clinical management is based on grading and clinical staging. However, the collection of additional data could be more valuable to define cytological criteria for accurate sarcoma typing.

Logistic regression analysis of high-grade spindle-cell sarcomas by Liu et al. [326] has shown that the presence of fibroblasts-like cells and giant cells were the key criteria of malignant fibrous histiocytoma. However, other authors [325,335] suggested that no cytologic features allow distinguishing malignant fibrous histiocytoma from other high-grade spindle and/or pleomorphic sarcomas. However, a consensus has been reached among other investigators that the storiform variant consists of an admixture of three cell types, pleomorphic/spindle-shaped, round, and giant multi-nucleated cells have been found [325,333,335,336].

In our previous study including myxoid malignant fibrous histiocytoma [325], the review of the original cytology diagnosis showed that 47 (49.5%) tumors were diagnosed as sarcoma not otherwise specified and as malignant fibrous histiocytoma in 23 (24.2%) cases. The remaining 21 (22.1%) cases were diagnosed as different types of sarcoma. Three (3.2%) samples were unsatisfactory and one (1%) sample was largely necrotic and classified as suspicious of sarcoma. When fine needle aspiration was used as a method of initial diagnosis in 44 primary tumors, the original diagnoses were sarcoma not otherwise specified in 25 (56.8%) tumors, malignant fibrous histiocytoma in 6 (13.6%) cases, and various sarcomas (four types) in 11 (25%) cases. One (2.3%) sample was suspicious and another sample (2.3%) was unsatisfactory.

6.7.1.5 *FNA Key Features.* The following are in favor of the diagnosis:

– Hypercellular smears with pleomorphic cells, giant cells, inflammatory cells
– Scant myxoid
– Mitotic figures or necrosis

The following are difficulties of the diagnosis:

– Some cases may lack cytonuclear atypia
– Aboundant myxoid

The following are evidence against the diagnosis:

– Osteoid, lipoblasts
– Muscular markers positive

6.7.2 Pleomorphic Liposarcoma

Pleomorphic liposarcoma is a rare, often deep-seated and aggressive neoplasm of late adulthood. It must be distinguished from dedifferentiated liposarcoma, which by virtue of its molecular genetic profile belongs to the well-differentiated liposarcoma. They are distributed equally between the retroperitoneum and deep somatic tissues of the extremities. Few collective data concern their biologic behavior. A recent study [337] has emphasized the aggressiveness behavior of pleomorphic liposarcoma whatever the grade and the histologic composition

6.7.2.1 *Histopathology.* The classical decription of pleomorphic liposarcoma includes two related but clearly distinguishable histologic forms. Both show a disorderly

growth pattern with bizarre giant cells (Figs 6.294 and 6.295). They differ by their intracellular component of lipid material. The first type resembles malignant fibrous histiocytoma admixed with giant lipoblasts, hyperchromtic, and scalloped nuclei, as well as deeply eosinophoilic cytoplasm containing hyaline droplets (Fig 6.296). The second

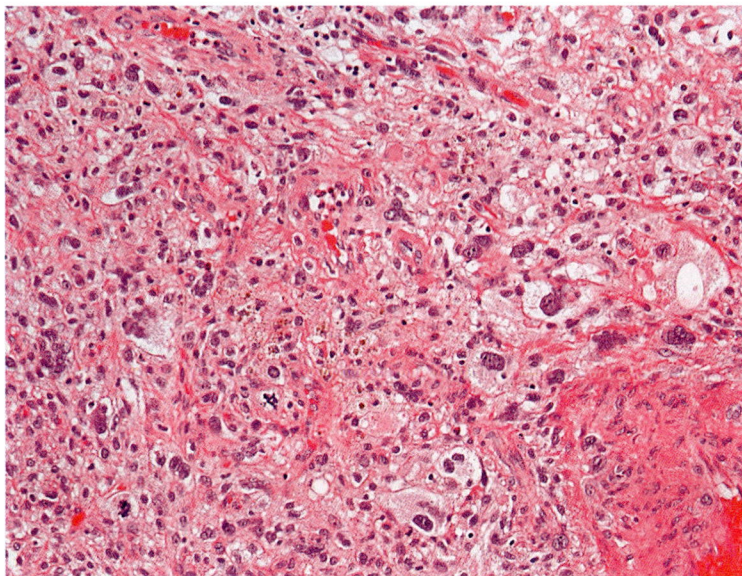

FIG 6.294 Pleomorphic liposarcoma, giant lipoblasts.

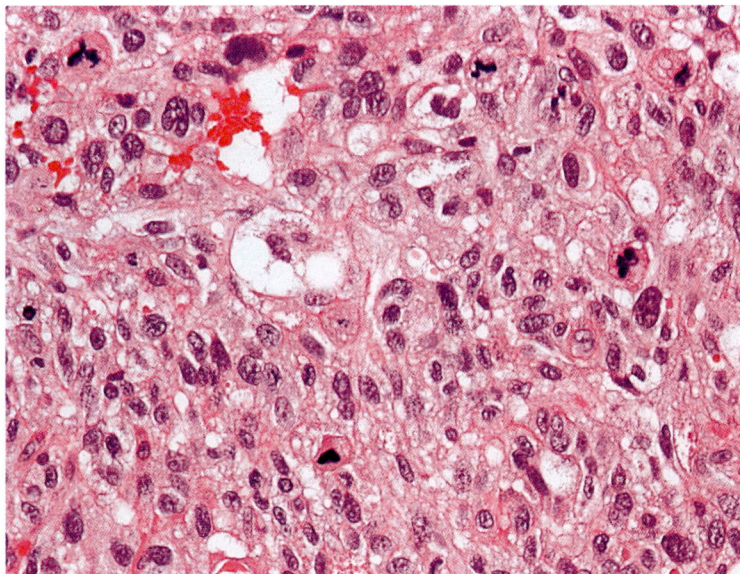

FIG 6.295 Pleomorphic liposarcoma, atypical mitosis admixed with recognizable lipoblasts.

type (less common) consists of sheets of large pleomorphic giant cells associated with smaller mononuclear cells (Figs 6.297 and 6.298). Both cells are vacuolated, lipid-rich and lipoblasts are identified readily. Tumors with a plethora of small round clear cells have been termed "epithelioid variant liposarcoma," which is debated and not accepted at

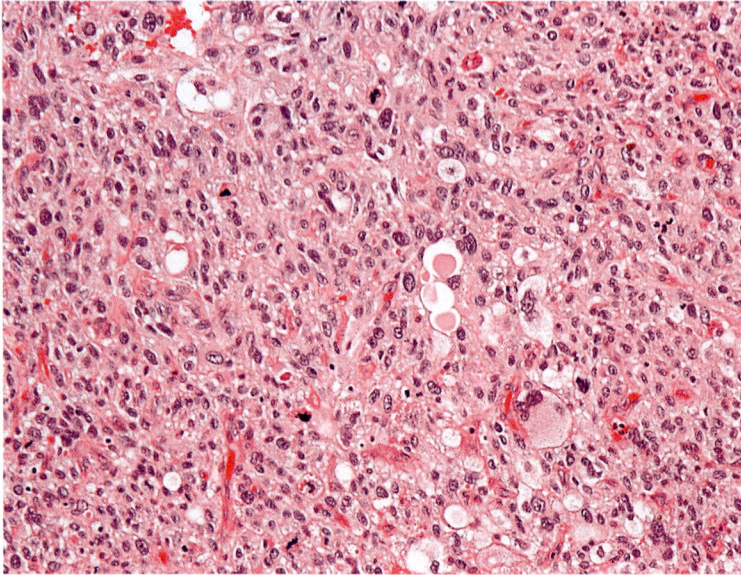

FIG 6.296 Pleomorphic liposarcoma, hyaline globules.

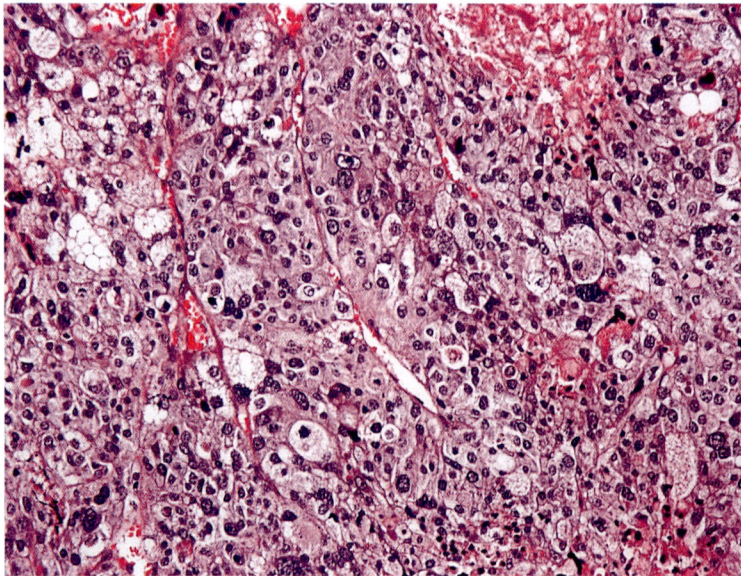

FIG 6.297 Pleomorphic liposarcoma, sheets of smaller vacuolar mononuclear cells and large pleomorphic cells.

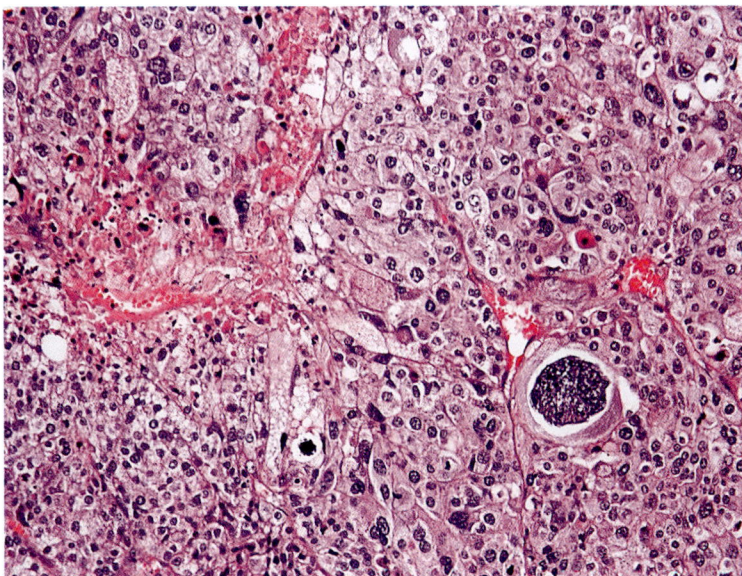

FIG 6.298 Pleomorphic liposarcoma, sheets of smaller vacuolar mononuclear cells and large pleomorphic cells.

present. An immunohistochemical profile of pleomorphic liposarcoma does not contribute to the precision of the diagnosis. Obviously, lipogenic areas express S-100 protein, whereas nonlipogenic areas do not. They rather depict a constellation of immunoreactivity including smooth muscle actin, desmin, CD34, S-100 protein, CD68, and EMA.

6.7.2.2 Cytopathology. Pleomorphic liposarcoma is characterized by the presence of polymorphous cells including spindle-shaped, roundish, round, and giant cells (Figs 6.299–6.301 and Fig 6.218). Occasionally, lipoblasts are present. Necrosis, mitotic figures, and prominent cytonuclear atypia are common.

6.7.2.3 Differential Diagnosis. Pleomorphic liposarcoma and dedifferentiated high-grade liposarcoma without lipoblasts may be misinterpreted as other high-grade sarcoma, especially pleomorphic malignant fibrous histiocytoma [325,338].

Table 6.14 illustrates the differential diagnosis of pleomorphic liposarcoma.

6.7.2.4 Comments. Pleomorphic liposarcoma is a high-grade malignant sarcoma. The clue to a correct diagnosis is the presence of highly atypical, often multinucleated lipoblasts [336,339–341]. In a previous review [338], no specific characteristics for this tumor type were found. The cytological material showed a polymorphous morphology comprising round or spindle cells with occasional lipoblasts. A myxoid matrix and arborizing vascular structures rarely were observed. Few studies have dealt with the cytologic findings of pleomorphic liposarcoma. Our own series [338] included eight such cases. Four were diagnosed accurately, one was misdiagnosed as malignant fibrous histiocytoma, two were suspicious of malignancy, and one was an unsatisfactory sample.

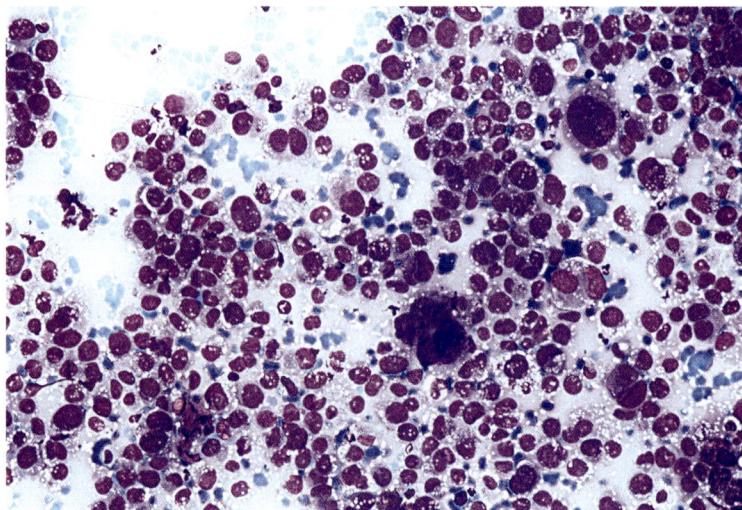

FIG 6.299 Pleomorphic liposarcoma, pleomorphic sarcoma showing occasional lipoblasts, allowing an accurate diagnosis.

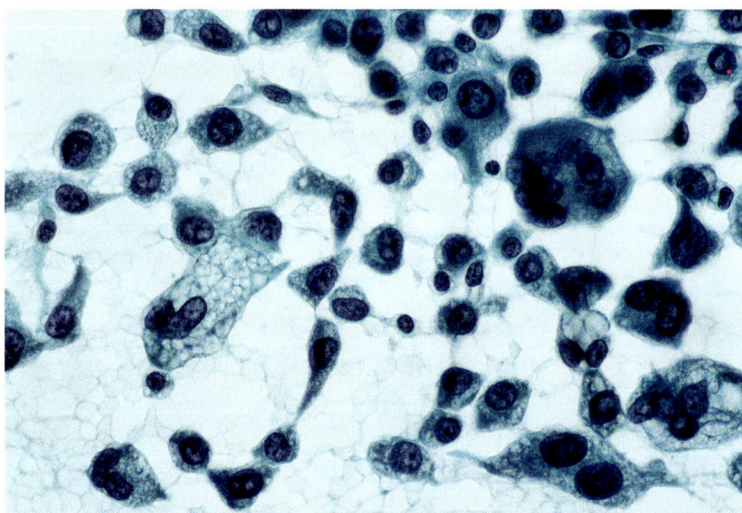

FIG 6.300 Pleomorphic liposarcoma, pleomorphic sarcoma showing occasional lipoblasts. Higher magnification, Papanicolaou.

6.7.2.5 FNA Key Features. The following is in favor of the diagnosis:

— Polymorphous sarcoma with lipoblasts

The following is a difficulty in the diagnosis:

— Lack of lipoblasts

The following are evidence against the diagnosis:

— Muscular markers positive
— Osteoid or chondroid

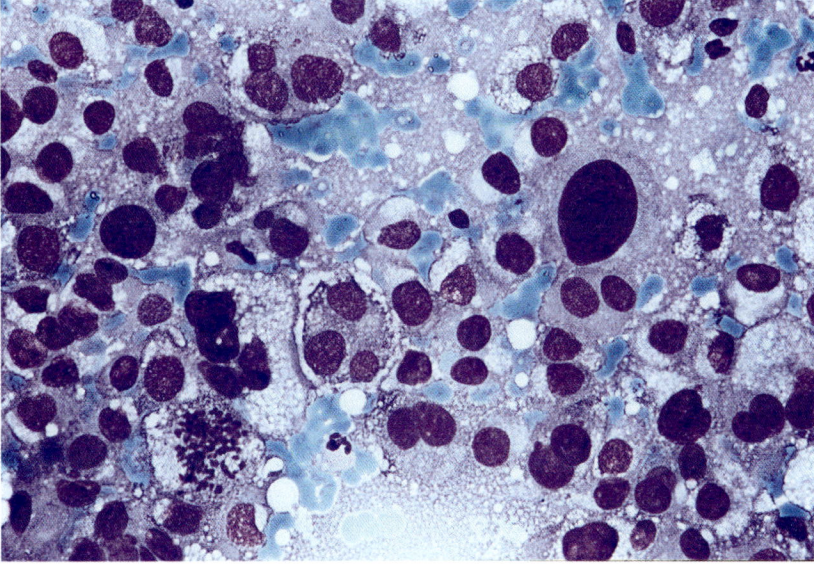

FIG 6.301 Pleomorphic liposarcoma, pleomorphic sarcoma showing lipoblasts, and numerous mitoses.

6.7.3   Pleomorphic Leiomyosarcoma and Rhabdomyosarcoma

In the past, ultrastructural and immunohistochemical studies have attempted to draw a distinction between pleomorphic sarcomas, in particular leiomyosarcoma, liposarcoma, and some variants of rhabdomyosarcoma. A reappraisal of pleomorphic myogenic soft tissue sarcomas of adulthood has been proposed [342]. Among a series of 325 diverse sarcomas, there were 38 rhabdomyosarcomas, and 135 leiomyosarcomas, of which 18 rhabdomyosarcomas and 14 leiomyosarcomas were of the pleomorphic variants. For comparison, the study included 24 malignant fibrous histiocytoma and 8 pleomorphic liposarcomas. All these neoplasms were studied by conventional histology and immunohistochemical methods with antibodies to intermediate filaments including vimentin, desmin, and actin isoforms (alpha smooth and alpha sarcomeric). The following conclusions have been reached: pleomorphic sarcomas are often indistinguishable by their histologic growth pattern; pleomorphic sarcomas are restricted to adults and are not uncommon neoplasms among pleomorphic sarcomas; the study defined desmin negative and alpha smooth muscle actin positive for pleomorphic rhabdomyosarcoma and desmin and alpha-actin negative for pleomorphic leiomyosarcoma. Thereafter, complementary studies have extracted pleomorphic rhabdomyosarcoma from the general group of pleomorphic sarcomas in view of its poor prognosis [343–345].

Similar studies have been conducted for pleomorphic leiomyosarcoma (346), although 100% of tumors examined showed histologically at least small foci of fascicular architecture consisting of smooth muscle cells, with the remainder of tumors being pleomorphic malignant fibrous histiocytoma. The importance of these findings is reflected by a rather aggressive biologic behavior of pleomorphic leiomyosarcoma in comparison with ordinary leiomyosarcoma. Thus, emphasis should be stressed on the clinical relevance for distinguishing entities encompassed in the group of pleomorphic sarcomas.

Rhabdomyosarcoma is the most common soft tissue sarcomas in children younger than 15 years of age as well as in adolescents and young adults. Most are of the embryonal and alveolar subtypes. Therefore, they are said to be rare in adults older than 45 years. Most rhabdomyosarcomas in adults are of the pleomorphic subtype, with a median age of 50–56 years. Correlation between location and histologic subtype is well established; for example, pleomorphic rhabdomyosarcoma originate in the deep soft tissues of the extremities. Because of the emergence of the malignant fibrous histiocytoma concept in the late 1960s and 1970s, the incidence of pleomorphic rhabdomyosarcoma has decreased significantly. They became rare if nonexistent. The advent of immunohistochemistry and the selection of appropriate panels of antibodies confirm the existence of pleomorphic rhabdomyosarcoma, as discussed.

6.7.3.1 *Histopathology.*

As already mentioined, large series dealing with pleomorphic leiomyosarcoma reveal that most cases have shown small foci of a better-differentiated tumor (Fig 6.302). However, the border between pleomorphic leiomyosarcoma and fascicular leiomyosarcoma is rarely sharp. Pleomorphic areas may mimick pleomorphic malignant fibrous histiocytoma and in some areas may mimick myxoid malignant fibrous histiocytoma. Obviously, these are high-grade tumors in the Fédéraion Nationale des Centres de Lutte Contre le Cancer (FNCLCC) system. Regarding the immunohistochemical profile, the fascicular areas express at least one of the three smooth muscle markers (desmin, alpha smooth muscle actin, and muscle-specific actin). In the pleomorphic areas, there is a significant decreased expression of those markers As a rule, only a few retroperitoneal leiomyosarcoma are pleomorphic tumors resembling malignant fibrous histiocytoma. They are described as comprising pleomorphic giant cells with deeply eosinophilic cytoplasm admixed with a component of more uniform-appearing spindle cells and round cells (Fig 6.303). Necrosis and hemorrhage are frequent.

Pleomorphic rhabdomyosarcomas are usually large tumors of >10cm, fleshy, well-circumscribed, and intramuscular masses. They are distinguished easily from other rhabdomyosarcoma subtypes by a composition of loosely arranged, pattern-less, haphazardly oriented large, and round pleomorphic cells with hyperchromatic nuclei and eosinophilic cytoplasms (Fig 6.304). Racket-shaped and tadepole-shaped cells occasionally are observed. Cross striations, which are indicative of sarcomeric cytoplasmic complexes, often are lacking in comparison with embryonal and alveolar rhabdomyosarcoma. A storiform pattern of malignant fibrous histiocytoma and a fascicular pattern of leiomyosarcoma can be present. The presence of large bizarre tumor cells with deeply eosinophilic cytoplasm should raise the presumption of pleomorphic rhabdomyosarcoma (Figs 6.305 and 6.306). When present, sarcomeric differentiation is revealed with the desmin antibody. Muscle-Specific actin, skeletal myogenein, fast-muscle myosin, and muscle-specific myogenin are other antibodie to test in such instances. MyoD1 is also useful because it stains striated muscle fibers in development. Pleomorphic rhabdomyosarcoma has to be differentiated from pleomorphic liposarcoma because it has similar histological features particularly in the absence of cytoplasmic cross striations. Howewer, unlike rhabdomyosarcoma, leiomyosarcoma usually displays, at least focally, foci of fascicular better-differentiated cells.

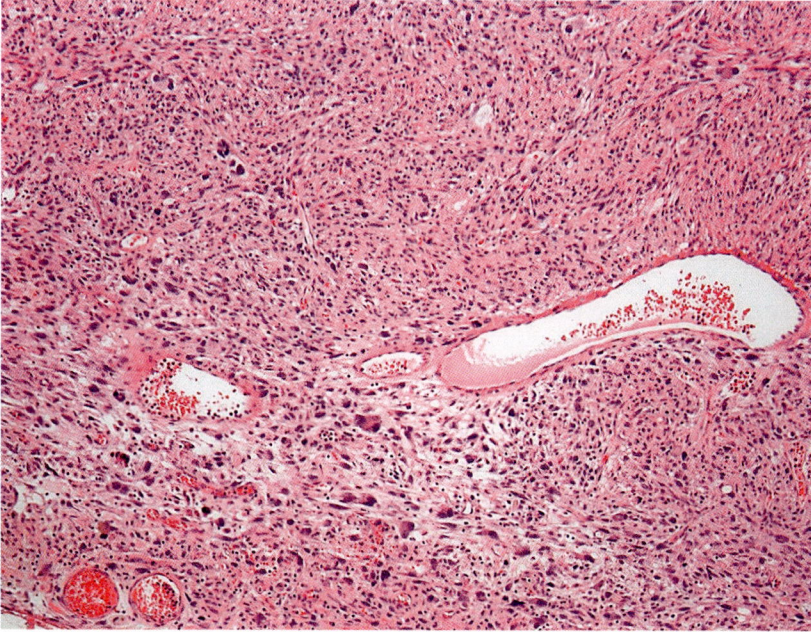

FIG 6.302 Pleomorphic leiomyosarcoma, small foci of pleomorphic sarcoma close to a better differentiated tumor component.

6.7.3.2 Cytopathology. Both, leiomyosarcoma and rhabdomyosarcoma have a similar cytomorphology. Neoplastic, polymorphous cells occur singly and in loose groups. Smears display marked cellular and nuclear pleomorphism (Figs 6.307 and 6.308). They show ovoid, elongated, or irregularly shaped nuclei with coarse clumpd chromatin and prominent nucleoli (Figs 6.309 to 6.312). Cells have scanty cytoplasm. Multinucleation frequently is present, and the multinucleated cells often contain small-to-moderate amounts of cytoplasm with cytoplasmic eosinophilic granules (Figs 6.313). Occasionally, cells are roundish (Figs 6.314 and 6.315). Mitotic figures are found frequently. Necrotic tumor debris also are often observed (Fig 6.316).

6.7.3.3 Differential Diagnosis. High-grade leiomyosarcoma manifests certain morphological similitude to low-grade tumors. Small spindle-shaped cells in parallel alignment with blunt-ended nuclei may be present, but high-grade variants show less small spindle-shaped cells in parallel alignment and fewer cells with blunt-ended nuclei than tumors of low grade. Inversely, background necrosis is much more frequent.

Given the presence of multinucleated and atypical spindle-shaped cells, poorly differentiated leiomyosarcomas are to be differentiated from pleomorphic rhabdomyosarcoma and pleomorphic malignant fibrous histiocytoma. Although malignant fibrous histiocytomas at one time were believed to represent a separate member of the soft tissue sarcoma family, it now is suggested [346] that malignant fibrous

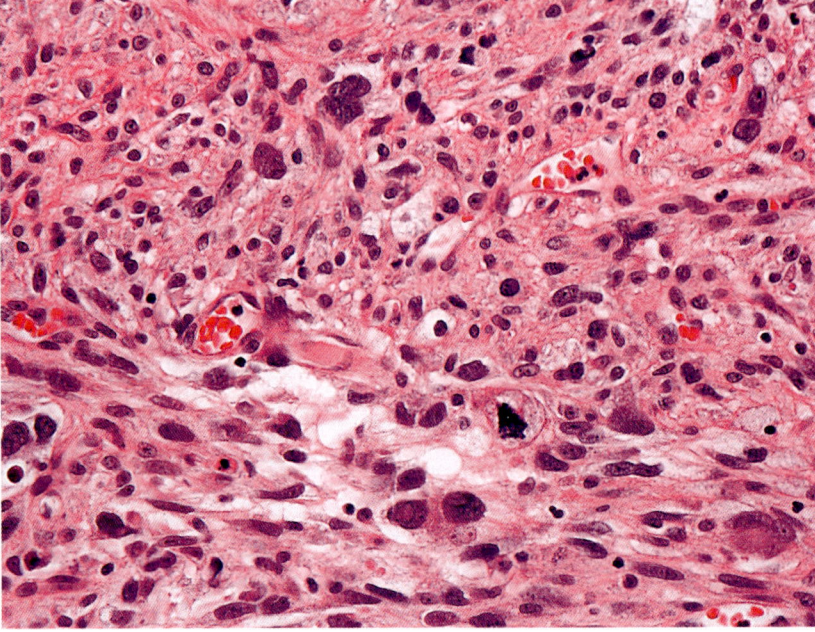

FIG 6.303 Pleomorphic leiomyosarcoma, pleomorphic area that could simulate a malignant fibrous histiocytoma.

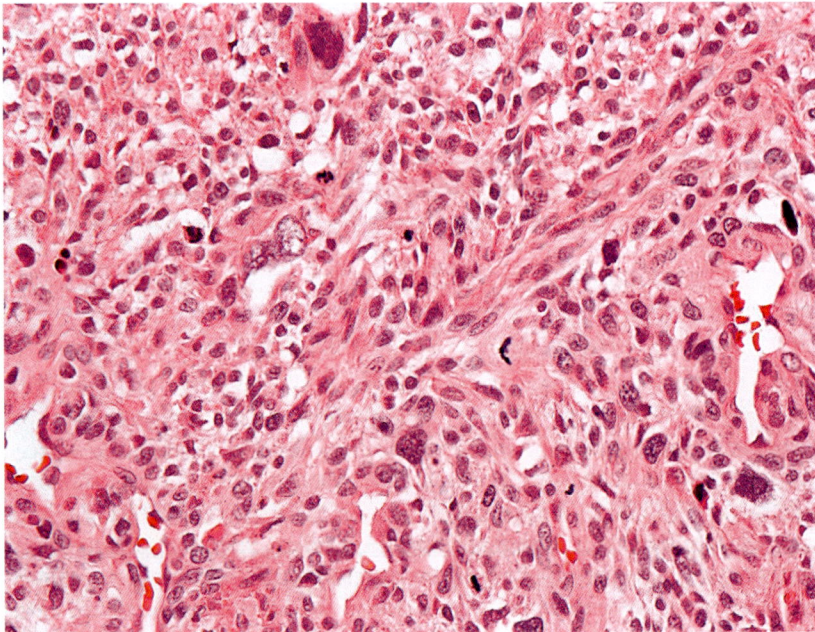

FIG 6.304 Pleomorphic rhabdomyosarcoma, area comprising round, spindle, and polygonal cells.

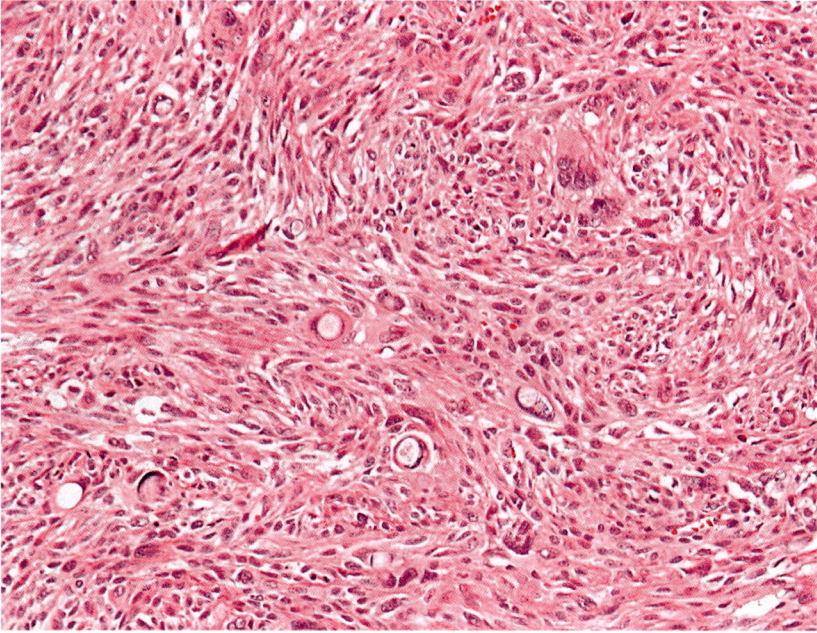

FIG 6.305 Pleomorphic rhabdomyosarcoma, large bizarre tumor cells with deeply eosinophilic cytoplasm raise the presumption of pleomorphic rhabdomyosarcoma.

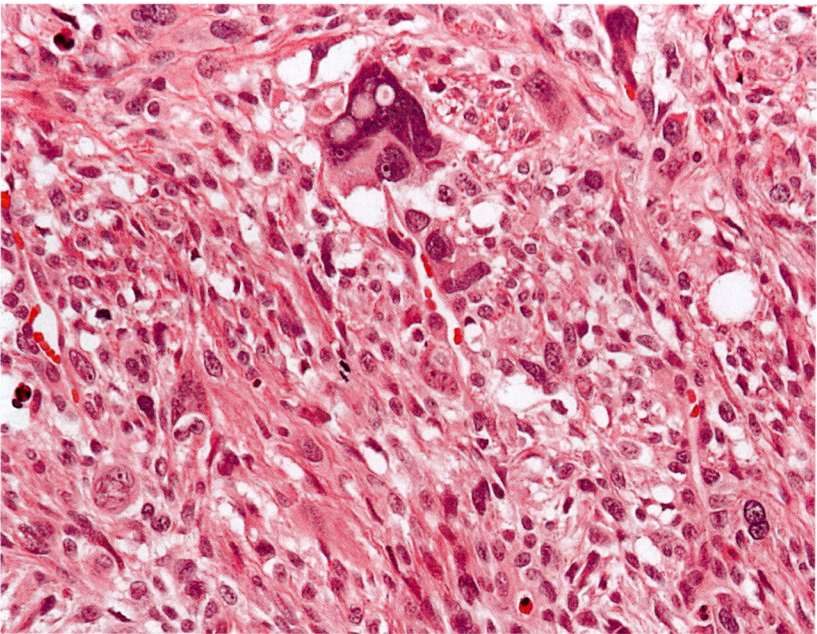

FIG 6.306 Pleomorphic rhabdomyosarcoma, higher magnification from the same tumor field.

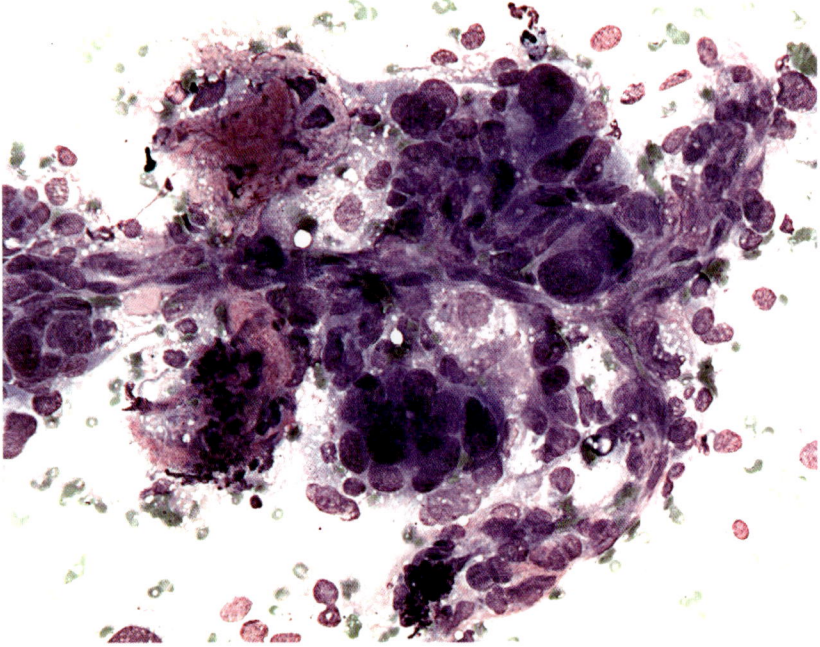

FIG 6.307 Pleomorphic leiomyosarcoma, polymorphous cells occur singly and in loose groupings.

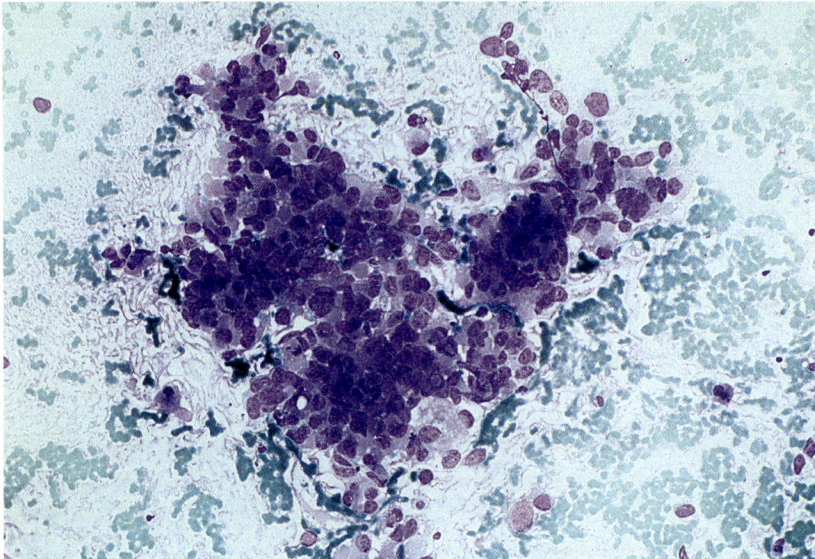

FIG 6.308 Pleomorphic rhabdomyosarcoma, polymorphous cells.

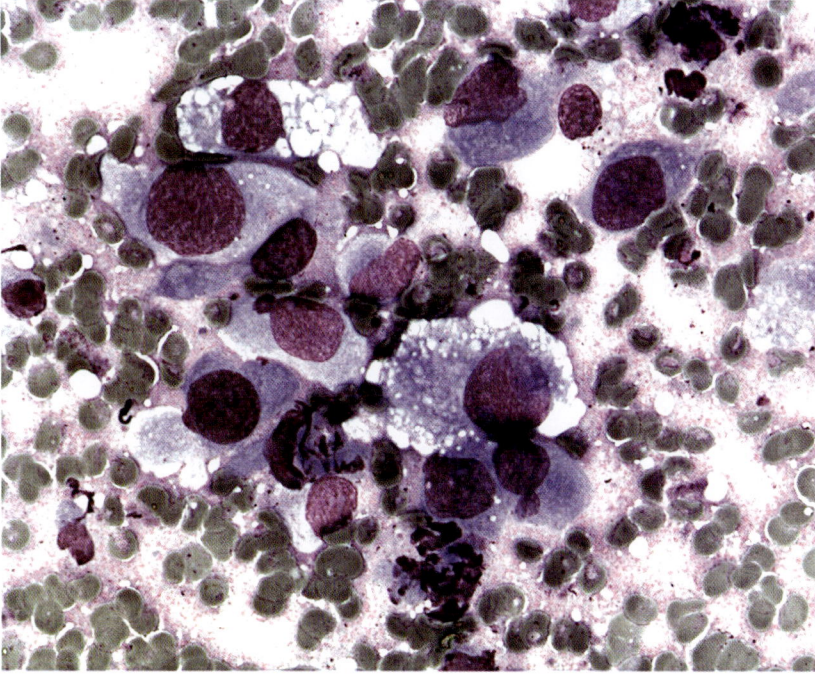

FIG 6.309 Pleomorphic leiomyosarcoma, polymorphous microvacuolated cells. Note mitotic figure.

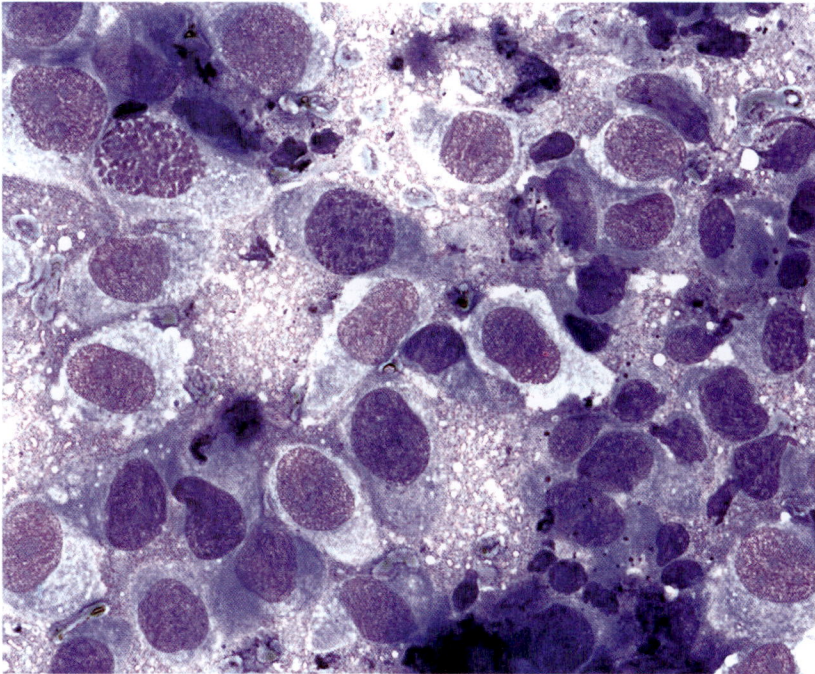

FIG 6.310 Pleomorphic rhabdomyosarcoma, polymorphous roundish and spindle cells. Rhabdomyoblastic origin is evident.

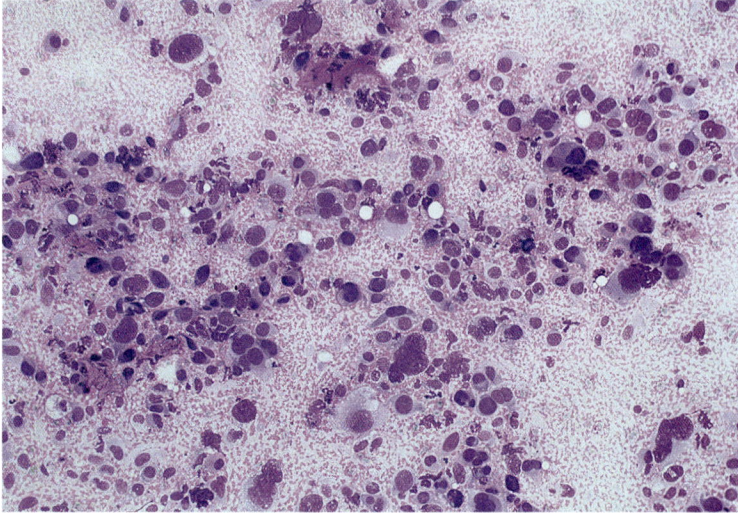

FIG 6.311   Pleomorphic rhabdomyosarcoma, polymorphous rhabdomyoblastic cells.

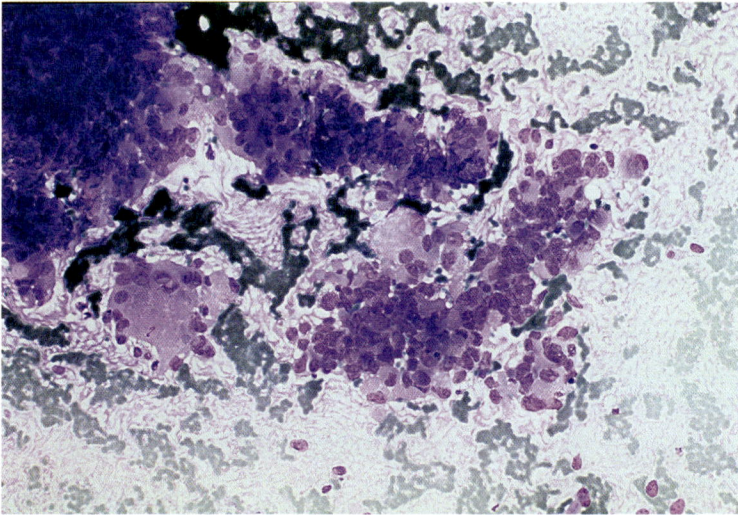

FIG 6.312   Pleomorphic rhabdomyosarcoma, polymorphous roundish and multinucleated cells.

histiocytoma are in fact a morphological variant of other sarcomas, particularly leiomyosarcoma [323,324,347–350].

This differential diagnosis is purely academic in terms of clinical management. Pleomorphic leiomyosarcoma shows various proportions of large spindle-shaped cells, as well as round, giant, and binucleated cells. However, cells with finely eosinophilic intracytoplasmic granulations, blunt-ended nuclei (cigar-like), intranuclear inclusions,

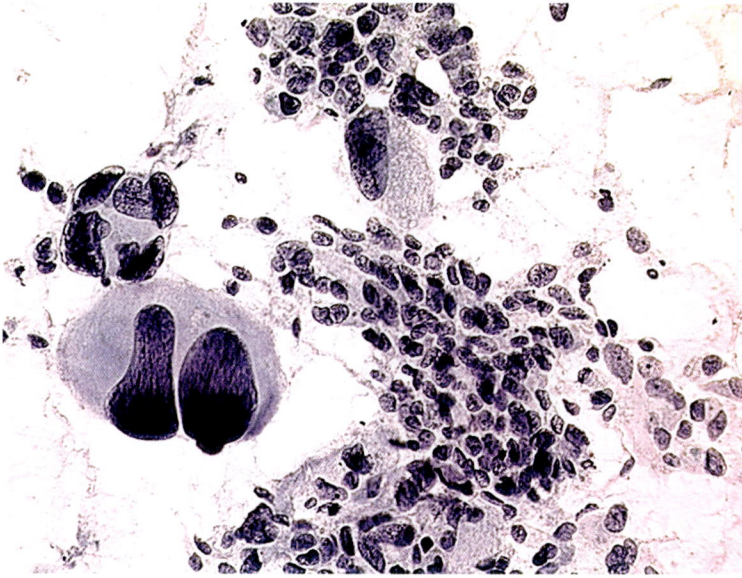

FIG 6.313 Pleomorphic leiomyosarcoma, giant cells.

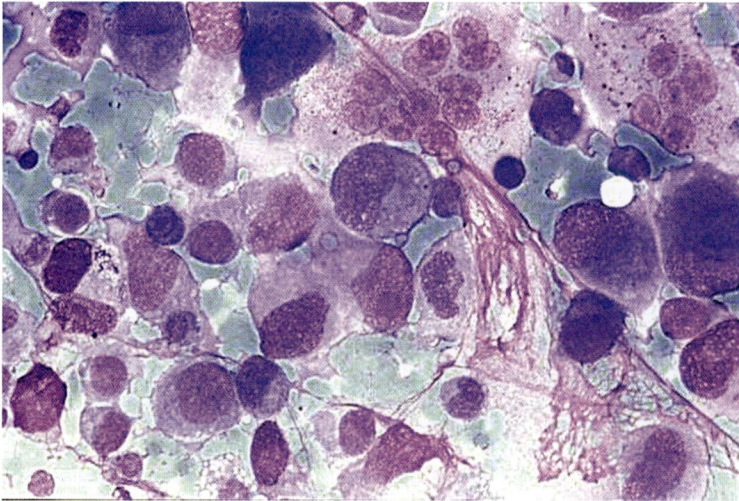

FIG 6.314 Pleomorphic leiomyosarcoma, roundish cells.

and fibrotic dense connective tissue fragments are more frequent features of the classical leiomyosarcoma.

Table 6.14 illustrates the differential diagnosis in pleomorphic sarcomas.

6.7.3.4 Comments. Several cytological studies of leiomyosarcoma with nearly 250 cases have been reported [324,333,347–350]. A comprehensive assessment of

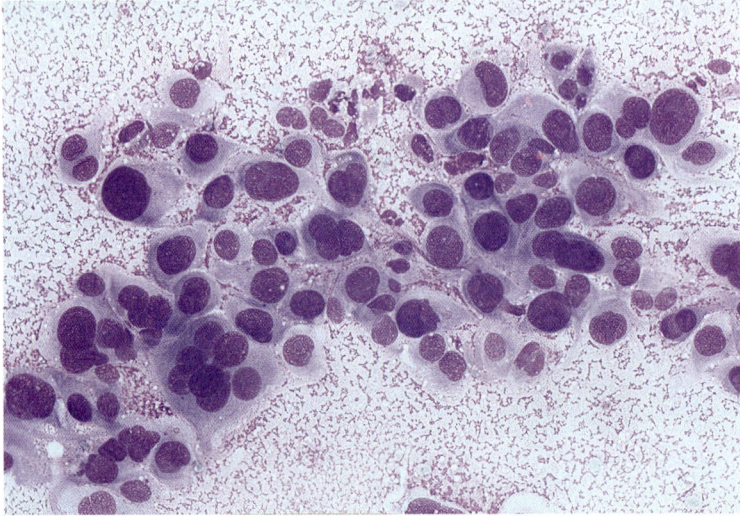

FIG 6.315 Pleomorphic rhabdomyosarcoma, roundish cells.

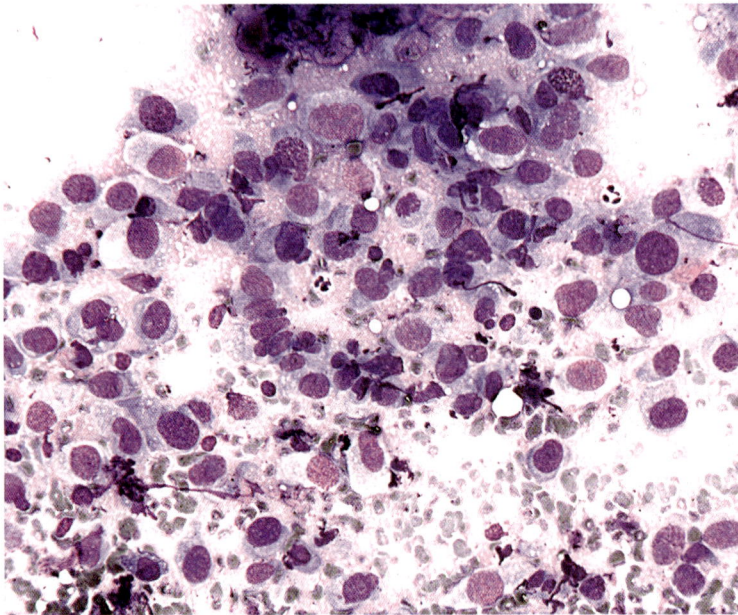

FIG 6.316 Pleomorphic leiomyosarcoma, necrosis.

the cytological findings representative of this entity is therefore difficult given the heterogeneity of the material and the variability of the criteria used for classifying leiomyosarcoma.

In a series of 38 pleomorphic rhabdomyosarcomas [344], three morphological variants of rhabdomyosarcoma, although all three shared a significant aggressive course, have been described; A - classical pleomorphic rhabdomyosarcoma comprising predominantly atypical rhabdomyoblasts in sheets; B - round cell pleomorphic rhabdomyosarcoma, comprising clusters of rhabdomyoblasts admixed with slightly atypical medium-sized, round blue cells; C - spindled-cell pleomorphic rhabdomyosarcoma, showing a predominance of atypical spindled-rhabdomyoblasts arranged in a storiform growth pattern. Other pleomorphic sarcomas also should be part of the differential diagnosis, and one cannot stress enough the importance of separating pleomorphic rhabdomyosarcoma from other pleomorphic malignant tumors included in this morphologic pattern

6.7.3.5 FNA Key Features. The following are in favor of the diagnosis:

- Polymorphous high-grade sarcoma
- Marked cellular and nuclear pleomorphism
- Cigar-like nuclei

The following is a difficulty of the diagnosis:

- Some tumors mat show less cytonuclear atypia

The following is evidence against the diagnosis:

- Osteoid, lipoblasts

6.7.4 Extraskeletal Osteosarcoma

The clinical features of extraskeletal osteosarcoma are not well documented because, in comparison with their osseous counterpart, extraskeletal osteosarcoma is a rare neoplasm. Strictly speaking, these tumors do not show by radiological examination any relation or attachment to the skeleton. They occur at several body sites with rare instances in the breast, the prostate, and visceral organs, although that raises the hypothesis of a morphological component of a sarcomatoid carcinoma/carcinosarcoma. In contrast to osteosarcoma of bone, extraskeletal osteosarcoma occurs principally in patients older than 40 years of age. Among reported cases, some extraskeletal osteosarcomas develop several years after radiotherapy for carcinoma or some other epithelial or mesenchymal malignancy. Data regarding their biological behavior are somewhat variable. Earlier series tend to show that they pursue a bad prognosis, with patients dying to metastatic growth within 2–3 years after the initial diagnosis [351,352]. Tumor size, histologic subtype, and proliferation index have been proposed as prognostic variables. However, two recent studies tend to show that the use of multimodal chemotherapy regimens similar to those used in conventional osteosarcoma can improve the prognosis. One of these was conducted by the Cooperative Oncology Study Group (COSS) in Germany, [353] and another one was supported by the Japanese Musculoskeletal Oncology Group [354].

6.7.4.1 Histopathology. The histologial spectrum of extraskeletal osteosarcoma parallels conventional bone osteosarcoma. They are defined better as neoplasms having in common the presence of neoplastic osteoid and bone admixed with a component of malignant stromal cells. All variants of conventional osteosarcoma can be observed; including tumors that resemble fibrosarcoma or malignant fibrous histiocytoma (Figs 6.317 and 6.318), tumors extremely cell-rich and others cell-poor with a predominant matrix component, a giant-cell variant, telangiectatic, and chondroid, although the latter is rarely a dominating feature. Architecturally, in comparison with myositis ossificans, extraskeletal osteosarcoma is characterized by a phenomenon of "inverted zone." Presently, there are few satisfactory commercially available antibodies to determine the phenotype of osteosarcoma, whatever its clinical setting, exclusive of osteocalcin. This antibody was reported in 82% to be sensitive for extraskeletal osteosarcoma (neoplastic cells in 91% and in 75% of bone matrix) [355].

6.7.4.2 *Cytopathology.*

Smears in extraskeletal osteosarcoma are cell- and stroma-rich. Tumors consist in various proportions of osteoblastic malignant cells (Figs 6.319–6.322), spindle-shaped cells (Fig 6.323), and osteoclastic cells. The matrix mainly consists of osteoid and is identified easily by its pinkish stain using MGG stain (Figs 6.324–6.326). In addition, naked nuclei, vacuolated cells, inflammatory cells, cytonuclear atypia, mitotic figures (Figs 6.327 and 6.328), necrotic background, chondroid matrix, vascular structures, and myxoid stroma also are observed in different proportions. Round cell extraskeletal osteosarcomas consist of monotonous roundish cells (Fig 6.329) and even in pseudoepithelial clusters (Fig 6.330).

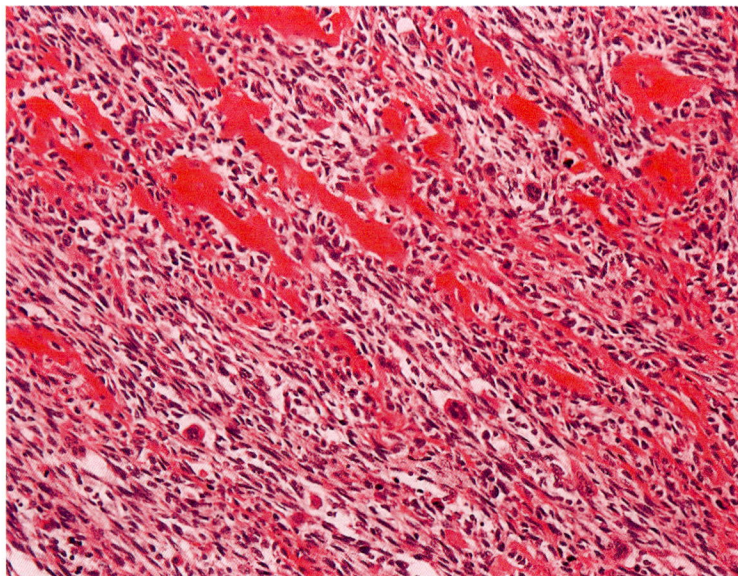

FIG 6.317 Extraskeletal osteosarcoma, spindle cells of fibroblastic type intermixed with osteoid matrix and giant cells of osteoclastic type.

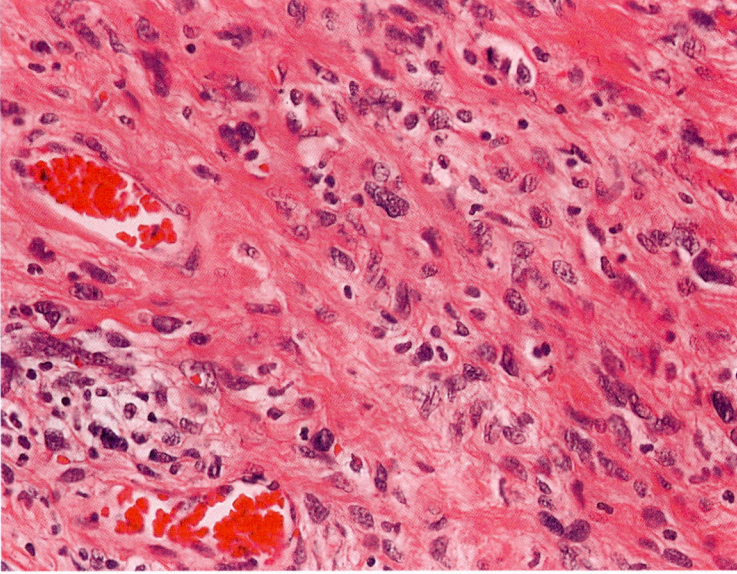

FIG 6.318 Extraskeletal osteosarcoma, pleomorphic cells component without a recognizable phenotype.

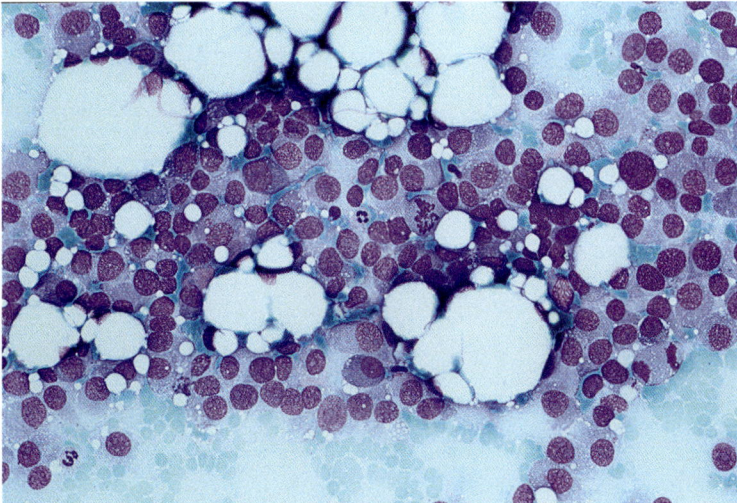

FIG 6.319 Extraskeletal osteosarcoma, osteoblasts.

6.7.4.3 Differential Diagnosis. The morphologic cytological data exclusive of Rx findings show that extraskeletal osteosarcoma should be differentiated from giant cell malignant fibrous histiocytoma and from myositis ossificans of soft tissues (Table 6.15). The smears of giant cell malignant fibrous histiocytomas are highly pleomorphic and similar to osteosarcoma. This entity consists of pleomorphic

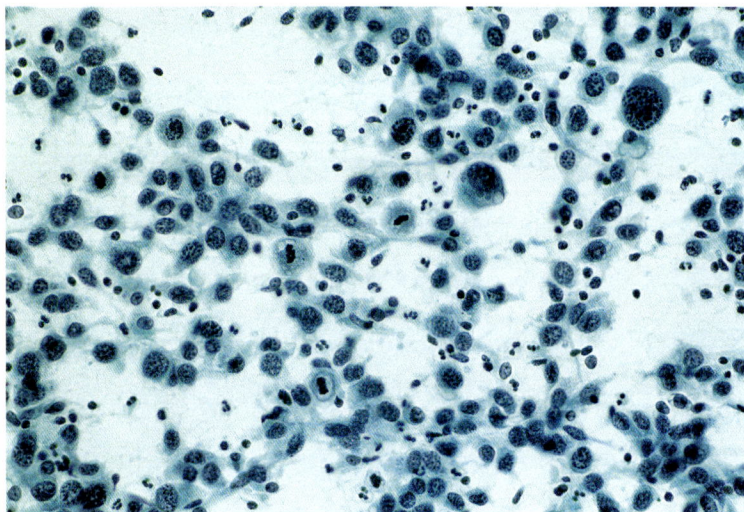

FIG 6.320 Extraskeletal osteosarcoma, various proportions of osteoblastic malignant cells, Papanicolaou.

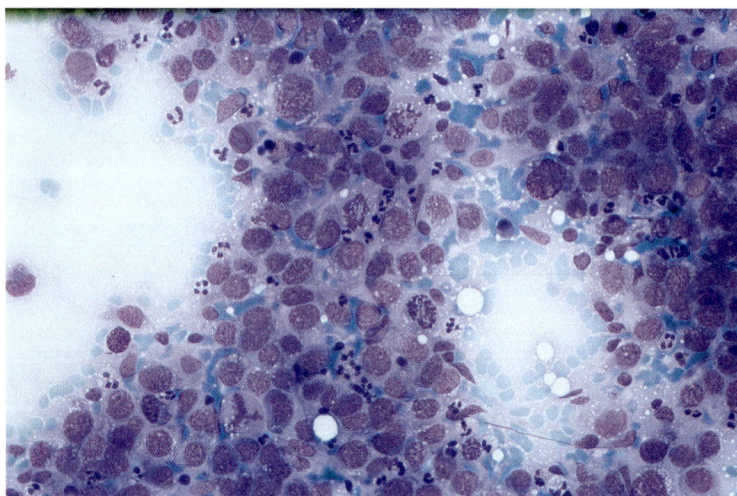

FIG 6.321 Extraskeletal osteosarcoma, osteoblastic malignant cells, note numerous mitoses.

sarcomatous cells within an abundant inflammatory background [325]. However, the presence of osteoclast-like giant cells with multiple bland nuclei has been suggested as a feature of these tumors. Myositis ossificans are to be distinguished from extraskeletal osteosarcoma. It is nearly impossible to diagnose both entities accurately on cytological grounds, save for the presence of numerous pleomorphic cells in extraskeletal osteosarcoma. Myositis ossificans are characterized by a zonal phenomenon, whereas soft tissue extraskeletal osteosarcomas depict an inverted zonal phenomenon, hence the importance of architectural characterization to

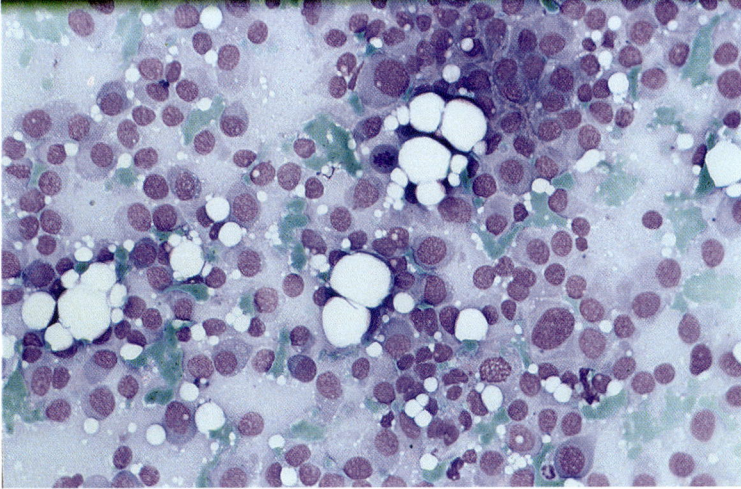

FIG 6.322 Extraskeletal osteosarcoma, various proportions of osteoblastic malignant cells. Going from round to oval or polyponal.

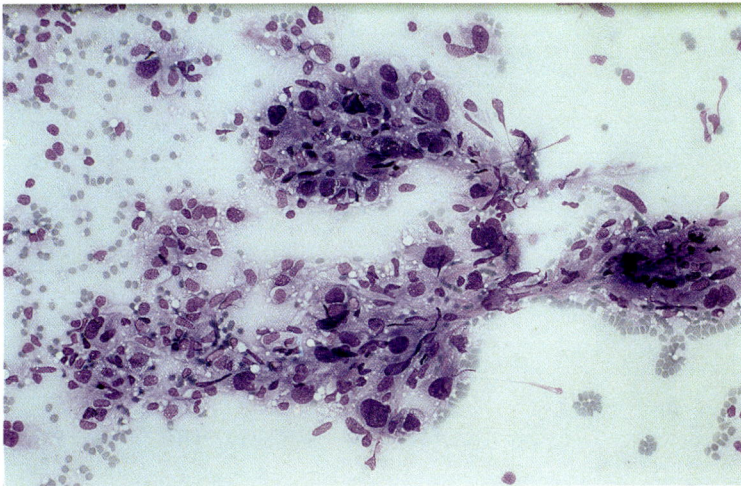

FIG 6.323 Extraskeletal osteosarcoma, spindle-shaped cells.

differentiate both entities [356]. Radiological findings are confirmatory of diagnosis with the observation of irregular peripheral calcifications [357] both on plain films and/or computed tomography [CT] scan.

6.7.4.4 Comments. Cytologic morphology is well known for extraskeletal osteosarcoma developing in the bones, whereas extraosseous osteosarcoma is less well defined. Netherthless, both types are morphologically identical [358]. Extraskeletal osteosarcoma is defined as a mesenchymal tumor in which the neoplastic cells produce a bone matrix. The histologic classification of extraskeletal osteosarcoma

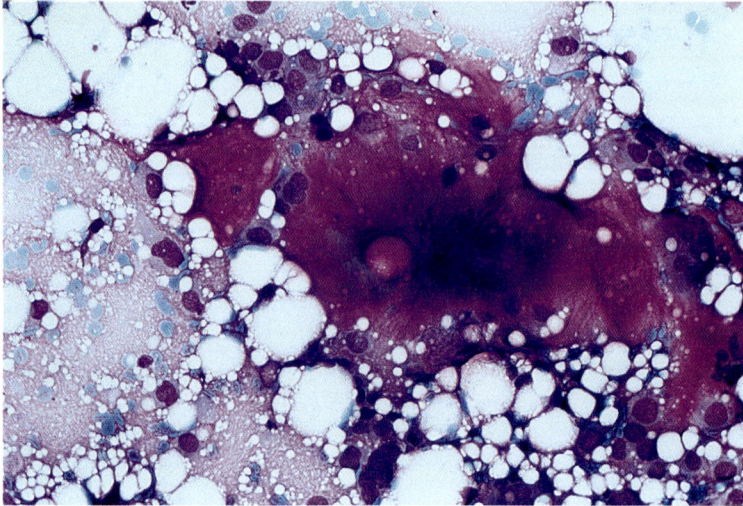

FIG 6.324 Extraskeletal osteosarcoma, pinkish osteoid.

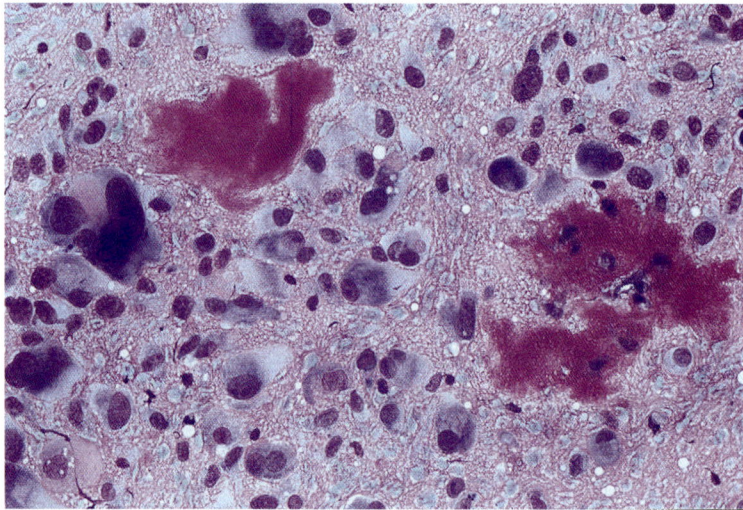

FIG 6.325 Extraskeletal osteosarcoma, pinkish osteoid allowing an accurate diagnosis, this pattern is characteristic.

such as that described by Dahlin and Unni [359] separating osteoblastic, chondroblastic, and fibroblastic types still is used widely for conventional osteosarcoma. Several subtypes of osteosarcoma also are recognized according to either histologic variants (telangiectatic, small cell, giant cell, low-grade intramedullary, etc.) or various clinical settings (multicentricity, association with preexisting conditions, localisation, etc.). A previous study [360] allowed identifying the following cytological patterns of osteosarcoma: pleomorphic (malignant fibrous histiocytoma -like), epithelioid, chondroblastic, small cell, and mixed, although considerable overlapping is observed frequently in the same tumor. In another study [358], no significant

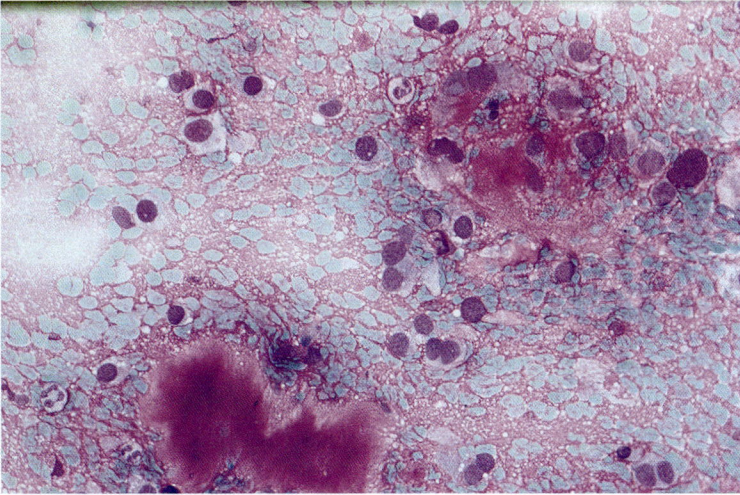

FIG 6.326   Extraskeletal osteosarcoma, pinkish chondxoid allowing an accurate diagnosis.

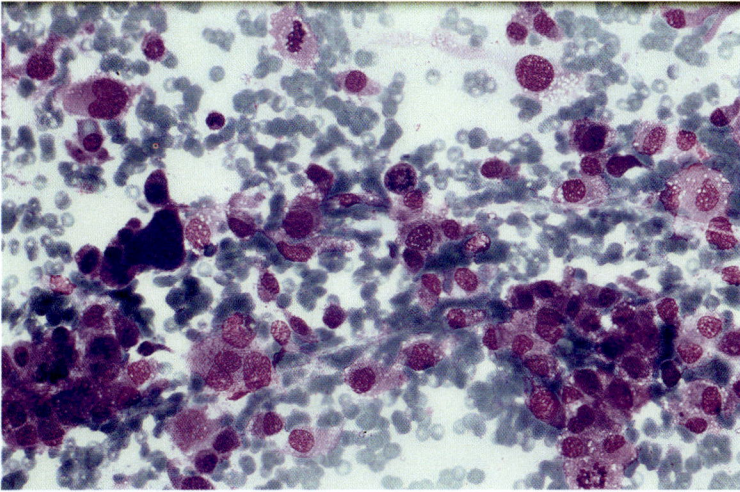

FIG 6.327   Extraskeletal osteosarcoma, cytonuclear atypia and mitotic figures.

difference was found in the stromal/matrix components in relation to the histologic subtype of osteosarcoma and to their grade.

Fine needle aspiration is a useful diagnostic tool in the multidisciplinary approach of extraskeletal osteosarcoma, given the high percentage of malignant tumors diagnosed by this method [361–364]. The limitation of the technique is more related to the material obtained either in terms of the volume of cells available for examination or to the difficulty in obtaining osteoid [360,365], which leads to under/misdiagnosis with other types of bone and soft tissue sarcomas. The finding of a pleomorphic sarcoma with characteristic clinical and radiological features is of

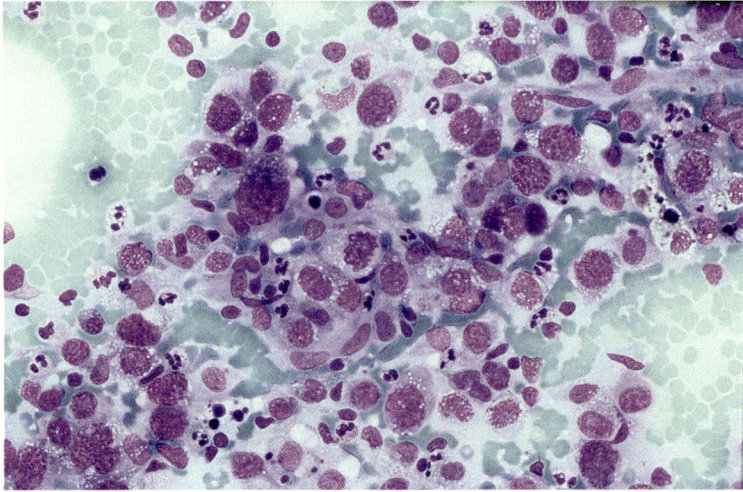

FIG 6.328 Extraskeletal osteosarcoma, cytonuclear mitotic figures, and inflammatory background.

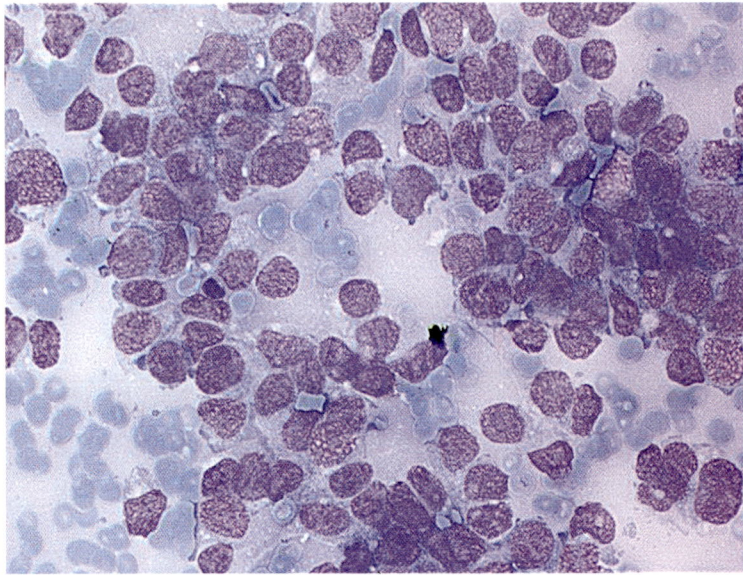

FIG 6.329 Round cell extraskeletal osteosarcoma, monotonous roundish cells. No osteoid is found.

more importance than the identification of osteoid in establishing a diagnosis of osteosarcoma [365–368].

The collected data of previous series or case reports concerning bone and extraskeletal osteosarcoma show that an accurate cytology diagnosis relies on the presence of characteristic osteoblasts and an osteoid or bone-producing matrix [360,367,369]. In a previous study [368], an osteoid matrix was found in only 58% of cases. Another study, using light microscopic polarization [370], allowed identifying

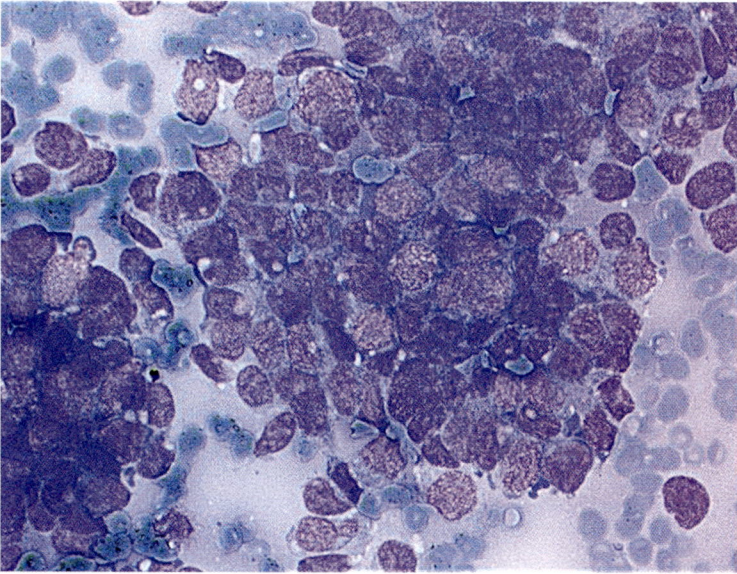

FIG 6.330 Round cell extraskeletal osteosarcoma, pseudoepithelial clusters.

TABLE 6.15   Principal cytological differential diagnosis of extraskeletal osteosarcoma

	Extraskeletal osteosarcoma	Giant cell malignant fibrous histiocytoma	Myositis ossificans
Atypical osteoblastic cells	++	+	−
Spindle cells	++	++	++
Osteoclastic-like cells	++	++	+
Mitotic figures	++	++	+
Necrosis	+	++	−
Osteoid	++	−	++
Chondroid	+/−	−	−

++; Frequent, +; rare, +/− occasionally seen, −; absent.

unequivocally osteoid in only 10% of cases, whereas other cases showed metachromatic matrix material indistinguishable from chondroid matrix. In our study, the absence of osteoid did not have a negative impact on the diagnostic accuracy, although we agree that the presence of osteoid is an important parameter to ascertain the diagnosis of osteosarcoma. Electron microscopy and immunohistochemistry are of limited value in establishing the diagnosis of osteosarcoma.

6.7.4.5   FNA Key Features. The following are in favor of the diagnosis:

- Roundish to spindle-shaped osteoblasts
- Chondroid substance, osteoid

The following is a difficulty in the diagnosis:

– Lack of stromal components

The following is evidence against the diagnosis:

– Rhabdomyoblasts, lipoblasts

6.7.5 Pleomorphic Malignant Peripheral Nerve Sheath Tumor

The wide histopathological diversity of malignant peripheral nerve sheath tumor is well recognized and has been well documented. A general overview has been presented in section 6.2, dealing with tumors of a fibrillary pattern. Malignant peripheral nerve sheath tumors with divergent/heterologous differentiation components are excluded from this discussion (i.e., liposarcoma, rhabdomyosarcoma, and epithelial sarcoma). Rather we will attempt to describe pleomorphic malignant peripheral nerve sheath tumor (i.e., tumors that simulate malignant fibrous histiocytoma-like features or other pleomorphic sarcomas). A previous correlative histological/cytological study of malignant peripheral nerve sheath tumor was attempted to define the morphological characteristics better that could support the diagnosis [371].

6.7.5.1 Histopathology. Anatomical and histological criteria to assume a sarcoma to be a malignant peripheral nerve sheath tumor already have been discussed (section 6.2). If most malignant peripheral nerve sheath tumor conform to the classical description, then some unusual cases seem to occur more often in NF1 and are morphologically different. Besides the low-grade malignant peripheral nerve sheath tumor originating in a neurofibroma, at the opposite end of the spectrum, there are so-called anaplastic malignant peripheral nerve sheath tumors, which may be difficult to distinguish from other pleomorphic sarcomas (Fig 6.331). These undifferentiated tumors have been documented in the setting of von Recklinghausen disease (Fig 6.332), hence the justified inclusion into malignant peripheral nerve sheath tumor despite their morphologic composition (i.e., plump, spindled, and giant cells with areas of necrosis and hemorrhage). Outside the setting of NF1, these tumors cannot be diagnosed with certainty, save for the identification in the same tumor of areas of typical low-grade malignant peripheral nerve sheath tumor.

6.7.5.2 Cytopathology. Cytologically, pleomorphic malignant peripheral nerve sheath tumors consist of polymorphous sarcomateous cells, anaplastic cells (Figs 6.333 and 6.334), and wavy nuclei. Fibrillary (Figs 6.335 and 6.336) and myxoid matrix also are observed in half of the cases that may allow a specific diagnosis. Rare cases may show epithelioid cells (Figs 6.337 and 6.338) and rhabdomyoblastic cells (Fig 6.339). We have reported 11 examples of anaplastic malignant peripheral nerve sheath tumor. They consisted of anaplastic giant and polymorphous cells. Mitoses were present. Spindle-shaped cells, comma-like naked nuclei, and myxoid background also were observed frequently.

Collective analysis from the literature and those of our series [371] show that all reported pleomorphic malignant peripheral nerve sheath tumor are in fact similar.

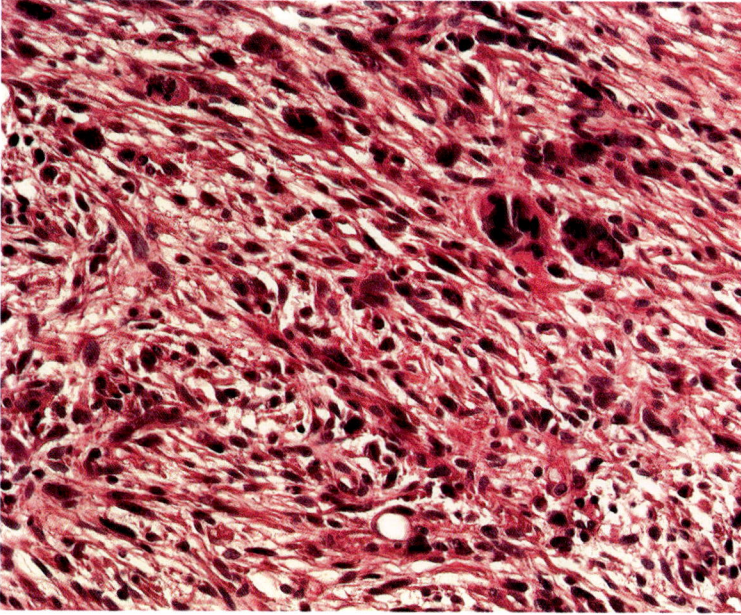

FIG 6.331 Pleomorphic malignant peripheral nerve sheath tumor, high-grade round and pleomorphic sarcoma in a setting of neurofibromatosis.

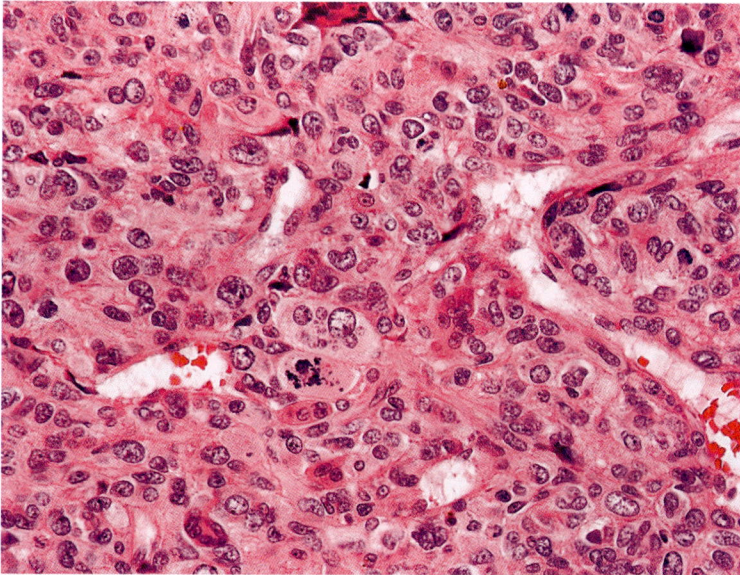

FIG 6.332 Pleomorphic malignant peripheral nerve sheath tumor, anaplastic focus simulating malignant fibrous histiocytoma.

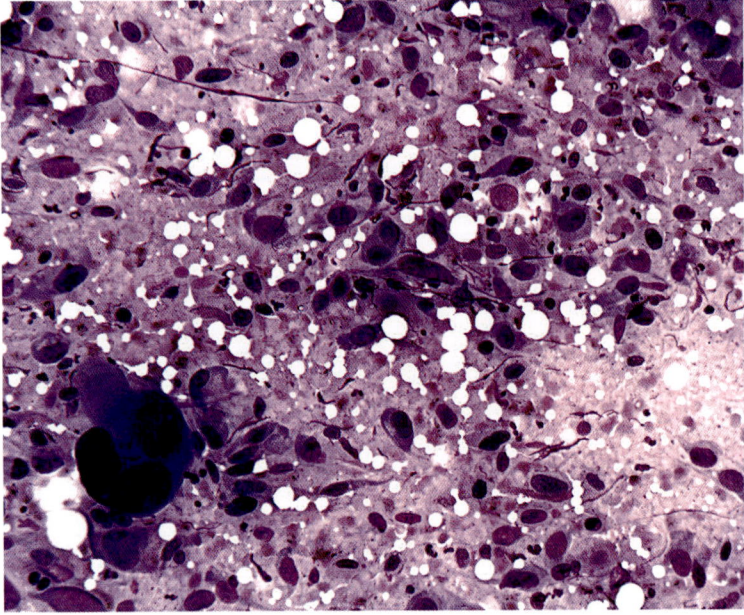

FIG 6.333 Pleomorphic malignant peripheral nerve sheath tumor, polymorphous, anaplastic cells.

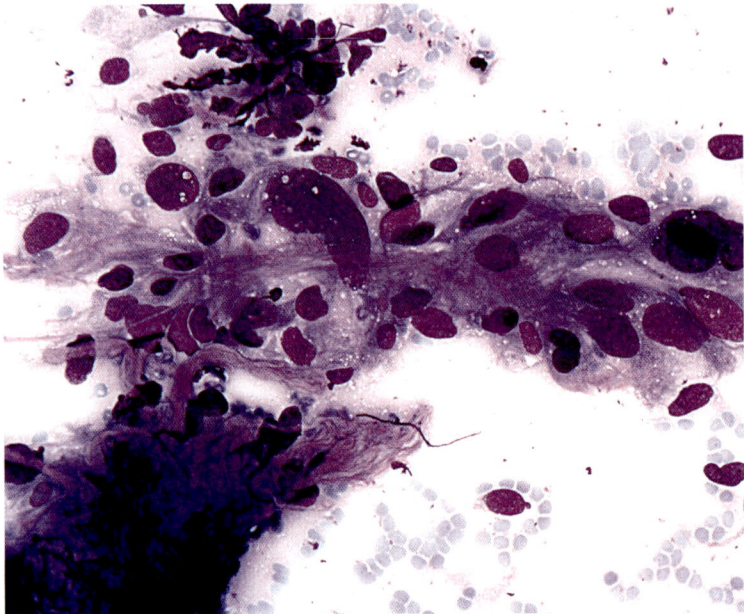

FIG 6.334 Pleomorphic malignant peripheral nerve sheath tumor, anaplastic cells and fibrillary matrix.

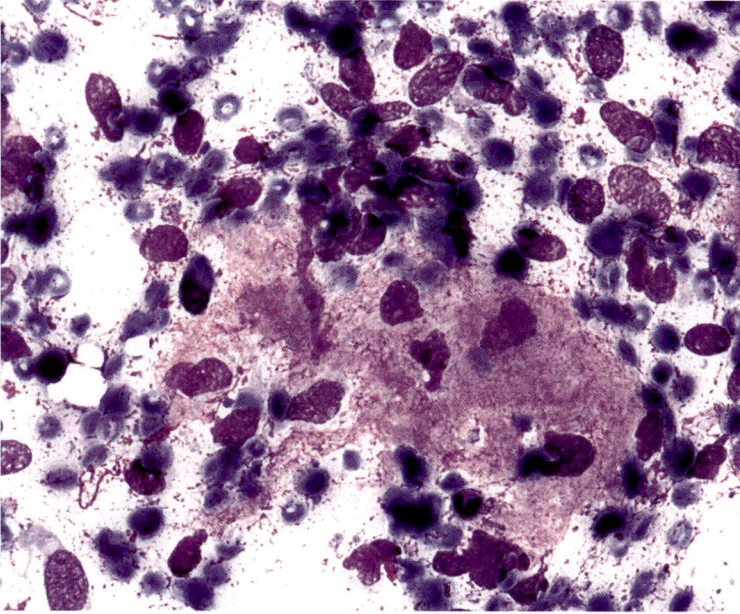

FIG 6.335 Pleomorphic malignant peripheral nerve sheath tumor, fibrillary stroma. Neural origin is evident.

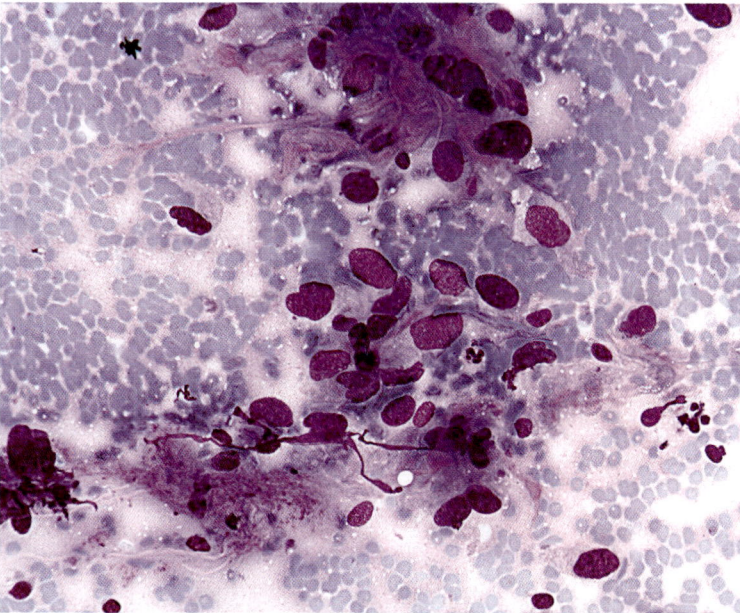

FIG 6.336 Pleomorphic malignant peripheral nerve sheath tumor delicate, fibrillary stroma.

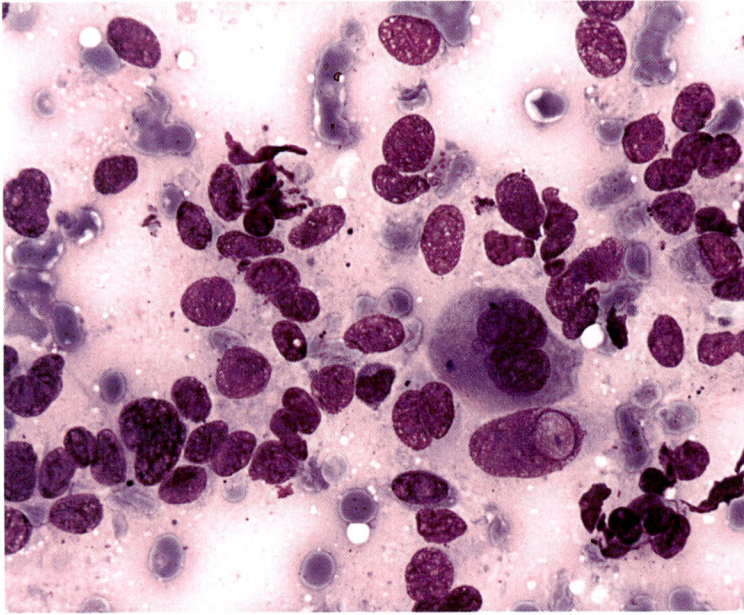

FIG 6.337 Pleomorphic malignant peripheral nerve sheath tumor, roundish and epithelioid cells.

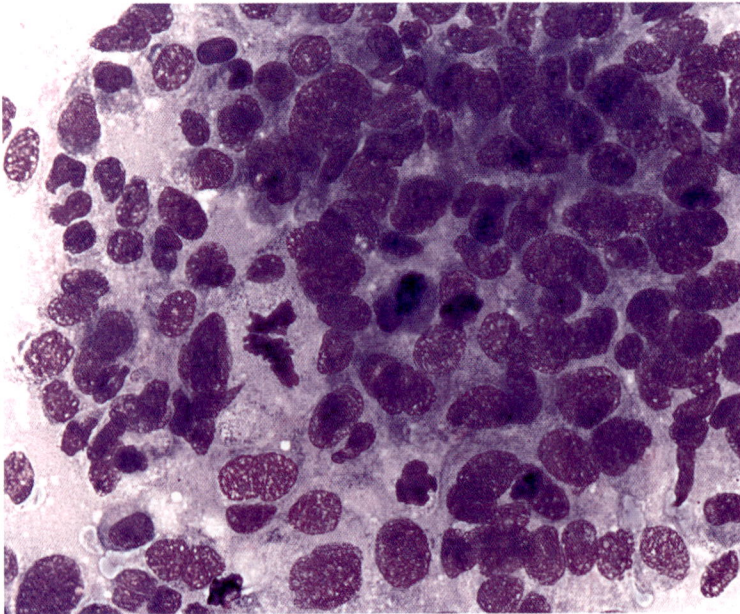

FIG 6.338 Pleomorphic malignant peripheral nerve sheath tumor, epithelioid cells.

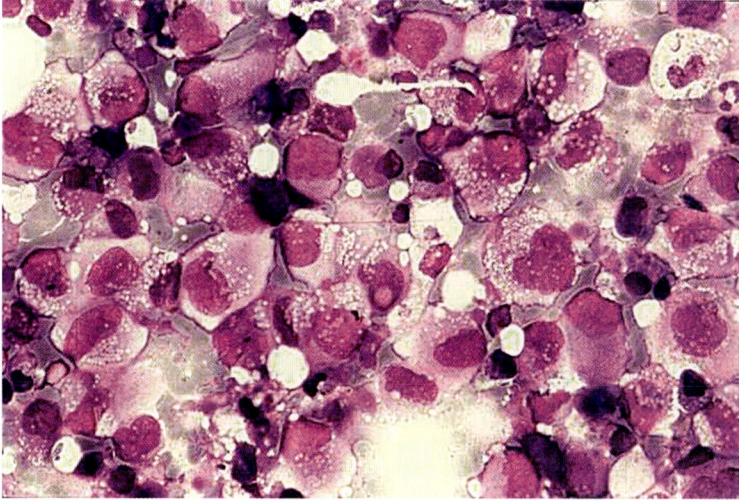

FIG 6.339 Pleomorphic malignant peripheral nerve sheath tumor, rhabdomyoblastic cells (Triton tumor).

We do not fully agree with the assertion that pleomorphic malignant peripheral nerve sheath tumor cannot be recognized by cytological examination because in many cases the accurate diagnosis is suggested by the presence of a fibrillary stroma.

6.8 ROUND CELL SARCOMAS

Round cell sarcomas largely affect the pediatric population, with few cases being observed in adults. Indeed, in latter circumstances, in assessing small round cell tumors, it is important to rule out entities such as small cell lymphoma and primary or metastatic small cell carcinoma. Among entities included in that category of sarcomas, some strongly are suspected by their clinical setting (e.g., mesenchymal chondrosarcoma, embryonal botryoid rhabdomyosarcoma, and desmoplastic small round cell tumor). Molecular genetics play a pivotal role in the precision of diagnosis because distinctive cytogenetic and molecular abnormalities allow the distinction of subtypes of a given phenotype of tumor and other round cell neoplasms. The emergence of new antibodies has widened the selected panel useful in the differentiation of round cell neoplasms of soft tissues.

6.8.1 Embryonnal and Alveolar Rhabdomyosarcoma

Embryonal rhabdomyosarcoma and alveolar rhabdomyosarcoma belong to this category of morphologic pattern. A solid variant of alveolar rhabdomyosarcoma is often of similar morphology to embryonal rhabdomyosarcoma and both are confused easily. In such cases, molecular genetics permit differentiating both entities because most alveolar type have a t(2;13)(q35;q14) translocation resulting in the breakpoint within the *PAX* gene on chromosome 2 and the *FKHR* on chromosome 13, which is not found in embryonal rhabdomyosarcoma [372]. In a few cases, a variant t(1;13)(p36;q14) translocation that juxtaposes the *PAX7* gene with the *FKHR* gene also is involved in the pathogenesis of alveolar rhabdomyosarcoma [373].

Embryonal rhabdomyosarcoma accounts for approximately 49% of all rhabdomyosarcomas. It affects children younger than 10 years of age and sometimes adolescents and young adults. The most common sites are head and neck followed by the genitourinary tract, deep soft tissues of the extremities, the pelvis, and the retroperitoneum. In comparison with alveolar rhabdomyosarcoma, the cytogenetic abnormalities are characterized by a consistent loss of heterozygocity for closely linked loci at chromosome 11p15.5 [374]. A spindle cell variant of embryonal rhabdomyosarcoma also has been characterized by virtue of its cellular component, mostly spindle cells, and its clinical setting (i.e., predilection for affecting males in paratesticular location, and it seems to pursue a more favorable clinical course).

The term "botryoid" polypoid grape-like growth embryonal rhabdomyosarcoma refers to neoplasms found in mucosa-lined hollow organs, (e.g., nasal cavity, nasopharynx, bile duct, urinary bladder, and the vagina). During the last 10 years, the clinical behavior of rhabdomyosarcomas has improved greatly particularly for the embryonal subtype because of a multidisciplinary therapeutic approach, including biopsy, surgical removal of the neoplasm, and chemotherapy with or without radiotherapy.

Alveolar rhabdomyosarcomas tend to occur at a slightly older age than the embryonal type. It develops in deep soft tissues of the extremities, accounting for 50% of all rhabdomyosarcomas in this location. In contrast to embryonal rhabdomyosarcoma, its prognosis did not improve in the last decades despite the institution of multidisciplinary therapeutic approaches.

6.8.1.1 *Histopathology.* Embryonal rhabdomyosarcoma shows similarities of histology with developing skeletal muscle, although under different patterns. The level of differentiation varies greatly, ranging from poorly differentiated small cell tumors difficult to diagnose without the help of immunohistochemistry and electron microscopy to better differentiated neoplasms resembling foetal muscle fibers. Consequently, features frequently observed in most tumors are varying degrees of cellular density, loosely myxoid areas (Fig 6.340), small hyperchromatic round/shaped cells (Fig 6.341), and varying numbers of rhabdomyoblasts recognized by their eosinophilic cytoplasm (Fig 6.342). The development of sarcomeric units is manifested by the presence of cytoplasmic cross striations. Pleomorphic embryonal rhabdomyosarcomas are difficult to distinguish from pleomorphic adult rhabdomyosarcomas. Embryonal spindle cell type predominantly consists of eleongated spindle cells resembling fetal myotubes at a late stage of cellular differentiation. The botryoid variant is characterized by a limited number of cells and by an abundance of myxoid stroma resembling a myxoma-like tumor (Fig 6.343). Densification of tumor cells under the intact overlying epithelium of affected organs realizes a "cambium layer."

Alveolar rhabdomyosarcoma consists of large ill-defined aggregates of round-to-oval cells (Fig 6.344) showing a central loss of cohesion, giving formation to irregular alveolar spaces (Fig 6.345). These aggregates are separated by strands of dense fibrous septa around dilated blood vascular channels. Not infrequently, cells in the center of alveolar spaces are arranged loosely and described as "freely

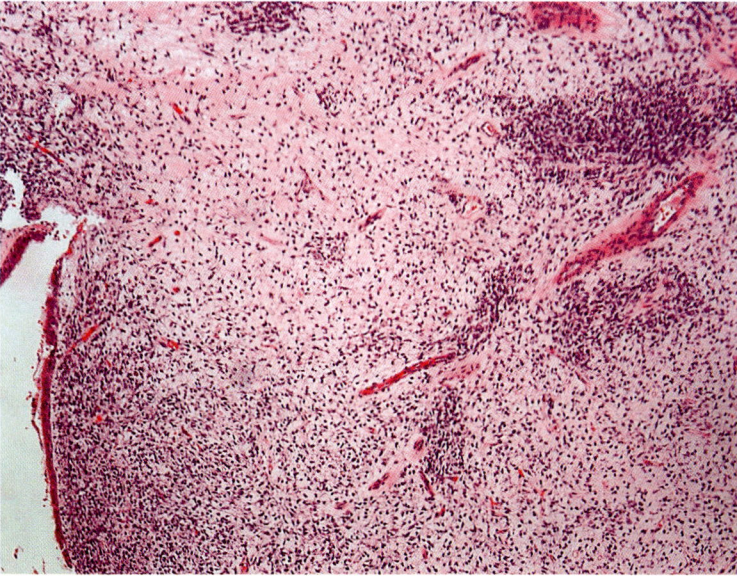

FIG 6.340 Embryonal rhabdomyosarcoma, varying degree of cellularity showing loosely myxoid zones and more solid areas.

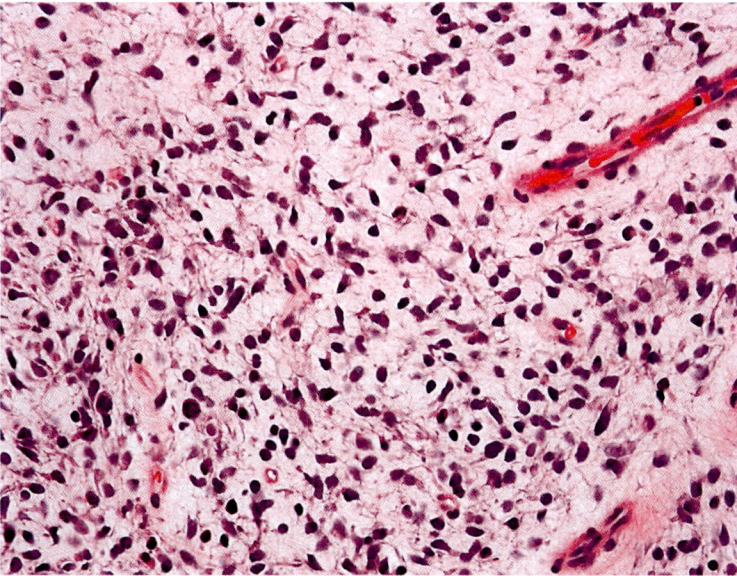

FIG 6.341 Embryonal rhabdomyosarcoma, hyperchromatic round and stellated cells in a loose stroma.

flooting" (Fig 6.346). As already mentioned, solid variants resemble embryonal rhabdomyosarcoma (Fig 6.347).

The immunohistochemical profiles of embryonal rhabdomyosarcoma and alveolar rhabdomyosarcoma are similar (see discussion in section 6.7 dealing with

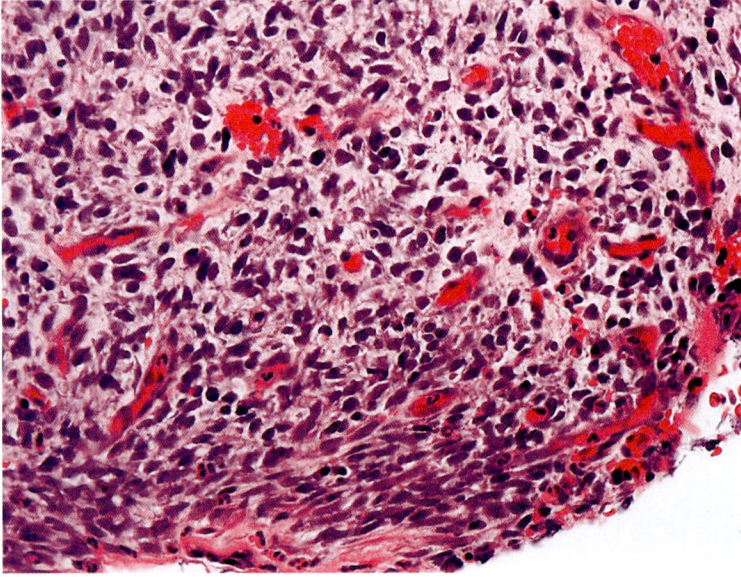

FIG 6.342   Embryonal rhabdomyosarcoma, mixture of round and spindle cells at different stages of maturation.

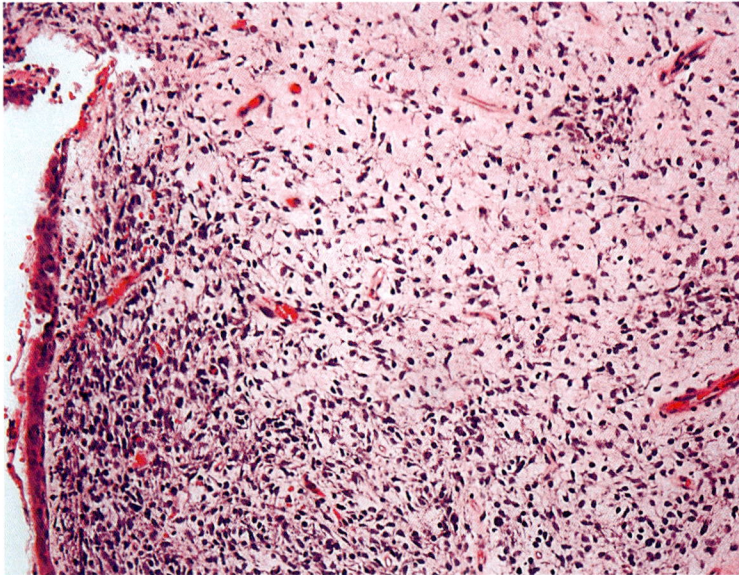

FIG 6.343   Embryonal rhabdomyosarcoma, botryoid variant.

leiomyosarcoma and rhabdomyosarcoma). It is worth mentioning that an antibody to myoglobin should be discarded from the selected panel because of its lack of sensibility and specificity. In contrast, myogenin, the best-studied member of the family of myogenic regulator genes, is an excellent marker for all subtypes of

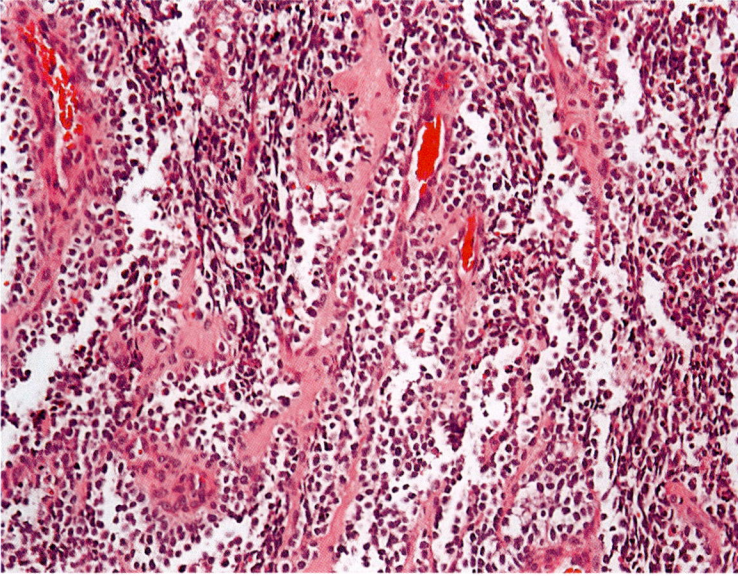

FIG 6.344 Alveolar rhabdomyosarcoma, irregular alveolar spaces with central loss of cohesion are typical.

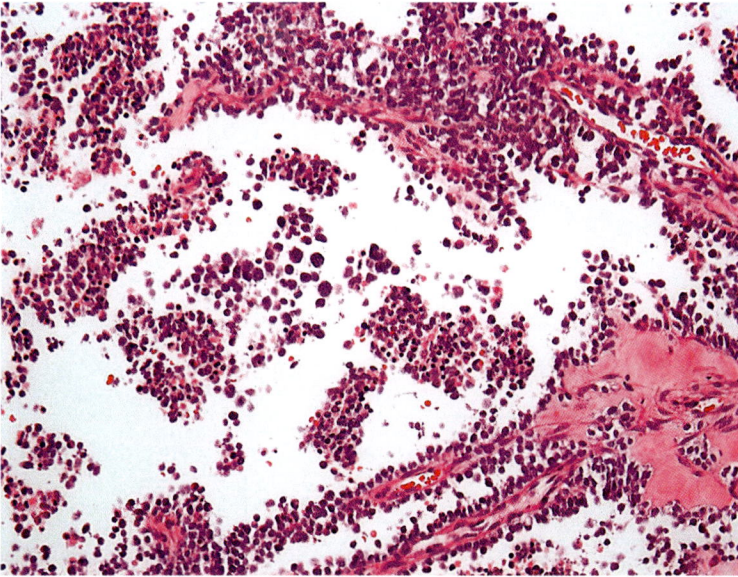

FIG 6.345 Alveolar rhabdomyosarcoma, aggregates of round cells "freely floating" in alveolar spaces.

rhabdomyosarcoma whose sensibility and specificity have been tested positively. Its interest relies on its capability to identify striated muscle fibers in differentiation.

6.8.1.2 Cytopathology. Smears from embryonal rhabdomyosarcomas and alveolar rhabdomyosarcoma are similar, but alveolar structures are lacking in

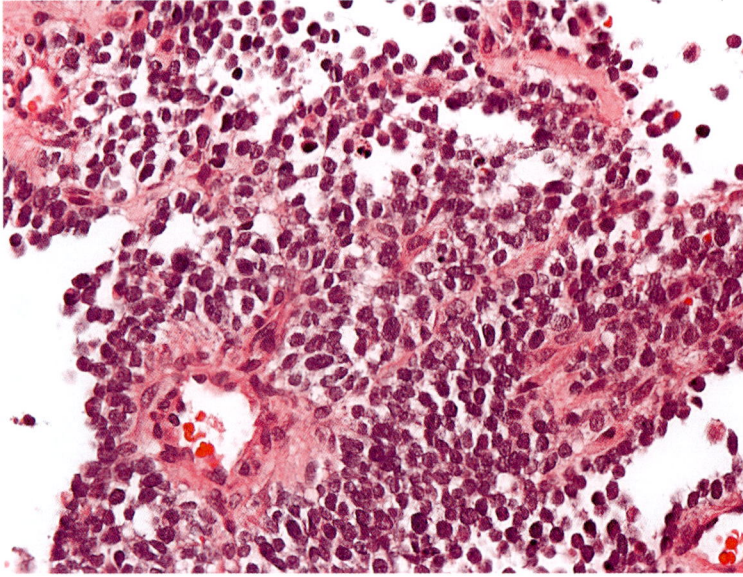

FIG 6.346   Alveolar rhabdomyosarcoma, higher magnification showing relative uniformity of tumor cells.

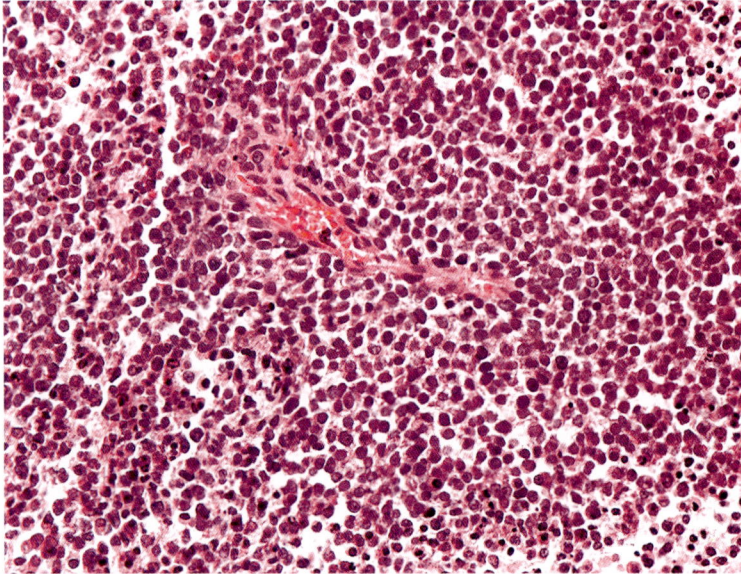

FIG 6.347   Alveolar rhabdomyosarcoma, solid variant simulating a tumor of the Ewing/PNET spectrum.

embryonal rhabdomyosarcoma. In embryonal rhabdomyosarcoma, smears are usually extremely cell-rich. Tumor cells are polymorphous (Fig 6.348), roundish (Fig 6.349), and spindle-shaped (Fig 6.350). However some embryonal rhabdomyosarcomas consist exclusively of small and regular spindle cells embedded in

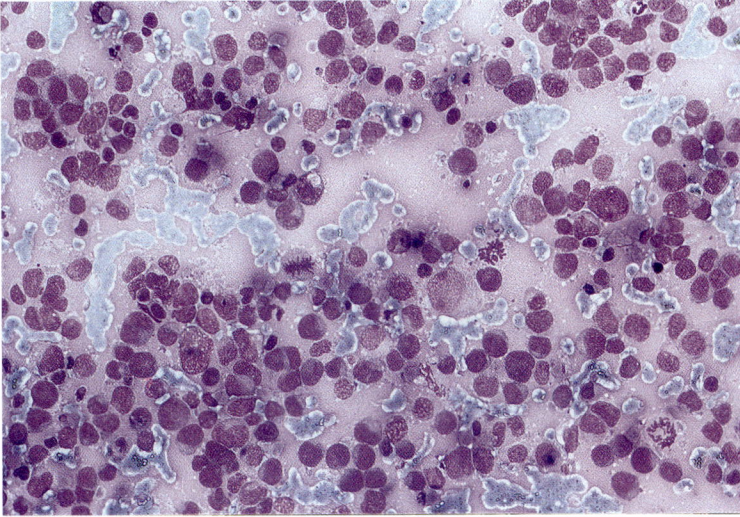

FIG 6.348 Embryonal rhabdomyosarcoma, polymorphous cells.

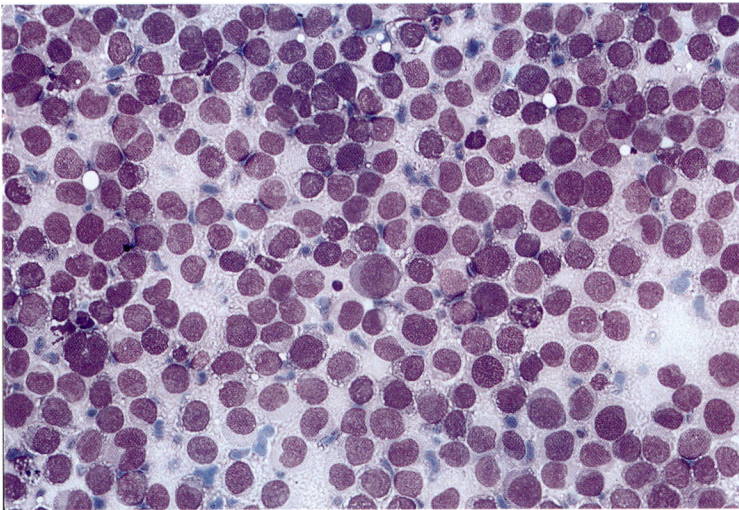

FIG 6.349 Embryonal rhabdomyosarcoma, roundish cells.

eosinophilic collagen. Smears from alveolar rhabdomyosarcoma are usually extremely cell-rich and stroma-poor. They consist of varieties of cells, including roundish (Fig 6.351), spindle-shaped, rhabdomyoblastic (Fig 6.352), and plasmacytoid, sometimes binucleated with excentric nuclei. Cells are arranged frequently in alveolar structures around connective septa or vascular structures (Figs 6.353 and 6.354). Numerous mitotic figures, prominent cytonuclear atypia, and sometimes and important necrotic background are observed.

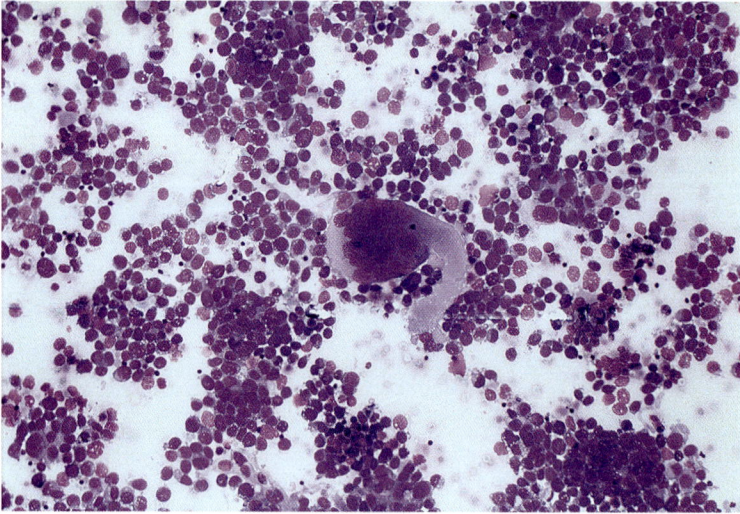

FIG 6.350 Embryonal rhabdomyosarcoma, spindle-shaped cells mixed with roundish cells.

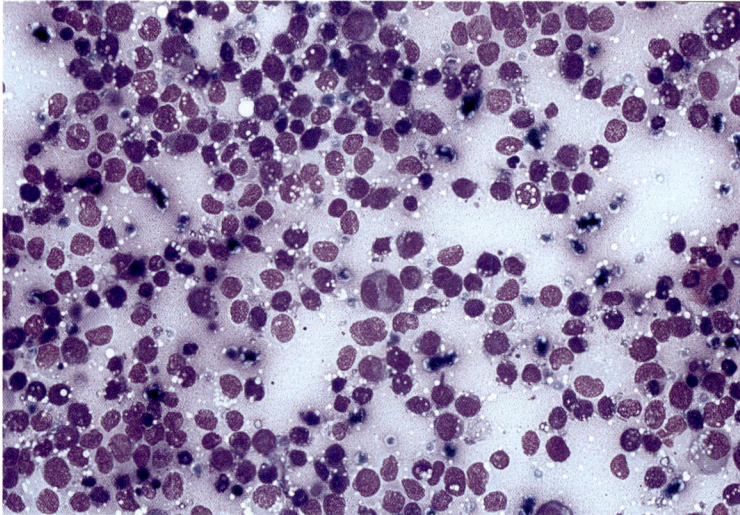

FIG 6.351 Alveolar rhabdomyosarcoma, roundish cells.

6.8.1.3 Differential Diagnosis. The following entities should be differentiated from embryonnal and alveolar rhabdomyosarcoma:

– Ewing sarcoma/ peripheral neuroectodermal tumor
– Rhabdoid tumor
– Desmoplastic round cell tumor
– Poorly differentiated synovial sarcoma

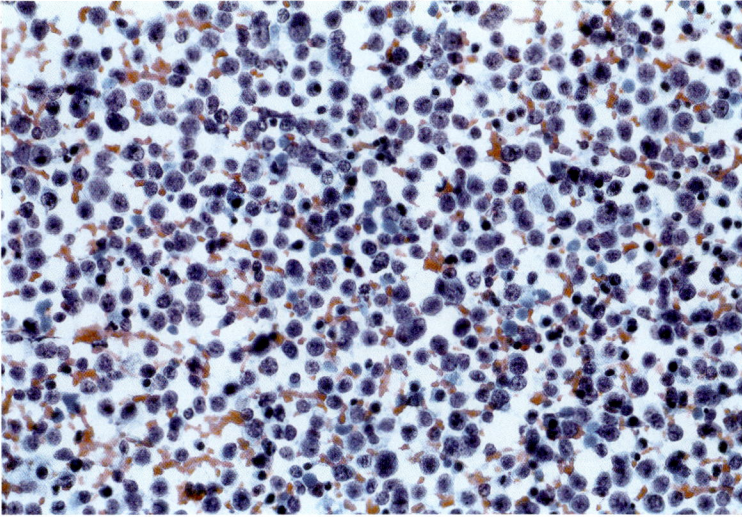

FIG 6.352 Alveolar rhabdomyosarcoma, rhabdomyoblastic cell, Papanicolaou.

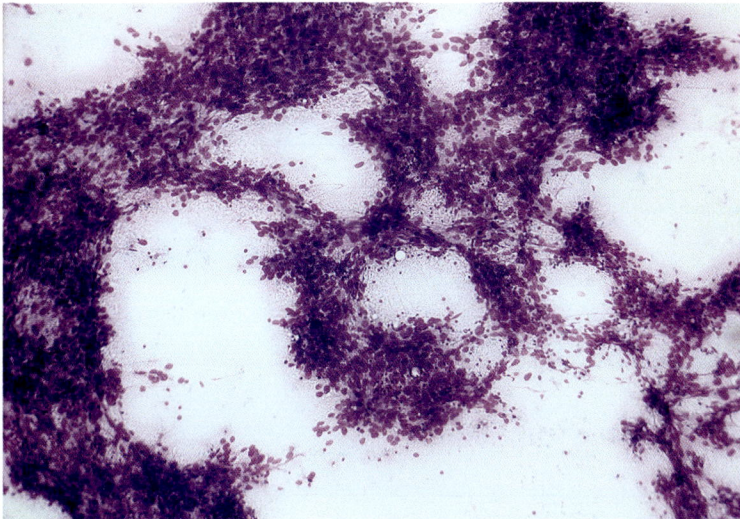

FIG 6.353 Alveolar rhabdomyosarcoma, alveolar structures observed in low-power field.

The morphologic cytological data of the different varieties of rhabdomyosarcoma should allow differentiatiation from Ewing sarcoma/peripheral neuroectodermic tumor, rhabdoid tumor, poorly differentiated synovial sarcoma, and desmoplastic small round cell tumor (Table 6.16). The presence of round cell soft tissue sarcoma with characteristic rhabdomyoblastic cells, specific chromosomal aberration, and muscular markers positivity is diagnostic of alveolar rhabdomyosarcoma. In rare instances of tumors that have no specific aberrations, core needle biopsy may be necessary to detect a morphological alveolar pattern. In our

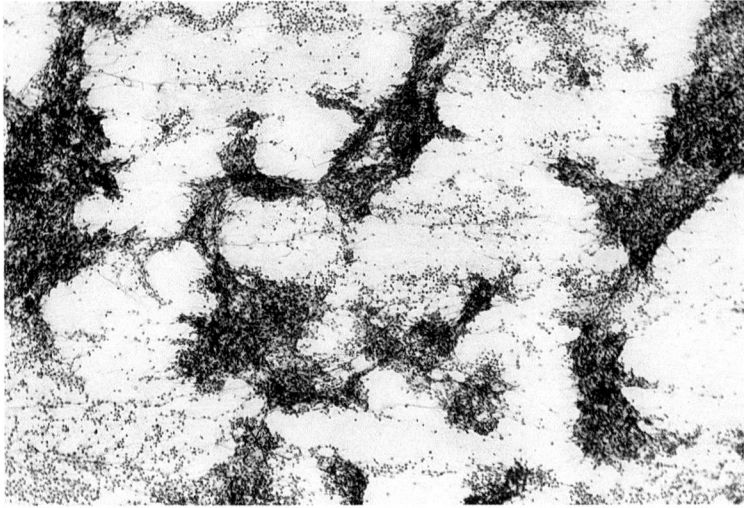

FIG 6.354   Alveolar rhabdomyosarcoma, alveolar structures observed in low-power field, Papanicolaou.

TABLE 6.16   Principal cytological differential diagnosis of rhabdomyosarcoma

	Rhabdomy osarcoma	Ewing sarcoma/ peripheral neuroectodermal tumor	Rhabdoid tumor	Poorly differentiated synovial sarcoma	Desmoplastic small round cell tumor
Roundish cells	++	++	++	++	++
Spindle-shaped cells	+	+/−	+/−	+	−
Rhabdomyoblastic- like cells	++	+/−	++	−	−
Pseudo alveolar structures	+	+/−	+/−	−	−
Giant cells	+	−	+	+/−	−
Mitotic figures	++	+/−	++	+	+
Cytonuclear atypia	++	+/−	++	+	+
Necrotic background	++	+	+/−	+	+
Collagenous component	−	+/−	−	−	++

++; Frequent, +; rare, +/− occasionally seen, −; absent.

previous study [375], we found that the alveolar rhabdomyosarcoma showed more frequently rhabdomyoblastic cells, alveolar structures, giant multinucleated cells, mitotic figures, and cytonuclear atypia, although these observations were not unique to this subtype. Cytomorphology alone is insufficient for an accurate diagnosis and should be supplemented by ancillary diagnostic methods and correlated with the histological findings.

Ewing sarcoma/peripheral neuroectodermal tumor family groups together with round with cell tumors with variable morphology but well-characterized transloca-tions t(11;22)(q24,q12) and t(21;22)(q22,q12) were found with an estimated pre-valence of 95%. The immunohistochemical reaction for antibody CD99 shows cell membrane positivity. Tumors characteristically consists of round, poorly differentiated cells with double cell population: larger cells with clarified cytoplasm and small, dark cells. Frequently, cellular clusters and rosettes are present.

Rhabdoid tumors could be confused with rhabdomyosarcoma [298]. The presence of perinuclear cytoplasmic globular inclusions is usually more characteristic of rhabdoid tumors. For the differential diagnosis of extrarenal tumors, hypercalcemia and cytokeratin positive/desmin negative immunostaining help in accurate tumor typing [376], although some cases with an expression of desmin and myofilaments have been described [377].

In poorly differentiated synovial sarcoma, smears are uniform, lack nuclear pleomorphism and mostly consist of ovoid-to-rounded tumor cells with scant tapering cytoplasm [378]. Branching papillary-like tumor tissue fragments with vessel stalks, acinar-like structures, and comma-like nuclei are also characteristic. Cytogenetic studies have shown a specific chromosomal translocation t(X;18)(p11.2;q11.2), with an estimated prevalence of 85% in synovial sarcoma [379]. Cytologic material also can be used for the analysis of specific transcripts using the RT-PCR technique to detect the SYT-SSX fusion transcripts whose estimated prevalence is 65% for SYT-SSX1 and 35% for SYT-SSX2 [378].

Smears in desmoplatic small round cell tumors are hypercellular and show numerous small cells with scant cytoplasm that are arranged primarily in loosely cohesive clusters. Nuclei are oval to round with evenly distributed, finely granular chromatin and inconspicuous nucleoli. Keratin and desmin usually are expressed strongly. Paranuclear aggregates of intermediate filaments may be observed on occasion. Nuclear molding is a predominant feature. The presence of rhabdomyoblastic cells is characteristic of rhabdomyosarcoma.

6.8.1.4 *Comments.* When FNA morphology is correlated with different histological subtypes, alveolar rhabdomyosarcomas are more cellular than embryonal tumors. They also show more rhabdomyoblastic cells, alveolar structures, giant cells, multinucleated cells, mitotic figures, and cytonuclear atypia. Inversely, spindle-shaped cells were observed more frequently in embryonal or adult rhabdomyosarcomas than in alveolar rhabdomyosarcomas.

A few studies, including 430 cases, have attempted to characterize the cytologic morphology of alveolar rhabdomyosarcoma [375,376,380–388]. Cytologic diagnosis in rhabdomyosarcoma seems to be of great value for an diagnosis of malignancy. Two studies [382,385] have reported 78–80% of diagnostic accuracy, and 100% for "malignant" diagnosis. An overview of other large series [381,384,387,389] have shown similar results; false negative and unsatisfactory samples were rare. During the last 20 years, the use of immunocytochemistry to identify muscular markers substantially improves the accuracy of diagnosis [390,391]. FNA material was used successfully in the ancillary techniques to detect the characteristic t(2;13)(q35;q14) chromosomal translocation and/or the gene fusion transcripts *PAX-FKHR* that are detected with an estimated prevalence of 80% in alveolar rhabdomyosarcoma.

It is now well established that cytogenetic and RT-PCR analyses are more objective and sensitive tools than conventional histologic and/or cytologic morphology, immuno(cyto)chemistry, or electron microscopic analysis for the diagnosis of soft tissue tumors [392]. The samples can be snap frozen in liquid nitrogen at bedside.

In the absence of facilities to analyze samples by these ancillary techniques, it could be impossible to diagnose the alveolar rhabdomyosarcoma accurately using only smears from FNA sampling. Smears from alveolar rhabdomyosarcoma tend to recapitulate the histologic architecture of the tumors [393]. It has been shown [376] that the embryonal rhabdomyosarcoma predominantly consists of primitive round cells with rounded nuclei resembling those of the alveolar rhabdomyosarcoma. The cells are larger than those of the alveolar rhabdomyosarcoma, and anisocytosis and anisokaryosis are more marked. Spindle-shaped cells are more often a component of embryonal rhabdomyosarcoma. In an analysis of 53 rhabdomyosarcoma [385], it was observed that the alveolar rhabdomyosarcoma exhibited the following major architectural patterns: one characterized by completely dissociated cells and the other containing many clustered formations; the embryonal rhabdomyosarcoma exhibited large tissue fragments with abundant eosinophilic material and various numbers of dissociated cells. The relative proportion of poorly differentiated and well-differentiated rhabdomyoblasts varied in both types and in all patterns. It was suggested that a reliable subclassification into alveolar and embryonal subtypes of rhabdomyosarcoma could not be reached with a high accuracy from cytologic smears. In a series of 37 aspirates and 6 touch prints [383] of the alveolar rhabdomyosarcoma, most tumor cells were small and lymphocyte-like, presenting fine granular chromatin. In contrast, in the embryonal rhabdomyosarcoma, two cell types, including large, tadpole, or ribbon-shaped cells and small round cells, were observed. It was concluded that, with sufficient experience, it was possible to subtype rhabdomyosarcoma by cytologic examination alone. In 17 aspirates and 3 touch prints from rhabdomyosarcoma [381] the subtypes were not specified; the morphologic findings most commonly observed were a uniform population of tumor cells arranged in single cells and cohesive aggregates. The cells were predominantly roundish with uniform nuclei and scant-to-moderate amounts of cytoplasm. Binucleated or multinucleated cells were found in 17 out of 20 smears. It was suggested that binucleate cells were important criteria for the diagnosis of rhabdomyosarcoma on FNA cytological material. In a series of 15 cases of rhabdomyosarcoma [389], including two alveolar subtypes, a variable mixture of cells were categorized as early, intermediate, or late rhabdomyoblasts according to differentiation grade. Embryonal rhabdomyosarcomas comprised mainly early rhabdomyoblasts. Hence, the recognition of these patterns could be helpful using FNA cytological material.

6.8.1.5 *FNA Key Features.* The following are in favor of the diagnosis:

- Roundish cells, rhabdomyoblastic cells, alveolar structures, positivity of muscular markers

The following is a difficulty in the diagnosis:

- Polymorphous morphology, spindle-shaped cells

The following are evidence against the diagnosis:

- Double round cell population
- Rosettes

 – Perinuclear inclusions
 – Papillary structures
 – Epithelial cells

6.8.2   Ewing Sarcoma/Peripheral Neuroectodermal Tumor

The concept of tumors of the Ewing sarcoma/peripheral neuroectodermal tumor (PNET) spectrum has evolved considerably in the last decades [394]. It allowed grouping in a specific category the extraskeletal Ewing tumor and peripheral neuroepithelioma (also reported as adult neuroblastoma and peripheral neuroepithelioma). Indeed, identification of a common cytogenetic abnormality t(11;22)(q24;q12) has been a strong argument to support the hypothesis that both neoplasms were linked histogenetically. Additional investigations revealed variations involving the 22q12 chromosome, the site of the EWS gene [379].

Most patients affected are adolescents, with most of the cohort being younger than 30 years of age. They orignate in the extremities for PNET and in the paravertebral areas for Ewing sarcoma. They are rapidly growing, deeply located large masses. Their prognosis has improved dramatically with the introduction of modern therapy including surgery and radiation therapy/multiagent chemotherapy. Key factors influencing prognosis are the presence of metastasis at initial diagnosis, large size of the tumor, extensive necrosis, and poor response to chemotherapy.

6.8.2.1   Histopathology. Classically, criteria distinguishing Ewing sarcoma from PNET were variable. Because it is accepted now that they are lesions histogenetically related, precise criteria to separate both entities are not critical [395]. Typical cases consist of solid areas of strong uniformity of round-to-ovoid individual cells with a distinct nuclear membrane, dusty chromatin, and minute nucleoli (Fig 6.355). Cytoplasm is ill-defined, scanty, pale-staining, and contains glycogen. Tumors are richly vascularized, which is not obvious at first sight with the vessels being compressed by closely packed tumor cells. Sometimes, a prominent vascular component depicts a pseudoalveolar pattern comprising small central fluid spaces surrounded by tumor cells in a peritheliomatous pattern, hence the initial designation of Ewing sarcoma as a "diffuse endothelioma" (Fig 6.356). In the peripheral neuroectodermal tumor variety, the cell composition formerly was described as "large cell" or atypical Ewing sarcoma (Fig 6.357). These tumors could contain fibrillary cytoplasmic extensions coalescing to form rosettes.

Besides the histochemical demonstration of glycogen, the immunohistochemical profile is now well precised, although for many years, it was an immunohistochemical diagnosis of exclusion. The product of the *MIC2* gene is recognized by antibodies CD99 whose sensibility has been tested [396,397]. However, this pattern of membrane immunoractivity is not specific because it has been recognized in various lymphomas, small cell carcinoma, and rhabdomyosarcoma. A plethora of neural markers also have been tested, including NSE, Leu-7, S-100 protein, and synaptophysin. CD99, although sensitive for recognizing Ewing sarcoma/peripheral neuroectodermal tumor family of tumors, is not expressed by neuroblastoma, an entity to consider in the differential diagnosis. Ewing sarcoma/PNET and neuroblastoma

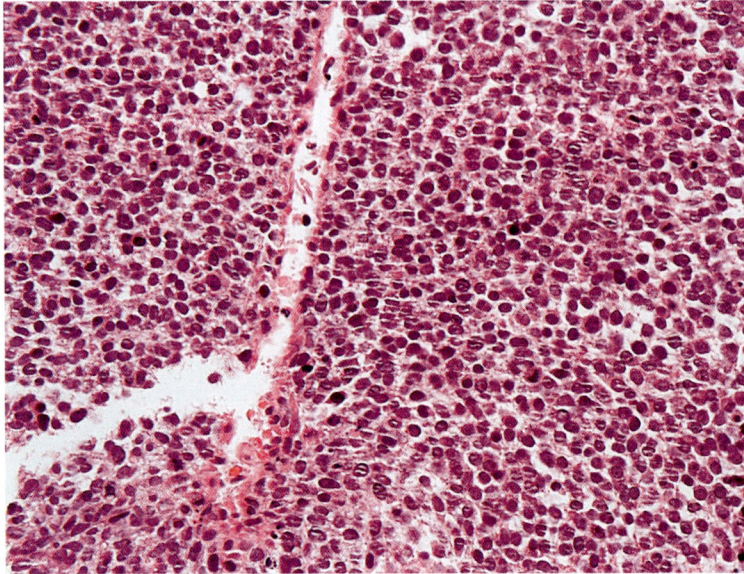

FIG 6.355 Ewing sarcoma/PNET, sheets of individual cells showing dusty chromatin and minute nucleoli.

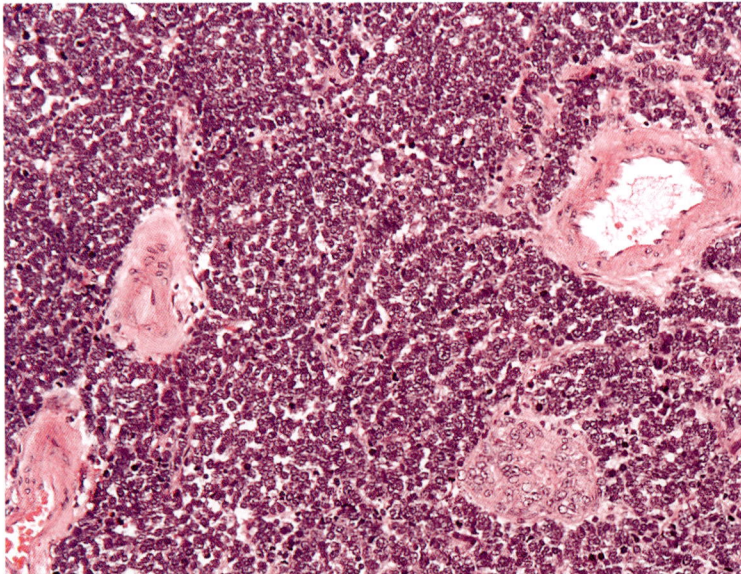

FIG 6.356 Ewing sarcoma/PNET, tumor cells are arranged in a peritheliomatous pattern.

could be confused easily because they occur in the young patients, because of the frequent paravertebral location of the tumor, and because of the histologic evidence of rosette-like structures in some tumors. Nevertheless, they differ by the average age of Ewing sarcoma/PNET which is older by a significant margin, by the presence by

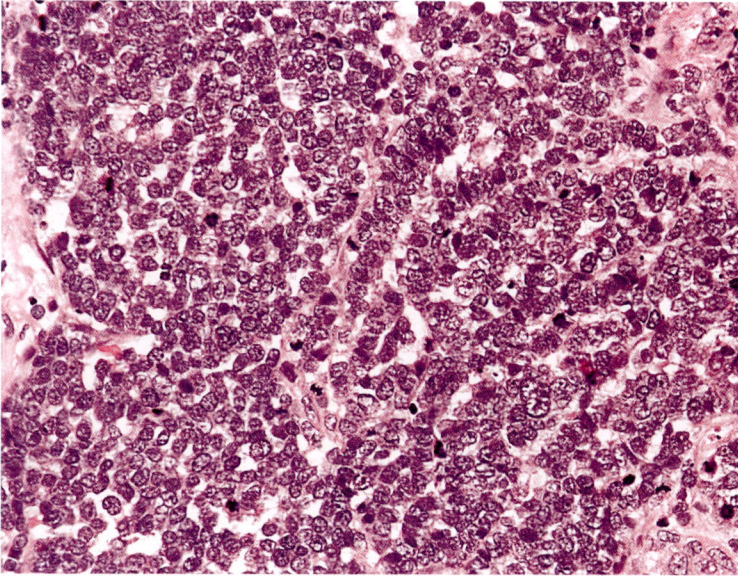

FIG 6.357 Ewing sarcoma/PNET, atypical Ewing sarcoma, formerly described as "large cell variant".

light microscopy of neuropil, by ganglionic differentiation, and finally, by the expression of CD99 and the cytogenetic profile.

Alveolar rhabdomyosarcoma and metastatic small cell carcinoma are candidates included in the differential diagnosis. Small cell osteosarcoma also is characterized by a population of small similar cells to those present in Ewing sarcoma/PNET. Identification of osteoid allows differentiating both entities, although it often is present only focally and is identified in biopsy specimens.

6.8.2.2 Cytopathology. Smears in Ewing sarcoma/PNET are hypercellular and stroma-poor and usually consist of round monomorphous cells (Fig 6.358) or roundish cells showing double population [398]. Darker and smaller cells represented the first population with a small, round nucleus with a rim of scant cytoplasm. The second population consists of lighter and larger cells with larger and clarified or microvacuolated cytoplasm (Fig 6.359) (microvacuolisations are PAS positive) (Fig 6.360). Rosette formations are observed in one third of cases (Figs 6.361 and 6.362). Some spindle cells also may be present in less differentiated tumors (Fig 6.363). They are small and elongated, but may present as longue cells with roundish nuclei and an elongated or rhabdomyoblastic-like shape. However, some smears may show morphologic variations like eosinophilic connective tissue fragments and pseudopapillary structures (Fig 6.364). Many cases show an abundant necrotic background and numerous mitotic figures (Fig 6.365).

6.8.2.3 Differential Diagnosis. In extraskeletal localization, the differential diagnosis with neuroblastoma, rhabdomyosarcoma, and poorly differentiated synovial sarcoma should be assessed (Table 6.17). In the absence of osteoid matrix, cytological differentiation of Ewing sarcoma from small cell osteosarcoma is not possible [399],

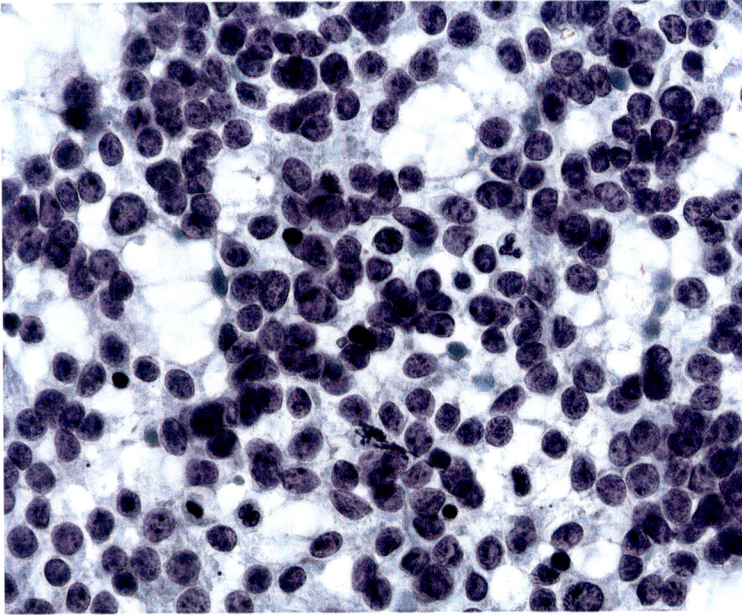

FIG 6.358 Ewing sarcoma/PNET, round monomorphous cells, Papanicolaou.

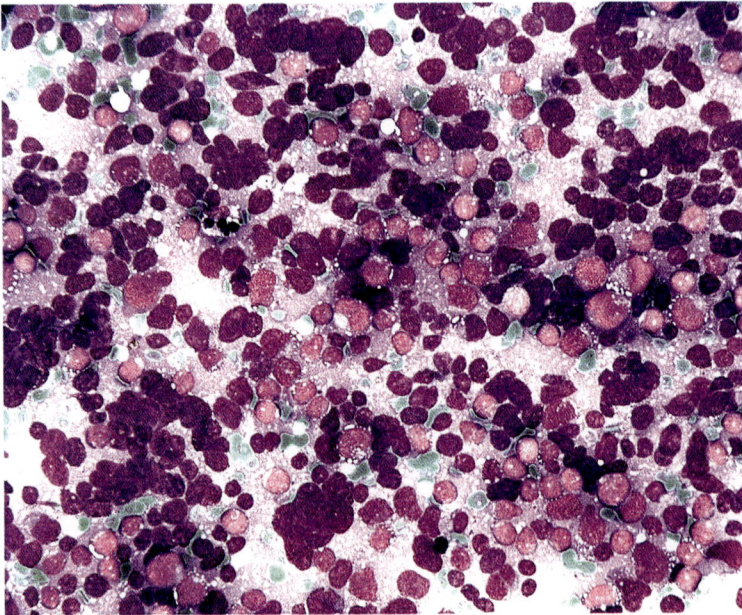

FIG 6.359 Ewing sarcoma/PNET, roundish cells showing double population, larger (lighter) and smaller (darker).

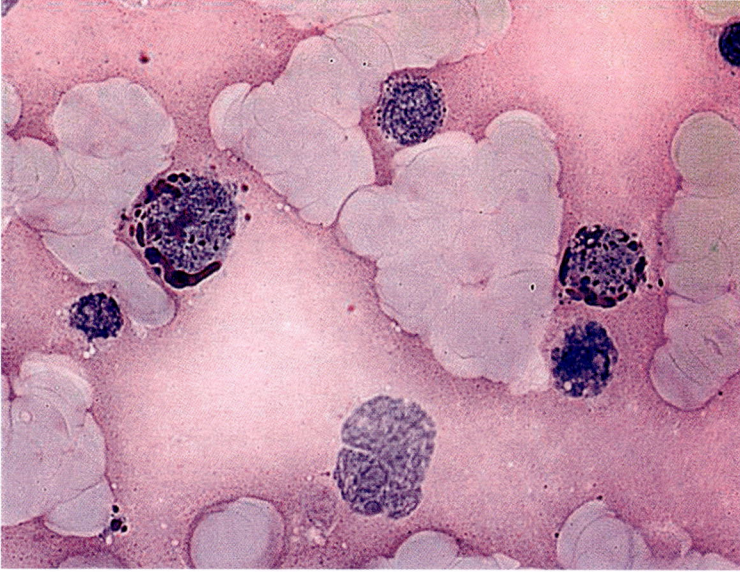

FIG 6.360 Ewing sarcoma/PNET, PAS is positive in cytoplasmic microvacuoles.

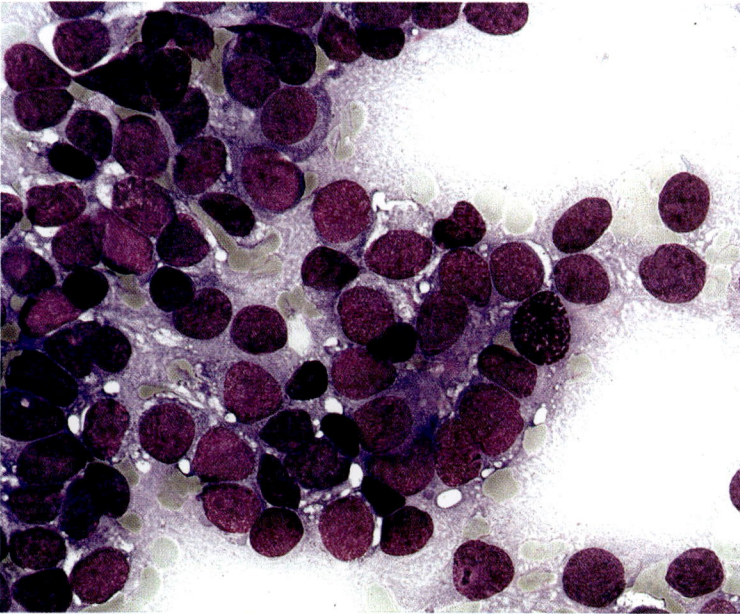

FIG 6.361 Ewing sarcoma/PNET, rosette formations.

unless special adjuvant techniques such as cytogenetic and molecular biology are performed, particularly by the demonstration or the absence of the typical transloca- tion found in a Ewing sarcoma with a prevalence of 100%. The presence of typical neuroblasts with fibrillary stroma is strongly in favor of neuroblastoma. For a poorly

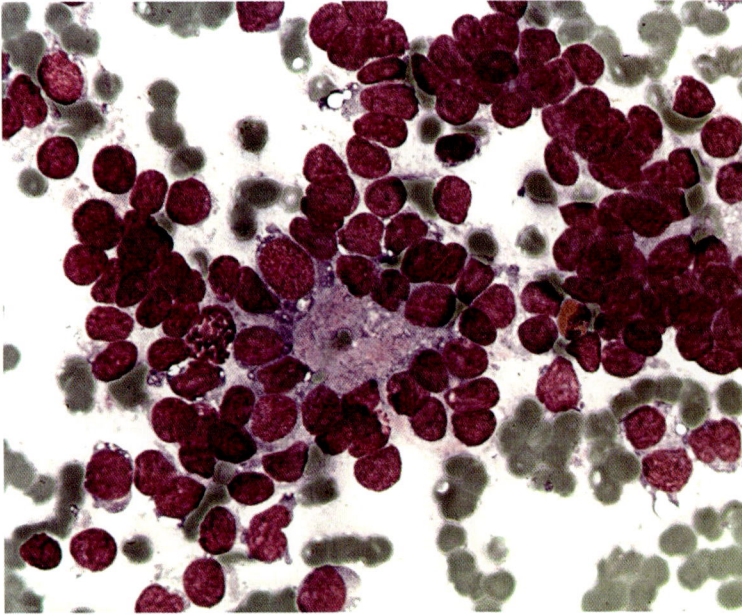

FIG 6.362 Ewing sarcoma/PNET, rosette formations.

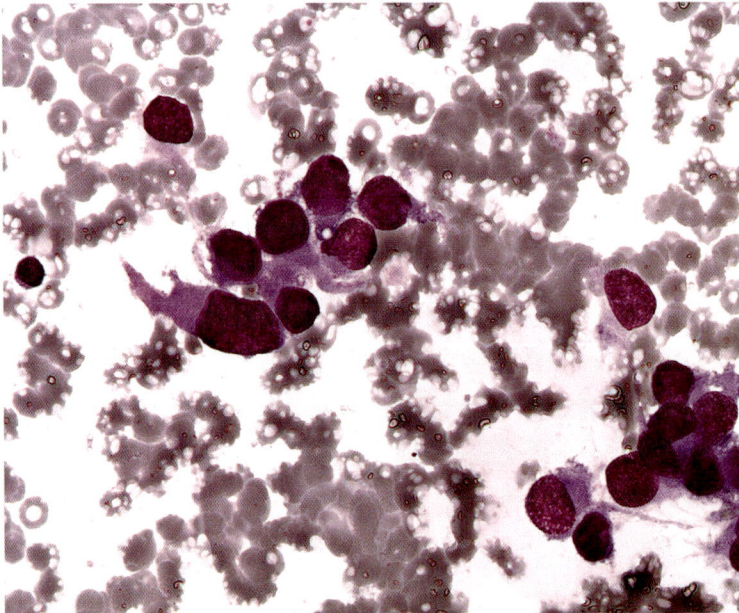

FIG 6.363 Ewing sarcoma/PNET, spindle cells.

differentiated neuroblastoma comprising uniform poorly differentiated roundish cells, the specific staining of anti-GD2 is essential [400].The presence of polymorphous cells with rhaddomyoblastic features is diagnostic of rhabdomyosarcoma. For polymorphous Ewing sarcoma/PNET with spindle cells, the immunocytochemical

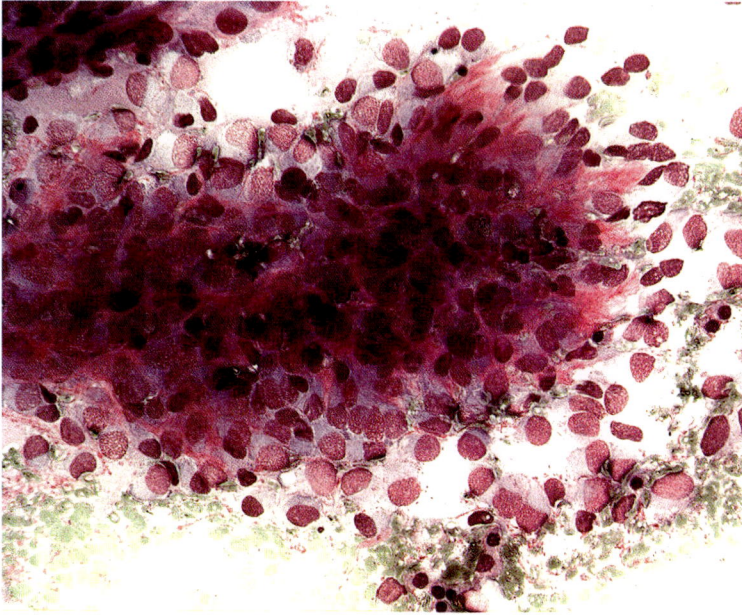

FIG 6.364 Ewing sarcoma/PNET, eosinophilic connective tissue fragments and pseudopapillary structures.

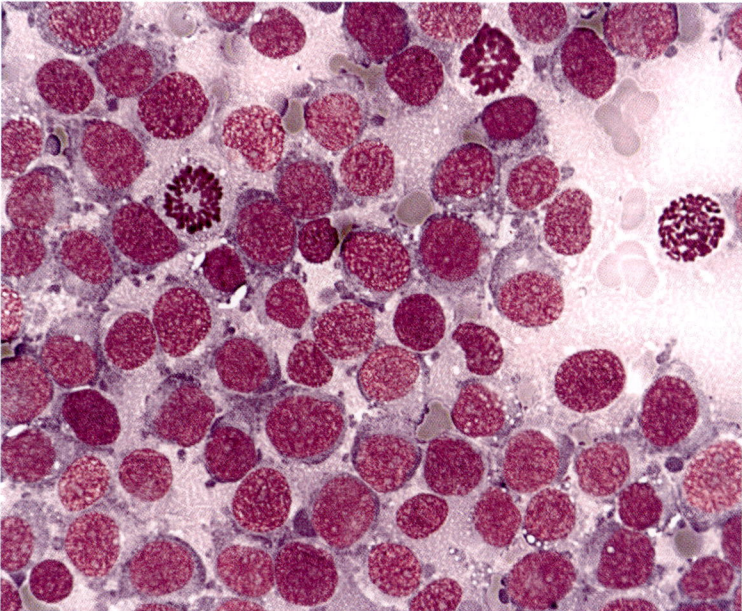

FIG 6.365 Ewing sarcoma/PNET, numerous mitotic figures.

TABLE 6.17 Cytological differential diagnosis of Ewing sarcoma/peripheral neuroectodermal tumor

	Ewing sarcoma/ PNET	Round cell osteosarcoma	Neuroblastoma	Rhabdomyo sarcoma	Poorly differentiated synovial sarcoma
Round cells	++	++	++	++	++
Double population	++	−	+/−	−	+/−
Spindle cells	+	−	−	+	++
Rosettes	++	−	++	−	Epithelial-like cells +/−
Fibrillary stroma	−	−	++	−	−
Osteoid	+/−	++	−	−	+/−
Cellular polymorphism	+	++	++	++	+
Mitotic figures	+/−	+	+	++	++
Necrosis	+	+	++	++	+/−
Specific site	++	+	++	+/−	+/−

++; Frequent, +; rare, +/− occasionally seen, −; absent.

positivity of muscular markers are in favor of rhabdomyosarcoma (375). Rare examples of poorly differentiated synovial sarcoma may simulate Ewing sarcoma/ PNET. The final differential diagnostic is based on molecular biology analysis [379].

6.8.2.4 *Comments.* Because of its high cellularity, Ewing sarcoma/PNET is diagnosed accurately on cytology smears. In our series, there were no false-negative results, and the insignificant rate was 4%. Similar results of a high accurate diagnosis were reported by other authors [396,401–407]. Despite the highly characteristic morphology, the diagnosis also may be confirmed using genomic techniques and immunocytochemistry on cytology material [396,398,405,407,408].

6.8.2.5 *Clinical and FNA Key Features.* The following are in favor of the diagnosis:

— Young adult
— Double population of large and small cells
— Rosette formation
— Specific molecular transcript and karyotypic translocation

The following are difficulties in the diagnosis:

— Spindle cells, necrosis
— Extraskeletal localizations
— No specific genomic abnormality or absence of abnormality

The following are evidence against the diagnosis:

— Fibrillary stroma
— Osteoid
— Epithelial cells

6.8.3 Desmoplastic Small Round Cell Tumor

Desmoplastic small round cell tumor (DSRCT) is the term most commonly used for this relatively rare malignant neoplasm whose most cases develop in the abdominal cavity and/or the pelvic peritoneum. Other cases occur in various anatomical sites including the parotid gland, thoracic region, and central nervous system. Most patients affected are males between 15 and 35 years of age, although it has been reported to occur in patients as young as 5 years and as old as 70–80 years. Most commonly, these tumors are large abdominal masses with extensive peritoneal involvement. So far, it is a highly malignant polyphenotypic neoplasm of unknown histogenesis.

They have a unique cytogenetic abnormality t(11;22)(p13;q12) translocation; hence, it constitutes a distinct nosologic and clinicopathologic entity [409,410]. The breakpoints involve the *EWS* gene on 22q12 and the Wilms tumor gene *WT1* on 11p13 [411]. *WT1* is a tumor suppressor gene that encodes a transcription factor that normally inhibits promoters of growth factors such as *PDGFA*. The fusion transcript is detected by RT-PCR. DSRCT pursues an aggressive biologic behavior with an extremely poor prognosis.

6.8.3.1 Histopathology. Microscopically, nests and groups of small-to-medium-sized cells embedded in a prominent hypervascularized desmoplastic stroma characterize the desmoplastic small round cell tumor (Fig 6.366). In larger nests, central necrosis is not infrequent. Tumor cells are similar to other round cell sarcomas, although foci are similar to rhabdoid tumor with large cells with abundant cytoplasm, and paranuclear inclusions may be found. The arrangement of tumor cells shows different patterns including tubular-like structures, cords of single cells reminiscent of infiltrating lobular carcinoma of the breast (Fig 6.367). The stroma consists of fibroblasts and myofibroblasts. The immunohistochemical profile is polyphenotypic, displaying a mixture of epithelial, mesenchymal, and neural markers. Keratin and desmin usually are expressed strongly. They include immunoreactivity for cytokeratin with a dot-like pattern, EMA, vimentin, and desmin, also with a dot-like pattern and with the latter being the most useful diagnostic marker in contrast to other small cell sarcomas. Entities to consider in the differential diagnosis include small round cell tumors, Ewing sarcoma family (Ewing sarcoma/PNET), rhabdomyosarcoma, lymphoma, poorly differentiated carcinoma, Merkel cell tumor, and because of its location, malignant mesothelioma, all of which present nevertheless different clinical settings.

6.8.3.2 Cytopathology. Smears are hypercellular and show numerous small cells with scant cytoplasm that are arranged primarily in loosely cohesive clusters (Fig 6.368). Nuclei are oval to round with evenly distributed, finely granular

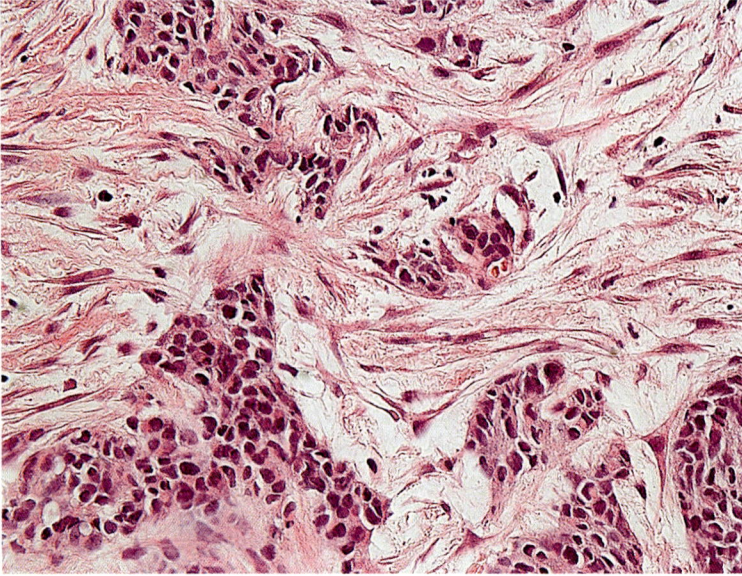

FIG 6.366 Desmoplastic small round cell tumor, nests of small to medium-size cells within a desmoplastic stroma are highly characteristic.

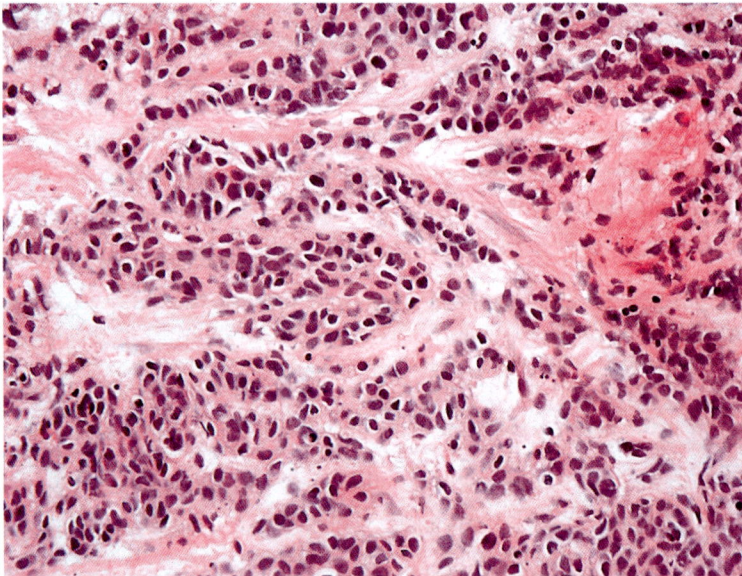

FIG 6.367 Desmoplastic small round cell tumor, cords of single tumor cells reminiscent of an infiltrating carcinoma of the breast.

chromatin and inconspicuous nucleoli (Fig 6.369). Paranuclear aggregates of inter-mediate filaments may be observed on occasion (Fig 6.370) that are positive with epithelial markers or desmin (Fig 6.371) [412,413]. Nuclear molding is a predominant feature. Smearing artifacts with poorly preserved nuclei, similar to small-cell

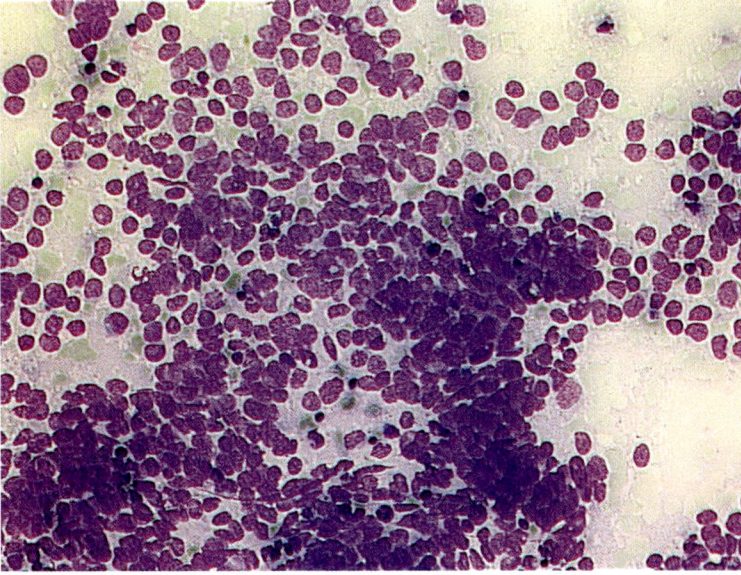

FIG 6.368 Desmoplastic small round cell tumor, small cells with scant cytoplasm that primarily are arranged in loosely cohesive clusters.

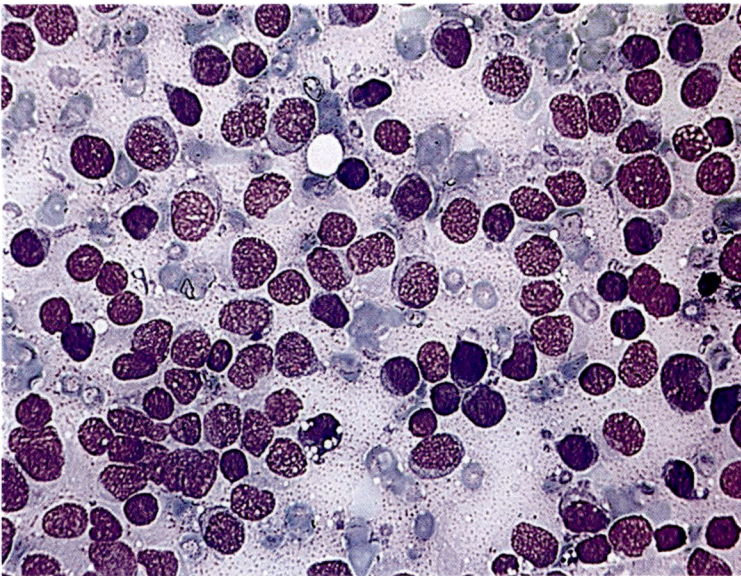

FIG 6.369 Desmoplastic small round cell tumor, oval-to-round nuclei.

carcinoma, may be present. Apoptosis and necrosis are frequent. Rosettes and neurofibrillary stroma are absent.

6.8.3.3 *Differential Diagnosis.* Desmoplastic small round cell tumor should be differentiated from other round cell tumors like rhabdomyosarcoma, Ewing sarcoma/ peripheral neuroectodermal tumor and neuroblastoma. The cytological differential

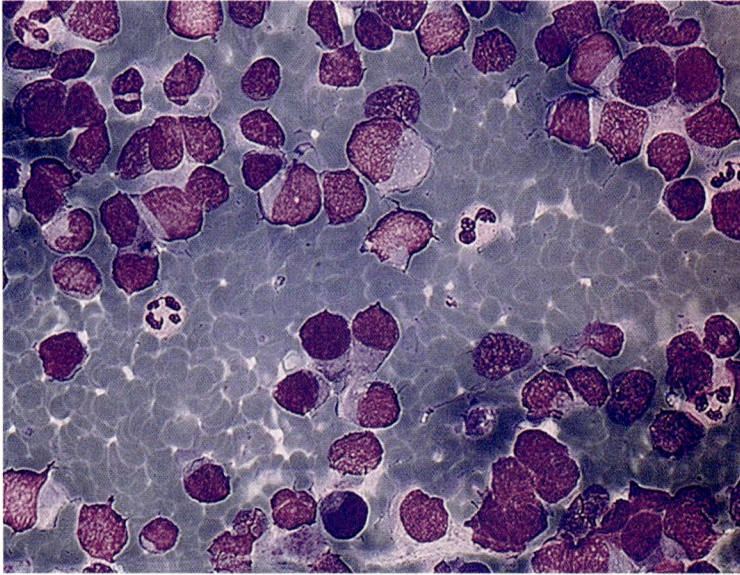

FIG 6.370 Desmoplastic small round cell tumor, paranuclear aggregates and cytoplasmic densities.

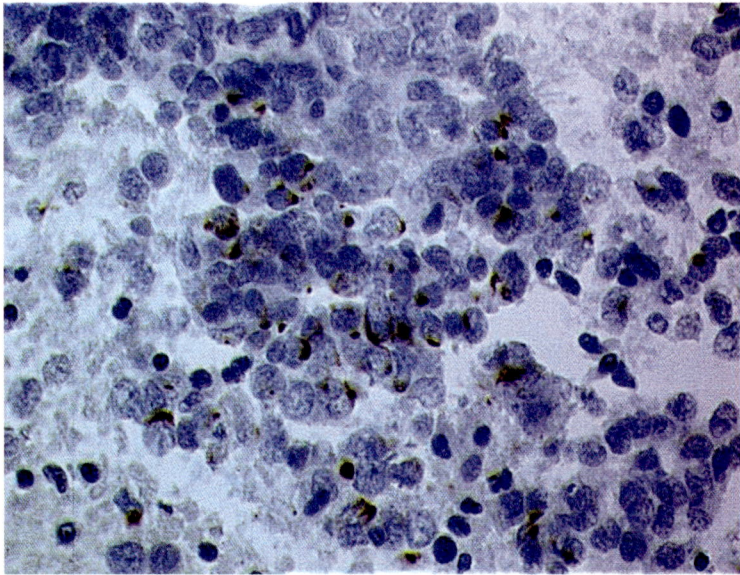

FIG 6.371 Desmoplastic small round cell tumor, desmin "dot-positivity".

diagnosis is shown in Table 6.16. The presence of rhabdomyoblasts, binucleated cells, and spindle-shaped cells are strongly in favor of rhabdomyosarcoma. Ewing sarcoma/ PNET characteristically consist of round, poorly differentiated cells with a double cell population: larger cells with clarified cytoplasm and small, dark cells. Frequently, cellular clusters and rosettes are present. Characteristic cytomorphology, CD99 expression, and specific chromosomal aberration allow differentiation from desmoplastic small round cell tumor. Neuroblastomas consist of characteristic neuro-blasts, and in better differentiated cases, fibrillary stroma and rosettes are present. Moreover, some neuroblastomas show a necrotic background and calcifications.

6.8.3.4 *Comments.* Desmoplastic small round cell tumors consist of round cells and connctive tissue fragments. The absence of the characteristic desmoplastic stroma in desmoplastic small round cell tumor aspirates and the nonspecific cytologic features of this small round cell tumor made cytologic interpretation difficult that required the use of ancillary diagnostic methods, such as immunohistochemistry, electron micro-scopy, and cytogenetic techniques. So far, 32 cases of desmoplastic small round cell tumor have been reported in the cytology literature [412–421]. All were diagnosed accurately as round cell sarcomas. Polymorphous sarcomatous and giant multi-nucleated cells also were reported [415]. In the few cases studied by electron micro-scopy, it was demonstrated that the cells were joined by small junctions and contained paranuclear aggregates of intermediate filaments [414]. A general consensus has been reached that the combination of poorly differentiated round cells on cytology documents, specific clinical context, young adult age, intraabdominal localization, suggestive immunocytochemical profile, and unique cytogenetic abnormality are highly specific and allow an accurate diagnosis.

6.8.3.5 *Clinical and FNA Key Features.* The following are in favor of the diagnosis:

- Age
- Intraabdominal site
- Poorly differentiated round cells with inconspitious cytoplasm
- Necrosis
- Paranuclear cytoplasmic densities

The following are difficulties of the diagnosis:

- Sarcomateous polymorphous cells
- Extensive necrosis.

The following is evidence against the diagnosis:

- Rhabdomyoblasts, fibrillary stroma, rosettes

6.8.4 Extraskeletal Mesenchymal Chondrosarcoma

Extraskeletal mesenchymal chondrosarcoma is a distinct entity of relatively recent identification. It is described as a cartilaginous tumor of bimorphic appearance comprising sheets of primitive mesenchymal cells and interspersed islands of well-differentiated cartilaginous tissue. Because of its undifferentiated cell composition, it is included in the category of small cell tumors. It is a rare malignant tumor that also could occur in bone and most commonly affects young adults and teenagers. In contrast with classical adult chondrosarcoma, the principal anatomic sites are the regions of head and neck, the orbit, the meninges, followed by the extremities, especially the thigh. When occurring in the bones, they are in different sites than conventional chondrosarcoma (i.e., the jaws, ribs, and spine) and have a minimal osseous participation with large tumoral extension into the surrounding soft tissues. Typical extraskeletal mesenchymal chondrosarcoma is not a difficult diagnosis if one excepts small biopsy specimens comprising only a small cell population indistinguishable from other small cell tumors. Extraskeletal mesenchymal chondrosarcoma is a malignant neoplasm that pursues a rapid clinical course and metastasizes in a high proportion of cases. So far, extraskeletal mesenchymal chondrosarcoma was included in the cartilaginous tumor, although the demonstration of t(11;22)(q24;q12) translocation has been documented raising the hypothesis of a close relationship to tumors of the Ewing sarcoma/PNET [422].

6.8.4.1   *Histopathology.*

Extraskeletal mesenchymal chondrosarcoma has a biphasic/bimorphic pattern comprising sheets of indifferentiated round or oval small cells grouped in well-defined islands or nodules (Fig 6.372) often separated by a vascular network of hemangiopericytoma-like pattern (Fig 6.373). The distribution and amount of cartilaginous matrix is variable. It may demonstrate calcifications and enchondral ossification (Fig 6.374). Usually, there is no evidence of a transition between both components, being rather a juxtaposition. The immunohistochemical profile shows strong positivity for S-100 protein in cartilagineous areas. The small cell component stains for Leu-7 and NSE, which is similar to other round cell sarcomas of the Ewing/PNET spectrum. Contradictory observations concern the expression of CD99, which does not allow distinction from tumors of the Ewing sarcoma/PNET spectrum.

6.8.4.2   *Cytopathology.*

Smears in extraskeletal mesenchymal chondrosarcoma are hypercellular and consist of two distinct cell populations: small, and oval-to-spindled cells with high nuclear-to-cytoplasmic ratios (Figs 6.375 and 6.376); the second population is an overtly malignant chondroid component scattered within an abundant myxoid/chondroid matrix (Fig 6.377) showing foamy cytoplasm, marked nuclear pleomorphism, and frequent multinucleation.

6.8.4.3   *Differential Diagnosis.*

Extraskeletal mesenchymal chondrosarcoma is characteristic. The differential diagnosis comprises all other round cell tumors (Table 6.18) as previously discussed [423,424] as well as the tumors depicting a pericytoma-like pattern such as poorly differentiated synovial sarcoma.

6.8.4.4   *Comments.*

Extraskeletal mesenchymal chondrosarcoma is diagnosed accurately if areas of cartilage are intermixed with a malignant small cell population. When chondroid is absent, extraskeletal mesenchymal chondrosarcoma is diagnosed as a round cell sarcoma not otherwise specified. Six cases of extraskeletal mesenchymal chondrosarcoma were studied cytologically [423–425]. Four tumors were primary and two were metastases. All cases were diagnosed accurately and consistently comprised a double component. We have observed seven such examples in three patients. Smears were hypercellular and always contained round-to-oval malignant cells. Chondroid was present in four cases.

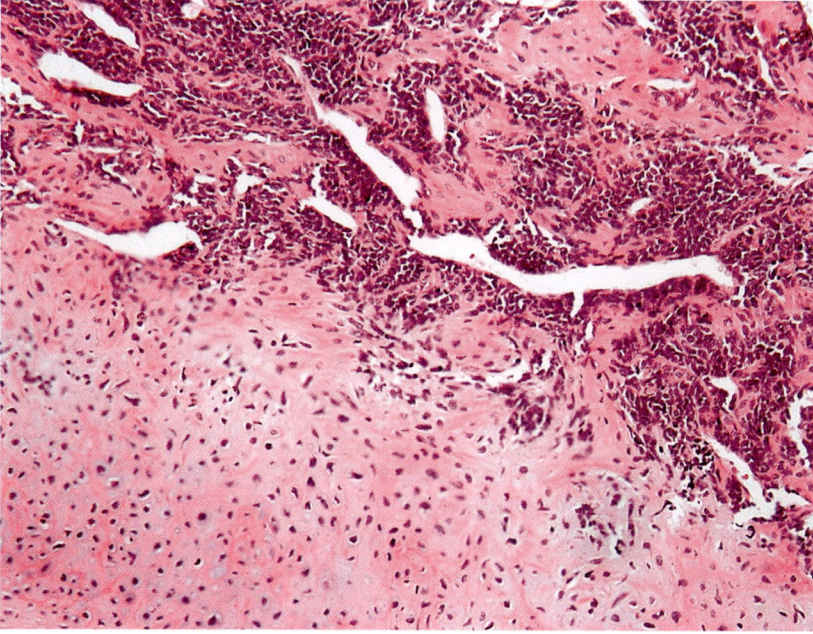

FIG 6.372 Extraskeletal mesenchymal chondrosarcoma, bimorphic pattern of islands of small cells in close contact with nodules of cartilage.

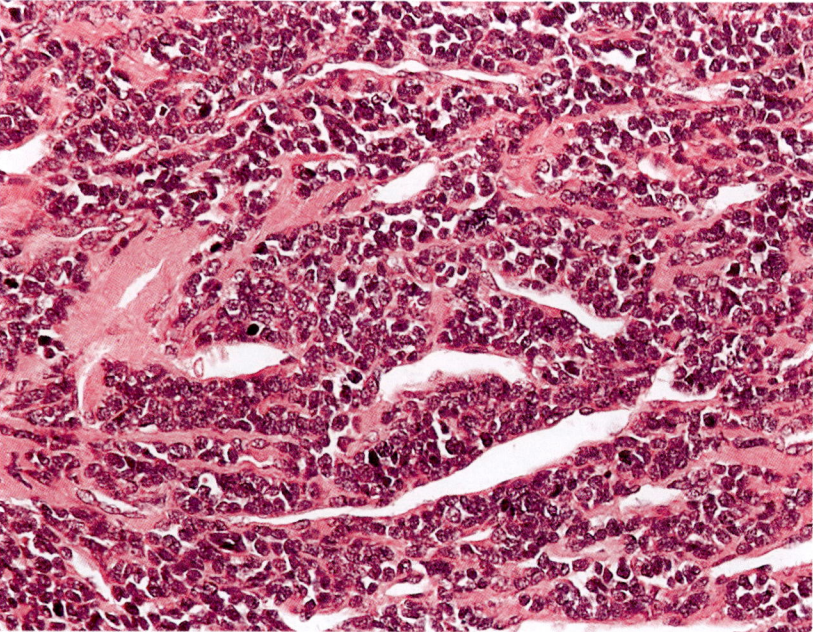

FIG 6.373 Extraskeletal mesenchymal chondrosarcoma, small cells often are grouped in islands separated by a vasculature of hemangiopericytoma-like pattern.

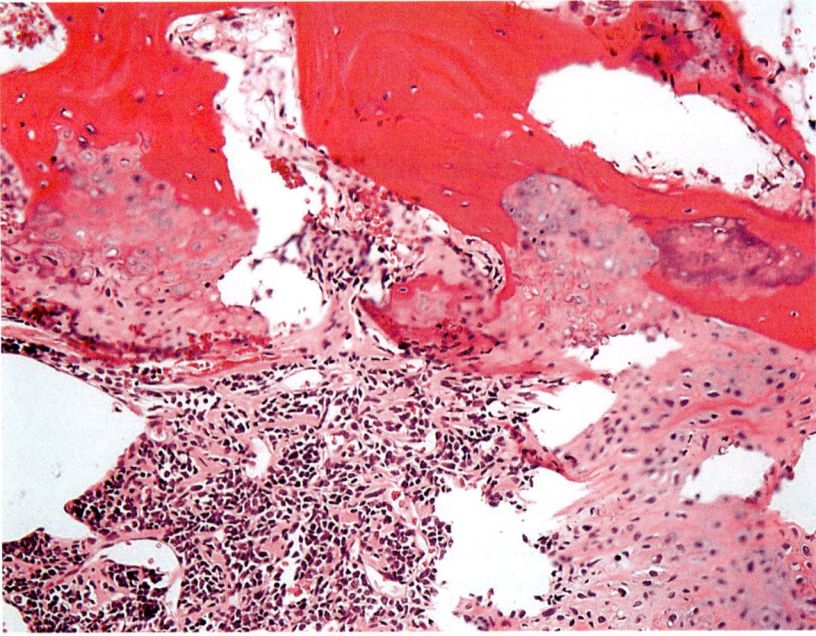

FIG 6.374 Extraskeletal mesenchymal chondrosarcoma, endochondral ossification.

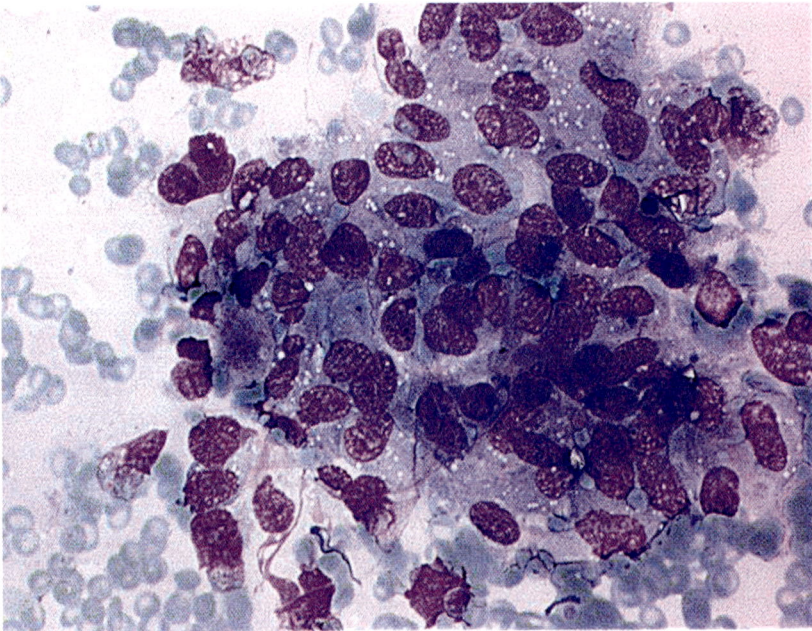

FIG 6.375 Extraskeletal mesenchymal chondrosarcoma, roundish cells.

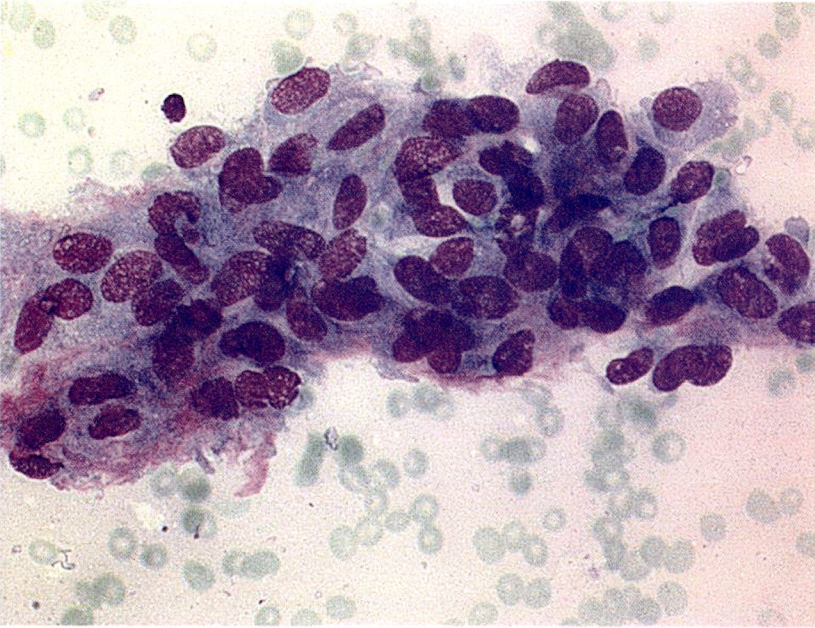

FIG 6.376 Extraskeletal mesenchymal chondrosarcoma, spindle-shaped cells.

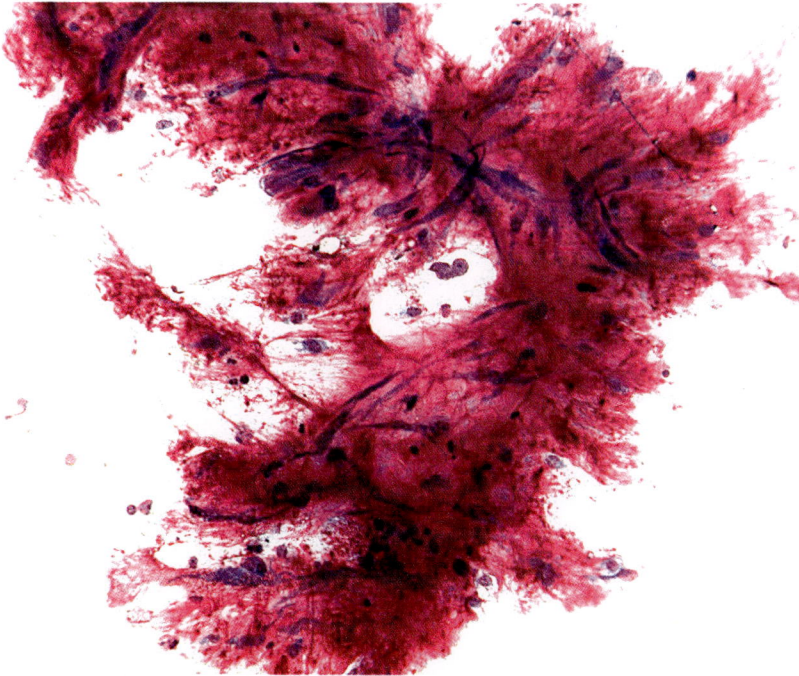

FIG 6.377 Extraskeletal mesenchymal chondrosarcoma, abundant chondroid matrix.

TABLE 6.18 Cytological differential diagnosis of extraskeletal mesenchymal chondrosarcoma

	Extraskeletal mesenchymal chondrosarcoma	Poorly differentiated synovial sarcoma	Ewing sarcoma/PNET
Round cells	++	++	++
Rosettes	−	−	++
Chondroid	+	−	−

++; Frequent, +; rare, +/− occasionally seen, −; absent.

6.8.4.5 *FNA Key Features*. The following is in favor of the diagnosis:

— Double component of small round cells and malignant chondroid

The following is a difficulty in the diagnosis:

— Lack of malignant chondroid component

The following is evidence against the diagnosis:

— Rosettes, physaliphorous cells

6.8.5 Poorly Differentiated Synovial Sarcoma

A general overview of synovial sarcoma has been discussed in a previous chapter. Of the four main histologic subtypes of synovial sarcoma, poorly differentiated synovial sarcoma is a high-grade small cell variant resembling a sarcoma of the Ewing sarcoma/PNET family. Its incidence is difficult to evaluate but probably will be increased since their molecular characterization. It originates in similar locations as other subtypes, is less frequent than the monophasic fibrous variety, and shows similar immunohisto-chemistry and cytogenetic features.

6.8.5.1 *Histopathology*. Poorly differentiated synovial sarcoma present under three different patterns: a large cell or epithelioid pattern comprising variable size rounded nuclei with prominent nucleoli, a small cell variant similar to the small round cell tumors (Figs 6.378–6.380), and a high-grade spindle cell pattern with high mitotic index and necrosis. The three variants depict a pericytomatous vascular pattern (Fig 6.381). A significant number of poorly differentiated synovial sarcoma have been diagnosed in the past as malignant hemangiopericytomas.

6.8.5.2 *Cytopathology*. Poorly differentiated synovial sarcoma share identical cytological features with the Ewing sarcoma/PNET group of tumors. Both entities consist of round and monomorphous cells (Fig 6.382). Inversely to poorly differentiated synovial sarcoma and tumors from the Ewing sarcoma/PNET family may show rosette formations and double round cell populations [378,398].

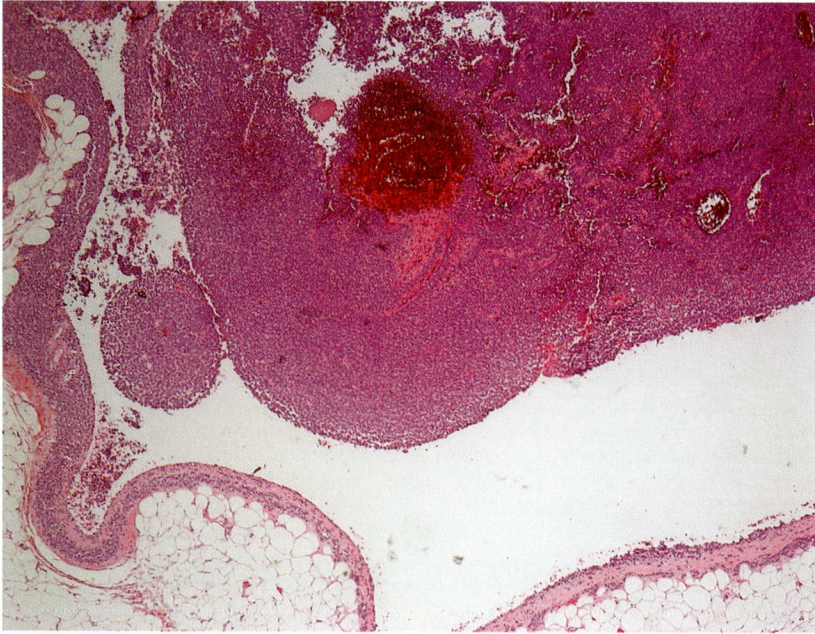

FIG 6.378   Poorly differentiated synovial sarcoma, protuding small round cell tumor into the joint space and proliferating along the synovial membrane.

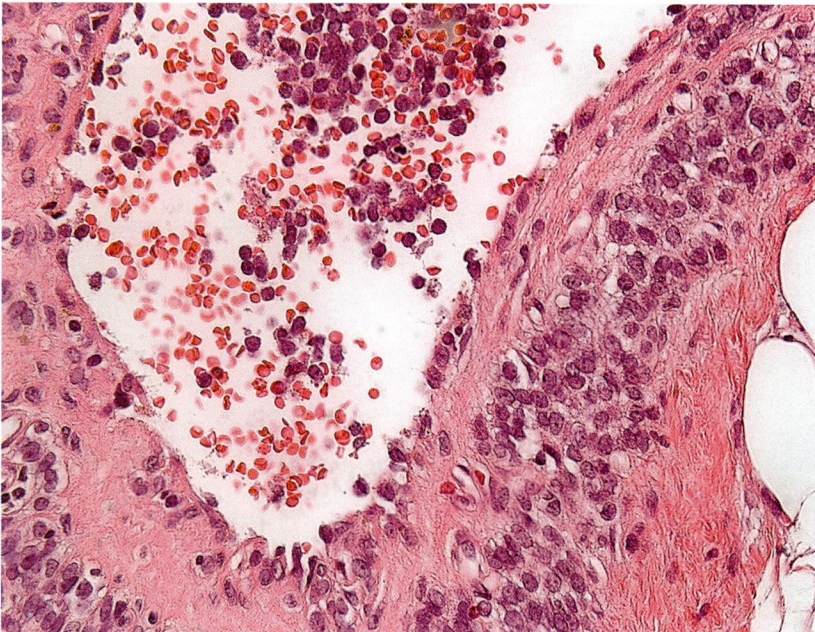

FIG 6.379   Poorly differentiated synovial sarcoma, higher magnification showing small round cells in the synovial membrane.

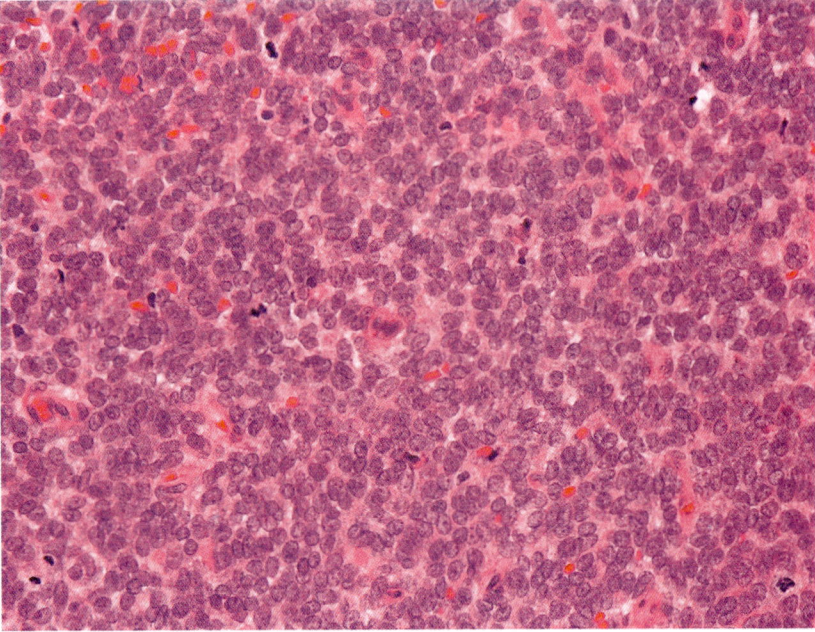

FIG 6.380   Poorly differentiated synovial sarcoma, solid area of monotonous small cells.

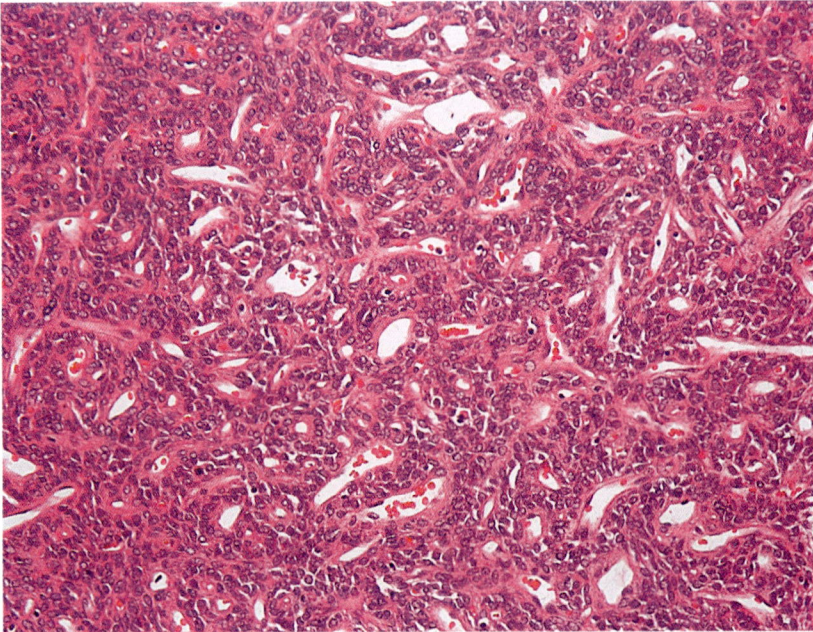

FIG 6.381   Poorly differentiated synovial sarcoma, pericytomatous vascular network.

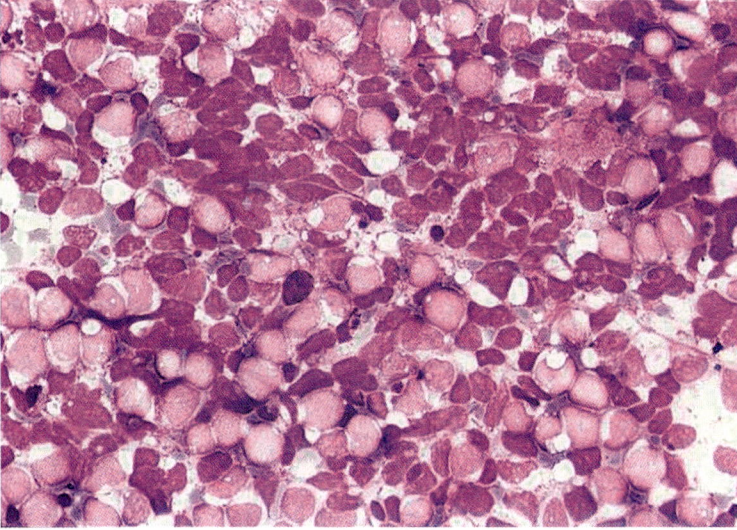

FIG 6.382 Smear from poorly differentiated synovial sarcoma, monomorphous roundish cells resembling Ewing sarcoma.

REFERENCES

1. Klijanienko J, Caillaud JM, Lagacé R. Fine-needle aspiration of primary and recurrent dermatofibrosarcoma protuberans. Diagn Cytopathol 2004, 30: 261–265.

2. Proppe KH, Scully RE, Rosai J. Postoperative spindle cell nodules of genitourinary tract resembling sarcomas. A report of eight cases. Am J Surg Pathol 1984, 2: 101–108.

3. Enzinger FM, Shiraki M. Musculo-aponeurotic fibromatosis of the shoulder girdle (extra-abdominal desmoid). Analysis of thirty cases followed up for ten or more years. Cancer 1967, 20: 1131–1140.

4. Pignatti G, Barbanti-Bròdano G, Ferrari D, et al. Extraabdominal desmoid tumor. A study of 83 cases. Clin Orthop Relat Res 2000, 375: 207–213.

5. Gronchi A, Casali PG, Mariani L, Lo Vullo S, et al. Quality of surgery and outcome in extra-abdominal aggressive fibromatosis: a series of patients surgically treated at a single institution. J Clin Oncol 2003, 2: 1390–1391.

6. Raab SS, Silverman JF, McLeod DL, Benning TL, Geisinger KR. Fine needle aspiration biopsy of fibromatoses. Acta Cytol 1993, 37: 323–328.

7. Kurtycz DF, Logrono R, Hoerl HD, Heatley DG. Diagnosis of fibromatosis colli by fine-needle aspiration. Diagn Cytopathol 2000, 23: 338–342.

8. Dalén BP, Meis-Kindblom JM, Sumathi VP, Ryd W, Kindblom LG. Fine-needle aspiration cytology and core needle biopsy in the preoperative diagnosis of desmoid tumors. Acta Orthop 2006, 77: 926–931.

9. Owens CL, Sharma L, Ali SZ. Deep fibromatosis (desmoid tumor): cytopathologic characteristics, clinicoradiologic features, and immunohistochemical findings on fine-needle aspiration. Cancer 2007, 111: 166–172.

10. Geethamani V, Ravindra S, Reddy VV. Fine needle aspiration cytology of juvenile hyaline fibromatosis: a case report. Acta Cytol 2007, 51: 624–626.

11. Dahl I, Åkerman M. Nodular fasciitis. A correlative cytologic and histologic study of 13 cases. Acta Cytol 1981, 25: 215–222.

12. Maly B, Maly A. Nodular fasciitis of the breast: report of a case initially diagnosed by fine needle aspiration cytology. Acta Cytol 2001, 45: 794–796.

13. Kong CS, Cha I. Nodular fasciitis: diagnosis by fine needle aspiration biopsy. Acta Cytol 2004, 48: 473–477.

14. Saad RS, Takei H, Lipscomb J, Ruzi B. Nodular fasciitis of parotid region: a pitfall in the diagnosis of pleomorphic adenomas on fine-needle aspiration cytology. Diagn Cytopathol 2005, 33: 191–194.

15. Plaza JA, Mayerson J, Wakely PE Jr. Nodular fasciitis of the hand: a potential diagnostic pitfall in fine-needle aspiration cytopathology. Am J Clin Pathol 2005, 123: 388–393.

16. Mentzel T, Beham A, Katenkamp D, Dei Tos AP, Fletcher CD. Fibrosarcomatous ("high-grade") dermatofibrosarcoma protuberans: clinicopathologic and immunohisto-chemical study of a series of 41 cases with emphasis on prognostic significance. Am J Surg Pathol 1998, 5: 576–587.

17. Layfield LJ. Cytopathology of bone and soft tissue tumors. Oxford, UK: Oxford University Press; 2002.

18. Domanski HA, Gustafson P. Cytologic features of primary, recurrent, and metastatic dermatofibrosarcoma protuberans. Cancer 2002, 25: 351–361.

19. Klijanienko J, Caillaud JM, Lagacé R, Vielh P. Comparative fine-needle aspiration and pathologic study in malignant fibrous histiocytoma. Cytodiagnostic features of 95 tumors in 71 patients. Diagn Cytopathol 2003, 29: 320–326.

20. Colin P, Lagacé R, Caillaud JM, Sastre-Garau X, Klijanienko J. Fine-needle aspiration in myxofibrosarcoma. Institut Curie experience. Diagn Cytopathol, 2010, 38: 343–346.

21. Klijanienko J, Caillaud J, Lagacé R, Vielh P. Cytohistologic correlations of 24 malignat peripheral nerve sheath tumors (MPNST) in 17 patients. The Institut Curie experience. Diagn Cytopathol 2002, 27: 103–108.

22. Kocjan G, Sams V, Davidson T. Dermatofibrosarcoma protuberans as a diagnostic pitfall in fine-needle aspiration diagnosis of angiosarcoma of the breast. Diagn Cytopathol 1996, 14: 94–95.

23. Aiba S, Tabuta N, Tagami H. Dermatofibrosarcoma protuberans is unique fibrohistio-cytic tumor expressing CD 34. Br J Dermatol 1992, 127: 79–84.

24. Henke AC, Salomao DR, Hughes JH. Cellular schwannoma mimics a sarcoma: an example of a potential pitfall in aspiration cytodiagnosis. Diagn Cytopathol 1999, 20: 312–316.

25. Mooney EE, Layfield LJ, Dodd LG. Fine-needle aspiration of neural lesions. Diagn Cytopathol 1999, 20: 1–5.

26. Dahl I, Åkerman M. Nodular fasciitis. A correlative cytologic and histologic study of 13 cases. Acta Cytol 1981, 25: 215–222.

27. Klijanienko J, Caillaud JM, Lagacé R. Fine-needle aspiration of primary and recurrent benign fibrous histiocytoma: classic, aneurysmal, and myxoid variants. Diagn Cytopathol 2004, 31: 387–391.

28. Filipowicz EA, Ventura KC, Pou AM, Logrono R. FNAC in the diagnosis of recurrent dermatofibrosarcoma protuberans of the forehead. A case report. Acta Cytol 1999, 43: 1177–1180.

29. Zee SY, Wang Q, Jones CM, Abadi MA. Fine needle aspiration cytology of dermatofi-brosarcoma protuberans presenting as a breast mass. A case report. Acta Cytol 2002, 46: 741–743.

30. Powers CN, Hurt MA, Frable WJ. Fine-needle aspiration biopsy: dermatofibrosarcoma protuberans. Diagn Cytopathol 1993, 9: 145–150.

31. Perry MD, Furlong JW, Johnston WW. Fine needle aspiration cytology of metastatic dermatofibrosarcoma protuberans. A case report. Acta Cytol 1986, 30: 507–512.

32. Powers CN, Berardo MD, Frable WJ. Fine-needle aspiration biopsy: pitfalls in the diagnosis of spindle-cell lesions. Diagn Cytopathol 1994, 10: 232–240.

33. Agiris A, Dardoufas C, Aroni K. Radiotherapy induced soft tissue sarcoma: an unusual case of a dermatofibrosarcoma protuberans. Clin Oncol (R Coll Radiol) 1995, 7: 59–61.

34. Fukushima H, Suda K, Matsuda M, Tanaka R, Kita H, Hanaoka T, Goya T. A case of dermatofibrosarcoma protuberans in the skin over the breast of a young woman. Breast Cancer 1998, 25: 407–409.

35. Trovik CS, Bauer HCF, Brosjo O, Skoog L, Soderlund V. Fine needle aspiration (FNA) cytology in the diagnosis of recurrent soft tissue sarcoma. Cytopathology 1998, 9: 320–328.

36. Maitra A, Ashfaq R, Hossein Saboorian M, Lindberg G, Gokaslan ST. The role of fine-needle aspiration biopsy in the primary diagnosis of mesenchymal lesions. A community hospital-based experience. Cancer 2000, 901: 178–185.

37. Palmer HE, Mukunyadzi P, Culbreth W, Thomas JR. Subgrouping and grading of soft-tissue sarcomas by fine-needle aspiration cytology: a histopathologic correlation study. Diagn Cytopathol 2001, 24: 307–316.

38. Bezabih M. Cytological diagnosis of soft tissue tumours. Cytopathology 2001, 12: 177–183.

39. Layfield LJ. Gopez EV. Fine-needle aspiration cytology of giant cell fibroblastoma: a case report and review of the literature. Diagn Cytopathol 2002, 26: 398–403.

40. Calonje E, Mentzel T, Fletcher CD. Cellular benign fibrous histiocytoma. Clinicopathologic analysis of 74 cases of a distinctive variant of cutaneous fibrous histiocytoma with frequent recurrence. Am J Surg Pathol 1994, 18: 668–676.

41. Kaddu S, McMenamin ME, Fletcher CD. Atypical fibrous histiocytoma of the skin: clinicopathologic analysis of 59 cases with evidence of infrequent metastasis. Am J Surg Pathol 2002, 26: 35–46.

42. Klijanienko J, Caillaud JM, Lagacé R. Fine-needle aspiration of primary and recurrent dermatofibrosarcoma protuberans. Diagn Cytopathol 2004, 30: 261–265.

43. Domanski HA, Gustafson P. Cytologic features of primary, recurrent, and metastatic dermatofibrosarcoma protuberans. Cancer 2002, 25: 351–361.

44. Dahl I, Åkerman M. Nodular fasciitis. A correlative cytologic and histologic study of 13 cases. Acta Cytol 1981, 25: 215–222.

45. Klijanienko J, Caillaud JM, Lagacé R, Vielh P. Cyto-histologic correlations in 56 synovial sarcomas in 36 patients. The Institut Curie experience. Diagn Cytopathol 2002, 27: 96–102.

46. Fiedman HD, Gonchoroff NJ, Jones CB, Tatum AH. Pleomorphic fibrohistiocytoma of the breast: a potential pitfall in breast biopsy interpretation. Virchows Arch 1994, 425: 199–203.

47. Bezabih M. Cytological diagnosis of soft tissue tumours. Cytopathology 2001, 12: 177–183.

48. Åkerman M. Supporting tissues. In: Orell SR, Sterrett GF, Walters MNI, Whitaker D, editors. Manual and atlas of fine needle aspiration cytology. 2nd edition. Edinburgh, Scotland: Churchill Livingstone; 1992, pp. 299–334.

49. Layfield LJ. Cytopathology of bone and soft tissue tumors. Oxford, UK: Oxford University Press; 2002.

50. Klemperer P, Robin CB. Primary neoplasms of the pleura: a report of 5 cases. Arch Pathol 1931, 11: 385–412.

51. Suster S, Nascimento AG, Miettinen M, Sickel JZ, Moran CA. Solitary fibrous tumors of soft tissue. A clinicopathologic and immnuhistochemical study of 12 cases. Am J Surg Pathol 1995, 19: 1257–1266.

52. Nascimento AG. Solitary fibrous tumor: an ubiquitous neoplasm of mesenchymal differentiation. Adv Anat Pathol 1996, 388–395.

53. Weiss SW, Goldblum JR. Hemangiopericytoma-solitary fibrous tumor. In: Strauss M editor. Enzinger and Weiss's soft tissue tumors. 5th edition. St. Louis, MO: Mosby; 2008, pp. 1120–1134.

54. Dal Cin P, Sciot R, Fletcher CD, Hilliker C, De Wever I, Van Damme B, Van den Berghe H. Trisomy 21 in solitary fibrous tumor. Cancer Genet Cytogenet 1996, 86: 58–60.

55. Nielsen GP, O'Connell JX, Dickersin GR, Rosenberg AE. Solitary fibrous tumor of soft tissue: a report of 15 cases including 5 malignant examples with light microscopic and ultrastructural data. Mod Pathol 1997, 10: 1028–1037.

56. Folpe AL, Devaney K, Weiss SW. Lipomatous hemangiopericytoma: a rare variant of hemangiopericytoma that may be confused with liposarcoma. Am J Surg Pathol 1999, 23: 1201–1207.

57. Carneiro SS, Scheithauer BW, Nascimento AG, Hirose T, Davis DH. Solitary fibrous tumor of the meninges a lesion distinct from meningioma: a clinicopathologic study. Am J Clin Pathol 1996, 106: 217–224.

58. Dei Tos AP, Seregard S, Calonje E, Chan JK, Fletcher CD. Giant cell angiofibroma. A distinctive orbital tumor in adults. Am J Surg Pathol 1995, 19: 1286–1293.

59. Guillou L, Gebhard S, Coindre JM. Orbital and extraorbital giant cell angiofibroma: a giant cell-rich variant of solitary fibrous tumor? Clinicopathologic and immunohisto-chemical analysis of a series in favour of a unifying concept. Am J Surg Pathol 2000, 24: 971–979.

60. Clayton AC, Salomao DR, Keeney GL, Nascimento AG. Solitary fibrous tumor: a study of cytologic features of six cases diagnosed by fine-needle aspiration. Diagn Cytopathol 2001, 25: 172–176.

61. Parwani AV, Galindo R, Steinberg DM, Zeiger MA, Westra WH, Ali SZ. Solitary fibrous tumor of the thyroid: cytopathologic findings and differential diagnosis. Diagn Cytopathol 2003, 28: 213–216.

62. Gerhard R, Fregnani ER, Falzoni R, Siqueira SA, Vargas PA. Cytologic features of solitary fibrous tumor of the parotid gland. A case report. Acta Cytol 2004, 48: 402–406.

63. Wiriosuparto S, Krassilnik N, Bhuta S, Rao J, Firschowitz S. Solitary fibrous tumor: report of a case with an unusual presentation as a spindle cell parotid neoplasm. Acta Cytol 2005, 49: 309–313.

64. Baliga M, Flowers R, Heard K, Siddiqi A, Akhtar I. Solitary fibrous tumor of the lung: a case report with a study of the aspiration biopsy, histopathology, immunohistochemistry, and autopsy findings. Diagn Cytopathol 2007, 35: 239–244.

65. Klijanienko J, Caillaud JM, Lagacé R, Vielh P. Cytohistologic correlations of 24 malignant peripheral nerve sheath tumor (MPNST) in 17 patients. The Institut Curie experience. Diagn Cytopathol 2002, 27: 103–108.

66. Zbieranowski I, Bedard YC. Fine needle aspiration of schwannomas. Value of electron microscopy and immunocytochemistry in the preoperative diagnosis. Acta Cytol 1989, 33: 381–384.

67. Akerman M, Domanski HA. Tumours of Peripheral Nerves. In: Orell SR editor. The cytology of soft tissue tumours. Monographs in clinical cytology. Volume 16, Basel, Switzerland: Karger; 2003, pp. 61–67.

68. Klijanienko J, Caillaud JM, Lagacé R. Cytohistologic correlations in schwannomas (neurilemmomas) including "ancient", cellular and epithelioid variants. Diagn Cytopathol 2006, 33: 517–522.

69. Ramzy I. Benign schwannoma: demonstration of Verocay bodies using fine needle aspiration. Acta Cytol 1977, 21: 316–319.

70. Dahl I, Hagmar B, Idwall I. Benign solitary neurilemoma (schwannoma). A correlative cytological and histological study of 28 cases. Acta Pathol Microbiol Immunol Scand 1984, 92: 91–101.

71. Resnick JM, Fanning CV, Caraway NP, Varma DG, Johnson M. Percutaneous needle biopsy diagnosis of benign neurogenic neoplasms. Diagn Cytopathol 1997, 16: 17–25.

72. Mooney EE, Layfield LJ, Dodd LG. Fine-needle aspiration of neural lesions. Diagn Cytopathol 1999, 20: 1–5.

73. Chong KW, Chung YF, Khoo ML, Lim DT, Hong GS, Soo KC. Management of intraparotid facial nerve schwannomas. Aust N Z J Surg 2000, 70: 732–734.

74. Hummel P, Cangiarella JF, Cohen JM, Yang G, Waisman J, Chhieng DC. Transthoracic fine-needle aspiration biopsy of pulmonary spindle cell and mesenchymal lesions: a study of 61 cases. Cancer 2001, 93: 187–198.

75. Gupta RK, Naran S, Lallu S, Fauck R. Fine-needle aspiration cytology in neurilemmoma (schwannoma) of the breast: report of two cases in a man and a woman. Diagn Cytopathol 2001, 24: 76–77.

76. Palmer HE, Mukunyadzi P, Culbreth W, Thomas JR. Subgruping and grading of soft-tissue sarcomas by fine-needle aspiration cytology: a histopathologic correlation study. Diagn Cytopathol 2001, 24: 307–316.

77. Henke AC, Salomao DR, Hughes JH. Cellular schwannoma mimics a sarcoma: an example of a potential pitfall in aspiration cytodiagnosis. Diagn Cytopathol 1999, 20: 312–316.

78. Laforga JB. Cellular schwannoma: report of a case diagnosed intraoperatively with the aid of cytologic imprints. Diagn Cytopathol 2003, 29: 95–100.

79. Ghossal N, Kapila K, Verma K. Fine needle aspiration cytology of epithelioid variant of schwannoma-a diagnostic dilemna. Indian J Pathol Microbiol 2003, 46: 73–76.

80. Weiss SW, Goldblum JR. Malignant tumors of the peripheral nerves. In: Strauss M editor. Enzinger and Weiss's soft tissue tumors. 5th edition, St. Louis, MO: Mosby, 2008, pp. 903–925.

81. Jiménez-Heffernan JA, López-Ferrer P, Vicandi B, Hardisson D, Gamallo C, Viguer JM. Cytologic features of malignant peripheral nerve sheath tumor. Acta Cytol 1999, 43: 175–183.

82. McGee RS, Ward WG, Kilpatrick SE. Malignant peripheral nerve sheath tumor: a fine-needle aspiration biopsy study. Diagn Cytopathol 1997, 17: 298–305.

83. Mooney EE, Layfield LJ, Dodd LG. Fine-needle aspiration of neural lesions. Diagn Cytopathol 1999, 20: 1–5.

84. Maitra A, Ashfaq R, Saboorian MH, Lindberg G, Gokaslan ST. The role of fine-needle aspiration biopsy in the primary diagnosis of mesenchymal lesions. A community hospital-based experience. Cancer 2000, 90: 178–185.

85. Molina CP, Putegnat BB, Logroño R. Fine-needle aspiration cytology and core biopsy of malignant peripheral nerve sheath tumor of the uterus: a case report. Diagn Cytopathol 2001, 24: 347–351.

86. Åkerman M, Willén H, Carlén B, Mandahl N, Mertens F. Fine-needle aspiration (FNA) of synovial sarcoma—a comparative histological-cytological study of 15 cases, including immunohistochemical, electron microscopic and cytogenetic examination and DNA-ploidy analysis. Cytopathology 1996, 7: 187–200.

87. Klijanienko J, Caillaud JM, Lagacé R, Vielh P. Cyto-histologic correlations in 56 synovial sarcomas in 36 patients. The Institut Curie experience. Diagn Cytopathol 2002, 27: 96–102.

88. Klijanienko J, Caillaud JM, Lagacé R, Vielh P. Fine-needle aspiration of leiomyosar-coma. A correlative cytohistopathological study of 96 tumors in 68 patients. Diagn Cytopathol 2003, 28: 119–125.

89. Vendraminelli R, Cavazzana AO, Poletti A, Galligioni A, Pennelli N. Fine needle aspiration cytology of malignant nerve sheath tumors. Diagn Cytopathol 1992, 8: 559–562.

90. Silverman JF, Weaver MD, Gardner N, Larkin EW, Park HK. Aspiration biopsy cytology of malignant schwannoma metastatic to the lung. Acta Cytol 1985, 29: 15–18.

91. Schwartz JG, Dowd DC. Fine needle aspiration cytology of metastatic malignant schwannoma. A case report. Acta Cytol 1989, 33: 377–380.

92. Dodd LG, Scully S, Layfield LJ. Fine-needle aspiration of epithelioid malignant peripheral sheath tumor (epithelioid malignant schwannoma). Diagn Cytopathol 1997, 17: 200–204.

93. Wojcik EM. Fine needle aspiration of metastatic malignant schwannoma to the thyroid gland. Diagn Cytopathol 1997, 16: 94–95.

94. Marco V, Sirvent J, Alvarez-Moro J, Clavel M, Muntal MT, Bauza A. Malignant melanotic schwannoma. Fine-needle aspiration biopsy findings. Diagn Cytopathol 1998, 18: 284–286.

95. Kilpatrick SE, Cappelari JO, Bos GD, Gold SH, Ward WG. Is fine-needle aspiration biopsy a practical alternative to open biopsy for the primary diagnosis of sarcoma? Experience with 140 patients. Am J Clin Pathol 2001, 115: 59–68.

96. Walker D, Gill TJ 3rd, Corson JM. Leiomyosarcoma in a renal allograft recipient treated with immunosuppressive drugs. JAMA 1971, 215: 2084–208.

97. Kingma DW, Shad A, Tsokos M, et al. Epstein-Barr virus (EBV)-associated smooth-muscle tumor arising in a post-transplant patient treated successfully for two PT-EBV-associated large-cell lymphomas. Case report. Am J Surg Pathol 1996, 12: 1511–1519.

98. Pérot G, Derré J, Coindre JM, et al. Strong smooth muscle differentiation is dependent on myocardin gene amplification in most human retroperitoneal leiomyosarcomas. Cancer Res 2009, 69: 2269–2278.

99. Klijanienko J, Caillaud JM, Lagacé R, Vielh P. Fine-needle aspiration of leiomyosar-coma. A correlative cytohistopathological study of 96 tumors in 68 patients. Diagn Cytopathol 2003, 28: 119–125.

100. Rubin BP, Fletcher CD. Myxoid leiomyosarcoma of soft tissue, an underrecognized variant. Am J Surg Pathol 2000, 24: 927–936.

101. Dahl I, Hagmar B, Angervall L. Leiomyosarcoma of the soft tissue. A correlative cytological and histological study of 11 cases. Acta Pathol Microbiol Immunol Scand A 1981, 89: 285–291.

102. Willén H, Åkerman H, Carlén B. Fine needle aspiration (FNA) in the diagnosis of soft tissue tumours; a review of 22 years experience. Cytopathology 1995, 6: 236–247.

103. Tao LC, Davidson DD. Aspiration biopsy cytology of smooth muscle tumors and cytologic approach to the differentiation between leiomyosarcoma and leiomyoma. Acta Cytol 1993, 37: 300–308.

104. Klijanienko J, Caillaud JM, Lagacé R, Vielh P. Cytohistologic correlations of 24 malignat peripheral nerve sheath tumors (MPNST) in 17 patients. The Institut Curie experience. Diagn Cytopathol 2002, 27: 103–108.

105. Klijanienko J, Caillaud JM, Lagacé R, Vielh P. Cytohistologic correlations in 56 synovial sarcomas in 36 patients. The Institut Curie experience. Diagn Cytopathol 2002, 27: 96–102.

106. Gonzalez-Campora R, Munoz-Arias G, Otal-Salaverri C, et al. Fine needle aspiration cytology of primary soft-tissue tumors. Morphologic analysis of the most frequent types. Acta Cytol 1992, 36: 905–917.

107. Palmer HE, Mukunyadzi P, Culbreth W, Thomas JR. Subgruping and grading of soft-tissue sarcomas by fine-needle aspiration cytology: a histopathologic correlation study. Diagn Cytopathol 2001, 24: 307–316.

108. Goel A, Gupta SK, Dey P, Radhika S, Nijhawan R. Cytologic spectrum of 227 fine-needle aspiration cases of chest-wall lesions. Diagn Cytopathol 2001, 24: 384–388.

109. Kilpatrick SE, Ward WG, Bos GD. The value of fine-needle aspiration biopsy in the differential diagnosis of adult myxoid sarcoma. Cancer 2000, 25: 167–177.

110. Kilpatrick SE, Cappelari JO, Bos GD, Gold SH, Ward WG. Is fine-needle aspiration biopsy a practical alternative to open biopsy for the primary diagnosis of sarcoma? Experience with 140 patients. Am J Clin Pathol 2001, 115: 59–68.

111. Inagaki H, Murase T, Otsuka T, Eimoto T. Detection of SYT-SSX fusion transcript in synovial sarcoma using archival cytologic specimens. Am J Clin Pathol 1999, 111: 528–533.

112. Jørgensen LJ, Lyon H, Myhre-Jensen O, Nordentoft A, Sneppen O. Synovial sarcoma. An immunohistochemical study of the epithelial component. APMIS 1994, 102: 191–196.

113. Weiss SW, Goldblum JR. Malignant tumors of uncertain type. In: Strauss M editor. Enzinger and Weiss's soft tissue tumors. 5th edition. St. Louis, MO: Mosby; 2008, p. 1176.

114. Terry J, Saito T, Subramanian S, et al. TLE1 as a diagnostic immunohistochemical marker for synovial sarcoma emerging from gene expression profiling studies. Am J Surg Pathol 2007, 31: 240–246.

115. Kilpatrick SE, Teot LA, Stanley MW, Ward WG, Savage PD, Geisinger KR. Fine-needle aspiration biopsy of synovial sarcoma. A cytomorphologic analysis of primary, recurrent, and metastatic tumors. Am J Clin Pathol 1996, 106: 769–775.

116. Jiménez-Heffernan JA, López-Ferrer P, Vicandi B, Hardisson D, Gamallo C, Viguer JM. Cytologic features of malignant peripheral nerve sheath tumor. Acta Cytol 1999, 43: 175–183.

117. Johnson TL, Lee MW, Meis JW, Zarbo RJ, Crissman JD. Immunohistochemical characterization of malignant peripheral nerve sheath tumors. Am J Surg Pathol 1991, 4: 121–135.

118. Weiss SW, Goldblum JR. Malignant soft tissue tumors of uncertain type. In: Strauss M editor. Enzinger and Weiss's soft tissue tumors. 5th edition. St. Louis, MO: Mosby; 2008, pp. 1161–1221.

119. Hummel P, Yang GCH, Kumar A, et al. PNET-like features of synovial sarcoma of the lung: a pitfall in the cytologic diagnosis of soft-tissue tumors. Diagn Cytopathol 2001, 24: 283–288.

120. Silverman JF, Landreneau RJ, Sturgis CD, et al. Small-cell variant of synovial sarcoma: fine-needle aspiration with ancillary features and potential diagnostic pitfalls. Diagn Cytopathol 2000, 23: 118–123.

121. Klijanienko J, Couturier J, Bourdeaut F, et al. Fine-needle aspiration as a diagnostic technique in 50 cases of primary Ewing sarcoma/peripheral neuroectodermal tumor (ES/PNET). Institut Curie's experience. Diagn Cytopathol, in press.

122. Srinivasan R, Gautam U, Gupta R, Rajwanshi A, Vasistha RK. Synovial sarcoma: diagnosis on fine-needle aspiration by morphology and molecular analysis. Cancer 2009, 117: 128–136.

123. Liu K, Layfield LJ, Coogan AC, Ballo MS, Bentz JS, Dodge RK. Diagnostic accuracy in fine-needle aspiration of soft tissue and bone lesions. Influence of clinical history and experience. Am J Clin Pathol 1999, 111: 632–640.

124. Molenaar WM, DeJong B, Buist J, et al. Chromosomal analysis and the classification of soft tissue sarcomas. Lab Invest 1989, 60: 266–274.

125. Saboorian MH, Ashfaq R, Vandersteenhoven JJ, Schneider NR. Cytogenetics as an adjunct in establishing a definitive diagnosis of synovial sarcoma by fine-needle aspiration. Cancer 1997, 81: 187–192.

126. Ryan MR, Stastny JF, Wakely PE. The cytopathology of synovial sarcoma. A study of six cases, with emphasis on architecture and histopathologic correlation. Cancer 1998, 84: 42–49.

127. Nilsson G, Wang M, Wejde J, et al. Reverse transcriptase polymerase chain reaction on fine needle aspirates for rapid detection of translocations in synovial sarcoma. Acta Cytol 1998, 42: 1317–1324.

128. Gonzáles-Cámpora R, Muñoz-Arias G, Otal-Salaverri C, et al. Fine needle aspiration cytology of primary soft tissue tumors. Morphologic analysis of the most frequent types. Acta Cytol 1992, 36: 905–917.

129. Åkerman M, Willén H, Carlén B, Mandahl N, Mertens F. Fine-needle aspiration (FNA) of synovial sarcoma – a comparative histological-cytological study of 15 cases, including immunohistochemical, electron microscopic and cytogenetic examination and DNA-ploidy analysis. Cytopathology 1996, 7: 187–200.

130. Viguer JM, Jiménez-Heffernan JA, Vicandi B, López-Ferrer P, Gamallo C. Cytologic features of synovial sarcoma with emphasis on the monophasic fibrous variant. A morphologic and immunocytochemical analysis of bcl-2 protein expression. Cancer 1998, 84: 50–56.

131. Kilpatrick SE, Ward WG, Cappellari JO, Bos GD. Fine-needle aspiration biopsy of soft tissue sarcomas. A cytomorphologic analysis with emphasis on histologic subtyping, grading, and therapeutic significance. Am J Clin Pathol 1999, 112: 179–188.

132. Maitra A, Ashfaq R, Saboorian MH, Lindberg G, Gokaslan ST. The role of fine-needle aspiration biopsy in the primary diagnosis of mesenchymal lesions. A community hospital-based experience. Cancer 2000, 90: 178–185.

133. Wakely PE, Kneisl JS. Soft tissue aspiration cytology. Diagnostic accuracy and limitations. Cancer 2000, 90: 292–298.

134. Palmer HE, Mukunyadzi P, Culbreth W, Thomas JR. Subgruping and grading of soft-tissue sarcomas by fine-needle aspiration cytology: a histopathologic correlation study. Diagn Cytopathol 2001, 24: 307–316.

135. Evans HL, Khurana KK, Kemp BL, Ayala AG. Heterologous elements in the dedifferentiated component of dedifferentiated liposarcoma. Am J Surg Pathol 1994, 18: 1150–1157.

136. Panagopoulos I, Storlazzi CT, Fletcher CD, et al. The chimeric FUS/CREB3l2 gene is specific for low-grade fibromyxoid sarcoma. Genes Chromosomes Cancer 2004, 40: 218–228.

137. Matsuyama A, Hisaoka M, Shimajiri S, et al. Molecular detection of FUS-CREB3L2 fusion transcripts in low-grade fibromyxoid sarcoma using formalin-fixed, paraffin-embedded tissue specimens. Am J Surg Pathol 2006, 30: 1077–1084.

138. Périgny M, Dion N, Couture C, Lagacé R. Low grade fibromyxoid sarcoma: a clinico-pathologic analysis of 7 cases. Ann Pathol 2006, 26: 419–425.

139. Guillou L, Benhattar J, Gengler C, et al. Translocation-positive low-grade fibromyxoid sarcoma: clinicopathologic and molecular analysis of a series expanding the morphologic spectrum and suggesting potential relationship to sclerosing epithelioid fibrosarcoma: a study from the French Sarcoma Group. Am J Surg Pathol 2007, 31: 1387–1402.

140. Meis-Kindblom JM, Kindblom LG, Enzinger FM. Sclerosing epithelioid fibrosarcoma. A variant of fibrosarcoma simulating carcinoma. Am J Surg Pathol 1995, 19: 979–993.

141. Tsuchido K, Yamada M, Satou T, Otsuki Y, Shimizu S, Kobayashi H. Cytology of sclerosing epithelioid fibrosarcoma in pleural effusion. Diagn Cytopathol 2010, 38: 748–753.

142. Kim K, Naylor B, Han IH. Fine needle aspiration cytology of sarcomas metastasizing to the lung. Acta Cytol 1986, 30: 688–694.

143. Logrono R, Filipowicz EA, Eyzaguirre EJ, Sawh RN. Diagnosis of primary fibrosarcoma of the lung by fine needle aspiration and core biopsy. Arch Pathol Lab Med 1999, 123: 731–735.

144. Lindberg GM, Maitra A, Gokasian ST, Saboorian MH, Albores-Saaverda J. Low grade fibromyxoid sarcoma: finee-needle aspiration cytology with histologic, cytogenic, immunohistochemical, and ultrastructural correlation. Cancer 1999, 25: 75–82.

145. Dawamneh MF, Amra NK, Amr SS. Low grade fibromyxoid sarcoma: report of a case with fine needle aspiration cytology and histologic correlation. Acta Cytol 2006, 50: 208–212.

146. Domanski H, Mertens F, Panagopoulos I, Akerman M. Low-grade fibromyxoid sarcoma is difficult to diagnose by fine needle aspiration cytology: a cytomorphological study of eight cases. Cytopathology 2009, 20: 304–314.

147. Derré J, Lagacé R, Nicolas A, et al. Leiomyosarcomas and most malignant fibrous histiocytomas share very similar comparative genomic hybridization imbalances: an analysis of a series of 27 leiomyosarcomas. Lab Invest 2001, 81: 211–215.

148. Sabah M, Cummins R, Leader M, Kay E. Leiomyosarcoma and malignant fibrous histiocytoma share similar allelic imbalance pattern at 9p. Virchows Arch 2005, 446: 251–8.

149. Idbaih A, Coindre JM, Derré J, et al. Myxoid malignant fibrous histiocytoma and pleomorphic liposarcoma share very similar genomic imbalances. Lab Invest 2005, 85: 176–181.

150. Coindre JM, Mariani O, Chibon F, et al. Most malignant fibrous histiocytomas developed in the retroperitoneum are dedifferentiated liposarcomas: a review of 25 cases initially diagnosed as malignant fibrous histiocytoma. Mod Pathol 2003, 16: 256–262.

151. Coindre JM, Hostein I, Maire G, et al. Inflammatory malignant fibrous histiocytomas and dedifferentiated liposarcomas: histological review, genomic profile, and MDM2 and CDK4 status favour a single entity. J Pathol 2004, 203: 822–830.

152. Klijanienko J, Caillaud JM, Lagacé R, Vielh P. Comparative fine-needle aspiration and pathologic study in malignant fibrous histiocytoma. Cytodiagnostic features of 95 tumors in 71 patients. Diagn Cytopathol 2003, 29: 320–326.

153. Akerman M, Domanski H. The cytology of soft tissue tumours. In: Orell SR, editor. Monographs in clinical cytology. Volume 16. Basel, Switzerland: Karger; 2003.

154. Hallor KH, Mertens F, Jin Y, et al. Fusion of the EWSR1 and ATF1 genes without expression of the MITF-M transcript in angiomatoid fibrous histiocytoma. Genes Chromosomes Cancer 2005, 44: 97–102.

155. Antonescu CR, Dal Cin P, Nafa K, Teot LA, Surti U, Fletcher CD, Ladanyi M. EWSR1–CREB1 is the predominant gene fusion in angiomatoid fibrous histiocytoma. Genes Chromosomes Cancer 2007, 46: 1051–1060.

156. Fleshman R, Mayerson J, Wakely PE Jr. Fine-needle aspiration biopsy of high-grade sarcoma: a report of 107 cases. Cancer 2007, 111: 491–498.

157. Klijanienko J, Caillaud JM, Lagacé R, Vielh P.Cytology in angiosarcoma including classic and epithelioid variants. Institut Curie's experience. Diagn Cytopathol 2003, 29: 140–145.

158. Hales M, Bottles K, Miller T, Donegan E, Ljung BM. Diagnosis of Kaposi's sarcoma by fine-needle aspiration biopsy. Am J Clin Pathol 1987, 88: 20–25.

159. Martin-Bates E, Tanner A, Suvarna SK, Glazer G, Coleman DV. Use of fine needle aspiration cytology for investigating lymphadenopathy in HIV positive patients. J Clin Pathol 1993, 46: 564–566.

160. al-Rikabi AC, Haidar Z, Arif M, al-Ajlan AZ, Ramia S. Fine-needle aspiration cytology of primary Kaposi's sarcoma of lymph nodes in an immunocompetent man. Diagn Cytopathol 1998, 19: 451–454.

161. Gamborino E, Carrilho C, Ferro J, et al. Fine-needle aspiration diagnosis of Kaposi's sarcoma in a developing country. Diagn Cytopathol 2000, 23: 322–325.

162. Poniecka A, Ghorab Z, Arnold D, Khaled A, Ganjei-Azar P. Kaposi's sarcoma of the thyroid gland in an HIV-negative woman: a case report. Acta Cytol 2007, 51: 421–423.

163. Morelli L, Pusiol T, Piscioli I, Del Nonno F, Brenna A, Licci S. Fine needle aspiration cytology determinants of the diagnosis of primary nodal Kaposi's sarcoma as the first sign of unknown HIV infection: a case report. Acta Cytol 2007, 51: 602–604.

164. Kilpatrick SE, Ward WG, Bos GD. The value of fine-needle aspiration biopsy in the differential diagnosis of adult myxoid sarcoma. Cancer 2000, 25: 167–177.

165. Layfield LJ, Liu K, Dodge RK. Logistic regression analysis of myxoid sarcomas: a cytologic study. Diagn Cytopathol 1998, 19: 355–360.

166. Klijanienko J, Caillaud JM, Lagacé, Vielh P. Comparative fine-needle aspiration and pathologic study in malignant fibrous histiocytoma: cytodiagnosis features of 95 tumors in 71 patients. Diagn Cytopathol 2003, 29: 320–326.

167. Klijanienko J, Caillaud JM, Lagacé R. Fine-needle aspiration in liposarcoma: cytohistologic correlative study including well-differentiated, myxoid and pleomorphic variants. Diagn Cytopathol 2004, 30: 307–312.

168. Klijanienko J, Caillaud JM, Lagacé R, Vielh P. Fine-needle aspiration of leiomyosarcoma. A correlative cytohistopathological study of 96 tumors in 68 patients. Diagn Cytopathol 2003, 28: 119–125.

169. Fletcher CD, Akerman M, Dal Cin P, et al. Correlation between clinicopathological features and karyotype in lipomatous tumors: a report of 178 cases from the Chromosomes and Morphology (CHAMP) Collaborative Study Group. Am J Pathol 1996, 148: 623–630.

170. Kilpatrick SE, Doyon J, Choong PF, Sim FH, Nascimento AG. The clinicopathologic spectrum of myxoid and round cell liposarcoma. A study of 95 cases. Cancer 1996, 77: 1450–1458.

171. Weiss SW, Goldblum JR. Liposarcoma. In: Strauss M editor. Enzinger and Weiss's soft tissue tumors. 5th edition. St. Louis, MO: Mosby; 2008, pp. 477–517.

172. Gonzalez-Campora R, Munoz-Arias G, Otal-Salaverri C, et al. Fine needle aspiration cytology of primary soft tissue tumors. Morphologic analysis of the most frequent types. Acta Cytol 1992, 36: 905–917.

173. Bennert KW, Abdul-Karim FW. Fine needle aspiration cytology vs. needle core biopsy of soft tissue tumors. A comparison. Acta Cytol 1994, 38: 381–384.

174. Kilpatrick SE, Doyon J, Choong PFM, Sim FH, Nascimento AG. The clinicopathologic spectrum of myxoid and round cell liposarcoma: a study of 95 cases. Cancer 1999, 77: 1450–1458.

175. Liu K, Layfield LJ, Coogan AC, Ballo MS, Bentz JS, Dodge RK. Diagnostic accuracy in fine-needle aspiration of soft tissue and bone lesions. Influence of clinical history and experience. Am J Clin Pathol 1999, 111: 632–640.

176. Maitra A, Ashfaq R, Hossein Saboorian M, Lindberg G, Tunc Gokasian S. The role of fine-needle aspiration biopsy in the primary diagnosis of mesenchymal lesions. A community hospital-based experience. Cancer 2000, 90: 178–185.

177. Wakely PE, Kneisl JS. Soft tissue aspiration cytopathology. Diagnostic accuracy and limitations. Cancer 2000, 90: 292–298.

178. Kilpatrick SE, Cappellari JO, Bos GD, Gold SH, Ward WG. In fine-needle aspiration biopsy a practical alternative to open biopsy for the primary diagnosis of sarcoma? Experience with 140 patients. Am J Clin Pathol 2001, 115: 59–68.

179. Palmer HE, Mukunyadzi P, Cilbreth W, Thomas JR. Subgrouping and grading of soft-tissue sarcomas by fine-needle aspiration cytology: a histopathologic correlation study. Diagn Cytopathol 2001, 24: 307–316.

180. Willén H, Åkerman H, Carlén B. Fine needle aspiration (FNA) in the diagnosis of soft tissue tumours; a review of 22 years experience. Cytopathology 1995, 6: 236–247.

181. Vicandi B, Jimenez-Heffernan J, Lopez-Ferrer P, Gonzalez-Peramato P, Viguier JM. Cytologic features of round cell liposarcoma. A report of 5 cases. Cancer 2003, 99: 28–32.

182. Nagira K, Yamamoto T, Akisue T, et al. Reliability of fine-needle aspiration biopsy in the initial diagnosis of soft-tissue lesions. Diagn Cytopathol 2002, 27: 354–361.

183. Layfield LJ. Cytopathology of bone and soft tissue tumors. Oxford, UK: Oxford University Press; 2002.

184. Angervall L, Kindblom LG, Merck C. Myxofibrosarcoma. A study of 30 cases. Acta Pathol Microbiol Scand A 1977, 85A: 127–140.

185. Weiss SW, Enzinger FM. Myxoid variant of malignant fibrous histiocytoma. Cancer 1977, 39: 1672–1685.

186. Mentzel T, Calonje E, Wadden C, et al. Myxofibrosarcoma. Clinicopathologic analysis of 75 cases with emphasis on the low-grade variant. Am J Surg Pathol 1996, 20: 391–405.

187. Huang HY, Lal P, Qin J, Brennan MF, Antonescu CR. Low-grade myxofibrosarcoma: a clinicopathologic analysis of 49 cases treated at a single institution with simultaneous assessment of the efficacy of 3–tier and 4–tier grading systems. Hum Pathol 2004, 35: 612–621.

188. Kilpatrick S, Ward W, Bos G. The value of fine-needle aspiration biopsy in the differential diagnosis of adult myxoid sarcoma. Cancer Cytopathology 2000, 90: 167–177.

189. Colin P, Lagacé R, Caillaud JM, Sastre-Garau X, Klijanienko J. Fine-needle aspiration in myxofibrosarcoma. Experience of Institut Curie. Diagn Cytopathol, 2010, 38: 343–346.

190. Lagacé R, Delage C, Seemayer TA. Myxoid variant of malignant fibrous histiocytoma: ultrastructural observations. Cancer 1979, 43: 526–534.

191. Hisaoka M, Moromitsu Y, Hashimoto H, et al. Retroperitoneal liposarcoma with combined well-differentiated and myxoid malignant fibrous histiocytoma-like myxoid areas. Am J Surg Pathol 1999, 12: 1480–1492.

192. Sirvant N, Maire G, Pedentour F. Genetics of dermatofibrosarcoma protuberans family of tumors: from ring chromosomes to tyrosine kinase inhibitor treatment. Genes Chromosomes Cancer 2003, 37: 1–19.

193. Kilpatrick S, Ward W. Myxofibrosarcoma of soft tissues: cytomorphologic analysis of a series. Diagn Cytopathol 1999, 20: 6–9.

194. Merck C, Hagmar B. Myxofibrosarcoma. A correlative cytologic and histologic study of 13 cases examined by fine-needle aspiration cytology. Acta Cytol 1980, 24: 137–44.

195. Trovik CS, Bauer HCF, Brosjo O, Skoog L, Soderlund V. Fine needle aspiration (FNA) cytology in the diagnosis of recurrent soft tissue sarcoma. Cytopathology 1998, 9: 320–328.

196. Rubin BP, Fletcher CD. Myxoid leiomyosarcoma of soft tissue, an underrecognized variant. Am J Surg Pathol 2000, 24: 927–936.

197. van Roggen JF, McMenamin ME, Fletcher CD. Cellular myxoma of soft tissue: a clinicopathological study of 38 cases confirming indolent clinical behaviour. Histopathology 2001, 39: 287–297.

198. Akerman M, Rydholm A. Aspiration cytology of intramuscular myxoma. A comparative clinical, cytologic and histologic study of ten cases. Acta Cytol 1983, 27: 505–510.

199. Caraway NP, Staerkel GA, Fanning CV, Varma DG, Pollock RE. Diagnosing intramuscular myxoma by fine-needle aspiration: a multidisciplinary approach. Diagn Cytopathol 1994, 11: 255–261.

200. Layfield LJ, Dodd LG. Fine-needle aspiration cytology findings in a case of aggressive angiomyxoma: a case report and review of the literature. Diagn Cytopathol 1997, 16: 425–429.

201. Wakely PE Jr, Bos GD, Mayerson J. The cytopathology of soft tissue myxomas: ganglia, juxta-articular myxoid lesions, and intramuscular myxoma. Am J Clin Pathol 2005, 123: 858–865.

202. Moriki T, Takahashi T, Wada M, Ueda S, Ichien M, Miyazaki E. Chondroid chordoma: fine-needle aspiration cytology with histopathological, immunohistochemical, and ultrastructural study of two cases. Diagn Cytopathol 1999, 21: 335–339.

203. Layfield LJ, Liu K, Dodd LG, Olatidoye BA. Dedifferentiated chordoma: a case report of the cytomorphologic findings on fine-needle aspiration. Diagn Cytopathol 1998, 19: 378–381.

204. Crapanzano JP, Ali SZ, Ginsberg MS, Zakowski MF. Chordoma: a cytologic study with histologic and radiologic correlation. Cancer 2001, 93: 40–51.

205. Chivukula M, Rao R, Macchi J, Ghazala F, Rao RN, Komorowski R, Shidham VB. FNAB cytology of chordoma masquerading as adenocarcinoma: case report. Diagn Cytopathol 2002, 26: 306–309.

206. Kay PA, Nascimento AG, Unni KK, Salomao DR. Chordoma. Cytomorphologic findings in 14 cases diagnosed by fine needle aspiration. Acta Cytol 2003, 47: 202–208.

207. Köybasioglu F, Simsek GG, Onal BU, Han U, Adabag A. Oropharyngeal chordoma diagnosed by fine needle aspiration: a case report. Acta Cytol 2005, 49: 173–176.

208. Dardick I, Lagacé R, Carlier MT, Jung RC. Chordoid sarcoma (extraskeletal myxoid chondrosarcoma). Virchows Arch 1983, 399: 61–78.

209. Sciot R, Dal Ciu P, Fletcher C, et al. t(9 ;22)(q22–31 ;q11–12) is a consistent marker of extraskeletal myxoid chondrosarcoma: evaluation of three cases. Mod Pathol 1995, 8: 765–768.

210. Huvos AG. Myxoid chondrosarcoma. In: Mitchel J editor. AG huvos. Bone tumors. Diagnosis, treatment and prognosis. 2nd edition. Philadelphia, PA: W.B. Saunders; 1991, pp. 366–367.

211. Oliveira AM, Sebo TJ, McGrory JE, Gaffey TA, Rock MG, Nascimento AG. Extraskeletal myxoid chondrosarcoma: a clinicopathologic, immunohistochemical, and ploidy analysis of 23 cases. Mod Pathol 2000, 13: 900–908.

212. Meis-Kindblom JM, Bergh P, Gunterberg B, Kindblom LG. Extraskeletal myxoid chondrosarcoma: a reappraisal of its morphologic spectrum and prognostic factors based on 117 cases. Am J Surg Pathol 1999, 23: 636–650.

213. Jakowski JD, Wakely PE Jr. Cytopathology of extraskeletal myxoid chondrosarcoma: report of 8 cases. Cancer 2007, 111: 298–305.

214. Layfield LJ. Cytologic differential diagnosis of myxoid and mucinous neoplasms of the sacrum and parasacral soft tissue. Diagn Cytopathol 2003, 28: 264–271.

215. Domanski HA, Carlén B, Mertens F, Akerman M. Extraskeletal myxoid chondrosarcoma with neuroendocrine differentiation: a case report with fine-needle aspiration biopsy, histopathology, electron microscopy, and cytogenetics. Ultrastruct Pathol 2003, 27: 363–368.

216. Niemann TH, Bottles K, Cohen MB. Extraskeletal myxoid chondrosarcoma: fine-needle aspiration biopsy findings. Diagn Cytopathol 1994, 11: 363–366.

217. Lucas DR, Nascimento AG, Sanjay BK, Rock MG. Well-differentiated liposarcoma. The Mayo Clinic experience with 58 cases. Am J Clin Pathol 1994, 102: 677–683.

218. Weiss SW, Rao VK. Well-differentiated liposarcoma (atypical lipoma) of deep soft tissue of the extremities, retroperitoneum, and miscellaneous sites. A follow-up study of 92 cases with analysis of the incidence of "dedifferentiation". Am J Surg Pathol 1992, 16: 1051–1058.

219. Fletcher CD, Akerman M, Dal Cin P, de Wever I, Mandahl N, Mertens et al. Correlation between clinicopathological features and karyotype in lipomatous tumors: a report of 178 cases from the Chromosomes and Morphology (CHAMP) Collaborative Study Group. Am J Pathol 1996, 148: 623–630.

220. Rosai J, Akerman M, Dal Cin P, et al. Combined morphologic and karyotypic study of 59 atypical lipomatous tumors. Evaluation of their relationship and differential diagnosis with other adipose tissue tumors (a report of the CHAMP Study Group). Am J Surg Pathol 1996, 20: 1182–1189.

221. Domanski HA, Carlen B, Jonsson K, Mertens F, Akerman M. Distinct cytologic features of spindle cell lipoma. A cytologic-histologic study with clinical, radiologic, electron microscopic, and cytogenetic correlations. Cancer 2001, 93: 381–389.

222. Lemos MM, Kindblom LG, Meis-Kindblom JM, Remotti F, Ryd W, Gunterberg B, Willen H. Fine-needle aspiration characteristics of hibernoma. Cancer 2001, 93: 206–210.

223. Bennert KW, Abdul-Karim FW. Fine needle aspiration cytology vs. needle core biopsy of soft tissue tumors. A comparison. Acta Cytol 1994, 38: 381–384.

224. Maitra A, Ashfaq R, Hossein Saboorian M, Lindberg G, Tunc Gokasian S. The role of fine-needle aspiration biopsy in the primary diagnosis of mesenchymal lesions. A community hospital-based experience. Cancer 2000, 90: 178–185.

225. Nagira K, Yamamoto T, Akisue T, Marui T, Hitora T, Nakatani T, Kurosaka M, Ohbayashi C. Reliability of fine-needle aspiration biopsy in the initial diagnosis of soft-tissue lesions. Diagn Cytopathol 2002, 27: 354–361.

226. Klijanienko J, Caillaud JM, Lagacé L. Fine-needle aspiration in liposarcoma. Cyto-histologic correlative study including well-differentiated, myxoid, and pleomorphic variants. Diagn Cytopathol 2004, 30: 307–312.

227. Gonzalez-Campora R, Munoz-Arias G, Otal-Salaverri C, et al. Fine needle aspiration cytology of primary soft tissue tumors. Morphologic analysis of the most frequent types. Acta Cytol 1992, 36: 905–917.

228. Palmer HE, Mukunyadzi P, Cilbreth W, Thomas JR. Subgrouping and grading of soft-tissue sarcomas by fine-needle aspiration cytology: a histopathologic correlation study. Diagn Cytopathol 2001, 24: 307–316.

229. Kilpatrick SE, Cappellari JO, Bos GD, Gold SH, Ward WG. In fine-needle aspiration biopsy a practical alternative to open biopsy for the primary diagnosis of sarcoma? Experience with 140 patients. Am J Clin Pathol 2001, 115: 59–68.

230. Wakely PE, Kneisl JS. Soft tissue aspiration cytopathology. Diagnostic accuracy and limitations. Cancer 2000, 90: 292–298.

231. Gonzalez-Campora R. Cytoarchitectural findings in the diagnosis of primary soft tissue tumors. Acta Cytol 2001, 45: 115–146.

232. Kilpatrick SE, Ward WG, Bos GD. The value of fine-needle aspiration biopsy in the differential diagnosis of adult myxoid sarcoma. Cancer 2000, 25: 167–177.

233. Åkerman M, Domanski HA. The cytological features of soft tissue tumours in fine needle aspiration smears classified according to histotype. Adipocytic tumors. In the cytology of soft tissue tumours. Monographs in clinical cytology. Vol. 16. S.R. Orell editor. Kaurger, Basel 2003, pp. 17–27.

234. Rioby HS, Wilson YG, Cawthorn SJ, Ibrahim NB. Fine-needle aspiration of pleomorphic lipoma. A potential pitfall of cytodiagnosis. Cytopathology 1993, 4: 55–58.

235. Thirumala S, Desai M, Kannan V. Diagnostic pitfalls in fine needle aspiration. Cytology of pleomorphic lipoma. A case report. Acta Cytol 2000, 44: 653–656.

236. Lopez-Rios F, Alberti N, Perrez-Barios A, De Agustin PP. Fine-needle aspiration in pleomorphic lipoma. Diagn Cytopathol 2001, 24: 296–297.

237. Chen X, Yu K, Tong G, Hood M, Storper I, Hamele-Bena D. Fine needle aspiration of pleomorphic lipoma of the neck: report of two cases. Diagn Cytopathol 2010, 38: 184–187.

238. Shmookler BM, Enzinger FM. Pleomorphic lipoma: a benign tumor simulating liposarcoma. A clinicopathologic analysis of 48 cases. Cancer 1981, 47: 126–133.

239. Guillou L, Wadden C, Coindre JM, Krausz T, Fletcher CD. "Proximal-type" epithelioid sarcoma, a distinctive aggressive neoplasm showing rhabdoid features. Clinicopathologic, immunohistochemical, and ultrastructural study of a series. Am J Surg Pathol 1997, 21: 130–146.

240. Hornick JL, Dal Cin P, Fletcher CD. Loss of INI1 expression is characteristic of both conventional and proximal-type epithelioid sarcoma. Am J Surg Pathol 2009, 33: 542–550.

241. Jogai S, Gupta SK, Goel A, Ahluwalia J, Joshi K. Epithelioid sarcoma. Report of a case with fine needle aspiration diagnosis. Acta Cytol 2001, 45: 271–273.

242. Ahmed NM, Feldman M, Seemayer TA. Cytology of epithelioid sarcoma. Acta Cytol 1974, 18: 459–461.

243. Pohar-Marinsek Z, Zidar A. Epithelioid sarcoma in FNAB smears. Diagn Cytopathol 1994, 11: 367–372.

244. Ikeda K, Tate G, Suzuki T, Mitsuya T. Fine needle aspiration cytology of primary proximal-type epithelioid sarcoma of the perineum: a case report. Acta Cytol 2005, 49: 314–318.

245. Zeppa P, Errico MF, Palombini L. Epithelioid sarcoma: report of two cases diagnosed by fine-needle aspiration biopsy with immunocytochemical correlation. Diagn Cytopathol 1999, 21: 405–408.

246. Hernandez-Ortiz MJ, Valenzuela-Ruiz P, Gonzalez-Estecha A, Santana-Acosta A, Ruiz-Villaespesa A. Fine needle aspiration cytology of primary epithelioid sarcoma of the vulva. A case report. Acta Cytol 1995, 39: 100–103.

247. Gonzales-Perazmato P, Jiménez-Heffernan JA, Cuevas J. Fine-needle aspiration cytology of "proximal-type" epithelioid sarcoma. Diagn Cytopathol 2001, 25: 122–125.

248. Bajaj P, Aiyer H, Sinha BK, Jain M, Ashok S. Pitfalls in the diagnosis of epithelioid sarcoma presenting in an unusual site: a case report. Diagn Cytopathol 2001, 24: 36–38.

249. Cardillo M, Zakowski MF, Lin O. Fine-needle aspiration of epithelioid sarcoma: cytology findings in nine cases. Cancer 2001, 93: 246–251.

250. Kitagawa Y, Ito H, Sawaizumi T, Matsubara M, Yokohama M, Naito Z, Maeda S, Sugisaki Y. Fine needle aspiration cytology of primary epithelioid sarcoma. A report of 2 cases. Acta Cytol 2004, 48: 391–396.

251. Fletcher CD, Berman JJ, Corless C, et al. Diagnosis of gastrointestinal stromal tumors: a consensus approach. Hum Pathol 2002, 33: 459–465.

252. Dong Q, McKee G, Pitman M, Geisinger K, Tambouret R. Epithelioid variant of gastrointestinal stromal tumor: diagnosis by fine-needle aspiration. Diagn Cytopathol 2003, 29: 55–60.

253. Kwon MS, Koh JS, Lee SS, Chung JH, Ahn GH. Fine needle aspiration cytology (FNAC) of gastrointestinal stromal tumor: an emphasis on diagnostic role of FNAC, cell block, and immunohistochemistry. J Korean Med Sci 2002, 17: 353–359.

254. Wieczorek TJ, Faquin WC, Rubin BP, Cibas ES. Cytologic diagnosis of gastrointestinal stromal tumor with emphasis on the differential diagnosis with leiomyosarcoma. Cancer 2001, 93: 276–287.

255. Tao LC, Davidson DD. Aspiration biopsy cytology of smooth muscle tumors and cytologic approach to the differentiation between leiomyosarcoma and leiomyoma. Acta Cytol 1993, 37: 300–308.

256. Li P, Wei J, West AB, Perle M, Greco MA, Yang GC. Epithelioid gastrointestinal stromal tumor of the stomach with liver metastases in a 12–year-old girl: aspiration cytology and molecular study. Pediatr Dev Pathol 2002, 386–394.

257. Klijanienko J, Caillaud JM, Lagacé R, Vielh P. Fine-needle aspiration of leiomyosarcoma. A correlative cytohistopathological study of 96 tumors in 68 patients. Diagn Cytopathol 2003, 28: 119–125.

258. Cheuk W, Lee KC, Chan JK. c-kit immunocytochemical staining in the cytologic diagnosis of metastatic gastrointestinal stromal tumor. A report of two cases. Acta Cytol 2000, 44: 679–685.

259. Schmitt FC, Gomes AL, Milanezi F, Reis R, Bardales RH. Mutations in gastrointestinal stromal tumors diagnosed by endoscopic ultrasound-guided fine needle aspiration. Minerva Med 2007, 98: 385–388.

260. Stelow EB, Murad FM, Debol SM, et al. A limited immunochtochemical panel for distinction of subepithelial gastrointestinal mesenchymal neoplasms sampled by endoscopic untrasound-guided fine-needle aspiration. Am J Pathol 2008, 129: 219–225.

261. Yoshida S, Yamashita K, Yokozawa M, et al. Diagnostic findings of ultrasound-guided fine-needle aspiration cytology for gastrointestinal stromal tumors: proposal of a combined cytology with newly defined features and histology diagnosis. Pathol Int 2009, 59: 712–719.

262. Elliott DD, Fanning CV, Caraway NP. The utility of fine-needle aspiration in the diagnosis of gastrointestinal stromal tumors: a cytomorphologic and immunohistochemical analysis with emphasis on malignant tumors. Cancer 2006, 108: 49–55.

263. Meara RS, Cangiarella J, Simsir A, Horton D, Eltoum I, Chhieng DC. Prediction of aggressiveness of gastrointestinal stromal tumours based on immunostaining with bcl-2, Ki-67 and p53. Cytopathology 2007, 18: 283–289.

264. Seidal T, Edvardsson H. Diagnosis of gastrointestinal stromal tumor by fine-needle aspiration biopsy: a cytological and immunocytochemical study. Diagn Cytopathol 2000, 23: 397–401.

265. Li SQ, O'Leary TJ, Sobin LH, Erozan YS, Rosenthal DL, Przygodzki RM. Analysis of KIT mutation and protein expression in fine needle aspirates of gastrointestinal stromal/ smooth muscle tumors. Acta Cytol 2000, 44: 981–986.

266. Boggino HE, Fernandez MP, Logroño R. Cytomorphology of gastrointestinal stromal tumor: diagnostic role of aspiration cytology, core biopsy, and immunochemistry. Diagn Cytopathol 2000, 23: 156–160.

267. Willmore-Payne C, Layfield LJ, Holden JA. c-KIT mutation analysis for diagnosis of gastrointestinal stromal tumors in fine needle aspiration specimens. Cancer 2005, 105: 165–170.

268. Padilla C, Saez A, Vidal A, Garcia L, Tolosa F, Andreu FJ, Combalia N. Fine-needle aspiration cytology diagnosis of metastatic gastrointestinal stromal tumor in the liver: a report of three cases. Diagn Cytopathol 2002, 27: 298–302.

269. Meis-Kindblom JM, Kindblom LG. Angiosarcoma of soft tissue: a study of 80 cases. Am J Surg Pathol 1998, 22: 683–697.

270. Weiss SW, Goldblum JR. Malignant vascular tumors. In: Strauss M editor. Enzinger and Weiss's soft tissue tumors. 5th edition. St. Louis, MO: Mosby; 2008, pp. 703–733.

271. Zeppa P, Errico ME, Palombini L. Epithelioid sarcoma: report of two cases diagnosed by fine-needle aspiration biopsy with immunocytochemical correlation. Diagn Cytopathol 1999, 21: 405–408.

272. Galindo LM, Shienbaum AJ, Dwyer-Joyce L, Garcia FU. Atypical hemangioma of the breast: a diagnostic pitfall in breast fine-needle aspiration. Diagn Cytopathol 2001, 24: 215–218.

273. Vielh P, Aurias A, Klijanienko J, Validire P, Zucker JM. Round cell tumors. In: Vielh P editor. Guides to clinical aspiration biopsy. Pediatrics. New York, NY: Igaku-Shoin Medical Publishers; 1993, 65–130.

274. Klijanienko J, Caillaud JM, Orbach D, et al. Cyto-histological correlations in primary, recurrent and metastatic rhabdomyosarcoma. The Institut Curie's experience. Diagn Cytopathol 2007, 35: 482–487.

275. Vesoulis Z, Cunliffe C. Fine-needle aspiration biopsy of postradiation epithelioid angiosarcoma of breast. Diagn Cytopathol 2000, 22: 172–175.

276. Boucher LD, Swanson PE, Stanley MW, Silverman JF, Raab SS, Geisinger KR. Cytology of angiosarcoma. Findings in fourteen fine-needle aspiration biopsy specimens and one pleural fluid specimen. Am J Clin Pathol 2000, 114: 210–219.

277. Wakely PE Jr, Frable WJ, Kneisl JS. Aspiration cytopathology of epithelioid angiosarcoma. Cancer 2000, 90: 245–251.

278. Lin O, Gerhard R, Coelho Siqueira SA, de Castro IV. Cytologic Findings of epithelioid angiosarcoma of the thyroid. A case report. Acta Cytol 2002, 46: 767–771.

279. Klijanienko J, Caillaud JM, Lagacé R, Vielh P. Cytology in angiosarcoma including classic and epithelioid variants. Institut Curie's experience. Diagn Cytopathol 2003, 29: 140–145.

280. Silverman JF, Lannin DL, Larkin EW, Feldman P, Frable WJ. Fine-needle aspiration cytology of postirradiation sarcomas, including angiosarcoma, with immunocytochemical confirmation. Diagn Cytopathol 1989, 5: 275–281.

281. Perez-Guillermo M, Sola Perez J, Garcia Rojo B, Hernandez Gil A. Fine-needle aspiration cytology of cutaneous vascular tumours. Cytopathology 1992, 3: 231–244.

282. Liu K, Layfield LJ. Cytomorphologic features of angiosarcoma on fine needle aspiration biopsy. Acta Cytol 1999, 43: 407–415.

283. Akatsu T, Kobayashi H, Uematsu S, Tamagawa E, Shinozaki H, Kase K, Kobayashi K, Otsuka S, Mukai M, Kitajima M. Granular cell tumor of the breast preoperatively diagnosed by fine-needle aspiration cytology: report of a case. Surg Today 2004, 34: 760–763.

284. Gibbons D, Leitch M, Coscia J, Lindberg G, Molberg K, Ashfaq R, Saboorian MH. Fine needle aspiration cytology and histologic findings of granular cell tumor of the breast: review of 19 cases with clinical/radiologic correlation. Breast J 2000, 6: 27–30.

285. Wieczorek TJ, Krane JF, Domanski HA, Akerman M, Caelén B, Misdraji J, Granter SR. Cytologic findings in granular cell tumors, with emphasis on the diagnosis of malignant granular cell tumor by fine-needle aspiration biopsy. Cancer 2001, 93: 398–408.

286. Pieterse AS, Mahar A, Orell S. Granular cell tumour: a pitfall in FNA cytology of breast lesions. Pathology 2004, 36: 58–62.

287. Liu Z, Mira JL, Vu H. Diagnosis of malignant granular cell tumor by fine needle aspiration cytology. Acta Cytol 2001, 45: 1011–1021.

288. Ng SB, Chuan KL. Fine needle aspiration cytology of metastatic malignant granular cell tumour: a case report and review of the literature. Cytopathology 2002, 13: 164–170.

289. Vielh P, Brisse H, Couturier J, de Cremoux P, Dellatre O, Klijanienko J, Michon J. Cytopathologie des tumeurs malignes du blastème de l'enfant. Ann Pathol 2004, 24: 568–573.

290. Yusuf Y, Belmonte AH, Tchertkoff V. Fine needle aspiration cytology of a recurrent malignant tumor of the kidney with rhabdoid features in an adult. A case report. Acta Cytol 1996, 40: 1313–1316.

291. Akhtar M, Ali MA, Sackey K, Bakry M, Burgess A. Fine-needle aspiration biopsy diagnosis of malignant rhabdoid tumor of the kidney. Diagn Cytopathol 1991, 7: 36–40.

292. Drut R. Malignant rhabdoid tumor of the kidney diagnosed by fine-needle aspiration cytology. Diagn Cytopathol 1990, 6: 124–126.

293. Obers VJ, Phillips JI. Fine needle aspiration of pediatric abdominal masses. Cytologic and electron microscopic diagnosis. Acta Cytol 1991, 35: 165–170.

294. Akhtar M, Kfoury H, Haider A, Sackey K, Ali MA. Fine-needle aspiration biopsy diagnosis of extrarenal malignant rhabdoid tumor. Diagn Cytopathol 1994, 11: 271–276.

295. Drut R, Drut RM. Renal and extrarenal congenital rhabdoid tumor: diagnosis by fine-needle aspiration biopsy and FISH. Diagn Cytopathol 2002, 27: 32–34.

296. Barroca HM, Costa MJ, Carvalho JL. Cytologic profile of rhabdoid tumor of the kidney. A report of 3 cases. Acta Cytol 2003, 47: 1055–1058.

297. Radhika S, Bakshi A, Rajwanshi A, Nijhawan R, Das A, Kakkar N, Joshi K, Marwaha RK, Rao KL. Cytopathology of uncommon malignant renal neoplasms in the pediatric age group. Diagn Cytopathol 2005, 32: 281–286.

298. Thomson TA, Klijanienko J, Conturier J, et al. Fine-needle aspiration of renal and extrarenal rhabdoid tumors. The experience of the institut curie regarding 20 tumors in 13 patients Cancer Cytopathol, in press.

299. Chritopherson WM, Foote FW Jr, Steward FW. Alveolar soft-part sarcoma: structurally characteristic tumors of uncertain histogenesis. Cancer 1952, 5: 100–111.

300. Ladanyi M, Lui MY, Antoncscu CR, et al. The der(17)t(X ;17)(p11 ;q25) of human alveolar soft part sarcoma fuses the TFE3 transcription factor gene ASPL, a novel gene 17q25. Oncogene 2001, 20: 48–57.

301. Sandberg A, Bridge J. Updates on the cytogenetics and molecular genetics of bone and soft tissue tumors: alveolar soft part sarcoma. Cancer Genet Cytogenet 2002, 136: 1–9.

302. Portera CA Jr, Ho V, Patel SR, et al. Alveolar soft part sarcoma: clinical course and patterns of metastasis in 70 patients treated at a single institution. Cancer 2001, 91: 585–591.

303. Kayton ML, Meyers P, Wexler LH, Gerald WL, LaQuaglia MP. Clinical presentation, treatment, and outcome of alveolar soft part sarcoma in children, adolescents, and young adults. J Pediatr Surg 2006, 41: 187–193.

304. Joyama S, Ueda T, Shimizu K, et al. Chromosome rearrangement at 17q25 and xp11.2 in alveolar soft-part sarcoma: a case report and review of the literature. Cancer 1999, 86: 1246–1250.

305. Bu X, Bernstein L. A proposed explanation for female predominance in alveolar soft part sarcoma. Noninactivation of X; autosome translocation fusion gene? Cancer 2005, 103: 1245–1253.

306. Shabb N, Sneige N, Fanning CV, Dekmezian R. Fine-needle aspiration cytology of alveolar soft-part sarcoma. Diagn Cytopathol 1991, 7: 293–298.

307. Logrono R, Wojtowycz MM, Wunderlich DW, Warner TF, Kurtycz DF. Fine needle aspiration cytology and core biopsy in the diagnosis of alveolar soft part sarcoma presenting with lung metastases. A case report. Acta Cytol 1999, 43: 464–470.

308. Machhi J, Kouzova M, Komorowski DJ, Asma Z, Chivukala M, Basir Z, Shidham VB. Crystals of alveolar soft part sarcoma in a fine needle aspiration biopsy cytology smear. A case report. Acta Cytol 2002, 46: 904–908.

309. Wakely P. Jr, McDermott JE, Ali SZ. Cytopathology of alveolar soft part sarcoma. A Report of 10 cases. Cancer 2009, 117: 500–507.

310. Lopez-Ferrer P, Jiménez-Heffernan JA, Vicandi B, Gonzalez-Peramato P, Viguer JM. Cytologic features of alveolar soft part sarcoma: report of three cases. Diagn Cytopathol 2002, 27: 115–119.

311. Husain M, Nguyen GK. Alveolar soft part sarcoma. Report of a case diagnosed by needle aspiration cytology and electron microscopy. Acta Cytol 1995, 39: 951–954.

312. Kawai A, Hosono A, Nakayama R, et al. Japanese Musculoskeletal Oncology Group. Clear cell sarcoma of tendons and aponeuroses: a study of 75 patients. Cancer 2007, 109: 109–116.

313. Antonescu CR, Tschernyavsky SJ, Woodruff JM, Jungbluth AA, Brennan MF, Ladanyi M. Molecular diagnosis of clear cell sarcoma: detection of EWS-ATF1 and MITF-M transcripts and histopathological and ultrastructural analysis of 12 cases. J Mol Diagn 2002, 4: 44–52.

314. Panagopoulos I, Mertens F, Dêbiec-Rychter M, et al. Molecular genetic characterization of the EWS/ATF1 fusion gene in clear cell sarcoma of tendons and aponeuroses. Int J Cancer 2002, 99: 560–567.

315. Langezaal SM, Graadt van Roggen JF, Cleton-Jansen AM, Baelde JJ, Hogendoorn PC. Malignant melanoma is genetically distinct from clear cell sarcoma of tendons and aponeurosis (malignant melanoma of soft parts). Br J Cancer 2001, 84: 535–538.

316. Almeida MM, Nunes AM, Frable WJ. Malignant melanoma of soft tissue. A report of three cases with diagnosis by fine needle aspiration cytology. Acta Cytol 1994, 38: 241–246.

317. Creager AJ, Pitman MB, Geisinger KR. Cytologic features of clear cell sarcoma (malignant melanoma) of soft parts: a study of fine-needle aspirates and exfoliative specimens. Am J Clin Pathol 2002, 117: 217–224.

318. Tong TR, Chow TC, Chan PW, Lee KC, Teung SH, Lam A, Yu CK. Clear-cell sarcoma diagnosis by fine-needle aspiration: cytologic, histologic, and ultrastructural features; potential pitfalls; and literature review. Diagn Cytopathol 2002, 26: 174–180.

319. Fletcher CD. Pleomorphic malignant fibrous histiocytoma: fact or fiction? A critical reappraisal based on 159 tumors diagnosed as pleomorphic sarcoma. Am J Surg Pathol 1992, 16: 213–228.

320. Mertens F, Fletcher CD, Dal Cin P, et al. Cytogenetic analysis of 46 pleomorphic soft tissue sarcomas and correlation with morphologic and clinical features: a report of the CHAMP Study Group. Chromosomes and Morphology. Genes Chromosomes Cancer 1998, 22: 16–25.

321. Idbaih A, Coindre JM, Derré J, et al. Myxoid malignant fibrous histiocytoma and pleomorphic liposarcoma share very similar genomic imbalances. Lab Invest 2005, 85: 176–181.

322. Chibon F, Mairal A, Fréneaux P, Terrier P, Coindre JM, Sastre X, Aurias A. The RB1 gene is the target of chromosome 13 deletions in malignant fibrous histiocytoma. Cancer Res 2000, 60: 6339–6345.

323. Derré J, Lagacé R, Nicolas A, et al. Leiomyosarcomas and most malignant fibrous histiocytomas share very similar comparative genomic hybridization imbalances: an analysis of a series of 27 leiomyosarcomas. Lab Invest 2001, 81: 211–215.

324. Klijanienko J, Caillaud JM, Lagacé R, Vielh P. Fine-needle aspiration of leiomyosarcoma. A correlative cytohistopathological study of 96 tumors in 68 patients. Diagn Cytopathol 2003, 28: 119–125.

325. Klijanienko J, Caillaud JM, Lagacé R, Vielh P. Comparative fine-needle aspiration and pathologic study in malignant fibrous histiocytoma. Cytodiagnostic features of 95 tumors in 71 patients. Diagn Cytopathol 2003, 29: 320–326.

326. Liu K, Dodge RK, Layfield LJ. Logistic regression analysis of high grade spindle cell neoplasms. A fine needle aspiration cytologic study. Acta Cytol 1999, 43: 593–600.

327. Ward WG Sr, Kilpatrick S. Fine needle aspiration biopsy of primary bone tumors. Clin Orthop 2000, 373: 80–87.

328. Jain M, Aiyer HM, Singh M, Naryla M. Fine-needle aspiration diagnosis of giant cell tumour of bone presenting at unusual sites. Diagn Cytopathol 2002, 27: 375–378.

329. Dodd LG, Scully SP, Cothran RL, Harrelson JM. Utility of fine-needle aspiration in the diagnosis of primary osteosarcoma. Diagn Cytopathol 2002, 27: 350–353.

330. Nagira K, Yamamoto T, Akisue T, Marui T, Hitora T, Nakatani T, Kurosaka M, Ohbayashi C. Reliability of fine-needle aspiration biopsy in the initial diagnosis of soft-tissue lesions. Diagn Cytopathol 2002, 23: 354–361.

331. Walaas L, Angervall L, Hagmar B, Save-Soderbergh J. A correlative cytologic and histologic study of malignant fibrous histiocytoma: an analysis of 40 cases examined by fine-needle aspiration cytology. Diagn Cytopathol 1986, 2: 46–54.

332. Gonzalez-Campora R, Otal-Salaverri C, Hevia-Vasquez A, Munoz-Munoz G, Garrido-Cintado A, Galera-Davidson H. Fine needle aspiration in myxoid tumors of the soft tissues. Acta Cytol 1990, 34: 179–191.

333. Gonzalez-Campora R, Munoz-Arias G, Otal-Salaverri C, Jorda-Heras M, Garcia-Alvarez E, Gomez-Pascual A, et al. Fine needle aspiration cytology of primary soft-tissue tumors. Morphologic analysis of the most frequent types. Acta Cytol 1992, 36: 905–917.

334. Willén H, Åkerman H, Carlén B. Fine needle aspiration (FNA) in the diagnosis of soft tissue tumours; a review of 22 years experience. Cytopathology 1995, 6: 236–247.

335. Berardo MD, Powers CN, Wakely PE Jr, Almeida MO, Frable WJ. Fine-needle aspiration cytopathology of malignant fibrous histiocytoma. Cancer 1997, 81: 228–237.

336. Kilpatrick SE, Cappelari JO, Bos GD, Gold SH, Ward WG. Is fine-needle aspiration biopsy a practical alternative to open biopsy for the primary diagnosis of sarcoma? Experience with 140 patients. Am J Clin Pathol 2001, 115: 59–68.

337. Gebhard S, Coindre JM, Michels JJ, et al. Pleomorphic liposarcoma: clinicopathologic, immunohistochemical, and follow-up analysis of 63 cases: a study from the French Federation of Cancer Centers Sarcoma Group. Am J Surg Pathol 2002, 26: 601–616.

338. Klijanienko J, Caillaud JM, Lagacé L. Fine-needle aspiration in liposarcoma. Cyto-histologic correlative study including well-differentiated, myxoid, and pleomorphic variants. Diagn Cytopathol 2004, 30: 307–312.

339. Bennert KW, Abdul-Karim FW. Fine needle aspiration cytology vs. needle core biopsy of soft tissue tumors. A comparison. Acta Cytol 1994, 38: 381–384.

340. Kilpatrick SE, Doyon J, Choong PFM, Sim FH, Nascimento AG. The clinicopathologic spectrum of myxoid and round cell liposarcoma: a study of 95 cases. Cancer 1999, 77: 1450–1458.

341. Wakely PE, Kneisl JS. Soft tissue aspiration cytopathology. Diagnostic accuracy and limitations. Cancer 2000, 90: 292–298.

342. Schürch W, Bégin LR, Seemayer TA, et al. Pleomorphic soft tissue myogenic sarcomas of adulthood. A reappraisal in the mid-1990s. Am J Surg Pathol 1996, 20: 131–147.

343. Gaffney EF, Dervan PA, Fletcher CD. Pleomorphic rhabdomyosarcoma in adulthood. Analysis of 11 cases with definition of diagnostic criteria. Am J Surg Pathol 1993, 17: 601–609.

344. Furlong MA, Mentzel T, Fanburg-Smith JC. Pleomorphic rhabdomyosarcoma in adults: a clinicopathologic study of 38 cases with emphasis on morphologic variants and recent skeletal muscle-specific markers. Mod Pathol 2001, 4: 595–603.

345. Franchi A, Massi D, Santucci M. The comparative role of immunohistochemistry and electron microscopy in the identification of myogenic differentiation in soft tissue pleomorphic sarcomas. Ultrastruct Pathol 2005, 29: 295–304.

346. Oda Y, Miyajima K, Kawaguchi K, et al. Pleomorphic leiomyosarcoma: clinicopathologic and immunohistochemical study with special emphasis on its distinction from ordinary leiomyosarcoma and malignant fibrous histiocytoma. Am J Surg Pathol 2001, 25: 1030–1038.

347. Dahl I, Hagmar B, Angervall L. Leiomyosarcoma of the soft tissue. A correlative cytological and histological study of 11 cases. Acta Pathol Microbiol Immunol Scand A 1981, 89: 285–291.

348. Hummel P, Cangiarella JF, Cohen JM, Yang G, Waisman J, Chhieng DC. Transthoracic fine-needle aspiration biopsy of pulmonary spindle cell and mesenchymal lesions. A study of 61 cases. Cancer 2001, 93: 187–198.

349. Tao LC, Davidson DD. Aspiration biopsy cytology of smooth muscle tumors and cytologic approach to the differentiation between leiomyosarcoma and leiomyoma. Acta Cytol 1993, 37: 300–308.

350. Klijanienko J, Caillaud JM, Orbach D, Brisse H, Lagacé R, Vielh P, Couturier J, Fréneaux P, Theocharis S, Sastre X. Cyto-histological correlations in primary, recurrent and metastatic rhabdomyosarcoma. The Institut Curie's experience. Diagn Cytopathol 2007, 35: 482–487.

351. Bane BL, Evans HL, Ro JY, Carrasco CH, Grignon DJ, Benjamin RS, Ayala AG. Extraskeletal osteosarcoma. A clinicopathologic review of 26 cases. Cancer 1990, 65: 2762–2770.

352. Lee JS, Fetsch JF, Wasdhal DA, Lee BP, Pritchard DJ, Nascimento AG. A review of 40 patients with extraskeletal osteosarcoma. Cancer 1995, 76: 2253–2259.

353. Goldstein-Jackson SY, Gosheger G, Delling G, et al. Extraskeletal osteosarcoma has a favourable prognosis when treated like conventional osteosarcoma. J Cancer Res Clin Oncol 2005, 131: 520–526.

354. Torigoe T, Yazawa Y, Takagi T, Terakado A, Kurosawa H. Extraskeletal osteosarcoma in Japan: multiinstitutional study of 20 patients from the Japanese Musculoskeletal Oncology Group. J Orthop Sci 2007, 12: 424–429.

355. Fanburg-Smith JC, Bratthauer GL, Miettinen M. Osteocalcin and osteonectin immunoreactivity in extraskeletal osteosarcoma: a study of 28 cases. Hum Pathol 1999, 30: 32–38.

356. Rösen B, Herrlin K, Rydholm A, Akerman M. Pseudomalignant myositis ossificans. Clinical, radiologic, and cytologic diagnosis. Acta Orthop Scand 1989, 60: 457–460.

357. Brisse H, Orbach D, Klijanienko J, Freneaux P, Neuenschwander S Imaging and diagnostic strategy of soft tissue tumors in children. Eur Radiol 2006, 16: 1147–1164.

358. Klijanienko J, Caillaud JM, Orbach D, Pacquement H, Lagacé R. Cyto-histological correlations in primary, recurrent and metastatic bone and soft tissue osteosarcoma. Institut Curie's experience. Diagn Cytopathol 2007, 35: 270–275.

359. Dahlin DC, Unni KK. Osteosarcoma of bone and its important recognizable varieties. Am J Surg Pathol 1977, 1: 61–72.

360. White VA, Fanning CV, Ayala AG, Raymond AK, Carrasco CH, Murray JA. Osteosarcoma and the role of fine-needle aspiration. A study of 51 cases. Cancer 1988, 62: 1238–1246.

361. Kilpatrick SE, Ward WG, Chauvenet AR, Pettenati MJ. The role of fine-needle aspiration biopsy in the initial diagnosis of pediatric bone and soft tissue tumors: an institutional experience. Mod Pathol 1998, 11: 923–928.

362. Ward WG Sr, Kilpatrick S. Fine needle aspiration biopsy of primary bone tumors. Clin Orthop 2000, 373: 80–87.

363. Kilpatrick SE, Ward WG, Bos GD, Chauvenet AR, Gold SH. The role of fine needle aspiration biopsy in the diagnosis and management of osteosarcoma. Pediatr Pathol Mol Med 2001, 20: 175–187.

364. Dodd LG, Scully SP, Cothran L, Harrelson JM. Utility of fine-needle aspiration in the diagnosis of primary osteosarcoma. Diagn Cytopathol 2002, 27: 350–353.

365. Peng XJ, Yan XC. Cytodiagnosis of bone tumors by fine needle aspiration. Acta Cytol 1985, 29: 570–575.

366. Layfield LJ, Glasgow BJ, Anders KH, Mirra JM. Fine needle aspiration cytology of primary bone lesions. Acta Cytol 1987, 31: 177–184.

367. Layfield LJ, Armstrong K, Zaleski S, Eckardt J. Diagnostic accuracy and clinical utility of fine-needle aspiration cytology in the diagnosis of clinically primary bone lesions. Diagn Cytopathol 1993, 9: 168–173.

368. Nicol KK, Ward WG, Savage PD, Kilpatrick SE. Fine-needle aspiration biopsy of skeletal versus extraskeletal osteosarcoma. Cancer Cytopathol 1998, 13: 176–185.

369. Layfield LJ. Osteoid-producing lesions. In: Cytopathology of bone and soft tissue tumors. Oxford, UK: 2002, Oxford University Press; pp. 193–211.

370. Dodd LG, Chai C, McAdams HP, Layfield LJ. Fine needle aspiration of osteogenic sarcoma metastatic to the lung. A report of four cases. Acta Cytol 1998, 42: 754–758.

371. Klijanienko J, Caillaud JM, Lagacé R, Vielh P. Cytohistologic correlations of 24 malignat peripheral nerve sheath tumors (MPNST) in 17 patients. The Institut Curie experience. Diagn Cytopathol 2002, 27: 103–108.

372. Turc-Carel C, Lizard-Nacol S, Justrabo E, et al. Consistent chromosomal translocation in alveolar rhabdomyosarcoma. Cancer Genet Cytogenet 1986, 19: 361–362.

373. Barr FG. Gene fusions involving PAX and FOX family members in alveolar rhabdomyosarcoma. Oncogene 2001, 20: 5736–5746.

374. Besnard-Guérin C, Newsham I, Winqvist R, et al. A common region of loss of heterozygosity in Wilms' tumor and rhabdomyosarcoma distal to be D11S988 locus on chromosome 11p15. Hum Genet 1996, 97: 163–170.

375. Klijanienko J, Caillaud JM, Orbach D, et al. Cyto-histological correlations in primary, recurrent and metastatic rhabdomyosarcoma: the institut Curie's experience. Diagn Cytopathol 2007, 35: 482–487.

376. Akerman M, Domanski HA. The cytological features of soft tissue tumours in fine needle aspiration smears classified according to histiotype. In: Orell SR editor. Monographs in clinical cytology. Volume 16, The cytology of soft tissue tumours. Switzerland: Kargel, Basel, 2003, pp. 17–84.

377. Fisher HP, Thomsen H, Altmannsberger M, Bertra U. Malignant rhabdoid tumour of the kidney expressing neurofilament proteins. Immunohistochemical findings and histogenetic aspects. Pathol Res Pract 1989, 184: 541–547.

378. Klijanienko J, Caillaud JM, Lagacé R, Vielh P. Cytohistologic correlations in 56 synovial sarcomas in 36 patients. The Institut Curie experience. Diagn Cytopathol 2002, 27: 96–102.

379. Peter M, Gilbert E, Delattre O. A multiplex real-time PCR assay for the detection of a gene fusions observed in solid tumors. Lab Invest 2001, 81: 905–912.

380. Seidal T, Walaas L, Kindblom LG, Angervall L. Cytology of embryonal rhabdomyo-sarcoma: a cytologic, light microscopic, electron microscopic, and immunohistochemical study of seven cases. Diagn Cytopathol 1988, 4: 292–299.

381. De Almeida M, Stastny JF, Wakely PE, Frable WJ. Fine-needle aspiration biopsy of childhood rhabdomyosarcoma: reevaluation of the cytologic criteria for diagnosis. Diagn Cytopathol 1994, 11: 231–236.

382. Frostad B, Bjork O, Skoog L. Fine needle aspiration cytology in the clinical management of childhood rhabdomyosarcomas. Int J Pediatr Hematol Onco 1996, 3: 89–94.

383. Atahan S, Aksu O, Ekinci C. Cytologic diagnosis and subtyping of rhabdomyosarcoma. Cytopathology 1998, 9: 389–397.

384. Layfield LJ, Liu K, Dodge RK. Logistic regression analysis of small round cell neoplasms: a cytologic study. Diagn Cytopathol 1999, 20: 271–277.

385. Pohar-Marinsek Z, Bracko M. Rhabdomyosarcoma. Cytomorphology, subtyping and differential diagnostic dilemmas. Acta Cytol 2000, 46: 787–789.

386. Udayakumar AM, Sundareshan TS, Appaji L, Biswas S, Mukkerjee G. Rhabdomyo-sarcoma: cytogenetics of five cases using fine-needle aspiration samples and review of the literature. Ann Genet 2002, 45: 33–37.

387. Das DK. Fine-needle aspiration (FNA) cytology diagnosis of small round cell tumors: value and limitations. Indian J Pathol Microbiol 2004, 47: 309–318.

388. Kilpatrick SE, Bergman S, Pettenati MJ, Gulley ML. The usefulness of cytogenetic analysis in fine needle aspirates for the histologic subtyping of sarcomas. Mod Pathol 2006, 19: 815–819.

389. Akhtar M, Ali MA, Hug M, Sackey K. Fine-needle aspiration biopsy diagnosis of rhabdomyosarcoma: cytologic, histologic, and ultrastructural correlations. Diagn Cyto-pathol 1992, 8: 465–474.

390. Brahmi U, Rajwanshi A, Joshi K, Ganguly NK, Vohra H, Gupta SK, Dey P. Role of immunocytochemistry and DNA flow cytometry in the fine-needle aspiration diagnosis of malignant small round-cell tumors. Diagn Cytopathol 2001, 24: 233–239.

391. Pohar-Marinsek Z, Anzic J, Jereb B. Value of fine needle aspiration biopsy in childhood rhabdomyosarcoma: twenty-six years of experience in Slovenia. Med Pediatr Oncol 2002, 38: 416–420.

392. Weiss SW, Goldblum JR. Rhabdomyosarcoma. In: Strauss M editor. Enzinger and Weiss's soft tissue tumors. 5th edition. St. Louis, MO: Mosby; 2008, pp. 595–633.

393. Gopez EV, Dauterman J, Layfield LJ. Fine-needle aspiration biopsy of alveolar rhabdomyosarcoma of the parotid: a case report and review of the literature. Diagn Cytopathol 2001, 24: 249–252.

394. Fletcher CDM, Unni KK, Mertens F. World Health Organization classification of tumors. pathology and genetics. Tumours of soft tissue and bone. Fletcher CDM, Unni KK, Mertens F. editors. Lyon, France: IARC Press; 2002.

395. Weiss SW, Goldblum JR. Ewing's sarcoma/PNET tumor family and related lesions. In: Weiss Sw, Goldblum JR editros. Enzinger and Weiss soft tissue tumors. 5th edition. St. Louis, MO: Mosby; pp. 945–988.

396. Halliday BE, Slagel DD, Elsheikh TE, Silverman JF. Diagnostic utility of MIC-2 immunocytochemical staining in the differential diagnosis of small blue cell tumors. Diagn Cytopathol 1997, 19: 410–16.

397. Jambhekar NA, Bagwan IZ, Chule P, Shet TM, Chinoy RF, Agarwal S, Joshi R, Amare Kadam PS. Comparative analysis of routine histology, immunohistochemistry, reverse transcriptase polymerase chain reaction, and fluorescence in situ hybridisation in diagnosis of Ewing family tumors. Arch Pathol Lab Med 2006, 130: 1813–1818.

398. Klijanienko J, Couturier J, Bourdeaut F, et al. Fine-needle aspiration as a diagnostic technique in 50 cases of primary Ewing/Peripheral Neuroectodermal Tumor (ES/PNET). Diagn Cytopathol, in press.

399. Klijanienko J, Caillaud JM, Orbach D, Brisse H, Lagacé R, Sastre-Garau X. Cyto-histological correlations in primary, recurrent and metastatic bone and soft tissue osteosarcoma. Institut Curie's experience. Diagn Cytopathol 2007, 35: 270–275.

400. Vielh P, Brisse H, Couturier J, De Cremoux P, Delattre O, Klijanienko J, Michon J. Cytopathology of malignant blastematous tumors. Ann Pathol 2004, 24: 568–573.

401. Willen H. Fine needle aspiration in the diagnosis of bone tumors. Acta Orthop Scand Suppl 1997, 273: 47–53.

402. Kilpatrick SE, Ward WG, Chauvenet AR, Pettenati MJ. The role of fine-needle aspiration biopsy in the initial diagnosis of pediatric bone and soft tissue tumors: an institutional experience. Mod Pathol 1998, 11: 923–928.

403. Guiter GE, Gamboni MM, Zakowski MF. The cytology of extraskeletal Ewing sarcoma. Cancer Cytopathol 1999, 87: 141–148.

404. Sahu K, Pai RR, Khadilkar U. Fine needle aspiration cytology of the Ewing's sarcoma family of tumors. Acta Cytologica 1999, 44: 332–336.

405. Udayakumar AM, Sundareshan TS, Goud TM, et al. Cytogenetic characterization of ewing tumors using fine needle aspiration samples. A 10–year experience and review of the literature. Cancer Genet Cytogenet 2001, 27: 42–48.

406. Fröstad B, Tani E, Brosjö O, Skoog L, Kogner P. Fine needle aspiration cytology in the diagnosis and management of children and adolescents with Ewing sarcoma and peripheral primitive neuroectodermal tumor. Med Pediatr Oncol 2002, 38: 33–40.

407. Sanati S, Lu DW, Schmidt E, Perry A, Dehner LP, Pfeifer JD. Cytologic diagnosis of Ewing sarcoma/peripheral neuroectodermal tumor with paired prospective molecular genetic analysis. Cancer 2007, 111: 192–199.

408. Kilpatrick SE, Bergman S, Pettenati MJ, Gulley ML. The usefulness of cytogenetic analysis in fine needle aspirates for the histologic subtyping of sarcomas. Modern Pathol 2006, 19: 815–819.

409. Biegel JA, Conard K, Brooks JJ. Translocation (11;22)(p13;q12): primary change in intra-abdominal desmoplastic small round cell tumor. Genes Chromosomes Cancer 1993, 7: 119–121.

410. Sawyer JR, Tryka AF, Lewis JM. A novel reciprocal chromosome translocation t(11;22) (p13;q12) in an intraabdominal desmoplastic small round-cell tumor. Am J Surg Pathol 1992, 16: 411–416.

411. Ladanyi M, Gerald W. Fusion of the EWS and WT1 genes in the desmoplastic small round cell tumor. Cancer Res 1994, 54: 2837–2840.

412. Caraway NP, Fanning CV, Amato RJ, Ordonez NG, Katz RL. Fine-needle aspiration of intra-abdominal desmoplastic small cell tumor. Diagn Cytopathol 1993, 9: 465–470.

413. Insabato L, Di Vizio D, Lambertini M, Bucci L, Pettinato G. Fine needle aspiration cytology of desmoplastic small round cell tumor. A case report. Acta Cytol 1999, 43: 641–646.

414. Akhtar M, Ali MA, Sabbah R, Bakry M, Al-Dayel F. Small round cell tumor with divergent differentiation: cytologic, histologic, and ultrastructural findings. Diagn Cytopathol 1994, 11: 159–164.

415. Drut R. Biphasic intraabdominal desmoplastic small round cell tumor: fine-needle aspiration cytology findings. Diagn Cytopathol 1995, 13: 325–329.

416. Ali SZ, Nicol TL, Port J, Ford G. Intraabdominal desmoplastic small round cell tumor: cytopathologic findings in two cases. Diagn Cytopathol 1998, 18: 449–452.

417. Crapanzano JP, Cardillo M, Lin O, Zakowski MF. Cytology of desmoplastic small round cell tumor. Cancer 2002, 96: 21–31.

418. Ferlicot S, Coué O, Gilbert E, Beuzeboc P, Servois V, Klijanienko J, Delattre O, Vielh P. Intraabdominal desmoplastic small round cell tumor: report of a case with fine needle aspiration, cytologic diagnosis and molecular confirmation. Acta Cytol 2001, 45: 617–621.

419. Dave B, Shet T, Chinoy R. Desmoplastic round cell tumor of childhood: can cytology with immunocytochemistry serve as an alternative for tissue diagnosis? Diagn Cytopathol 2005, 32: 330–335.

420. Presley AE, Kong CS, Rowe DM, Atkins KA. Cytology of desmoplastic small round-cell tumor: comparison of pre- and post-chemotherapy fine-needle aspiration biopsies. Cancer 2007, 111: 41–46.

421. Waugh MS, Dash RC, Turner KC, Dodd LG. Desmoplastic small round cell tumor: using FISH as an ancillary technique to support cytologic diagnosis in an unusual case. Diagn Cytopathol 2007, 35: 516–520.

422. Sciot R, Dal Cin P, Fletcher C, et al. t(9;22)(q22–31;q11–12) is a consistent marker of extraskeletal myxoid chondrosarcoma: evaluation of three cases. Mod Pathol 1995, 7: 765–768.

423. Gonzalez-Campora R, Otal Salaverri C, Gomez Pascual A, Hevia Vazquez A, Galera Davidson H. Mesenchymal chondrosarcoma of the retroperitoneum. Report of a case diagnosed by fine needle aspiration biopsy with immunohistochemical, electron microscopic demonstration of S-100 protein in undifferentiated cells. Acta Cytol 1995, 39: 1237–1243.

424. Trembath DG, Dash R, Major NM, Dodd LG. Cytopathology of mesenchymal chondrosarcomas: a report and comparison of four patients. Cancer 2003, 99: 211–216.

425. Doria MI Jr, Wang HH, Chinoy MJ. Retroperitoneal mesenchymal chondrosarcoma. Report of a case diagnosed by fine needle aspiration cytology. Acta Cytol 1990, 34: 529–532.

FURTHER READING

Ryd W, Mugal S, Ayyash K. Ancient neurilemmoma: a pitfall in the cytologic diagnosis of soft-tissue tumors. Diagn Cytopathol 1986, 2: 244–247.

Dodd LG, Marom EM, Dash RC, Matthews MR, McLendon RE. Fine-needle aspiration cytology of "ancient" schwannoma. Diagn Cytopathol 1999, 20: 307–311.

Hruban RH, Shiu MH, Senie RT, Woodruff JM. Malignant peripheral nerve sheath tumors of the buttock and lower extremity. A study of 43 cases. Cancer 1990, 66: 1253–65.

Hood IC, Qizilbash AH, Young JE, Archibald SD. Needle aspiration cytology of a benign and malignant schwannoma. Acta Cytol 1984, 28: 157–164.

Khalbuss WE, Teot LA, Monaco SE. Diagnostic accuracy and limitations of the fine-deelde aspiration cytology of bone and soft tissue lesions: a review of 1114 cases with cytological-histological correlation. Cancer 2010, 118: 24–32.

Thomson TA, Klijanienko J, Couturier J, et al. Fine-needle aspiration of renal and extrarenal rhabdoid tumors: the experience of the Institut Curie regarding 20 tumors in 13 patients. Cancer Cytopathol 2010.

Index